ESSENTIAL PEDIATRIC CARDIOLOGY

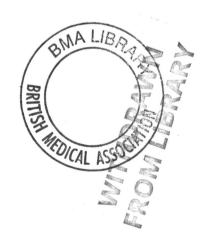

NOTICE

Medicine is an ever-changing science. As new research and clinical experience broaden our knowledge, changes in treatment and drug therapy are required. The authors and the publisher of this work have checked with sources believed to be reliable in their efforts to provide information that is complete and generally in accord with the standards accepted at the time of publication. However, in view of the possibility of human error or changes in is in every respect accurate or complete, and they disclaim all responsibility medical sciences, neither the authors nor the publisher nor any other party who has been involved in the preparation or publication of this work warrants that the information contained herein for any errors or omissions or for the results obtained from use of the information contained in this work. Readers are encouraged to confirm the information contained herein with other sources. For example and in particular, readers are advised to check the product information sheet included in the package of each drug they plan to administer to be certain that the information contained in this work is accurate and that changes have not been made in the recommended dose or in the contraindications for administration. This recommendation is of particular importance in connection with new or infrequently used drugs.

ESSENTIAL PEDIATRIC CARDIOLOGY

Peter Koenig, MD

Assistant Professor of Pediatrics
University of Chicago Pritzker School of Medicine and
University of Chicago Children's Hospital
Chicago, Illinois

Ziyad M. Hijazi, MD, MPH, FACC

Professor of Pediatrics and Medicine
Chief, Section of Pediatric Cardiology
University of Chicago Pritzker School of Medicine and
University of Chicago Children's Hospital
Chicago, Illinois

Frank Zimmerman, MD

Assistant Professor of Pediatrics and Medicine
University of Chicago Pritzker School of Medicine and
University of Chicago Children's Hospital
Chicago, Illinois

McGraw-Hill
Medical Publishing Division

New York / Chicago / San Francisco / Lisbon / London
Madrid / Mexico City / Milan / New Delhi / San Juan
Seoul / Singapore / Sydney / Toronto

The McGraw·Hill Companies

Essential Pediatric Cardiology

1 2 3 4 5 6 7 8 9 0 DOC/DOC 0 9 8 7 6 5 4

ISBN 0-07-140919-X

This book was set in Times Roman by International Typesetting and Composition.
The editors were James Shanahan and Michelle Watt.
The production supervisor was Richard Ruzycka.
Project management was provided by International Typesetting and Composition.
RR Donnelley was printer and binder.
This book was printed on acid-free paper.

Library of Congress Cataloging-in-Publication Data

Essential pediatric cardiology / edited by Peter Koenig, Ziyad Hijazi.
  p. ; cm.
 Includes bibliographical references and index.
 ISBN 0-07-140919-X
 1. Pediatric cardiology.   I. Koenig, Peter, 1960-   II. Hijazi, Ziyad.
 [DNLM: 1. Heart Diseases—Child.   2. Heart Diseases—Infant.
 3. Cardiovascular Abnormalities—Child.   4. Cardiovascular
Abnormalities—Infant.   5. Diagnostic Techniques, Cardiovascular—Child.
 6. Diagnostic Techniques, Cardiovascular—Infant. WS 290 E78 2004]
 RJ421.E85 2004
 618.92'12—dc22
                                          2003064889

We would like to dedicate this textbook to our wives, families, colleagues, and friends, for all the support they have given us over the years.

CONTENTS

CONTRIBUTORS

RA-ID ABDULLA, MD
Associate Professor of Pediatrics
Director, Pediatric Cardiology Fellowship Program
University of Chicago Pritzker School of Medicine and
University of Chicago Children's Hospital
Chicago, Illinois

BROJENDRA AGARWALA, MD
Professor of Pediatrics
University of Chicago Pritzker School of Medicine and
University of Chicago Children's Hospital
Chicago, Illinois

ERNERIO ALBOLIRAS, MD
Associate Professor of Pediatrics
University of Chicago Pritzker School of Medicine and
University of Chicago Children's Hospital
Chicago, Illinois

EMILE BACHA, MD
Assistant Professor of Surgery and Pediatrics
Director, Congenital and Pediatric Cardiac Surgery
University of Chicago Pritzker School of Medicine and
University of Chicago Children's Hospital
Chicago, Illinois

ANDREW S. BENSKY, MD
Sanger Clinic
Charlotte, North Carolina

WILLIAM BONNEY, MD
Pediatric Resident
Rush University
Chicago, Illinois

SUANNE DAVES, MD
Associate Professor of Pediatrics and Anesthesia
University of Chicago Pritzker School of Medicine and
University of Chicago Children's Hospital
Chicago, Illinois

S. BRUCE GREENBERG, MD
Associate Professor of Radiology
Department of Radiology
University of Arkansas for Medical Sciences and
Arkansas Children's Hospital
Little Rock, Arkansas

JOEL T. HARDIN MD
Assistant Professor of Pediatrics
Director, Cardiac Intensive Care Program
University of Chicago Pritzker School of Medicine and
University of Chicago Children's Hospital
Chicago, Illinois

ZIYAD M. HIJAZI, MD, MPH, FACC
Professor of Pediatrics and Medicine
Chief, Section of Pediatric Cardiology
University of Chicago Pritzker School of Medicine and
University of Chicago Children's Hospital
Chicago, Illinois

PETER KOENIG, MD
Assistant Professor of Pediatrics
University of Chicago Pritzker School of Medicine and
University of Chicago Children's Hospital
Chicago, Illinois

TRACY K. KOOGLER, MD
Assistant Professor of Anesthesia
Department of Anesthesia and Critical Care
Department of Pediatrics
MacLean Center for Clinical Ethics
University of Chicago Pritzker School of Medicine and
University of Chicago Children's Hospital
Chicago, Illinois

CHARLES MARCUCCILLI, MD, PhD
Assistant Professor of Pedatrics and Neurology
University of Chicago Pritzker School of Medicine and
University of Chicago Children's Hospital
Chicago, Illinois

JOHN MARCINAK, MD
Associate Professor of Pediatrics
University of Chicago Pritzker School of Medicine and
University of Chicago Children's Hospital
Chicago, Illinois

DONALD I. MOEL, MD, MM
Associate Professor of Pediatrics
University of Chicago Pritzker School of Medicine and
University of Chicago Children's Hospital
Chicago, Illinois

HITENDRA T. PATEL, MBBS, MRCP
Pediatric Cardiology Medical Group-East Bay, Inc.
Children's Hospital of Oakland
Oakland, California

RUTH RETONDO RUDINSKY, MD
Assistant Professor of Pediatrics
University of Chicago Pritzker School of Medicine and
University of Chicago Children's Hospital
Chicago, Illinois

DAVID G. RUSCHHAUPT, MD
Associate Professor Pediatrics
University of Chicago Pritzker School of Medicine and
University of Chicago Children's Hospital
Chicago, Illinois

MARGARET M. SAMYN, MD FAAP FACC
Associate Professor of Pediatrics
Director, Outpatient Pediatric Cardiology Clinic
University of Florida College of Medicine
Gainesville, Florida

JOEL SCHWAB, MD
Associate Professor of Pediatrics
Director Medical Student Education, Department of
    Pediatrics
University of Chicago Pritzker School of Medicine and
University of Chicago Children's Hospital
Chicago, Illinois

LAURA SCHWAB, MD
Clinical Instructor in Pediatrics
Northwestern University School of Medicine
Erie Family Health Center
Chicago, Illinois

PATRICIA SMITH, RN, MN, CPNP
Nurse Practitioner
University of Chicago Children's Hospital
Chicago, Illinois

JOANNE P. STARR, MD
Assistant Professor of Surgery and Pediatrics
University of Chicago Pritzger School of Medicine and
University of Chicago Children's Hospital
Chicago, Illinois

DAVID J. WAIGHT, MD, FAAP
Assistant Professor of Pediatrics
Northeastern Ohio Universities College of Medicine
Director, Cardiac Catheterization Lab and Interventional
    Cardiology
The Heart Center
Akron Children's Hospital
Akron, Ohio

DARREL WAGGONER, MD
Assistant Professor of Human Genetics and Pediatrics
Medical Director, Department of Human Genetics
Medical Genetics Residency Program Director
University of Chicago Pritzger School of Medicine and
University of Chicago Hospitals
Chicago, Illinois

FRANK ZIMMERMAN, MD
Assistant Professor of Pediatrics and Medicine
University of Chicago Pritzger School of Medicine and
University of Chicago Children's Hospital
Chicago, Illinois

PREFACE

Pediatricians and other primary care providers taking care of infants, children, and adolescents have two very important roles: that of the medical care giver, and of the patient advocate. In order to achieve both, a good fund of knowledge in pediatric subspecialties is desirable and necessary. However, especially in the field of pediatric cardiology, this experience is often lacking. The purpose of this book is not to teach the primary care provider to become a pediatric cardiologist, but to help the clinician understand what issues are within the realm of primary care management; when to refer patients to specialist; and how to interact with the specialist in pediatric cardiology.

The order of chapters in this book reflects the issues of highest relevance in primary care pediatric cardiology. Chapters 1 through 10, addressing common presentations, will aid the reader in understanding the manifestations of cardiac disease in the pediatric patient, as well as how to differentiate cardiac from other sources of those presentations.

Chapter 11 provides a succinct review of physiology, essential in helping the primary care clinician understand normal cardiac function and the derangements that take place in abnormal function.

Chapters 12 through 36 focus on common cardiovascular diseases in children, with a particular emphasis on the causes of each, the approach to diagnosis, and the approach to therapy. Concise reviews of pathophysiology further aid the clinician's understanding of these diseases and disorders.

Chapters 37 through 45 address diagnostic methods and tests, those available to the primary clinician and those that may be commonly used by specialists. A review of treatment interventions and methods, special issues in pediatric cardiology, and a very useful summary of pharmacological approaches to pediatric cardiac disease concludes the book.

In addition to focusing on issues commonly encountered and managed by general pediatricians, this book presents issues and controversies that are beyond the scope of primary care. Understanding of these issues is important to make the primary care provider a better patient advocate, who can guide informed choices for his/her patient, and to practice using the techniques of evidence-based medicine. In addition, relative risks of procedures are pointed out so that the primary care provider will have a better understanding of the standard of care, which is increasingly becoming less region specific. The latter will no doubt change with time.

We have taken care to cover all subjects in the required and suitable scope and depth, but also to present information that can be read and used quickly. Wide use of algorithms, tables, lists, and other summary features, in addition to the narrative text, is appropriate for today's busy practices and hospital settings

ESSENTIAL PEDIATRIC CARDIOLOGY

1

CHEST PAIN

Joel T. Hardin

INTRODUCTION

Chest pain is a common somatic complaint in child-hood and is a frequent basis for emergency room evaluation and/or referral to a pediatric cardiologist.[1] While most physicians recognize a low probability of important heart disease behind such complaints, symptomatic children and their parents frequently believe the exact opposite to be true. Equating chest pain with "heart pain" is often the presumption, either stated or unstated. This chapter will review the epidemiology and differential diagnosis of child-hood chest pain, focusing on the majority noncar-diac etiologies and ending with a discussion of the rare but important cardiogenic causes.

EPIDEMIOLOGY

At least 5% of children will report symptoms of chest pain. Although the majority of complaints occur dur-ing the adolescent years, a significant minority of patients under the age of 12 years will seek medical attention. There is no sex predilection related to the complaint itself, nor is there such a predilection as relates to cardiac causes. Most patients present with acute complaints and self-limiting chest pain, rarely lasting more than 1–2 months. Thirty to 40% of patients with chronic chest pain are likely to receive multiple medical evaluations; however, these more extensive (and expensive) diagnostic investigations do not increase the yield of cardiac or other serious diagnoses.

DIFFERENTIAL DIAGNOSIS

Although not intended to be exhaustive, Table 1-1 lists the most common causes of chest pain during childhood and adolescence. Idiopathic chest pain accounts for 20–40% of all clinical presentations, even after thorough medical evaluation and follow-up. When a diagnosis can be clinically established, musculoskeletal or costochondral chest pain syn-dromes are by far the most common, representing 50–75% of all diagnoses. Exercise-induced bron-chospasm and other respiratory disorders account for another 10–15%, gastrointestinal disorders rep-resent 5–10%, and less than 5% are appropriately attributed to psychogenic causes. Importantly, most research has identified an extremely low incidence of heart disease in children with chest pain, gener-ally less than 1%, even in selected populations referred for cardiology consultation.

TABLE 1-1

DIFFERENTIAL DIAGNOSIS OF CHILDHOOD
CHEST PAIN

Idiopathic
Musculoskeletal or Costochondral
Precordial catch syndrome
Direct trauma
Overuse/stress injury
Costochondritis (Tietze's syndrome)
Slipping rib syndrome
Collagen vascular disorders
Respiratory
Exercise-induced asthma
Pleuritis/pleural effusion
Pneumonia
Pneumothorax/pneumomediastinum
Pulmonary embolism
Sickle cell acute chest syndrome
Gastrointestinal
Gastritis
Duodenitis
Esophagitis
Esophageal foreign body
Psychogenic
Anxiety or panic disorder
Conversion disorder
Hyperventilation
Cardiac
Pericarditis
Myocarditis
Cardiac arrhythmia
Mitral valve prolapse
Ventricular outflow tract obstruction
Pulmonary hypertension
Marfan syndrome aortic dissection
Drug-induced
Coronary artery anomalies
Myocardial infarction
Other
Referred pain from thoracic spine

Musculoskeletal and Costochondral Disorders

Arguably the most common clinical presentation of childhood chest pain, the so-called precordial catch syndrome has a highly characteristic history and physical examination. Patients (typically adolescents) report unpredictable but brief episodes of sharp and easily localized chest pain. The pain is often subjectively described as severe, but unrelated to strenuous exercise. Pain exacerbated by inspiration is almost universal, and pain that radiates elsewhere is uncommon. The physical examination often corroborates point tenderness over the symptomatic area, but is otherwise normal. Diagnosis is predicated on history and physical examination, with no additional requirement for laboratory testing or referral. There is no particularly worrisome prognosis conferred by variable descriptions of pain frequency, intensity, or chronicity.

Successful treatment of the precordial catch syndrome centers on effectively acknowledging the patient's complaint as real (i.e., not imagined or psychogenic), and educating the patient/parents regarding the common occurrence of this syndrome— focusing on the well-described, benign, and ultimately self-limiting natural history. The physician must successfully convey confidence in the diagnosis, even in the absence of a specific confirmatory diagnostic study, and without relying on a panel of "rule-out" investigations. There is generally no role for oral analgesic medications, especially since episodes of chest pain occur unpredictably and are rapidly self-limiting. Applying a warm compress over the area is sometimes helpful with no untoward effects. Finally, validation of this diagnosis requires continued doctor-patient dialogue after the initial evaluation. The patient should be cautioned on the potential hazards and cost-ineffectiveness of embarking on a diagnostic fishing expedition, and they should receive specific instructions to report new or unusual symptoms for reconsideration.

Children may experience chest pain secondary to direct trauma (usually evident by history), stress or overuse myofascial injuries, and occasionally stress fractures (ribs or sternum). Not surprisingly, most of these symptoms will wax and wane until effective treatment begins and/or time for recovery is allotted. Pain exacerbated by inspiration is also characteristic in these patients. Physical examination usually discloses tenderness over the symptomatic area. Other than radiography or bone scans for diagnosis of sternal or rib fractures, no specific diagnostic studies are indicated. Oral nonsteroidal anti-inflammatory drug therapy and rest are the mainstays of effective treatment.

Costochondritis is another common and self-limiting cause of chest pain. It is rarely associated with obvious signs of inflammation surrounding a particular costosternal articulation (Tietze's syndrome). Unlike the patient with precordial catch syndrome, episodes of pain are more sustained, and often follow nonspecific and presumably viral illness. Similar to other musculoskeletal disorders, there is exacerbation of pain with deep breathing, and there is point tenderness on examination. Laboratory testing is unnecessary for these patients, and treatment recommendations center on reassurance, warm compresses, oral analgesics, and rest. In contrast, collagen vascular disorders such as rheumatoid arthritis are relatively rare and usually suggested from the history, system review, and physical examination. The typical chest pain of rheumatoid arthritis is localized to the sternoclavicular articulations, providing a clue to the underlying diagnosis.

The very rare "slipping rib syndrome" usually presents with severe pain along the costal margin. Ruptured or otherwise inadequate interchondral fibrous attachments allow portions of the 8th, 9th, or 10th ribs and their costal cartilages to slip and compress adjacent intercostal nerves. These lax interchondral attachments can be easily subluxed on palpation during physical examination. A sensation of popping or snapping is often reported by both patient and examiner. Most affected patients can be managed conservatively with reassurance and oral analgesics, although a minority of patients may require surgical excision of the subluxing rib and costal cartilage.

Respiratory Disorders

Among the respiratory disorders listed in Table 1-1, exercise-induced asthma (EIA) is the most common cause of chest pain. Associated symptoms usually include coughing, wheezing, and shortness of breath, but absence of these symptoms at rest does not exclude a diagnosis of EIA. Patients with EIA have greater problems with activities that involve short and intense bursts of exertion (e.g., running), more so than other exercise (e.g., swimming or bicycling). Diagnosis of EIA is facilitated by exercise testing coupled with pulmonary function tests. Treatment with inhaled bronchodilators (e.g., albuterol) is generally quite effective.

Spontaneous pneumothorax and/or pneumomediastinum presenting as chest pain is seen in patients with severe asthma, prior air leak syndromes, Marfan syndrome, and even some previously healthy individuals. Diagnosis is predicated on clinical grounds (dyspnea, reduced breath sounds/hyperresonance over the affected lung field, subcutaneous crepitus), as well as radiographic findings. Pneumonia and pleural effusion are likewise diagnosed on clinical and radiographic findings, with a predilection for scapular or back pain referred from phrenic nerve irritation.

Pulmonary embolism is rare during childhood, and often associated with prothrombotic conditions (e.g., indwelling venous catheters, prior cardiac surgery, malignancy, nephrotic syndrome, antiphospholipid syndromes, or systemic lupus erythematosus). Diagnosis of pulmonary embolism can be difficult to diagnose on routine clinical examination in children. Unexplained tachypnea, more so than chest pain or even significant hypoxemia, may be the most important clue to pulmonary embolism, especially in children at risk. Diagnosis is confirmed with radionuclide ventilation-perfusion scan, high resolution computed tomography, and occasionally pulmonary arteriography.

Gastrointestinal Disorders

Gastritis, duodenitis, and/or esophagitis are often underdiagnosed causes of childhood chest pain. Symptoms related to specific food ingestion, reclining position, and which include description of a burning sensation are classic but not universal, especially in young children. On physical examination, presence of epigastric tenderness should increase suspicion for one of these diagnoses. Accurate diagnosis and treatment is facilitated by referral for gastroenterology consultation and subsequent endoscopy.

Psychogenic Disorders

Psychogenic chest pain is probably overdiagnosed, especially when the clinical encounter is hurried or frankly viewed as purely a nuisance. Clues to psychogenic chest pain include obvious anxiety or emotional stress, sleep disorders, recent death or separation in the family, multiple and otherwise unexplained somatic complaints, or hyperventilation. The latter is usually unrecognized by the patient, but there are usually clues such as lightheadedness, headache, and/or paresthesias. In general, it is not wise to attribute a psychogenic etiology simply as a diagnosis of exclu-

sion in children with otherwise unexplained chest pain. In the absence of corroborating clinical history such as that described above, it would be better to simply acknowledge uncertainty about the diagnosis (i.e., idiopathic chest pain) than to forward a poorly substantiated diagnosis of psychogenic disorder.

Cardiac Disorders

Unlike the spectrum of cardiac disease in adults, the majority of congenital and acquired heart disease in children does not present with chest pain. Fortunately, those heart conditions that can present with chest pain are generally associated with useful clues in the personal and family history, physical examination, and/or 12-lead electrocardiogram (ECG) (Figure 1-1).

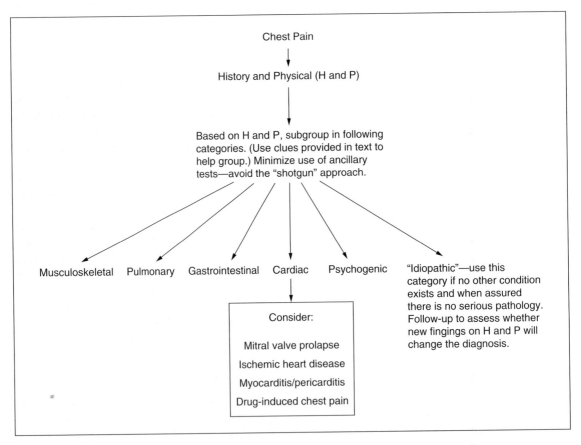

FLOW DIAGRAM FOR THE DIAGNOSIS AND MANAGEMENT OF CHEST PAIN IN CHILDREN

Pericarditis and Myocarditis

Pericarditis, and to a lesser extent myocarditis, can complicate otherwise benign respiratory or gastrointestinal illnesses, and occasionally develops after cardiac surgery (the postpericardiotomy syndrome). Myopericarditis is also seen in Kawasaki's disease, which now exceeds the incidence of acute rheumatic fever in developed countries. Historic attributes of chest pain in patients with myopericarditis include incessant chest discomfort, aggravated by recumbent positioning, and often associated with significant dyspnea. Palpitations or syncope may indicate associated cardiac arrhythmia. Physical examination signs include respiratory distress, tachycardia, narrowed pulse pressure with an increased pulsus paradoxus, neck vein distention, distant heart sounds, murmurs of valvar regurgitation, a pericardial friction rub, arrhythmia, and occasionally hemodynamic collapse. Chest radiography may or may not show cardiomegaly, depending on the size of any associated pericardial effusion. Temporal changes of pericarditis on the 12-lead ECG include PR segment depression and ST segment elevation early in the course (i.e., first few days), later evolving to T-wave flattening, then T-wave inversion, and finally reversion to normal (weeks to months later). Serum myocardial enzymes can be elevated in myocarditis, and markers of systemic inflammation (e.g., C-reactive protein or erythrocyte sedimentation rate) are usually elevated in pericarditis. Echocardiography is the diagnostic test of choice for both conditions, and in the case of pericarditis, can be useful in guiding pericardiocentesis. With appropriate management, the majority of patients with acute pericarditis completely recovers, while a minority may have relapsing chronic pericarditis, and less than 10% will go on to develop constrictive pericarditis.

Cardiac Arrhythmia

The most common arrhythmias in childhood are re-entrant supraventricular tachycardias. Ventricular arrhythmias are comparatively rare. Most children with an important cardiac arrhythmia are more likely to complain of palpitations, subjective tachycardia,

dizziness, or syncope, as compared to reporting chest pain as the sole manifestation. Exercise-related syncope is an ominous historic indicator of potentially serious ventricular arrhythmia, with or without a history of associated chest pain. Inquiry on family history should include unexplained syncope, sudden death, or resuscitated cardiac arrest. A 12-lead ECG is central to the subsequent evaluation, and even in sinus rhythm may provide clues to an arrhythmia mechanism (e.g., ventricular preexcitation seen in patients with Wolff-Parkinson-White syndrome; repolarization abnormalities in the congenital long QT syndromes). When cardiac arrhythmia is suspected on the basis of history, but not immediately evident on initial examination or ECG, ambulatory monitoring with a patient-activated event recorder can be diagnostic. An event recorder is preferable to a single 24-h ambulatory Holter monitor if symptoms are not occurring on a daily basis.

Congenital Heart Disease

With a few noteworthy exceptions, congenital heart disease rarely presents with chest pain. These exceptions include moderate-to-severe forms of valvar or subvalvular ventricular outflow tract obstruction (e.g., aortic valve stenosis) and congenital coronary anomalies (e.g., aberrant coronary artery origin from the contralateral sinus of Valsalva). Chest pain with moderate-strenuous exercise, and/or chest pain associated with palpitations, dizziness, or syncope should heighten index of suspicion. Physical examination should focus on identifying abnormal precordial activity and pathologic heart murmurs. A chest radiograph and ECG are relatively insensitive tools for investigating congenital heart disease, whereas echocardiography has high sensitivity and specificity for virtually all forms of congenital heart disease.

Mitral Valve Prolapse

Few disorders have provoked as much controversy as mitral valve prolapse (MVP). Whereas there is little doubt regarding the importance of MVP in terms of risk for endocarditis, progressive mitral regurgitation, and atrial arrhythmias, it is much less clear how often a direct cause-effect link between chest pain and MVP exists. Studies in adults have shown similar incidences of chest pain between subjects with and without MVP.[2] The diagnosis is best confirmed by echocardiography, as reliance on clinical auscultation (e.g., clicks and/or murmurs) yields excessive false-positive diagnoses. Using established echocardiographic criteria for MVP diagnosis is essential if overdiagnosis based on more ambiguous images is to be avoided. Finally, beta-adrenergic blockade treatment of chest pain in patients with MVP is akin to treating with placebo, and should be discouraged.

Drug-Induced Chest Pain

Cocaine abuse is a well-recognized cause of chest pain and acute cardiac ischemia in adult patients presenting for emergency care. Like their adult counterparts, many adolescents will fail to self-report cocaine use during an evaluation for chest pain. In other cases, over-the-counter drugs (e.g., ephedrine) may cause chest pain. ECG changes induced by cocaine or other drugs can be nonspecific, and assays for myocardial enzyme release are not always positive. A presumptive diagnosis of drug-induced chest pain should still be considered likely when the urine drug screen is positive in the absence of another plausible explanation for the symptom. Under these circumstances, a period of observation in a specialized chest pain unit or inpatient facility is usually recommended.

Chest Pain, Athletes, and Sudden Death

Heightened concerns are often raised when a young athlete complains of chest pain. There is statistical evidence that mortality is higher during exercise compared to resting time, and among athletes the incidence of sudden cardiac death is approximately five times higher during exercise. Even though the annual incidence of sudden cardiac death in athletes is very low (approximately 1:200,000),[3] it is important for physicians to develop skills to effectively screen the athlete for this risk. A complete discus-

sion of this topic is beyond the scope of this review, but as relates to a sentinel complaint of chest pain, a few important points are worth noting.

The most common cause of sudden death in athletes is hypertrophic cardiomyopathy (HC), and chest pain (during exercise or at rest) can be the presenting complaint. Chest pain is not, however, the most useful clue to stratifying risk of sudden death. History of recurrent unexplained syncope and family history of sudden death are much more predictive. The importance of a family medical history must be underscored. Many patients with HC have murmurs of left ventricular outflow tract obstruction, and some will have overt signs of heart failure. The electrocardiogram in patients with HC is almost always abnormal, and echocardiography is currently the best means of confirming the diagnosis.

Another important cause of sudden death among athletes is aberrant course of the left or right coronary artery, and affected patients often report chest pain during exercise. This diagnosis can also be established by echocardiography, but may also require additional testing such as MRI or coronary arteriography.

CONCLUSION

The vast majority of childhood chest pain complaints are secondary to idiopathic and relatively benign musculoskeletal conditions. Thorough history and physical examination are sufficient to diagnose virtually all cases of musculoskeletal chest pain, making "rule-out" cardiac testing unnecessary. Likewise, history and physical examination will provide reliable indicators of respiratory (e.g., exercise-induced asthma) or gastrointestinal (e.g., gastritis) etiologies of chest pain. Psychogenic chest pain is uncommon in childhood, and should not be considered merely a diagnosis of exclusion.

The important cardiac causes of chest pain are pericarditis, myocarditis, cardiac arrhythmia, hypertrophic cardiomyopathy, congenital coronary anomalies, and drug-induced acute cardiac ischemia. MVP, on the other hand, is not as important a cause of chest pain as previously considered. The physician should have an increased suspicion of heart disease on eliciting a history of chest pain associated with moderate-strenuous exercise, dyspnea, palpitations, and/or syncope. Investigating the family history for heart disease or sudden death, identifying abnormalities on cardiovascular physical examination, and a screening 12-lead ECG will further assist in discriminating children with cardiogenic chest pain. These principles are especially important in terms of screening young athletes during routine preparticipation examinations. Although most complaints of chest pain are self-limiting and best handled with reassurance, referral to a pediatric cardiologist should be a priority if any of the aforementioned clues to potential heart disease are discovered (see Figure 1-1).

References

1 Selbst SM: Chest pain in children. *Pediatrics* 75:1068–1070, 1985.

2 Freed LA, Levy D, Levine RA, et al: Prevalence and clinical outcome of mitral-valve prolapse. *N Engl J Med* 1:341:1–7, 1999.

3 Maron BJ, Goldman TE, Aeppli D: Prevalence of sudden cardiac death during competitive sports activities in Minnesota high school athletes. *J Am Coll Cardiol* 32:1881–1884, 1998.

2

MURMURS

David G. Ruschhaupt

Proper auscultation of the heart and interpretation of the findings are essential to assessing the general good health of the pediatric patient. Often, even the most senior of clinicians seem confused by the frequent presence of heart murmurs in newborns and young children. Expensive but unnecessary testing is frequently ordered to avoid missing a serious problem. The converse also happens. No follow-up may be organized because the findings have been misinterpreted as innocent. It is hoped that the following discussion will be a practical guide to the interpretation of murmurs in the pediatric patient.

THE PATHOPHYSIOLOGY OF HEART MURMURS

Heart murmurs are, by definition, noises created by the turbulence of blood flow. Furthermore, they are in the cardiac area of the chest (outside this area, blood flow turbulence is known as a *bruit*). They may occur as part of systole or diastole whenever normal laminar blood flow within the cardiac chambers or the great vessels is interrupted. The quality of the murmur depends on the amount of turbulence generated, which in turn is defined by

the Reynolds number (Reynolds number = RVD/v, where R is radius of the tube; V is mean velocity of blood flow; D is density of fluid; and v is viscosity). The Reynolds number needs to be greater than 2000 in order to generate audible sound. Of note is that a pressure gradient or flow through a narrowed orifice leads to an exponential increase in the amount of turbulence. Thus, increasing cardiac output, reducing viscosity, or the presence of a stenotic valve will increase turbulence.

The presence of a heart murmur does not require or imply cardiac pathology. For example, increased cardiac output that occurs in hypermetabolic conditions, anemia, infection, or anxiety may be associated with a heart murmur. A murmur without cardiac pathology is called an innocent or functional heart murmur. Typically these murmurs have an even harmonic sound, are of low intensity with a cycle length of about 200 cps, occur in midsystole, and are maximally appreciated at the third left intercostal space, often with radiation toward the apex of the heart. Not infrequently such murmurs may be loud. Loudness, however, is not a criterion for pathology. The murmur created in structurally abnormal hearts is related to increased volume of blood flow, as in shunting lesions, or to increased velocity of blood flow created by obstructive or regurgitant lesions. As will be discussed, these pathologic murmurs may be separated from innocent murmurs by their specific sound qualities, associated sounds or other physical findings.

THE BASIC CARDIAC EXAMINATION

In order to fully understand the significance of a heart murmur, it is necessary to perform a complete cardiac examination. Murmurs are ubiquitous in the pediatric patient population. Identification of the pathologic murmur requires not only proper characterization of its sound quality, not to be confused with loudness, but the appreciation of systolic and diastolic sounds that may accompany the murmur.

Palpation of the Precordium

Palpation of the precordium, especially in the newborn where physiologic adaptations may prevent the occurrence of heart murmurs, can provide a very useful clue to the presence of congenital heart defects and should, therefore, be the first step in the cardiac exam. Generally, when the clinician palpates the area of the xyphoid process, there is no awareness of

cardiac activity. A palpable impulse will be felt in this location with volume overload associated with large left-to-right shunts or with the increased cardiac activity produced by hypoplastic left heart syndrome or coarctation of the aorta. This type of hyperdynamic activity, even without a cardiac murmur, is abnormal and requires careful examination and follow-up.

Heart Sounds

Prior to listening for heart murmurs, it is very important to mentally scan both systole and diastole for heart sounds and clicks (Figures 2-1 and 2-2). The importance of making this effort first cannot be over emphasized. The systolic heart sounds are created by the closure of the various heart valves and abrupt directional change in blood flow. Diastolic heart sounds are created when the atrio-ventricular (AV) valves are open and there is blood filling the ventricles (Figure 2-1).

The first heart sound (S1) is created by the closure of the mitral and tricuspid valves. This sound is best appreciated at the left lower sternal border and the apex of the heart. Since the left ventricle is electrically depolarized before the right ventricle, contraction of the ventricles is not synchronous. The

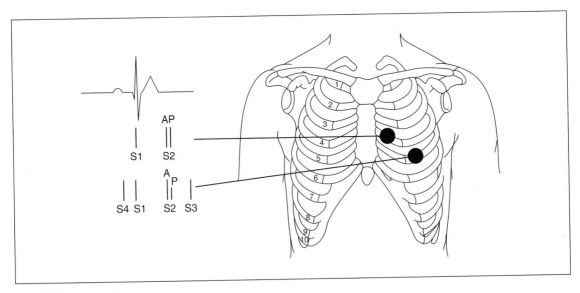

FIGURE 2-1

LOCATION OF HEART SOUNDS

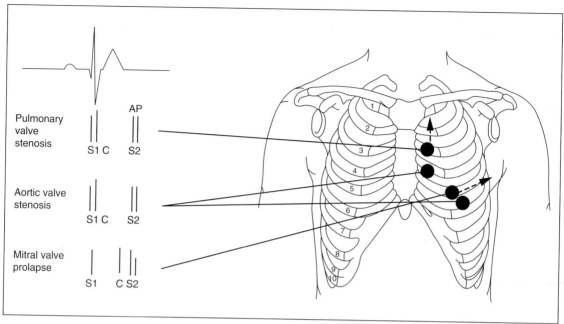

FIGURE 2-2

LOCATION OF CLICKS

mitral valve closure precedes tricuspid valve closure. Often this discrepancy in closure time creates an audible splitting of the first heart sound. This splitting is normal but it needs to be distinguished from an ejection click.

The second heart sound (S2) is created by the closure of the semilunar valves. Similar to S1, S2 is also split with the aortic valve closure preceding the pulmonary valve closure. There is respiratory variation in the degree of splitting for S2. Inhalation increases right ventricular volume with corresponding delay of the completion of right ventricular systole and pulmonary valve closure. With exhalation, the volume load on the right ventricle is removed. S2 becomes narrowed or even single to the human ear. Widened and fixed splitting of S2 is classically described in right ventricular volume overload conditions such as an atrial septal defect (ASD) or total anomalous drainage of the pulmonary veins; however, so-called fixed splitting of S2 is not pathognomic of an ASD. Other conditions such as pulmonary valve stenosis

or right bundle branch block in the electrocardiogram may create fixed splitting of S2. Fixed splitting of S2 is not normal. The observation needs further evaluation with an electrocardiogram (ECG) or possibly an echocardiogram. Separate from the splitting of the second heart sound, the clinician should also consider the intensity of the sound. This sound is best heard at the second left intercostal space using the diaphragm of the stethoscope. Increased intensity of the sound may indicate the presence of pulmonary hypertension. In the newborn, a loud, single S2 may suggest transposition of the great arteries because the high pressure aorta is now anterior to the pulmonary artery and directly under the stethoscope.

The third heart sound (S3) is a low-frequency diastolic sound occurring approximately 0.10 s after the second heart sound and is related to blood flowing into the ventricles. Since the S3 is a low-frequency sound, it is best heard with the bell of the stethoscope lightly placed on the precordium at the left lower sternal border or midway between the left sternal border and the apex of the heart. Particularly in younger children, a third heart sound commonly reflects normal ventricular filling; however, the clinician ought to be aware that this sound may be an indicator of increased blood flow across an AV valve, as seen with left-to-right shunting lesions or with significant AV valve regurgitation. When an S3 is unusually prominent and associated with tachycardia, it may be an indication of congestive heart failure and is referred to as a "gallop" sound. A prominent S3, with or without a murmur, may reflect a thickened and noncompliant left ventricle such as is found in constrictive or restrictive diseases of the heart in which there is rapid ventricular filling. Thus, while likely to be a normal finding, the appreciation of a diastolic S3 should alert the clinician to further possibilities.

The fourth heart sound (S4) is very infrequently heard in children. Like the S3, it is a low-frequency sound heard late in diastole, and is associated with blood flow during atrial contraction. A prominent S4 may reflect altered compliance (relaxation) of either the right or left ventricle. If owing to left-sided lesions, it may be seen in coronary artery disease, hypertrophic obstructive cardiomyopathy, aortic stenosis, or systemic hypertension. An S4 owing to right-sided lesions may be seen in children with elevated right atrial pressure as seen in pulmonary artery hypertension, tricuspid valve stenosis, or Ebstein's anomaly of the tricuspid valve.

Clicks

Clicks are systolic heart sounds that, when present, indicate cardiac pathology. They are sharp sounds that are not felt to be owing to blood flow but rather mechanical sounds of valves. Clicks may be classified as ejection or nonejection and are representative of valve pathology (as seen with obstruction, thickening, or abnormal structure) or vessel dilatation (as seen with connective tissue disorders or hypertension). The timing as well as the location of clicks is the key to their proper interpretation (Figure 2-2). Early systolic clicks (ejection systolic click) that combine with S1 are related to semilunar valve abnormalities. Systolic opening of the semilunar valves requires that the AV valves have

closed, generating S1. Therefore, an ejection click occurs after S1. The timing of the click may be such that the human ear will not separate it from the first sound. Ejection clicks, therefore, are sharp sounds that are appreciated simultaneously with or very narrowly separated from S1. Location is very important to interpretation (Figure 2-2). An ejection click at the third left intercostal space and/or just at the apex of the heart is indicative of aortic stenosis or a bicuspid aortic valve. The associated heart murmur will indicate the presence and severity of obstruction or insufficiency of the valve. An ejection click at the second left intercostal space that varies with breathing (intensity increases with inhalation and decreases with exhalation) is indicative of pulmonary valve stenosis. Again the nature of the murmur will suggest the severity of the abnormality. A constant click in the pulmonary area may represent pulmonary hypertension. Ejection clicks observed in the newborn have special significance, indicating pulmonary valve atresia, aortic valve atresia, or truncus arteriosus. The common abnormality in these lesions is a dilated and hemodynamically altered semilunar valve, or dilated arterial root.

Late systolic clicks, also known as nonejection clicks, occur one-half to two-thirds of the way into systole. The clicks may be multiple. When present they indicate AV valve prolapse, most commonly mitral valve prolapse. The presence or absence of a murmur will indicate whether there is associated mitral valve insufficiency.

Friction Rubs

Friction rubs are a special set of sounds that may be heard in various locations. Unlike murmurs, which are caused by turbulent blood flow, friction rubs are sounds caused by the friction between serosal surfaces such as the pleura and pericardium. These rubs are usually caused by friction between the parietal and visceral portions because of inflammation. Since they are not generated within the cardiovascular system, they do not have a typical systolic and diastolic component; however, they may be confused with cardiac murmurs, as the surfaces may be adjacent to the heart and thus influenced by the cardiac cycle. They may be heard in both systole and diastole, and can be described as having a "to and fro" or "shuffling" quality resembling the noise made by rubbing two pieces of sandpaper together.

Heart Murmurs

Heart murmurs can be described in detail as shown in Table 2-1 and Figures 2-3 and 2-4. The accurate and detailed description of a heart murmur is a disciplined process, which allows the clinician (especially the student) to learn and properly diagnose it. Furthermore, the detailed description will allow appropriate communication among clinicians as well as comparison of the murmur over time. In the future, digital recordings of a murmur noted on examination may obviate the need for this type of detailed documentation. The most obvious

and well-documented description is the loudness, graded on a familiar scale of 1-6 (Table 2-1). Murmurs can also be described in terms of location and radiation. The former is the location where the murmur is loudest, and the latter the location where the murmur is noted just as loud assuming known patterns of blood flow.

Most heart murmurs are described as ejection systolic, pansystolic, early diastolic, middiastolic, presystolic, or continuous. The timing, sound quality, location as well as other descriptors (as noted above) of the murmur on the chest are all considered in making a proper interpretation (Figures 2-3 and 2-4 and Tables 2-1 through 2-3). The "shape" of the murmur can be described (crescendo-decrescendo, decrescendo, plateau) as well as the quality. The latter is an adjective that is derived by the examiner to help describe the sound heard (e.g. vibratory, musical, honking, clanking, whistling, buzzing, blowing, puffy, squeaky). Finally, the response of the murmur to maneuvers can be described. A simple maneuver is the change in body position from lying supine, sitting, standing, and squatting and noting the difference in the murmur with each. Physiologically, the venous return and stroke volume are greater supine than sitting and standing. Squatting increases afterload and further increases venous return (preload). Thus, innocent murmurs (owing to blood flow with a normal heart) will typically be noticeably louder with lying supine versus standing, while a pathologic murmur willl be unchanged (since the change in turbulence due to the change in the amount of blood flow is trivial compared to the turbulence created from the cardiac pathology) or behave differently (as seen with mitral valve prolapse and hypertrophic obstructive cardiomyopathy as described in those chapters).

Ejection systolic murmurs begin after S1 when the ventricles have generated sufficient pressure to open the semilunar valves. The peak intensity of the murmur is in midsystole and then the intensity fades and ends before the closure of the semilunar valves. The most common ejection murmur is the innocent (functional) murmur with an even harmonic quality. Murmurs created by an increased blood volume flowing across an outflow tract and semilunar valve as occurs in atrial septal defects, anemia, or increased metabolic states will also have an even harmonic

TABLE 2-1

DESCRIPTORS IN MURMUR EVALUATIONS

Loudness (grade)
  No thrills
    I—soft
    II—louder
    III—loud
  Thrills
    IV—loud
    V—loud—can hear with the stethoscope partly off the chest
    VI—loud—can hear with the stethoscope completely off the chest
Location
Radiation
Phase—systole, diastole, both, continuous
Length—shot, medium, long, pan, or holo
Timing—early, mid, late—only pertains to short or medium length murmurs
Shape—crescendo/decrescendo, decrescendo, plateau
Quality—special adjective
Affect of maneuvers—supine, sitting, standing, squatting

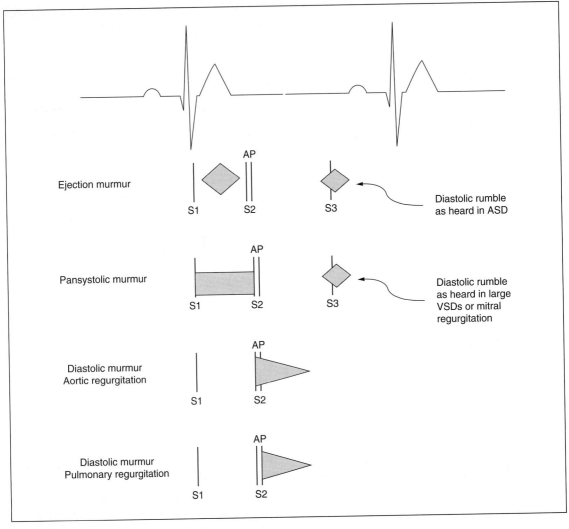

F I G U R E   2 - 3

THE "SHAPE," PHASE, TIMING, AND LENGTH OF MURMURS

quality similar to an innocent murmur. In contrast, a murmur with a rough quality heard best at the third left intercostal space with radiation to the right upper sternal border where it may actually be loudest, is no longer in the innocent category. This type of murmur represents increased turbulence across a stenotic aortic valve. A similar type of rough murmur, appreciated best in the second left intercostal space with radiation to the left infraclavicular area, follows the direction of the pulmonary artery and indicates

abnormal turbulence across the pulmonary valve. Therefore, with careful auscultation of the entire precordium and making proper observations regarding the maximum location of a murmur and searching for the presence and location of ejection clicks, one may decide if a systolic ejection murmur is innocent or created by an abnormality of the aortic or pulmonary valve.

Pansystolic (or holosystolic) murmurs are not usually confused with innocent murmurs. By

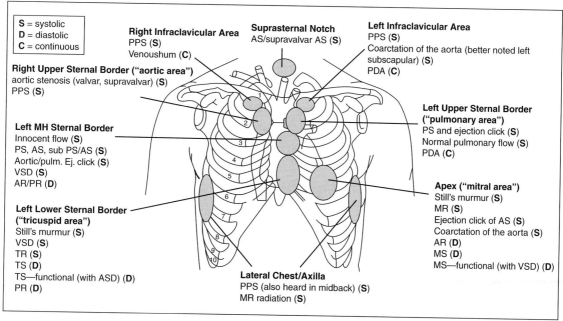

S = systolic
D = diastolic
C = continuous

Right Infraclavicular Area
PPS (**S**)
Venoushum (**C**)

Suprasternal Notch
AS/supravalvar AS (**S**)

Left Infraclavicular Area
PPS (**S**)
Coarctation of the aorta (better noted left subscapular) (**S**)
PDA (**C**)

Right Upper Sternal Border ("aortic area")
aortic stenosis (valvar, supravalvar) (**S**)
PPS (**S**)

Left MH Sternal Border
Innocent flow (**S**)
PS, AS, sub PS/AS (**S**)
Aortic/pulm. Ej. click (**S**)
VSD (**S**)
AR/PR (**D**)

Left Upper Sternal Border ("pulmonary area")
PS and ejection click (**S**)
Normal pulmonary flow (**S**)
PDA (**C**)

Left Lower Sternal Border ("tricuspid area")
Still's murmur (**S**)
VSD (**S**)
TR (**S**)
TS (**D**)
TS—functional (with ASD) (**D**)
PR (**D**)

Apex ("mitral area")
Still's murmur (**S**)
MR (**S**)
Ejection click of AS (**S**)
Coarctation of the aorta (**S**)
AR (**D**)
MS (**D**)
MS—functional (with VSD) (**D**)

Lateral Chest/Axilla
PPS (also heard in midback) (**S**)
MR radiation (**S**)

FIGURE 2-4

TYPICAL LOCATION OR LISTENING AREAS FOR MURMURS

TABLE 2-2

EPONYMS

Innocent murmur	Benign heart murmur because of normal blood flow
Carey Coombs murmur	A low-frequency diastolic murmur at the apex of the heart. It resembles the murmur of mitral stenosis but is created by increased diastolic blood flow across the mitral valve in the presence of significant mitral insufficiency
Austin Flint murmur	A low-frequency diastolic murmur with presystolic accentuation heard at the apex of the heart in the presence of aortic valve insufficiency
Machinery murmur	A continuous murmur at the left upper sternal border that represents a patent ductus arteriosus
Graham Steell murmur	The murmur of pulmonary valve insufficiency in the presence of pulmonary artery hypertension
Gallop sound	An abnormally loud third heart sound created by the filling of the left ventricle in heart failure
Rumble	Low-frequency diastolic murmur created by increased diastolic flow across the mitral valve in a VSD
Seagull murmur	High-frequency apical murmur caused by mitral insufficiency

TABLE 2-3

SYSTOLIC MURMURS AND SOUNDS

Defect	Murmur Type	Murmur Location
ASD	Ejection systolic	2nd–3rd LICS
		Both infraclaviular areas
	S3, diastolic rumble	3rd–4th LICS
Aortic stenosis	Ejection systolic	3rd LICS to RUSB
	Ejection click, constant	3rd LICS and apex
Pulmonary stenosis	Ejection systolic	2nd LICS
	Ejection click, variable	2nd LICS
VSD	Pansystolic	3rd–4th LICS
	S3, diastolic rumble	4th LICS, LSB to apex
Mitral insufficiency	Pansystolic, blowing	Apex to axilla
	S3, Diastolic rumble	4th LICS near apex
PDA	Continuous "machinery"	2nd LICS
	S3, diastolic rumble	4th LICS near apex
Mitral valve prolapse	Pansystolic, blowing	4th LICS near apex
	Late systolic click	
Hypertrophic Cardiomyopathy	Variable; no murmur	
	Short systolic, S3;	LLSB to apex
	harsh, longer systolic	Toward apex

LICS = left intercostal space
LLSB = left lower sternal border

definition, pansystolic timing of a heart murmur means that there is abnormal blood flow occurring over the entirety of systole, i.e., from the time of AV valve closure (S1) to the time of semilunar valve closure (S2). This pathophysiology indicates that a pressure difference exists between the ventricle and the receiving chamber throughout systole. This can happen with ventricular septal defect (VSD), mitral valve regurgitation, and tricuspid valve regurgitation. The pansystolic murmur of a VSD is a relatively harsh sound that is best heard at the third and fourth left intercostal space at the left sternal border. This murmur, when present, is distinctive and is not mistaken for an innocent murmur. The pansystolic murmur of mitral valve insufficiency has a blowing quality, and may sound similar to a VSD. Frequently, mitral insufficiency murmurs have a high-frequency "squeal" buried in them creating the nickname of "seagull type murmur." The location of the murmur is at the apex area of the heart with radi-

ation toward the left axilla (unlike a VSD). Because it is a high-frequency murmur, it is best appreciated with the diaphragm of the stethoscope. Murmurs of tricuspid valve insufficiency are also typically soft and blowing in quality. The diaphragm of the stethoscope picks this sound up best at the third and fourth left intercostal space in the midsternal area.

Early, high-frequency diastolic murmurs are the most difficult to hear. They tend to be very soft and may require positioning the patient in a forward leaning direction in full exhalation while listening with the diaphragm of the stethoscope. When this murmur is caused by aortic valve insufficiency, it will be heard best at the third left intercostal space. The murmur of significant aortic insufficiency may radiate toward the apex of the heart. Since pulmonary artery pressure is lower than aortic pressure, pulmonary valve insufficiency murmurs are slightly lower pitched. They are appreciated best in the second and third left intercostal space, often radiating toward the left lower sternal border. As the murmur follows pulmonary valve closure, splitting of S2 will be appreciated.

Middiastolic murmurs are frequently referred to as "rumbling" because of their low frequency. They will be best heard with the bell of the stethoscope and reflect diastolic flow across an AV valve. An apical diastolic murmur in the presence of a VSD indicates significant increase in diastolic blood flow across the mitral valve and correlates with a measured increase in pulmonary blood flow that is at least twice the amount of systemic blood flow. In the presence of significant mitral valve insufficiency, there will be increased diastolic flow back across the mitral valve, creating an apical diastolic murmur (Carey Coombs murmur—Table 2-2). Significant aortic valve incompetence may create diastolic blood flow along the septal leaflet of the mitral valve, forcing the opened leaflet back into the flow pattern of that orifice. This will create a low-frequency rumble at the apex of the heart that resembles that of mitral valve stenosis (Austin Flint murmur—Table 2-2). Mitral valve stenosis is not very common in the pediatric patient. When it occurs, there will be a low-frequency middiastolic murmur with presystolic (very late diastolic) accentuation that relates to atrial contraction against the stenotic valve. Finally, the left-to-right shunting of an atrial septal defect volume loads the right ventricle. The increased diastolic flow across the tricuspid valve produces low-frequency turbulence and a diastolic murmur. Because the right ventricle is dilated, this murmur may be heard midway between the left lower sternal border and the apex of the heart. Appreciation of this murmur is the key to separating atrial septal defect patients from those with innocent murmurs. Increasing cardiac output with mild exercise such as sit-ups on the examining table may make this murmur more easily heard.

Continuous (systolic/diastolic) murmurs occur in situations where a vascular communication has a pressure difference through the entire cardiac cycle. The classic continuous murmur is referred to as a "machinery" murmur and is heard at the left upper sternal border because of a patent ductus arteriosus (PDA). Frequently children between the ages of 3 and 10 years may have a continuous murmur in this same area that is called a "venous hum." This particular murmur is heard mainly in the upright position, changes with head position and is obliterated by compression on the neck venous system. This is a benign condition and is important only in that it is confused with the murmur of a patent ductus. A continuous murmur away from this area indicates some other type of arterial-venous fistula involving the lungs, the coronary arteries, the liver, or the brain.

THE INNOCENT MURMURS

There are a number of innocent murmurs that are frequently noted and well described (Table 2-4). It is worthwhile mentioning these with detailed descriptions. Clinicians taking care of children should become familiar with these murmurs and be able to recognize them as normal. Future digital "textbooks" will no doubt contain digital audio clips to enhance learning these murmurs. The reader is referred to audiotapes and CDs containing these sounds (listed in Suggested Readings section).

Still's Murmur

A Still's murmur is an innocent murmur first described by George Frederick Still in the early 1900s. The exact origin is unclear, though it is felt to possibly originate from within the left ventricle or outflow tract owing to vibration of the chordae tendinae. It is usually grade 1–2, though may sometimes be grade 3 (never greater). This murmur is typically described as vibratory or musical. It is a medium to long systolic ejection-type murmur best heard between the left lower sternal border and the apex. There is slight radiation to the upper sternal border. As with other innocent murmurs, it is best heard while lying supine and decreases with standing.

Pulmonary Flow Murmur

An innocent pulmonary flow is because of normal flow into the pulmonary arteries. The pulmonary arteries are the most anterior structure of the cardiac anatomy, thus blood flow is most likely to be heard in this area. Since children usually have smaller statures than adults, blood flow turbulence

TABLE 2-4

INNOCENT HEART MURMURS

Name or Eponym	Murmur Type	Murmur Description
Still's	Systolic, ejection	Grades 1–3, vibratory Between LLSB and apex
Pulmonary flow	Systolic, ejection	Grades 1–3, soft, nonharsh LUSB
PPS	Systolic, ejection short	Soft, grades 1–2, LUSB Radiates to axilla/back
Venous hum	Continuous	Heard at right clavicle Varies with neck position
Carotid/cranial bruits	Systolic	Soft, grades 1–2 Heard over appropriate artery
Cardiorespiratory	Continuous	Not really a murmur An airway sound Disappears when not breathing

is more likely to be heard. This murmur is medium to long, systolic, ejection and usually grade 1–2, and rarely (but never greater than) grade 3. It is best heard in the left upper sternal border with slight radiation in a pulmonary artery distribution. It is not harsh, and is medium to low pitched. It is also louder when supine and softer with standing.

Peripheral Pulmonary Stenosis

The murmur of peripheral pulmonary stenosis (PPS) is not always innocent. It is because of narrowing and/or distortion/acute angulation of the branch pulmonary arteries. In infants, this narrowing of an acute angulation is part of the normal anatomy. With normal development of the pulmonary arteries, this condition no longer occurs after approximately 6 months of age. Thus, this murmur will no longer be present at that time. If there is a pathologic narrowing of distortion of the pulmonary arteries, the murmur will persist. The murmur of PPS is typically grade 1–2, systolic, ejection type and best heard at the left upper sternal border with radiation to the axillae and out to the back (distribution of pulmonary blood flow). It is usually short to medium

length and in midsystole. It is usually soft (nonharsh) and may have a blowing or "puffy" quality to it when heard in the back. The pitch is similar to a breath sound and may be difficult to hear because of the noise of breathing. It is best heard between breaths. When pathologic, it lasts beyond 6 months, is longer in length, and is harsher in quality. Maneuvers such as standing and lying supine are not useful in infants. If the PPS is pathologic, there will be no change with maneuvers.

Cardiorespiratory Murmur

This term is a misnomer, as the sound called a "cardiorespiratory murmur" is not a murmur at all. It is because of airway noise rather than blood flow. Since the airways are close to the heart and great vessels, noise in them may have a systolic and diastolic cycle to them reflecting pulsation of the heart and great vessels next to the airways. This sound is soft and may be continuous. It is best heard near the sternum, where the large airways are located. It is differentiated from a cardiac murmur by the fact that it disappears when the patient holds his/her breath.

Venous Hum—Supraclavicular Bruit

The murmur of a venous hum is produced by turbulent blood flow in the great vein (superior vena cava and the like). It is a soft, continuous murmur of grade 1–2 (never greater than 3). It is best heard in the right clavicular area and is present with the neck in extension (compression and distortion of the veins causing turbulence) and becomes softer or disappears with the neck in flexion. It is not heard while lying supine.

Carotid and Cranial Bruits

Although not murmurs, owing to their location, carotid and cranial bruits should also be mentioned in a discussion of innocent heart sounds. Similar to normal turbulence in the heart and great vessels, there is turbulence in the carotid and temporal arteries. The sound created is a grade 1–2, soft, systolic ejection sound over the artery.

SUMMARY AND EVALUATION OF MURMURS

The logical approach to auscultation of the heart, listening to both systole and diastole with specific attention to heart sounds, clicks and their primary location area on the chest will aid in the accurate interpretation of most cardiac murmurs. There is no substitute for a complete examination by an experienced clinician. Admittedly, some findings may be subtle, leaving doubt whether a murmur is innocent. The most commonly overlooked congenital cardiac conditions are ASD and hypertrophic cardiomyopathy. Therefore, there is a role for auxiliary testing.

The ECG is probably the most useful initial screening test. Right ventricular hypertrophy will be present in ASD or significant pulmonary valve stenosis. Electrographic left or biventricular hypertrophy may be present in large ventricular septal defects; however, the correlation of voltage and hypertrophy or enlargement is poor and these findings may be present in children with no pathology. T-wave abnormalities and/or abnormal initial electrical forces are very likely in hypertrophic cardiomyopathy. It must be underscored that a

normal ECG may be seen in the presence of underlying cardiac pathology and an abnormal ECG may be seen in normal children. This is discussed further in Chapter 37. Thus, there is no substitute for the examination, and this needs to be correlated with any tests obtained.

Echocardiography has rendered routine chest radiographs less useful than they once were in the routine evaluation of patients with suspected congenital heart defects. An exception to this may be in the nursery setting, where the presence of cyanosis or tachypnea may be diagnosed on the chest film as obvious pulmonary pathology. Again, it must be underscored that neither chest radiography nor echocardiography can substitute for auscultation by an experienced clinician. In each case, the test may be normal in the presence of underlying pathology, or the test may show abnormalities that do not reflect the physical findings (e.g., the echocardiographic finding of a PDA in the absence of a PDA murmur but the presence of a Stills murmur). The specific laboratory findings for each congenital heart lesion will be addressed in detail by subsequent chapters.

The focus of the murmur evaluation changes with age, but the examination should stand alone, with no test or scheme as an adequate substitute. If the clinician determines that a murmur is pathologic, then referral to a more experienced clinician (usually a pediatric cardiologist) is in order and the clinician should learn from the final findings and gain additional experience in auscultation; however, the management of clearly pathologic or innocent murmurs is usually not of concern to most clinicians. The cause for concern is the "not-so clearly innocent murmur." For these, an initial "referral" to a more experienced colleague or partner may prove helpful and a valuable source of ongoing education for the less experienced or junior physician. The following provide a framework and clinical considerations in the evaluation of the not-so-clearly-innocent murmur.

A suggested scheme for the evaluation of murmurs is given in Figure 2-5. The age of the patient becomes important in terms of possible diagnoses and the effect of underlying physiology, namely, pulmonary vascular resistance (PVR), as it changes

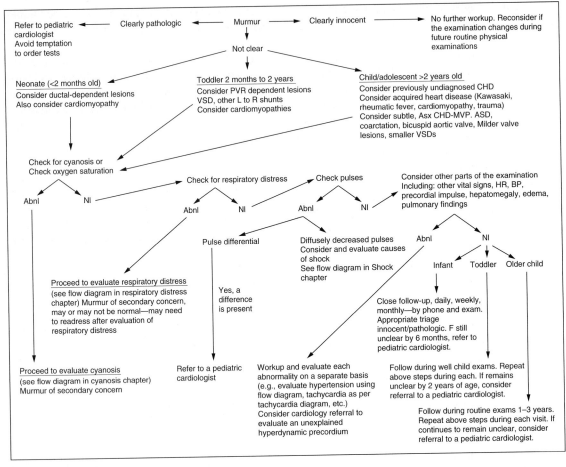

FIGURE   2 - 5

FLOW DIAGRAM IN THE EVALUATION OF MURMURS

with age. In the newborn, the greatest concern is over critical, ductal-dependent, and life-threatening heart defects. Many of these defects do not have a clearly pathologic murmur as the presenting feature; rather, cyanosis, respiratory distress, or shock are the important features. After the newborn period (4–6 weeks), ductal-dependent lesions are usually no longer a concern. At this time, PVR-dependent lesions become important. Lesions such as ASDs, VSDs, PDAs, and anomalous coronary arteries become manifest as the PVR decreases and the shunt to the lungs (and steal from the systemic circulation or coronary arterial circulation) produces clinical signs and symptoms with

associated murmurs. Left untreated, a large left-to-right shunt may lead to pulmonary vascular disease; however, this does not occur for many months to years. Lesions that do not cause significant symptoms may be more difficult to detect and should be the focus of the examination in older children and adolescents. The latter lesions include ASDs, valve lesions, bicuspid aortic valve, mitral valve prolapse, coarctation of the aorta, hemodynamically insignificant PDAs and VSDs, and electrical or muscle abnormalities.

Thus, the clinician should consider above possibilities in the evaluation and management of a murmur realizing that the final determination is based on the clinical examination; however, the age of the patient may determine how soon and carefully the clinician follows the patient. For instance, a murmur in the newborn will require a more intense examination of pulses, saturations, and general state to help exclude ductal-dependent lesions. Follow-up evaluations should be scheduled sooner than routine, and instructions to the parents should include the possibility of underlying cardiac concerns. If clinical doubt continues, a cardiology consultation should be obtained.

In the nonneonatal age, the clinician should be cognizant of the underlying possible cardiac conditions. In the absence of symptoms (including growth and weight gain), the urgency for follow-up is not as great as in the neonate. There are usually multiple well child visits to allow reexamination and diagnosis of pathology. The important point is to not allow a large left-to-right shunt to escape detection within the first 6 months to a year of life with the possible consequence of irreversible pulmonary vascular disease. The murmurs associated with these lesions are usually clearly pathologic and may be associated with other symptoms.

In the older child and adolescent, the considerations of ductal-dependent lesions and large left-to-right shunts are rarely of concern (irreversible pulmonary vascular disease may already be present if a large left-to-right shunt were missed). Thus, the urgency of the prior two age groups is no longer present. In the asymptomatic patient, the clinician may allow reevaluation during the next routine physical examination. A number of reevaluations will probably not cause harm; however, the clinician should eventually commit to a diagnosis of pathologic or innocent heart murmur. If unable to make the diagnosis after a number of reevaluations during routine physical examinations, the clinician should consider referral to a more experienced clinician (usually a pediatric cardiologist). An initial "referral" to a more experienced colleague or partner may be valuable and allow for ongoing learning for a less experienced physician. The temptation to obtain tests to help or make the diagnosis should be avoided as there are many false positives and negatives that have to be dealt with.

In summary, the evaluation of a cardiac murmur requires a disciplined approach by an experienced clinician with the procedure in turn leading to more experience. With a disciplined examination and strategy, including other findings on the history and physical examination, the proper diagnosis can be made or the appropriate management can be undertaken.

Suggested Readings

Ainsworth S, Wyllie JP, Wren C: Prevalence and clinical significance of cardiac murmurs in neonates. *Arch Dis Child Fetal Neonatal Ed* 80(1):F43–F45, 1999.

Arlettaz R, Archer N, Wilkinson AR: Natural history of innocent heart murmurs in newborn babies:controlled echocardiographic study. *Arch Dis Child Fetal Neonatal Ed* 78:F166, 1998.

Bensky, et al: Primary care physician's use of screening echocardiography. *Pediatrics* 103:e40, 1999.

Castello-Herbreteau B, Vaillant MC, Magontier N, Pottier JM, Blond MH, Chantepie A: Diagnostic value of physical examination and electrocardiogram in the initial evaluation of heart murmurs in children. *Arch Pediatr* 7(10):1041–1049, 2000.

Conti RC: The stethoscope: the forgotten instrument in cardiology? *Clin Cardiol* 20:911–912, 1997.

Craige E: Should auscultation be revisited? *N Engl J Med* 318:1611–1613, 1988.

Danford D, Nasir A, Guminer C. Cost assessment of the evaluation of heart murmurs in children. *Pediatrics* 91:365–368, 1993.

Danford DA, McNamara DG: Innocent murmurs in childhood, in: *The Science and Practice of Pediatric Cardiology*, Chap. 109. Philadelphia, Pa: Lea & Febiger, 1990.

Danford, et al: Children with heart murmurs—can specific defects be reliably diagnosed without an echocardiogram? *J Am Coll Cardiol* 30:243–246, 1997.

Davidson, et al: Cardiomegaly—what does it mean? A comparison of echocardiographic to radiologic cardiac dimensions in children. *Pediatr Cardiol* 11:181–185, 1990.

Driscoll D, et al: Guidelines for evaluation and management of common congenital cardiac problems in infants, children and adolescents. A statement for healthcare professionals from the committee on congenital heart defects of the council on cardiovascular disease in the young, American Heart Association. *Circulation* 90(4):2180–2188, 1994.

Du ZD, Roguin, Barak M: Clinical and echocardiographic evaluation of neonates with heart murmurs. *Acta Paediatr* 86(7):752–756, 1997.

Geva, et al: Reappraisal of the approach to the child with heart murmurs: is echocardiography necessary? *Int J Cardiol* 19:107–113, 1988.

Glascock, et al: Should the primary care physician or pediatric cardiologist be the gatekeeper for echocardiographic testing in the evaluation of heart murmurs? *J Am Soc Echocardiogr* p. 448–abstract 2000.

Haney I, et al: Accuracy of clinical assessment of heart murmurs by office-based (general practice) paediatricians. *Arch Dis Child* 81:409–412, 1999.

Hanson, et al: Initial evaluation of children with heart murmurs by the nonspecialized paediatrician. *Eur J Pediatr* 154:15–17, 1995.

Kandah, et al: When is echocardiography unreliable in patients undergoing catheterization for pediatric cardiovascular disease? *J Am Soc Echocardiogr* 4:51–56, 1991.

Mangione, et al: Cardiac auscultatory skills of internal medicine and family practice trainees. A comparison of diagnostic accuracy. *JAMA* 278:717–722, 1997.

McCrindle BW, Shaffer KM, Kan JS, Zahka KG, Rowe SA, Kidd L: An evaluation of parental concerns and misperceptions about heart murmurs. *Clin Pediatr (Phila)* 34(1):25–31, 1995.

Newburger, et al: Noninvasive tests in the initial evaluation of heart murmurs in children. *N Engl J Med* 308:61–64, 1983.

Pelech AN: The cardiac murmur. When to refer? *Pediatr Clin North Am* 45:107–122, 1998.

Rein AJ, Omokhodion SI, Nir A: Significance of a cardiac murmur as the sole clinical sign in the newborn. *Clin Pediatr (Phila)* 39(9):511–520, 2000.

Roldan CA, Crawford MH: *Cardiol Rev* 14:51–54, 1997.

Rosenthal A: How to distinguish between innocent and pathologic murmurs in childhood. *Pediatr Clin North Am* 31:1229, 1984.

Sapin SO: Recognizing normal heart murmurs: a logic-based mnemonic. *Pediatrics* 99(4):616–619, 1997.

Shaver JA: Cardiac auscultation: a cost effective diagnostic skill. *Curr Probl Cardiol* 20:442–530, 1995.

Skelton R, Evans N, Smythe J: A blinded comparison of clinical and echocardiographic evaluation of the preterm infant for patent ductus arteriosus. *J Pediatr Child Health* 30(5):406–411, 1994.

Smythe, et al: Initial evaluation of heart murmurs are laboratory tests necessary? *Pediatrics* 86:497–500, 1990.

Steinberger, et al: Echocardiographic diagnosis of heart disease in apparently healthy adolescents. *Pediatrics* 105;815–818, 2000.

Still GF: *Common Disorders and Diseases in Childhood.* London, Frowdder: Hadder & Stoughton, 1915.

Stranger P, et al: Diagnostic accuracy of pediatric echocardiograms performed in adult laboratories. *Am J Cardiol* 83:908–914, 1999.

Swenson JM, et al: Are chest radiographs and electrocardiograms still valuable in evaluating new pediatric patients with heart murmurs or chest pain. *Pediatrics* 99:1–3, 1997.

Tworetzky, et al: Echocardiographic diagnosis alone for the complete repair of major congenital heart defects. *J Am Coll Cardiol* 33:228–33, 1997.

Van Oort, et al: The vibratory innocent heart murmur in school children: difference in auscultatory findings between school medical officers and a pediatric cardiologist. *Pediatr Cardiol* 15:282–287, 1994.

Xu M, McHaffie DJ: Nonspecific systolic murmurs: an audit of the clinical value of echocardiography. *N Z Med J* 106(950):54–56, 1993.

Audio CDs

Criley JM, Criley D, Zalace C: *The Physiologic Origins of Heart Sounds and Murmurs: The Unique Interactive Guide to Cardiac Diagnosis.* Philadelphia, PA: Lippincott Williams & Wilkins, 1997.

Altman CA, Nihill MR, Bricker JT: *Pediatric Cardiac Auscultation CD-ROM.* Philadelphia, PA: Lippincott Williams & Wilkins.

3

PALPITATIONS

Frank Zimmerman

INTRODUCTION

Palpitations are a common symptom in the pediatric population. It is defined as a feeling or awareness of an irregular or rapid beating of the heart. It may also be described as pounding in the chest, skipped beats, fluttering, or heart beating out of the chest. This symptom may occur in isolation or may be associated with symptoms of chest pain, dizziness, blurred vision, or a feeling of panic. While often benign in nature, symptoms of palpitations may be disruptive to daily activities and debilitating in some patients. In older patients with palpitations, 19% report work impairment, 37% report decreased functioning at home, and 75–84% have recurrent symptoms.

INCIDENCE

The incidence of symptoms of palpitations in a primary care setting is reported to be approximately 16%. Despite the frequency of this complaint, most patients with palpitations do not have associated cardiac arrhythmias with their symptoms. In reports using 24-h Holter monitors to record the cardiac rhythm during symptoms, less than 10% of patients with palpitations had associated cardiac arrhythmias. Other studies have shown that a high percentage of patients with palpitations either have psychiatric causes ranging from 28 to 31% of patients, or have an unknown etiology.

DIFFERENTIAL DIAGNOSIS

The differential diagnosis of palpitations can be seen in Table 3-1. The pathophysiology of palpitations depends on the etiology. Diagnoses include cardiac arrhythmias (Chapter 36). Sinus tachycardia is found in the majority of patients with palpitations.

Sinus Tachycardia

The etiology of sinus tachycardia is quite broad and can be categorized as compensatory, physiologic, and owing to external influences. Compensatory sinus tachycardia occurs with hypovolemia, anemia, pregnancy, cardiac failure, aortic or mitral regurgitation, large ventricular septal defect, or other lesions with significant left-to-right shunting. This is because of the fact that cardiac output is related to the product of heart rate and stroke volume. Physiologic sinus tachycardia occurs with exertion, emotion, or fever. The goal is to determine if the cause of physiologic sinus tachycardia is appropriate (exercise) or inappropriate (anxiety). Sinus tachycardia can be owing

T A B L E   3 - 1

DIFFERENTIAL DIAGNOSIS OF PALPITATIONS

1. Sinus tachycardia
   a. Compensatory (hypovolemia, anemia, pregnancy, cardiac failure)
   b. Physiologic (exertion, emotion, fever)
   c. External (fever, stimulant use, drug side effects, metabolic causes)
2. Single palpitations
   a. Atrial or ventricular premature beats
   b. Escape beats after a pause or blocked beat
3. Paroxysmal tachycardia
   a. Supraventricular tachycardia
   b. Ventricular tachycardia

to external influences such as fever, stimulant use, drug side effects, or metabolic causes (insulin reaction, pheochromocytoma, or hyperthyroidism).

Single Palpitations

Palpitations characterized by irregular or single skipped beats are often because of premature atrial or ventricular beats. They may also occur with the escape beat following a pause or blocked beat.

Paroxysmal Tachycardia

When episodes are described as having an abrupt onset and resolution, they are often because of paroxysmal tachycardia, such as supraventricular tachycardia or ventricular tachycardia. Occasionally patients may describe an abrupt onset of symptoms with a gradual resolution. In reality, this may owe to an abrupt termination of tachycardia followed by sinus tachycardia owing to increased adrenergic tone following the tachycardia. Episodes with less abrupt onset or resolution are suggestive of automatic atrial tachycardia or sinus tachycardia.

DIAGNOSTIC APPROACH

History

A complete description of the patient's symptoms frequently helps lead to the diagnosis; however,

many patients may be unable to give an accurate or detailed account of their symptoms. Important features of the history include the mode of onset of palpitations, the frequency and duration of symptoms, and any associated symptoms such as dizziness or syncope. The situations associated with symptoms of palpitations may also be important in guiding further diagnostic testing. For instance, symptoms with exercise or stress may be best evaluated by an exercise stress test in order to reproduce the symptoms in a controlled environment. A thorough review of systems is also important and should include any history of weight loss, sleep problems, drug or medication use, and social or emotional situations. Family history of any cardiac disorders or psychiatric disorders should be ascertained. A complete detailed medication use is imperative, especially medicines that contain stimulants (such as over-the-counter cold medicines) or medications associated with QT prolongation (such as antiarrhythmic agents).

Physical Examination

A. Vital signs: Attention to the heart rate in reference to the normal values for age in both the supine and standing position should be noted. An increase in heart rate greater than 20 beats per minute associated with standing can be associated with postural orthostatic tachycardia syndrome, or POTS (see Chapter 4). This may also be a sign of dehydration. Likewise, blood pressure measurements should also be obtained in the supine and standing position with a decrease in systolic blood pressure of 10 mmHg consistent with orthostatic hypotension. A baseline resting tachycardia may be seen in patients with compensatory sinus tachycardia.
B. Skin: The skin should be examined for color or signs of hyperthyroidism and anemia.
C. HEENT: The eyes should be examined for exophthalmus and the neck for goiter.
D. Lungs: The lungs should be examined for any evidence of rales that would be suggestive of congestive heart failure.
E. Cardiovascular: The cardiac exam should be assessed for any heart murmur, gallop, click, rhythm irregularities, and splitting in intensity of the second heart sound. The extremities

palpitations are disruptive to the patient's lifestyle, then treatment can be initiated with beta-blockers or calcium channel-blockers. In rare circumstances, if the symptoms are severe or the premature beats occur frequently and do not respond to medications, then radiofrequency catheter ablation may be offered as more definitive treatment. The role of caffeine in precipitating these arrhythmias is debatable, and the current recommendation is for avoidance of excessive caffeine intake, i.e., greater than five cups of coffee per day, unless the patient has specific symptoms related to any lesser amounts of caffeine intake.

Paroxysmal Supraventricular Tachycardia (PSVT)

The therapy for PSVT is based on the specific type of arrhythmia as well as the frequency and duration of symptoms. In general, the treatment options are conservative management (observation), antiarrhythmic medical therapy, or definitive treatment with radiofrequency catheter ablation. Detailed management of the specific types of PSVT can be found in Chapter 36.

Ventricular Tachycardia

The finding of ventricular arrhythmias as the cause of palpitations prompts an extensive evaluation to assess for underlying cardiac disease. Management is directed at controlling the arrhythmia and treating any underlying pathology. A common cause for ventricular arrhythmias in the pediatric population is benign right ventricular outflow tract tachycardia. This tachycardia occurs in the setting of a structurally normal heart, and treatment is based on symptomatic relief with medications or more definitive therapy with radiofrequency catheter ablation.

SUMMARY

Palpitations are a common complaint in the pediatric population; however, this symptom is rarely associated with cardiac abnormalities. A thorough history and physical exam can often lead to the etiology of the symptoms.

Suggested Readings

Barsky AJ: Palpitations, arrhythmias, and awareness of cardiac activity. *Ann Intern Med* 134:832–837, 2001.

Braunwald E: Examination of the patient—the history, in: Braunwald E, et al. (eds): *Heart Disease: A Textbook of Cardiovascular Medicine*, 6th ed. New York, NY, WB. Saunders, pp. 37–39, 2001.

Daniels CJ, Franklin WH: Common cardiac disease in adolescents. *Pediatr Clin North Am* 44(6): 1591–1604, 1997.

Zimetbaum P, Josephson ME: Current concepts: evaluation of patients with palpitations. *N Engl J Med* 338(19):1369–1373, 1998.

4

SYNCOPE

Frank Zimmerman

INTRODUCTION

Syncope, or fainting, is characterized by a brief period of loss of consciousness that resolves spontaneously or rarely may require resuscitation. The reported incidence of syncope in the general population is varying, ranging from 1:2000 emergency room visits up to 47% of all college students. In the pediatric population, syncope accounts for approximately 0.125% of all patients seeking medical attention. Syncope occurs more often in females than in males, with a peak incidence of 15–19 years of age. Of those with a syncopal episode, approximately 50% will go on to have another episode in the future. Because of the often sudden and dramatic circumstances associated with syncope as well as the possibility of associated risk factors for sudden death, the amount of time and resources devoted to the evaluation of syncope is often significant. This chapter will discuss the etiology, mechanisms, evaluation, and management of syncope in the pediatric population.

THE ETIOLOGY OF SYNCOPE

The broad differential diagnosis of syncope can be divided into three subcategories: neurocardiogenic, cardiac, and noncardiac (Table 4-1).

Neurocardiogenic Syncope

The most common cause of syncope in children is neurocardiogenic syncope, also known as vasovagal syncope or simple fainting. It is characterized by an abrupt onset of symptoms usually occurring with the patient in the upright position either sitting or standing. There may be a prodrome of dizziness, nausea, palpitations, vision changes, pallor, or diaphoresis, but in some, the episodes occur without the prodrome. Loss of consciousness is brief, lasting no more than 1–2 min, and resolves spontaneously. It may be followed by a period of fatigue lasting for up to 24 h after the syncopal episode. There may be associated tonic-clonic activity during the episode because of cerebral hypoperfusion. It is important to determine if the seizure activity occurs at the onset or after loss of consciousness, as this helps to differentiate neurocardiogenic syncope from a primary seizure disorder. Despite this typical clinical description and course, the physiology leading to neurocardiogenic syncope remains debatable. The most common hypothesis suggests that the series of events leading to neurocardiogenic syncope begins with a decrease in the volume of blood filling the right or left ventricles of the heart. This can occur at times of dehydration or during position changes from sitting to standing. The heart responds to the decrease in filling by increasing

TABLE 4-1
CAUSES OF SYNCOPE

1. Neurocardiogenic
2. Cardiac
   Tachyarrhythmias (SVT, VT)
   Bradyarrhythmias (heart block, sinus node dysfunction)
   LV or RV outflow obstruction (aortic stenosis, hypertrophic cardiomyopathy, pulmonary hypertension)
   Coronary disease (Kawasaki's, anomalous coronary artery)
   Primary cardiac dysfunction (dilated or restrictive cardiomyopathy)
   Secondary cardiac dysfunction (myocarditis, metabolic)
3. Noncardiac
   Orthostatic hypotension
   Neurologic (seizures, central nervous system (CNS) abnormality, migraine, dysautonomia)
   Breath-holding spells
   Situational (micturation, cough, swallow)
   Psychogenic (hysteria, hyperventilation)
   Carotid sinus hypersensitivity
   Metabolic abnormality (hypoglycemia, anemia)
   Drugs, medications

contractility. This activates nerves within the ventricular muscle called C-fibers, sending afferent signals to the brain via the vagus nerve.

The brain in turn sends efferent signals to the body and to the heart, making adjustments in sympathetic and parasympathetic tone. These include a dramatic decrease in sympathetic tone with an increase in parasympathetic tone resulting in hypotension and bradycardia, ultimately leading to syncope. It is the abnormal exaggerated response of this normal reflex that leads to neurocardiogenic syncope. The exaggerated response occurs either because of increased vagal sensitivity or exaggerated changes in contractility and C-fiber activation in response to the decrease in ventricular filling. Once the patient becomes supine, increased venous flow to the heart occurs, the reflex mechanism is stopped and syncope resolves. This hypothesis has been challenged; however, mainly based on the finding that patients who have undergone heart transplantation, where the transplanted heart is completely denervated, continue to have episodes of vasovagal syncope. This has led to the speculation that higher neural centers participate in this reflex and either endogenous opioids or serotonin production may play a role in neurocardiogenic syncope.

Cardiac Syncope

Cardiac syncope occurs when the heart is unable to meet the demands of the body, particularly during times of exertion. This may occur with obstruction to flow such as with aortic stenosis, left ventricular (LV) outflow tract obstruction, or pulmonary hypertension. Limited cardiac output can occur with cardiomyopathy or myocarditis. Abrupt decrease in cardiac output may occur with tachyarrhythmias, bradyarrhythmias, or following myocardial infarction.

Noncardiac Syncope

This category includes a wide variety of causes of syncope such as seizures, migraines, drugs, metabolic causes, hyperventilation, hypoglycemia, situational syncope leading to a vasovagal-type reaction, dysautonomia, hysteria, and orthostatic hypotension. Breath-holding spells are a common cause of syncope in young children with a peak incidence occurring at 2–3 years of age. There are two forms of breath-holding spells that have been described and both are thought to represent a form of vasovagal syncope. Cyanotic breath-holding spells are characterized by an episode of crying followed by apnea and cyanosis resulting in a brief period of loss of consciousness. Pallid breath-holding spells are characterized by an initiating event such as injury or startling followed by an acute loss of consciousness.

EVALUATION OF SYNCOPE

Figure 4-1 details steps in the evaluation of syncope.

History

Pertinent information gathered during the history should include as many details as possible about the

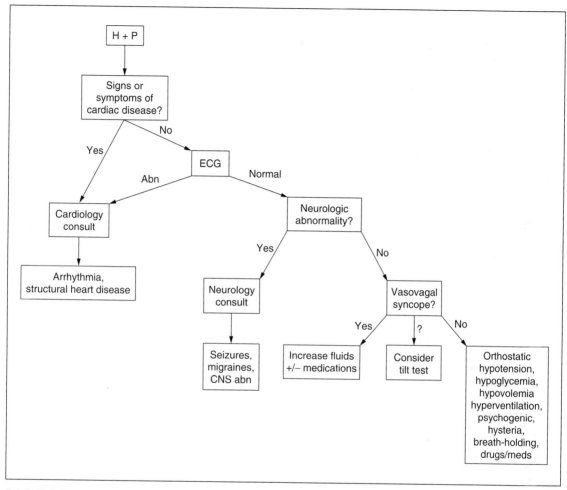

FIGURE 4-1

EVALUATION OF SYNCOPE

episode either from the patient, parent, or from any witnesses. This should include the presence of any triggers initiating the event such as stress, anxiety, position changes, or situations such as micturition or injury. One should also elicit any history of a prodrome of headache, nausea, dizziness, diaphoresis, or visual or auditory hallucinations. Details about other episodes of syncope or near-syncope, especially if the patient becomes symptomatic when standing from a sitting position, may suggest a propensity toward neurocardiogenic syncope. An extensive family history regarding sudden death, arrhythmias, seizures, migraine headaches, sudden

infant death syndrome (SIDS), or congenital deafness (which can be seen in patients with long QT syndrome) should be sought.

Physical Examination

Pertinent findings on the physical exam include assessment of the blood pressure in the supine position and standing position. Orthostatic hypotension is defined as a decrease in blood pressure of 20 mmHg with position changes. The cardiac exam should assess for murmurs suggestive of LV outflow tract obstruction, clicks suggestive of mitral valve prolapse or aortic valve disease and splitting and intensity of the second heart sound that may be increased in intensity in cases of pulmonary hypertension. In older patients, carotid sinus massage can be performed, once carotid bruits have been ruled out with auscultation, to assess for carotid sinus hypersensitivity.

Laboratory Testing

Laboratory testing is guided by the history and physical exam. It may include assessment of serum glucose if hypoglycemia is suspected. Hemoglobin level can be used for patients with suspected anemia and a urine toxicity screen can be performed at the time of presentation to assess for illicit drug use. Further testing and diagnostic procedures are given below.

12-Lead Electrocardiogram (ECG)

The ECG is an easy, quick, and noninvasive test that is essential for the evaluation of syncope. The baseline heart rhythm as well the corrected QT interval is assessed in patients with suspected long QT syndrome. The ECG is also used to screen for conduction disturbances or ventricular preexcitation that may predispose patients to orthodromic reciprocating tachycardia (the Wolff-Parkinson-White syndrome). Detection of left ventricular hypertrophy (which may be a marker for hypertrophic cardiomyopathy) by ECG is limited by low sensitivity and specificity in children.

24-Hour Ambulatory Monitoring

This may be performed for patients with suspected arrhythmias as the cause of their syncope; however, studies have shown that only 13% of adults demonstrate arrhythmias as the cause of their syncope with this type of monitoring. Event recorder monitoring has been shown to have a slightly higher yield than 24-h ambulatory monitoring especially in patients with infrequent symptoms. Because of the low incidence of arrhythmias in the pediatric population, event monitoring is useful for select patients whose history or physical exam is suggestive of arrhythmias as a cause of their syncope.

Exercise Stress Testing

Patients whose primary symptoms of syncope occur either during exercise or immediately following exercise may benefit from formal exercise stress testing. Blood pressure and heart rate abnormalities as well as ECG signs of ischemia or arrhythmias can be determined. It should be noted that recent studies show that the majority of patients with syncope immediately following exercise have neurocardiogenic syncope rather than a cardiac etiology such as LV outflow tract obstruction, ischemia, or arrhythmias.

Echocardiogram

This procedure is performed if the patient has any abnormalities on cardiac exam or if there is a family history of congenital or acquired cardiac disease. It is used to assess for any cardiac structural anomalies and also to determine cardiac function either in the baseline state or with exercise.

Head-up Tilt Table Test

Tilt testing is performed to confirm the diagnosis of neurocardiogenic syncope or to assess the autonomic nervous system function. It is limited by variable sensitivity and specificity of the test and is complicated by the poor reproducibility of results. It is not considered the gold standard for diagnosing neurocardiogenic syncope but may be used in conjunction with the history, physical exam, and other tests mentioned.

Intracardiac Electrophysiology (EP) Study

Invasive evaluation with EP testing is usually reserved for patients who are highly suspected of having arrhythmias or conduction disturbances as the cause of their syncope. Intracardiac EP studies have been shown to have a low yield of positive results in patients with structurally normal hearts and normal cardiac function undergoing evaluation for syncope.

MANAGEMENT OF SYNCOPE

Neurocardiogenic Syncope

The management of neurocardiogenic syncope begins with patient education regarding the avoidance or minimization of the causes or triggers of symptoms. Several maneuvers may prevent the development of neurocardiogenic syncope. These include sitting or lying down once the patient feels any premonitory symptoms in an attempt to stop the reflex leading to syncope. Intermittent leg crossing promotes blood flow back to the heart and avoids venous pooling in the lower extremities. Other prophylactic measures include increasing total daily fluid intake and avoidance of a low-salt diet in hopes of maintaining an adequate intravascular volume. If these maneuvers are ineffective, then medications may be useful. Medical therapies are given below.

Florinef

Florinef is a mineralocorticoid used to expand plasma volume. In uncontrolled studies, it has been shown to result in 78% improvement of symptoms. It is often used as a first-line medication in patients with neurocardiogenic syncope.

Beta-Blockers

The acute and long-term benefits of the use of beta-blockers have been shown in multiple studies as well as in one randomized, placebo-controlled study. The mechanism of action is unknown, although it is thought that beta-blockers decrease or limit the force of contraction of the left ventricle, thus decreasing C-fiber activation and avoiding initiation of the reflex.

Midodrine

This is an alpha-1 agonist that increases peripheral vascular tone and decreases peripheral pooling of blood. The efficacy of midodrine for treatment of syncope and near-syncope has been shown in nonrandomized studies in children.

Sertraline

The use of serotonin uptake inhibitors such as sertraline was first shown to be effective in young patients resistant to other medical therapies, with up to 53% of patients responding to this medication; however, there have been reports of exacerbation of dizziness or syncope with the use of serotonin uptake inhibitors and the time to respond is longer because of the delayed time to action of these medications.

Pacemakers

The efficacy of pacemakers for prevention or decrease in frequency of syncope was demonstrated in the North American vasovagal pacemaker study in adults. The patients who benefited with this form of therapy were those found to have significant cardioinhibitory response on tilt table testing and who were resistant to other forms of medical therapy. The pacemakers used a feature called rate-drop response, which detects sudden drops in heart rate (as seen during a vasovagal episode) and responds by increasing the heart rate above the normal resting rate to counter the vasovagal reaction. This study demonstrated an 85–89% reduction of symptoms in previously refractory patients with syncope.

Disopyramide

This class IA antiarrhythmic medication has strong anticholinergic properties thought to be useful for the treatment of vasovagal syncope; however, disopyramide is poorly tolerated because of anticholinergic side effects of the medication. Furthermore, no clinical studies have shown any significant change in symptoms when disopyramide is compared to placebo.

Scopolamine

This anticholinergic agent was thought to be useful for the treatment of vasovagal syncope but again is poorly tolerated because of frequent side effects of urinary retention, dry mouth, constipation, nausea, or blurred vision. Also, there have been no studies to show any significant change in symptoms with scopolamine compared to placebo.

Cardiac Syncope

Cardiac etiologies of syncope are managed based on the underlying pathology and the frequency of symptoms. It is important to correlate the abnormal finding such as an arrhythmia with the episode of syncope before initiating therapy. Since this may be difficult in patients with life-threatening or infrequent symptoms, exercise stress testing or intracardiac EP testing is often used to assess the likelihood of the etiology of syncope and the risk for future events.

Noncardiac Syncope

Noncardiac etiologies of syncope are managed based on the etiology. Breath-holding spells are often managed conservatively with the knowledge that these will resolve within 1–2 years. Patients may, however, be at risk for later development of vasovagal syncope at older ages. Concomitant neurologic evaluation is often necessary in cases of atypical syncope or when seizures are the main symptom.

SUMMARY

Syncope in the pediatric population is predominantly a result of benign causes such as neurocardiogenic syncope and can be readily managed in most patients with simple maneuvers or medications. A thorough history and physical exam are essential to assess for the rare situation of syncope because of a potentially life-threatening cause. A 12-lead ECG, while acknowledging its limitations, is the most useful screening tool to assess for cardiac causes of syncope such as the long QT syndrome.

Suggested Readings

Connolly SJ, Sheldon R, Roberts RS, Gent M: The North American Vasovagal Pacemaker Study (VPS): A randomized trial of permanent cardiac pacing for the prevention of vasovagal syncope. *J Am Coll Cardiol* 33(1):16–20, 1999.

Lombroso CT, Lerman P: Breathholding spells (cyanotic and pallid infantile syncope). *Pediatrics* 39:563–581, 1967.

Tanel RE, Walsh EP: Syncope in the pediatric patient. *Cardiol Clin* 15(2):277–294, 1997.

Wolff GS, Young ML, Tamer DF: Syncope—diagnosis and management, in: Deal B, Wolff G, Gelband H (eds): *Current Concepts in Diagnosis and Management of Arrhythmias in Infants and Children.* Armonk, NY, Futura Publishing Co., pp. 223–240, 1998.

5

CYANOSIS

Peter Koenig

OVERVIEW OF CYANOSIS

Cyanosis is a bluish discoloration of the skin. In order to understand the medical implications of cyanosis, it may be best to ascertain all the determining factors (as trivial as they may be). Once the determining factors are recognized, a more appropriate differential diagnosis may be made, with an appreciation of false positives and false negatives in diagnosing pathology. The fact that a color is involved implies that there is a reflected color source, light, a light receptor, and a manner in which the light is analyzed. Although intuitive, dividing the components of cyanosis in this fashion allows each to be examined and its sources understood.

The first component, a color source, can be broken down into several subcomponents. The first is the actual source of the blue color, desaturated hemoglobin. It is reported that the clinically recognizable amount of desaturated hemoglobin is 5 g/dL. Less than this will not be noticeable. The fact that there is a minimal quantity of hemoglobin to create the appearance of cyanosis implies that no cyanosis will exist in the absence of hemoglobin. In other words, a severely anemic patient may be less noticeably cyanotic despite desaturation. In contrast to this, since there is always a small percentage of desaturated hemoglobin, cyanosis may be present in someone with a greater than the normal hemoglobin concentration (polycythemia). This will occur if the product of hemoglobin concentration and the percent desaturation is greater than 5 g/dL. Thus, false positives and negatives may occur with variations in hemoglobin concentration.

In order for the hemoglobin to cause a blue reflection, the reflected light must travel through layers of the skin. This implies that skin characteristics may influence the detection of cyanosis. Lightly pigmented or fair-skinned individuals are more likely to appear cyanotic than darkly pigmented individuals. In the latter, cyanosis may go unrecognized. Thus, false positives and negatives may occur with varying skin color.

The second component, light, is frequently taken for granted. The physical examination may frequently be performed with suboptimal lighting conditions such as a darkened room. This will lead to the underappreciation (false negative) of cyanosis. In a similar fashion, certain types of light such as fluorescent lighting (without a full spectrum of white light) may lead to the overappreciation of cyanosis (false positive). Ideally, white sunlight is best to assess for blue discoloration of a patient.

The next component in the recognition of cyanosis is the color receptor. In this case, it is the human eye and more specifically the cones in the retina, which are responsible for color reception. It is known that some individuals have a reduced sensitivity for color detection or color blindness. Thus, cyanosis may be underappreciated in these individuals.

The next component of cyanosis is the analysis of the sensed color. In this case, it is the human brain and implies cortical function and experience. As discussed above, 5 g/dL of desaturated hemoglobin is the usual amount to cause a bluish discoloration that we term cyanosis. In the presence of normal lighting conditions and normal color reception, it may still be possible for examiners to disagree on the presence of cyanosis. The 5 g/dL most likely represents a bell shaped curve which will reflect the differences in experience and thus perception of a blue color.

In summary, there are many factors that may influence the detection or perception of cyanosis. In the current era, it may be more useful to measure and diagnose oxyhemoglobin saturation rather than cyanosis. This would eliminate the bias of anemia/polycythemia, skin pigmentation, lighting conditions, color reception, and examiner experience. Since oxygen saturation is not yet a standard measurement in all patients (5th vital sign), the finding of cyanosis should lead to further investigation, the first being the assessment of saturation. Depending on these results, further evaluation may be indicated.

PULSOXIMETRY

Oxyhemoglobin saturation is calculated using spectrophotometry to measure light absorbance and the differences in it resulting from pulsatile arterial blood flow. The actual pulsoximeter sensor/probe is placed on a well-perfused portion of the body in which the blood flow is close to the surface of the skin such as the fingers, toes, or ears. Two wavelengths (600 nm [red] and 930 nm [infrared]) of light are transmitted through the skin and are differentially absorbed by oxyhemoglobin (which is red and absorbs infrared light) and deoxyhemoglobin (which is blue and absorbs red light). There is a photodetector on the other side of the light transmitter that receives and converts the transmitted light into electrical signals proportional to the absorbance. The signal is then sent to a microprocessor, which derives a saturation reading and sends an alarm if the saturation value is outside a range of preset limits. Pulsatile blood flow is required as each pulse results in a cycle of expanding and relaxing capillary beds. This cycle creates a variation in the path length of transmitted light. This allows the sensor to distinguish between pulsating (arterial) hemoglobin saturation and venous blood and surrounding tissue components because (1) there is no pulse from the surrounding tissue and (2) in the absence of motion, the pulse of venous blood flow is insignificant. The microprocessor compares the relationship of the absorbance values of pulsatile arterial blood with stored "normal" data from prior invasive studies in humans to calculate and display the oxygen saturation. One of the problems with these machines is motion artifact. This can be improved by synchronizing the absorbance measurements with the R wave on the ECG thus preventing motion artifact signals being mistaken for pulsatile flow. The machines may include memory to display trends, and may use algorithms in order to average data, which may also reduce the number of false values from artifactual waveforms. Additional features of pulsoximeters may include alarms, pulse rate, pulse amplitude bar graphs, error messages, and digital output which may be entered into patient monitors and databases. Advances in signal processing may continue to decrease the effect of motion and low perfusion states. Overall, clinical correlation as oversight is still required to recognize false readings. Once other factors are ascertained as noncontributory, the measurement is taken as accurate.

PERIPHERAL
VERSUS CENTRAL CYANOSIS

One important branch point in the evaluation of cyanosis is whether or not there is peripheral cyanosis versus central cyanosis. Peripheral (e.g., fingers, toes) cyanosis is seen in the less-well-perfused capillary beds, while central cyanosis (e.g., lips) is seen in well-perfused capillary beds. The former will be seen when there is sluggish blood flow in those vascular beds because of increased oxygen extraction. This will occur with vasoconstriction during shock (with all the causes associated with this) or with physiologic compensations such as heat conservation in a cold individual. Shock and hypothermia should be easily differentiated from one another by history and physical examination. Central cyanosis is owing to desaturated arterial blood with the differential diagnosis listed below.

THE CLINICAL IMPLICATIONS OF CYANOSIS OR DESATURATION

One of the common clinical questions, especially in patients with known diseases causing desaturation, is what the appropriate saturation should be. First, a brief review of oxygen physiology is in order. Oxygen is needed for aerobic metabolism (the tricarboxylic acid cycle or TCA cycle) which is required for generating the energy containing molecular ATP required to maintain life processes. This biochemical process occurs mainly in the mitochondrion of the cell. Oxygen diffuses across the cell membrane and into the mitochondrion where this can occur. Oxygen reaches cells via the vascular system and is mainly carried in red blood cells bound to hemoglobin. Very little is dissolved in the blood itself. Each volume of blood has a certain oxygen carrying capacity, which is the amount of dissolved blood plus the amount carried via hemoglobin. The latter is a product of the hemoglobin concentration and percent hemoglobin saturation. The cardiac system is responsible for maintaining an appropriate flow of oxygen carrying blood to the cells. The amount of oxygen delivered to the cell is thus a product of blood flow (cardiac output) and oxygen carrying capacity. Cellular oxygen-requiring metabolism is dependent on the latter oxygen delivery. Of note is that the delivery can be increased by increasing cardiac output, increasing hemoglobin concentration, or increasing the ability of hemoglobin to release the bound oxygen. (Oxygen delivery is minimally influenced by the amount of dissolved oxygen, though this may be important in

times of decreased reserve). The ability of hemoglobin to release oxygen is described by the hemoglobin dissociation curve. Release will be enhanced with acidosis, and in the presence of 2,3-diphosphoglycerate (an intermediary metabolite in glycolysis, which will be increased in the presence of low oxygen concentrations and a shift of metabolism from aerobic to anaerobic—lactate-producing—metabolism). If inadequate oxygen is released despite these compensations (in oxygen delivery or hemoglobin oxygen release), increased anaerobic metabolism and lactic acid production will occur. This will result in compensatory tachypnea to normalize blood pH.

In the neonate, hemoglobin oxygen dissociation is different than in children and adults in that there is a higher concentration of fetal hemoglobin. Fetal hemoglobin has a higher affinity for oxygen, meaning that it will be highly saturated, even in a low oxygen (fetal-like) environment. Thus, the neonate will be better able to tolerate low oxygen environments. Other compensations in the neonate also occur so that the neonate is able to handle lower oxygen saturations. In fact, tachypnea in a neonate with desaturation may not be because of the desaturation. Instead, it may be because of decreased lung compliance or difficulty in ventilation if there is associated lung disease.

Given this background in oxygen metabolism and physiology, the question again becomes what an appropriate oxygen saturation should be. This can be subdivided into four categories: (1) desired oxygen saturation, (2) expected oxygen saturation, (3) acceptable oxygen saturation or a level of saturation that is tolerated, and (4) unacceptable oxygen saturation. The first and last categories are easily defined. The desired oxygen saturation (or content) is always normal. An oxygen saturation that is unacceptable is that which causes lactic acidosis or other derangements and will lead to death. The latter can be clinically seen with tachypnea and other signs of shock, as well as the abnormal direct measurement of an arterial blood gas (ABG). Unacceptable oxygen saturations are usually in the range of 30–40% but can vary with clinical scenarios and are somewhat dependent on the accuracy of pulsoximeters when measuring low oxygen saturations.

Evaluation of the patient should occur when there is a difference between the measured oxygen saturation and the expected oxygen saturation. (Rapid assessment and resuscitation should occur if the saturation is accurately measured as incompatible with life.) Evaluation should proceed as discussed below and outlined in Figure 5-1. After evaluation, a conclusion should be reached as to the cause of the discrepancy between the measured and expected oxygen saturation. If there is a pulmonary or hematologic explanation, the disorder is appropriately treated. This is because the expected oxygen saturation (although lower than normal) is not acceptable. In these cases, unless there is an untreatable disease, the desired (and only acceptable) saturation is normal. In the case of cyanotic heart disease, the desired saturation (normal) cannot be reached without surgery (if at all), and a decision is made whether or not the measured and expected (based on underlying physiology) oxygen saturation is acceptable. If acceptable, then no further therapy is instituted. If unacceptable, or felt to be unacceptable in the near future (i.e., ductal-dependent cyanotic heart lesion), interventions are performed in order to make the oxygen normal or acceptable.

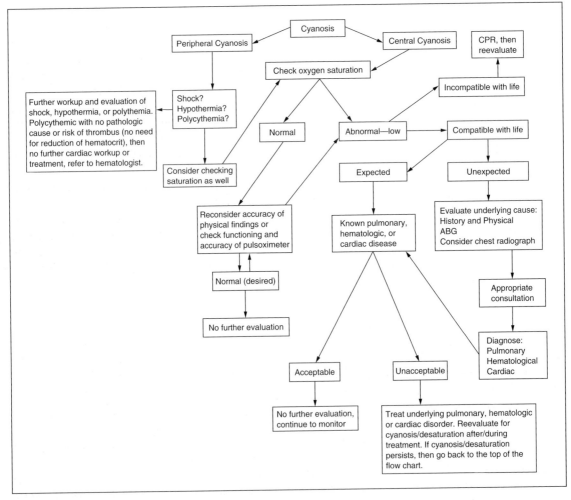

FIGURE 5 - 1

FLOW DIAGRAM IN THE EVALUATION OF CYANOSIS

DIFFERENTIAL DIAGNOSIS OF DESATURATION—APPROACH TO WORKUP

The basic evaluation of cyanosis is outlined in Figure 5-1. The three major organ categories of oxy-hemoglobin desaturation are hematological, cardiac, and pulmonary. Physiologically, the major processes can be grouped into those with hypoventilation, ventilation/perfusion (V/Q) mismatching or localized hypoventilation, pulmonary diffusion abnormalities, and nonpulmonary right-to-left shunting. The first three physiologic categories fit into the pulmonary differential diagnoses, and the fourth fits into the cardiac and hematologic differential diagnoses. These three major organ systems can be rapidly evaluated with a combination of history, physical examination, and a few laboratory tests.

The history and physical examination may lead to the suspicion of a pulmonary cause of cyanosis if there is respiratory distress, tachypnea, hyper or hypoventilation, abnormal breath sounds, and the like. A cardiac cause may be suspected if there are historical and physical features of a critical (ductal dependent) heart lesion, such as desaturation, shock, respiratory distress, or a pathologic murmur; however, pathologic murmurs are not frequently a major presenting feature of critical or cyanotic heart disease. Both cardiac and hematologic causes of desaturation tend to be diagnoses of exclusion.

A chest radiograph may give further information on the possibility of a pulmonary cause or lead to suspicion of a cardiac cause. An ABG may lead to a suspicion of a hemoglobinopathy in the presence of a normal PO_2 with a low measured saturation (i.e., if the saturation is not calculated based on the PO_2). The latter may be seen with methemoglobinemia. In addition, an ABG during a hyperoxia test may help distinguish between the obligatory right-to-left shunt of a cyanotic heart defect and a diffusion abnormality with lung disease. A hyperoxia test is performed by obtaining an ABG after breathing 100% FiO_2 for 5–10 min, and comparing the ABG with the baseline ABG. With an oxygen diffusion problem (pulmonary disease), the PO_2 will typically rise above 300 mmHg, which will not occur with an obligatory intracardiac right-to-left shunt; however, in some intracardiac lesions such as total anomalous pulmonary venous connection, the PO_2 may increase substantially (to 150 mmHg). Thus, monitoring saturations alone during the hyperoxia test is insufficient. If the saturation does not increase (above 90%) with the hyperoxia test, then the follow-up ABG will add little additional information. Of note during the hyperoxia test: careful monitoring is required as the oxygen may stimulate ductal closure, or cause increased systemic steal in the case of a ductal-dependent systemic circulation. In both cases, clinical deterioration and lactic acidosis may occur.

After the history and physical examination, and these simple lab tests, the basic underlying cause of cyanosis or desaturation can usually be deduced; however, this is not absolute and diagnoses such as persistent fetal circulation (persistent pulmonary hypertension of the newborn (PPHN)), hyaline membrane disease or pneumonitis, or pulmonary arteriovenous malformations may still be confused with an underlying congenital heart defect. Clinical behavior (i.e., improvement of desaturation and other parameters with hyperventilation in the case of PPHN) may help deduce the cause of desaturation. Otherwise, the general cause (via exclusion) of the desaturation is most likely an underlying congenital heart defect with the differential diagnosis as outlined in the chapter on right-to-left shunts. The specific diagnosis is made with a combination of clinical examination and laboratory studies of which the most useful is an echocardiogram. The differential diagnosis of cyanotic heart disease is discussed in the chapter on right-to-left shunting.

Suggested Readings

Green M: *Pediatric diagnosis, Interpretation of Symptoms and Signs in Different Age Periods*, 4th ed. Philadelphia, PA, WB Saunders, 1986.

Garson A, Bricker JT, Fisher DJ, Neish SR: *The Science and Practice of Pediatric Cardiology*, 2nd ed. Baltimore, MD, Williams and Wilkins, 1998.

Gessner IH, Victoria BE: *Pediatric cardiology. A Problem-Based Approach*. Philadelphia, PA, WB Saunders, 1993.

Szocik J, Barker S, Tremper KK: *Fundamental Principals of Monitoring*, in: Miller R (ed): *Anesthesia*, 5th ed. New York, NY, Elsevier, Chap. 28, pp. 1073–1075, 2000.

6

DYSPNEA

David J. Waight

INTRODUCTION

Dyspnea is defined as "shortness of breath, a subjective difficulty or distress in breathing usually associated with serious disease of the heart or lungs and occurring in health during intense physical exertion or at high altitude." Dyspnea is often referred to as shortness of breath. Dyspnea is a complaint or a symptom that must be voiced by the patient. Common complaints include "cannot get enough air," "trouble breathing," "chest tightness," and "breathless." All of these terms are efforts of the patient to describe unpleasant or uncomfortable breathing. This is a perception that the patient has, that is fairly easy to discern for older children and adults, but is very difficult for younger children to express properly and is impossible for very small children and infants to convey.

The term *dyspnea* cannot be properly applied to infants and small children, but the obvious difficulty in breathing and/or respiratory distress that is often described by physicians, nurses, or other examiners is essentially equivalent to the adult complaint of dyspnea. Signs that suggest dyspnea include a fast respiratory rate, labored breathing, intercostal, suprasternal or subcostal retractions, nasal flaring, and head bobbing with each breath. Older patients may also have difficulty speaking as

they are struggling to catch their breath. Any of these findings on exam may lead to a medical description of dyspnea. This has also been described as "increased work of breathing."

A person's perception of their own breathing is a result of the feedback mechanism of the mechanical work of breathing and the physiologic results of that respiratory effort. The feedback from oxygen saturation and carbon dioxide concentration through chemoreceptors in the body automatically controls respiratory rate and depth of respiration. There is further feedback of the mechanical work of breathing by receptors in the airways, lungs, and chest wall. When the feedback of the mechanical work of breathing does not correlate with the feedback from the chemoreceptors, the sensation of dyspnea may be described. The patient feels that respiratory effort is out of proportion to the resulting level of ventilation, leading to the complaint of dyspnea, or shortness of breath.

It is important to differentiate dyspnea from tachypnea, or rapid breathing. Tachypnea is the normal physiologic result of increasing respiratory demand associated with any increased metabolic state, such as exercise or fever. Tachypnea is simply a more rapid than normal rate of breathing without any respiratory distress or perceived increased respiratory effort. In the field of pediatric cardiology, there are many forms of cyanotic heart disease that are described elsewhere in this book. Many infants who have cyanotic heart disease have tachypnea associated with their cyanosis but no respiratory distress and no observed signs consistent with dyspnea. This hyperventilation is described as "comfortable tachypnea" and can be a clinical marker for congenital heart disease in cyanotic infants. These infants do not have an elevated carbon dioxide level and usually have a normal pH. They have a lower oxygen saturation that is similar to the physiologic desaturation present in fetal life and this does not lead to distress. These infants also have normal gas exchange, no pulmonary edema, normal airways, and normal lung parenchyma.

THE PATHOPHYSIOLOGY OF DYSPNEA

The original stimulus that often causes a patient to experience dyspnea is either a decreased level of oxygen in the blood, known as hypoxia, or an increased level of carbon dioxide within the blood stream, which is known as hypercapnia. Both of these abnormalities chemically induce an increase in respiratory motor activity. If the hypoxia or hypercapnia is not corrected by the increased respiratory motor activity, there will be a mismatch between the central respiratory motor activity stimulation from the incoming signals from sensors in the airway, lungs and chest wall (that sense the rate and depth of respiration), and the incoming chemoreceptor signals. This mismatch can induce the symptom of dyspnea. There are many causes of both hypoxia and hypercapnia (Table 6-1). The differential diagnosis of hypoxia/cyanosis is included in Chapters 5 and 11. A complete differential of hypercapnia is beyond the scope of this chapter, but includes the general processes of poor gas exchange in the lungs and increased production of carbon dioxide owing to metabolic acidosis.

The Differential Diagnosis of Dyspnea Based on Underlying Pathophysiology

The pathophysiology of dyspnea can be divided into four general categories that can produce hypoxia and/or hypercapnia. These categories physiologically range from normal, to environmental abnormalities,

TABLE 6-1

PATHOPHYSIOLOGIC CONSIDERATIONS WHEN EVALUATING CARDIOPULMONARY FUNCTION

Hypoxia
a. Hypoventilation
b. Oxygen diffusion abnormalities
c. Ventilation-perfusion mismatch
d. Right-to-left shunting

Hypercapnia
Increased CO_2 Production
a. Metabolic acidosis—usually initially compensated by increased ventilation.
  Metabolic derangements resulting in increased acid production (e.g., DKA), cardiogenic shock
b. Decreased gas exchange
  Hypoventilation
    Decreased rate of ventilation
    Decreased volume of ventilation
      Obstruction
      Decreased depth of ventilation
      Restrictive lung disease
  Ventilation-perfusion mismatch—Hypoxia is usually more pronounced.

to mechanical air exchange, to the alveolar/capillary interface.

Category I is increased ventilatory demand secondary to exercise. This is a normal physiologic response and is generally not perceived as abnormal by the exercising individual. At very high levels of activity, people experience shortness of breath, but do not describe it as an abnormal or uncomfortable phenomenon. This may not produce either hypoxia or hypercapnia, but the increased work of breathing generates respiratory muscle fatigue.

Category II is hypoxia secondary to a decreased partial pressure of oxygen in the ambient air. The decreased oxygen is noted at increasing altitude and is the reason many people experience some shortness of breath, or dyspnea, when traveling to a mountainous area or exercising at altitude. This is a normal physiologic response but will be perceived as increased work of breathing and may be described as dyspnea by the individual. When significant symptoms are present at rest, the individual likely has significant pulmonary edema that may progress to life-threatening high altitude pulmonary edema (HAPE) if they do not descend to a lower altitude with increased partial pressure of oxygen. This is commonly referred to as HAPE and is a frequent problem for alpine trekkers or climbers. Hypercapnia does not occur because of the increased diffusion capacity of carbon dioxide compared to the diffusion capacity of oxygen.

Category III is respiratory muscle disease or dysfunction, which produces hypoventilation and results in hypoxia and hypercapnia (neuro/mechanical pulmonary disease). This includes severe kyphoscoliosis, which is a severe deformity of the chest wall that is likely to cause significant dyspnea. Respiratory muscle disease is often a late finding of other muscle disease that generally presents with peripheral weakness with forms of muscular dystrophy. In the field of congenital heart disease, the most common respiratory muscle disease is an acute diaphragm paralysis that is a known complication of thoracic surgery. This can present as failure to progress to extubatable settings in a patient postcardiothoracic surgery or noted postextubation with significant respiratory distress. This is often easily diagnosed with a simple chest x-ray, which demonstrates one diaphragm significantly higher than the other. Further evaluation can be performed with ultrasound to observe the motion of the diaphragm during the normal respiratory cycle. Hypoventilation owing to suppressed respiratory stimulation or abnormal control may be a result of sedation, anesthesia, or neurologic disease.

Within Category III are mechanisms of abnormal ventilatory impedance that are frequently noted in children with asthma or reactive airway disease. A similar phenomenon is found in older adults with chronic obstructive pulmonary disease. Other diseases of the parenchyma of the lung can present with similar findings and the feeling of dyspnea. Pulmonary fibrosis secondary to frequent pulmonary parenchymal infections or radiation damage of the lungs may also present with dyspnea. These patients also have elements of ventilation/perfusion mismatch that contribute to hypoxia and hypercapnia.

Category IV is a decrease in effective gas exchange secondary to a large dead space in the airways or decreased gas diffusion producing ventilation/perfusion mismatch. Dead space is that quantity of air that does not provide effective ventilation to the alveoli but is involved in passage of air through the upper airways, bronchi, and any sections of the lung that do not have normal perfusion or gas exchange. This enlarged dead space is commonly secondary to parenchymal lung disease or pulmonary vascular disease. It is associated with pulmonary congestion resulting from infections including bronchitis or pneumonia. The increased airway secretions associated with infection also increase the effective dead space.

Pulmonary congestion with pulmonary edema and resultant decreased gas diffusion is often a result of cardiac disease. It can also occur because of recurrent pulmonary embolism that may be associated with hypercoagulable states or low flow systems such as the Fontan circulation, which is a common palliation for patients with single ventricle physiology. In addition to the above, intrapulmonary right-to-left shunts owing to pulmonary arteriovenous malformations, as well as intracardiac right-to-left shunts are included in Category IV. *Congenital heart disease and acquired cardiac dysfunction are included in Category IV.*

The two primary causes of dyspnea and respiratory distress in the field of pediatric cardiology are right-to-left shunts and lung disease secondary to heart disease. Right-to-left shunts and the resultant hypoxia are discussed elsewhere in this book. Lung disease most commonly results from the pathophysiologic mechanism of pulmonary edema. Pulmonary edema is a secondary response to increasing pulmonary capillary pressure. This most commonly occurs with increased left atrial pressure. Increased left atrial pressure can be the result of mitral stenosis, left ventricular dysfunction, or a significantly increased left-sided volume load secondary to left-to-right shunting. Large shunts cause a greatly increased pulmonary blood flow and increased pulmonary venous return leading to increased left atrial pressure. Increased pulmonary capillary pressure can occur without increased left atrial pressure if there are obstructed pulmonary veins. Pulmonary venous obstruction may also lead to isolated increased pulmonary venous pressure and pulmonary edema.

From the causes noted above, the end result is an increased pulmonary venous pressure and resultant increased capillary pressure. This increased pulmonary venous pressure leads to engorgement of the pulmonary vasculature, which decreases lung compliance and increases the resistance in the small airways. This can lead to hyperexpansion of the lungs and flattened diaphragms. There is also an increase in the lymphatic flow within the lungs, which works to maintain a constant pulmonary extravascular fluid volume. In the early stages, there may be mild tachypnea but no significant respiratory distress. If

the heart disease is uncorrected, there will be a further increase in intravascular pressure with a net increase in extravascular fluid that will exceed the ability of the lymphatic system to drain the fluid and lead to edema of the alveolar walls. This will result in increasing tachypnea with a decreasing PO_2 and an initial unchanged (later increasing) PCO_2. The chest radiograph may correlate with these findings with what is described as Kerley B lines. This is still an early stage with interstitial edema. If there is no change in the cardiac physiology, the increasing edema will progress to alveolar

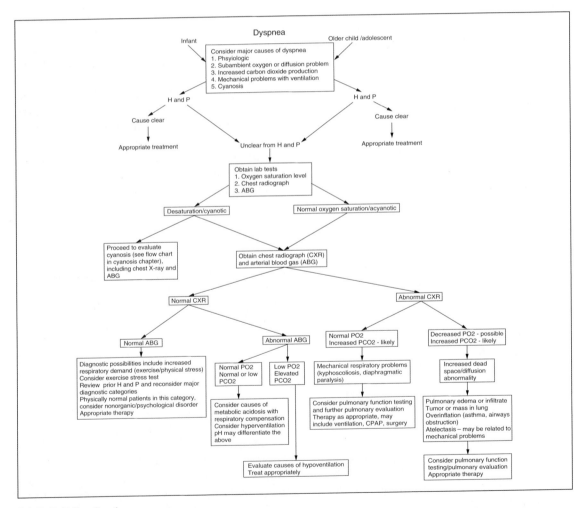

FIGURE 6-1

EVALUATION OF DYSPNEA

edema. At this time, the patient will have tachypnea and respiratory distress with abnormal physical findings including rales (felt to be due to alveolar fluid). The latter findings are not typically seen in infants and small children. The chest radiograph will now demonstrate a diffuse haziness of the lung fields consistent with significant pulmonary alveolar edema. Hyperexpansion and flattened diaphragms may also be noted (owing to decreased lung compliance). Gas exchange is compromised with increasing hypoxia and hypercapnia. Most forms of cardiac disease do not progress to severe life-threatening respiratory distress unless ignored or unrecognized for a prolonged time. Exceptions to this generalization include acutely obstructed pulmonary venous return or acute left ventricular dysfunction that can occur with severe myocarditis or myocardial infarction.

Dyspnea not because of pulmonary edema may also be part of the presentation of severe cardiac disease. Respiratory distress and tachypnea may also be seen with severe cardiac dysfunction and resultant circulatory collapse and shock. This is a result of metabolic acidosis from poor cardiac output. Significant cyanosis may progress beyond comfortable tachypnea and also lead to dyspnea and respiratory distress as the degree of cyanosis progresses and metabolic acidosis becomes severe.

EVALUATION OF DYSPNEA

Preliminary testing of patients with respiratory distress or dyspnea should include a complete history and physical examination with particular emphasis on the cardiac, pulmonary, and neuromuscular systems (Figure 6-1). Additional testing usually includes a chest radiograph and may include lung function testing. Spirometry and lung volume measurements may be important to diagnose obstructive airway problems, restrictive pulmonary disease, increased dead space, and parenchymal disease. The addition of bronchodilators with this testing can help to diagnose reactive airway disease. Arterial blood gas analysis may also be helpful by determining the partial pressure of oxygen and carbon dioxide to determine if the patient has significant hypoxia, hypercapnia, or metabolic acidosis (accompanying major categories in Table 6-2). Exercise stress testing may demonstrate dysnpea associated with exercise-related hypoxia and hypercapnia.

TABLE 6-2

EVALUATION OF DYSPNEA

Category	Chest Radiograph (CXR)	Lung Function Tests	Blood Gas	Exercise Test
I. Increased ventilatory demand	Normal	Normal	Normal	Normal
II. Decreased FiO_2 at altitude	Pulmonary edema	Normal—after recovery	Decreased PO_2 ±Decreased PCO_2	Normal—after recovery
III. Respiratory muscle disease	Normal ±Kyphoscoliosis ±Elevated diaphragm	±Decreased tidal volume ±Increased functional residual volume	±Increased PCO_2 Normal PO_2	Decreased duration
IV. Increased dead space-pulmonary edema	±Pulmonary edema ±Infiltrate ±Overinflation	Increased dead space ±Decreased forced expiratory volume in 1 second (FEV1)	±Increased PCO_2 ±Decreased PO_2	Decreased duration ±Desaturation

Suggested Readings

American Thoracic Society: Dyspnea. Mechanisms, assessment, and management: a consensus statement. *Am J Respir Crit Care Med* 159(1):321–340, 1999.

Ingram RH, Braunwald E: Dyspnea and pulmonary edema. *Harrison's Principles of Internal Medicine*, 11th ed. New York, NY, McGraw-Hill, 1987.

Stedman's Medical Dictionary, 24th ed. Baltimore, MD, Williams & Wilkins, 1982.

Scano G, Ambrosino N: Pathophysiology of dyspnea. *Lung* 180(3):131–148, 2002.

7

EXERCISE INTOLERANCE

Peter Koenig*

INTRODUCTION

Exercise intolerance is a relatively frequent complaint in the pediatric age group. It is a broad term that encompasses both pathologic and benign physiologic conditions. To the pediatric cardiologist, the term denotes the possibility of heart disease, since exercise is a nonpharmacologic stress on the cardiovascular system. Exercise can be thought of as any physical exertion beyond the resting state. In infants, crying or feeding is exertion. In older infants, exertion is in the form of crawling, standing, and walking. In children and adolescents, exertion is in the form of more usual types of exercise such as running and other sports.

DIFFERENTIAL DIAGNOSIS OF EXERCISE INTOLERANCE BASED ON THE UNDERLYING PATHOPHYSIOLOGY

In order to understand the causes of exercise intolerance, it may be easiest to divide this symptom into components. In order to exercise, the following organ systems are required: the nervous, musculoskeletal, hematologic, pulmonary, and cardiovascular systems. Other organ systems, such as the renal and endocrine systems, are required to a lesser

extent and participate mainly via their affects on the main organ systems noted above. Abnormalities involving these latter organ systems usually present with other symptoms, although fatigue can be one of them. The main organ systems involved in exercise may be further subdivided.

The central nervous system obviously plays an important role in exercise. Although a discussion of the neuroanatomic circuitry involved in voluntary movement is beyond the scope of this chapter, a few important concepts are worth mentioning. Cortical output is required to initiate voluntary actions, while the basal ganglia and cerebellum help to coordinate these movements. Normal function of the spinal cord, peripheral nervous system, and neuromuscular junction is required to deliver the electric output to the muscles. In addition, the limbic system plays a role in motor control. The emotional state of the individual influences overall somatic motor control, as a lack of motivation or interest may result in complaints of fatigue even though the capability of exercise remains intact. The limbic system may also influence respiration and swallowing. Finally, the autonomic nervous system helps to regulate the cardiovascular response to exercise. For example, withdrawal of parasympathetic activity during the

*The author gratefully acknowledges the contributions of Charles Marcuccilli to portions of this chapter.

early stages of the exercise state results in an increased heart rate, while increased sympathetic outflow may be responsible for further increases in heart rate with continued exercise. Derangements in any of these systems may result in an inability to exercise, hence, exercise intolerance; however, unlike cardiovascular derangements, the history and physical examination (i.e., constant weakness) will suggest that the intolerance results from the *inability to begin to exercise* rather than an inability to reach higher levels of exertion. It is important to note that neurologic disorders that present with fluctuating muscle weakness, such as myasthenia gravis, Lambert-Eaton syndrome, and periodic paralysis may be exacerbated by exercise leading to the diagnosis. Confirmation of the diagnosis for these conditions may be aided by electrophysiologic, serologic, and genetic studies. Hence, in most cases, the clinical history and physical examination should raise suspicion of a neurologic disorder.

The next organ system involved is the musculoskeletal system. An obvious gross skeletal abnormality (e.g., limb abnormality) will clearly result in an inability to exercise. This inability will be at the onset of exercise and not necessarily related to the amount of physical exertion. In a similar fashion, a gross muscle abnormality (e.g., traumatic injury) will result in an inability to exercise normally from the onset. Abnormalities of the muscle tissue itself (myocyte abnormalities—myopathies) may be manifest by the inability to engage in increasing amounts of physical exertion. Physical examination may reveal weakness or hypotonia; however, the findings may be subtle, with only complaints of difficulty with exertion. The complaints may be more of muscle fatigue rather than overall fatigue, which may include shortness of breath. A myopathy requires differentiation from a lack of physical fitness.

Physical fitness consists of improvements in cardiac, pulmonary and muscular function on a gross and cellular level. Grossly, there is muscular hypertrophy and increased lung capacity. On a cellular level are increased numbers of mitochondrion, an adaptive change to make the cell more efficient. The findings to differentiate a myopathy from poor muscular fitness are given in Table 7-1.

The next organ involved in exercise is the hematologic system. In order for muscles to function

TABLE 7-1

FEATURES TO SUGGEST A MYOPATHY RATHER THAN POOR PHYSICAL FITNESS

History
1. History of fatigue of muscles usually not fatigued
2. Fatigability with activities of daily living
3. Dyspnea to suggest respiratory muscle weakness
4. Muscle pain (to suggest inflammation)
5. Lack of improvement or worsening with an exercise program

Physical Examination
1. Abnormal neuromuscular examination in general
2. Opthalmoplegia
3. Hypotonia
4. Fasciculations
5. Abnormal reflexes

Laboratory Testing
1. Abnormal muscle enzymes
2. Abnormal invasive studies: Electromyography (EMG), muscle biopsy

efficiently, there needs to be adequate oxygen delivery. This is directly proportional to the hematocrit. Lack of hemoglobin, or abnormalities causing an inability of the hemoglobin to deliver oxygen, will result in exercise intolerance and fatigue. The history may reveal a prior diagnosis of a hemoglobinopathy, or a predisposition for anemia (lack of iron supplementation, heavy menstrual bleeding, recent blood loss). Historical features of hemolysis should be sought in the review of systems (jaundice, abnormal urine color). With a significant hemoglobinopathy or anemia, fatigue will be present at rest. With less severe abnormalities, symptoms may be present only with exercise. Physical findings may be subtle and include pallor with anemia or cyanosis with methemoglobinemia. Laboratory testing is diagnostic.

The next organ system involved with exercise is the pulmonary system. In order to exercise, normal pulmonary function is required to supply muscles with oxygen, and eliminate accumulating carbon dioxide. This includes gross mechanical components (the thoracic wall, muscles of ventilation such as the diaphragm and intercostal muscles, lungs, and large and small airways). Abnormal function or lack of one of these may result in decreased ventilation/oxygenation via hypoventilation or ventilation/perfusion mismatch. There are neural and muscular components involved; thus neuromuscular diseases may also affect pulmonary function. In addition to gross mechanical components, cellular gas exchange at the alveolar level is required. Thus, pneumonia or infiltration of the lungs may lead to decreased oxygen diffusion and cyanosis. Symptoms related to the lungs such as shortness of breath, coughing, wheezing, or cyanosis should be sought after. Greater complaints—shortness of breath greater than actual fatigue with exercise—should increase the suspicion of a primary pulmonary abnormality.

The last organ system in the list of major systems involved in exercise is the cardiovascular system. In order to deliver oxygen and eliminate carbon dioxide, a pump is needed as well as vessels to deliver blood and oxygen to the muscles and allow carbon dioxide to be delivered to the lungs for elimination. In order for this to occur, the vascular system needs to be intact with proper vascular tone in order to maintain pressure. There should be no sources of runoff such as a vascular malformation, which will steal from the systemic cardiac output. In addition to the vascular system, a pump is required. Components of the pump include heart rate, volume of blood in the heart, and contractility. The pump is influenced by afterload, which is partly determined by vascular tone. The volume of blood in the heart (preload), myocyte function (contractility), and afterload determine the volume of blood the heart ejects or stroke volume. The stroke volume multiplied by the heart rate or beats per minute determines the total cardiac output per minute. There are mechanical (based on underlying anatomy and muscle function) and electrical components of the heart, which can influence preload, contractility and afterload and thus the net function or cardiac output.

A slow heart rate may reach limits in which the stroke volume may not be increased enough to maintain cardiac output. In contrast, a very elevated heart rate may not allow enough time for the heart to fill (decreased preload) to generate an adequate stroke volume. Etiologies of bradycardia to consider in exercise intolerance include drugs, injury to the sinus node, and injury to the arterial-venous (AV) node (resulting in a slow junctional or ventricular escape rhythm). These etiologies can be obtained as part of the medical history. The nature of the bradycardia and rhythm disturbance can be ascertained with an electrocardiogram (ECG) or similar electrophysiologic study.

Mechanical heart dysfunction can be a result of anatomic abnormalities or muscle dysfunction. Both of these can influence one another (e.g., a cardiomyopathy causes cardiac dilation which causes valvar regurgitation, or valve stenosis or regurgitation causes abnormal loading conditions and long-term changes in cardiac muscle). There are primary cardiac muscle diseases (e.g., familial dilated or hypertrophic cardiomyopthy, restrictive cardiomyopathy) and secondary cardiac muscle diseases (e.g., hypertensive hypertrophic cardiomyopathy, dilated cardiomyopathy owing to renal, vascular diseases, drugs, infections or arrhythmias). The cardiomyopathies have a component of diastolic and systolic dysfunction, with one usually being predominant. The end result is the inability of the heart to meet the demands of the body (heart failure). This is a dynamic relation between the severity of the myopathy and the intensity of the demand. Theoretically, a normal heart can be made to "fail" if the demands (exercise) are great enough. Usually, a normal person will recognize personal limitations and stop exercising before this happens. A person with a cardiomyopathy will usually not be able to exercise to the same extent as a normal person, hence, complaints of exercise intolerance. If there is pulmonary edema associated with the cardiomyopathy, shortness of breath may be the first symptom during exercise rather than decreased duration. Since exercise requires increasing stroke volume (via increasing contractility and heart rate, and to an extent preload), a person with a cardiomyopathy will not be able to increase cardiac contractility normally, and the increased preload will result in an increased left ventricular diastolic pressure transmitted to the lungs, causing pulmonary edema. If diastolic dysfunction is the primary problem, left atrial pressures will rise to a greater extent and pulmonary edema will occur earlier than in a patient with primarily systolic dysfunction.

Anatomic abnormalities can be subdivided into those that cause cyanosis or desaturation, and those that have no desaturation (unless pulmonary edema occurs). The latter can be further subdivided into those that cause pressure loading of the heart and those that cause volume loading of the heart. Volume loading can be a result of regurgitation or a shunt. With lesions that cause desaturation, the level of oxygenation and the ability of the heart to increase it are the determining factors of how much exercise is tolerated. The degree of exercise intolerance is a significant determinant of the timing of cardiac interventions to increase oxygen saturation. With lesions that cause pressure loading (stenosis, coarctation of the aorta), the heart is usually able to adequately increase the end-systolic pressure to overcome the obstruction at the expense of increasing end-diastolic pressures and compensatory hypertrophy. As long as the myocytes are not injured (e.g., fibrosis) cardiac function will be near normal and exercise intolerance may not be present. As end-diastolic pressures increase further, pulmonary edema and shortness of breath with exercise may occur. With long-standing pressure overload, myocardial injury and dysfunction may occur with accompanying signs and symptoms of heart failure (systolic and diastolic), including exercise intolerance. Volume loading does not immediately cause exercise intolerance unless there is systemic (e.g., arteriovenous malformation) or

TABLE 7-3

DIFFERENTIAL DIAGNOSIS OF EXERCISE INTOLERANCE

CNS (pathology vs. motivational)
Musculoskeletal (primary muscle or skeletal disorder vs. poor physical fitness)
Hematologic (anemia, hemoglobinopathy)
Pulmonary (parenchymal or airway diseases, mechanical because of thoracic, muscle, or CNS problem)
Cardiac
- Electrical
  - Bradyarrhythmias
  - Tachyarrhythmias
- Mechanical
  - Anatomic
    Cyanotic
    Acyanotic
      Pressure loading
      Volume loading
        Regurgitant lesions
        Shunts
  - Muscle
    Primary
    Secondary
Other organ system abnormality (renal failure, hypothyroidism, etc.).

myocardial steal (e.g., aortic valve regurgitation). The latter may cause ischemia of the heart via decreased coronary artery perfusion at a time of increased myocardial demand because of volume loading. The ischemia will lead to decreased myocardial performance. With volume loading, there will be an increased ventricular end-diastolic pressure, which is minimal in a normal heart. Normal ventricles can accommodate increases in volume and deliver increased output during exercise with minimal ill effect unless the volume loading is severe. In abnormal hearts, or with severe volume loading, the increase in end-diastolic volume may lead to pulmonary edema and shortness of breath with exercise as a first symptom. With long-standing volume overload, myocyte dysfunction and decreased

TABLE 7-2

NYHA CLASSIFICATION OF HEART FAILURE

Grade 1: No limitations of physical activity—no exercise intolerance with normal activities
Grade 2: Slight limitations of physical activity—fatigue with ordinary activities
Grade 3: Marked limitations of physical activity—Comfortable at rest, fatigue with less than ordinary activities
Grade 4: Inability to carry on any physical activity without symptoms. In bed

contractility may occur, with signs and symptoms of heart failure.

For all the cardiac lesions, there is a classification of heart failure known as the New York Heart Association (NYHA) classification, shown in Table 7-2. This emphasizes the dynamic nature of heart failure. Exercise intolerance is implied. A summary of the differential diagnosis of exercise intolerance is given in Table 7-3.

WORKUP/EVALUATION OF EXERCISE INTOLERANCE

The evaluation of exercise intolerance begins with a history. Primary symptoms such as shortness of breath may prompt evaluation in the pulmonary pathway. A complaint of constant fatigue may lead to the possible diagnosis of a motivational problem, myopathy, or anemia. Palpitations, lightheadedness, or syncope may lead to consideration of an arrhythmia as a primary problem. The physical examination should further differentiate the major organ systems, usually to one or two major categories. Simple testing such as a CBC, chest radiograph, and ECG (as indicated by the history and physical) may further narrow the possibilities. Once narrowed, consultation with a pediatric neurologist, hematologist, or cardiologist may be the most cost-effective next step. Figure 7-1 shows a flow diagram of the workup of exercise intolerance.

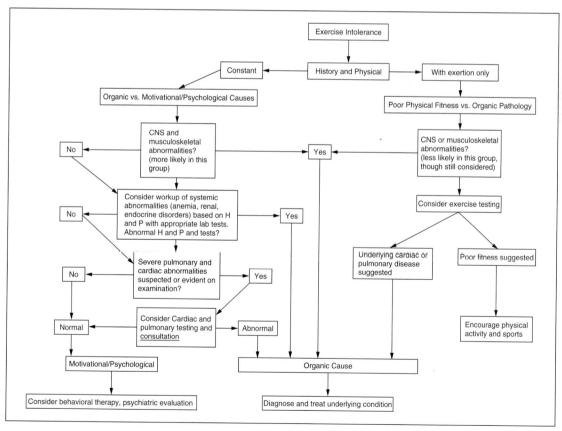

FIGURE 7-1

EXERCISE INTOLERANCE

CONTROVERSIES
IN THE EVALUATION
OF EXERCISE INTOLERANCE

There are few, if any, controversies in the evaluation of exercise intolerance. The timing of further testing is not clear, though an exercise test may help differentiate poor motivation from poor physical fitness or myocardial dysfunction. The latter may disclose exercise-induced asthma. An echocardiogram is diagnostic for cardiomyopathies, though it should not be a first screening test because of the expense. The ECG is usually abnormal in patients with cardiomyopathy.

Suggested Readings

Allen HD, Gutgesell HP, Clark EB, Driscoll DJ: *Moss and Adams' Heart Disease in Infants, Children and Adolescents Including the Fetus and Young Adult*, 6th ed. Philadelphia, PA, Lippincott Williams & Wilkins, 2001.

Garson A, Bricker JT, Fisher DJ, Neish SR: *The Science and Practice of Pediatric Cardiology*, 2nd ed. Baltimore, MD, Williams & Wilkins, 1998.

Rowland TW: *Pediatric Laboratory Exercise Testing. Clinical Guidelines*. Champaign, IL, Human Kinetics, 1993.

Wasserman K. Hansen JE, Sue DY, Casaburi R, Whipp BJ: *Principles of Exercise Testing and Interpretation*, 3rd ed. Philadelphia, PA, Lippincott Williams & Wilkins, 1999.

8

CARDIOGENIC SHOCK

Joel T. Hardin

INTRODUCTION

Shock represents a clinical and physiologic state of inadequate tissue oxygen and metabolic substrate delivery leading to cellular hypoxia, anaerobic metabolism, tissue acidosis, and organ failure. No single clinical finding defines shock. Instead one must integrate multiple elements of history, examination, laboratory results, and frequent clinical reassessments in order to recognize and manage shock effectively. If not recognized and subsequently treated, shock ultimately results in cardiopulmonary failure and either immediate or delayed death. As shown in Table 8-1, shock can be caused by reduced cardiac preload, abnormal distribution of circulating blood volume, and/or cardiac failure. This chapter reviews the pathophysiology, common etiologies, clinical presentation, and priorities for management in shock, with an emphasis on the pathophysiology and clinical manifestations of cardiogenic shock.

PATHOPHYSIOLOGY

Recognizing shock as a state of inadequate tissue oxygen delivery, there are two primary variables that define oxygen delivery: *arterial oxygen content* and *cardiac output* (CO).

Arterial oxygen content is defined by hemoglobin concentration, hemoglobin affinity for oxygen, and unbound or dissolved oxygen. As red blood cells circulate through the pulmonary alveolar capillaries, oxygen diffuses across the alveolar/capillary membrane and is bound to hemoglobin. Many intracellular factors affect the relative affinity of hemoglobin for oxygen, including concentrations of hydrogen ion, carbon dioxide, and 2,3-diophosphoglycerate (2,3-DPG). Tissue oxygen delivery, the unloading of oxygen from hemoglobin, is characterized by a sigmoid-shaped dissociation curve, and is facilitated (i.e., curve shifted to the right) when pH decreases or when the concentration of 2,3-DPG increases.

Cardiac output can be defined by the following relationship: CO = heart rate × stroke volume. Stroke volume varies according to changes in preload, afterload, and myocardial contractility. Preload is most accurately defined by the volume of blood filling the systemic ventricle (usually left ventricle). Invasive measures of preload include left atrial pressure, pulmonary arterial pressure, and right atrial or central venous pressure which can be estimated clinically as shown in Table 8-2. Cardiac preload and stroke volume are related by

TABLE 8-1

DIFFERENTIAL DIAGNOSIS OF SHOCK

Hypovolemic Shock—Reduced Preload/Reduced Cardiac Output
Hemorrhage
Extracellular fluid loss (e.g., vomiting/diarrhea)
Iatrogenic (e.g., diuretics, fluid restriction) Venodilator overdose

Distributive Shock—Normal Preload/Normal or Increased Cardiac Output
Sepsis
Anaphylaxis
Neurogenic injury (spinal shock)
Vasodilator overdose (e.g., ACE inhibitor)

Cardiogenic Shock—Normal or Increased Atrial Pressure/Volume "Preload" With

1. Low Cardiac Output
   a. Rhythm disturbances
      Bradycardia
      Tachycardia—can be grouped with diastolic dysfunction
   b. Systolic muscle dysfunction (myopathy)
      Obstructive disease (increased afterload)
         Critical semilunar valve/outflow obstruction
         Coarctation of the aorta
         Pulmonary hypertensive crisis
         Systemic hypertensive crisis
         Total anomalous pulmonary venous connection with pulmonary venous obstruction
      Primary muscle disease—cardiomyopathy
      Secondary cardiomyopathy—(ischemic—anomalous coronary artery), myocarditis
   c. Diastolic muscle dysfunction or problems
      Restrictive/constrictive diseases/tamponade
      Pneumothorax
      Critical AV valve or inflow obstruction
2. High Cardiac Output
   Steal or maldistribution of blood flow
      Cardiac disease—shunts
      Cardiac disease—valvar regurgitation
      Arteriovenous malformations

the Frank-Starling relationship, wherein (up to a physiologic limit) increasing ventricular end-diastolic volume leads to increased stroke volume. Contractility is a complex interplay of cardiac fiber shortening velocity, length of displacement, and actual contractile element forces. There is no sim-ple clinical measure of contractility, and it is a common mistake to assume measurements derived from echocardiography such as ejection fraction or fractional shortening are solely related to contrac-tility. Afterload is what modulates cardiac work, and is a composite of vascular resistance, blood

TABLE 8-2

CLINICAL AND LABORATORY MARKERS FOR PRELOAD (ATRIAL PRESSURE/VOLUME), AFTERLOAD AND CONTRACTILITY

Preload (increased)

Increased right ventricular "preload" (descreased will be absence or opposite of findings listed)
Physical findings—hepatomegaly, jugular venous distension, peripheral edema
Lab findings—increased CVP, direct measurement of right ventricular end-diastolic pressure, echocardiographic estimation of ventricular and atrial volumes.

Increased left ventricular "preload" (decreased will be absence or opposite of findings listed)
Physical findings—pulmonary edema (rales, wheezing, tachypnea)
Lab findigs—cardiomegaly (left atrial enlargement), increased wedge pressure, direct measurement of LVEDP, echo estimation of ventricular and atrial volumes.

Afterload

Decreased
Physical findings—increased pulse pressure, bunding pulses, vasodilation
Lab findings—decreased resistance via direct measurement (Chapter 44).

Increased
Physical findings—increased blood pressure, murmurs of outflow obstruction
Lab findings—increased of resistance via direct measurement (Chapter 44).

Contractility

Decreased
Physical findings—tachycardia with decreased pulse pressure, combined with hepatomegaly or pulmonary edema
Lab findings—decreased ejection fraction in the face of normal estimated afterload and normal preload, direct measurement of contractility (Chapter 43).

Increased
Physical findings—tachycardia (if generalized response) or bradycardia (with heart block), wide pulse pressure
Lab findings—increased ejection fraction in the face of normal estimated afterload and normal preload, direct measurement of contractility (Chapter 43).

viscosity, and vascular capacitance. A further relationship exists between cardiac output and vascular resistance such that CO = pressure gradient/vascular resistance. Thus, as vascular resistance increases and cardiac output decreases, blood pressure may remain relatively constant.

Factors that reduce arterial oxygen content and/or cardiac output will, *if not compensated for,* result in reduced tissue oxygen delivery, cellular hypoxia, tissue lactic acidosis, and ultimately decompensated shock. Additionally, tissue metabolic demands are dynamic such that when oxygen delivery is at the threshold for cellular hypoxia, relatively small changes in arterial oxygen content or cardiac output can result in precipitous decompensation. Early in the shock state, there are *compensatory mechanisms* that offset decreasing cardiac output and tissue oxygen delivery. In the face of decreased stroke volume, heart rate will normally increase and attenuate changes in cardiac output. Conversely, if heart rate decreases, stroke volume increases via changes in preload, afterload, and contractility, thereby stabilizing cardiac output. Low cardiac output results in fluid retention to increase the cardiac preload, and increased systemic resistance to maintain mean arterial pressure. The latter compensatory vasorestriction affects organs such as the skin, muscle systems, and so forth but spares organs such as the brain and the heart.

As compensatory mechanisms reach physiologic limits, any unmet metabolic demands lead to depletion of cellular energy stores, anaerobic metabolism, tissue hypoxia, and organ dysfunction. Vasoactive peptides are subsequently released into the circulation, inducing increased vascular permeability and edema (capillary leak syndrome). As blood flow to brain, kidneys, and the coronary circulation becomes further and critically reduced, a state of *decompensated* shock ensues marked by multiple organ system failure and ultimately death.

Many of these factors assume greater importance or have unique susceptibilities in neonates compared to older children and adults. In neonates, for example, the relatively immature myocardium has minimal contractility reserve, such that heart rate becomes the major determinant of cardiac output. Bradycardia and extreme tachycardia are poorly tolerated in this population. Neonates may also have critical or ductal-dependent structural abnormalities, each with a unique physiology. Left atrial filling may be dependent on an atrial level right-to-left shunt, and systemic perfusion may be dependent on ductal flow to the aorta.

ETIOLOGIES OF SHOCK

Hypovolemic Shock

Hypovolemia is the most common cause of shock in pediatrics. Hemorrhage, vomiting, diarrhea, capillary leak syndromes, and iatrogenic problems

(e.g., excessive diuresis or fluid restriction) are typical examples, and clues are almost always immediately evident on history or physical examination. Hypovolemia primarily reduces cardiac output via decreased stroke volume (low preload), and increased vascular resistance mediates redistribution of limited cardiac output to major viscera (brain, kidneys, and heart). Compensatory measures of increased heart rate and contractility are insufficient to overcome a profound reduction in preload in hypovolemic shock.

Distributive Shock

Sepsis, anaphylaxis, and neurogenic injury are the common causes of distributive shock. In this category, the mechanism of shock is abnormal distribution of blood flow and blood volume. These conditions share characteristics of markedly reduced systemic vascular resistance with normal or even raised cardiac output. Profound vasodilation is the hallmark of septic shock, and results in relative hypovolemia compared to the increased vascular capacitance. Additionally, endotoxins and low diastolic coronary perfusion pressure can induce secondary cardiac dysfunction, further complicating clinical interpretation and management. The physiologic derangement in distributive shock is one of normal or decreased preload with normal or increased cardiac output. The cardiac output is maintained or increased because of increased heart rate and contractility; however, compensatory measures of increased heart rate and contractility are insufficient to overcome the maldistribution of blood flow and maintain appropriate organ perfusion.

Cardiogenic Shock

Cardiogenic shock is usually secondary to extremes of systolic dysfunction, heart rate, diastolic dysfunction, or elevated afterload. Clinical examples include myocarditis, complete heart block, hypertrophic cardiomyopathy, and hypertension, respectively. Systolic dysfunction generally implies a problem with cardiac contractility, while diastolic dysfunction results in reduced stroke volume via decreased preload. The common physiologic denominator is a reduced cardiac output. With cardiogenic shock, unlike hypovolemic shock, preload is expected to be normal, based on indirect measures of preload (e.g., atrial volume and pressure). With diastolic dysfunction or extreme tachycardia, however, atrial volume and pressure may be normal (or elevated), while ventricular filling is inadequate. Thus, indirect measures of ventricular preload indicate that it is normal while it is actually inadequate.

The negative consequences of bradycardia on cardiac output have already been discussed. Extreme tachycardia limits diastolic filling time, thereby reducing preload and thus stroke volume. Therefore, tachycardia can be considered akin to diastolic dysfunction.

Other causes of diastolic dysfunction include cardiomyopathies, pericardial diseases and tamponade, mitral or tricuspid stenosis, and tension pneumothorax. In each of these cases, indirect measurements of ventricular preload (atrial pressure and volume) can be normal with decreased stroke volume owing to decreased ventricular preload.

Elevated afterload implies raised vascular resistance and is especially deleterious in those with reduced contractility reserve (e.g., dilated cardiomyopathy). It usually does not cause shock unless the heart is unable to increase contractility or heart rate. The physiology is similar to systolic failure in that stroke volume can be decreased in the presence of adequate preload. Increased afterload may be in the form of increased vascular resistance (systemic or pulmonary hypertension), or fixed anatomic obstruction (critical aortic or pulmonary stenosis). Extreme pulmonary hypertension may not only cause right ventricular failure, but can also result in inadequate loading (preload) of the left ventricle. In this case, there may be steal from pulmonary blood flow with right-to-left shunting through an atrial septal defect (ASD), patent foramen ovale (PFO), or ventricular septal defect (VSD), with resultant cyanosis.

Another form of cardiogenic shock is systemic steal owing to a shunting lesion such as a large VSD, aortopulmonary window, large patent ductus arteriosus (PDA), or aortic valve regurgitation. These lesions are similar to distributive shock as

cardiac output is normal or elevated with a normal preload. Cardiac output may be insufficient to compensate for the shunt or regurgitation and thus shock occurs. Lesions with a large drop in diastolic pressure (such as aortic regurgitation or an aortopulmonary window) may also cause decreased cardiac function because of decreased coronary artery blood flow and myocardial ischemia. Thus, the typical features of cardiogenic shock owing to systolic dysfunction are seen (decreased cardiac output with a normal preload).

The congenital heart defects at greatest risk of cardiogenic shock include critical left heart valve obstruction (e.g., hypoplastic left heart syndrome), severe coarctation of the aorta, interrupted aortic arch, tetralogy of Fallot, critical pulmonary stenosis, transposition of the great arteries, total anomalous pulmonary venous connection, and congenital coronary anomalies (e.g., anomalous origin of left coronary artery from pulmonary artery). In contrast, the much more common left-to-right shunt defects (e.g., VSD, ASD, and PDA) generally present a low risk of cardiogenic shock. There are important exceptions, however, usually involving a combination of left-to-right shunt defect *and* left heart valve obstruction or aortic arch obstruction (e.g., VSD and coarctation of the aorta).

Cardiac arrhythmias at risk for cardiogenic shock include incessant or extremely rapid supraventricular tachycardia, complete heart block, ventricular tachycardia, and ventricular fibrillation. Myocarditis, pericarditis with tamponade, dilated cardiomyopathy, cardiac trauma, and acute myocardial infarction (e.g., Kawasaki's disease) are the most common acquired heart diseases at risk for cardiogenic shock.

CLINICAL PRESENTATION IN SHOCK

Recognizing shock in its earliest manifestations is critical if adverse outcomes are to be avoided. As described above, blood pressure can be maintained even in the face of significant reduction in cardiac output, primarily through a compensatory increase in vascular resistance. Thus, hypotension is not a useful early sign of shock. Prodromal symptoms of shock should be detected early and include tachycardia, altered mental status, oliguria, discrepant proximal versus distal pulses, prolonged capillary refill time, and mental status changes. Hypotension is an ominous sign of impending decompensation and usually coexists with other late manifestations of shock including bradycardia, irregular breathing, and coma. Sinus tachycardia is almost universally present early in shock. Tachycardia is nonspecific, however, and may also result from other stressors such as anxiety, fever, and pain. As a shock state evolves, compensatory shunting of blood flow away from the peripheral circulation results in discrepancy between central and peripheral pulses. Skin temperature decreases and skin color progresses from normal to mottled, and then pale to cyanotic. Tachypnea reflects compensatory effort to increase oxygen uptake and also serves to stabilize acid-base equilibrium in metabolic acidosis. The reduction in renal blood flow with resulting oliguria (urine production <1 mL/kg/h) is an important and potentially ominous sign that compensation mechanisms may soon fail. Mental status changes reflect the severity of brain hypoperfusion, including confusion or irritability in early stages of shock, progressing to lethargy, agitation, stupor, and ultimately coma in decompensated shock. Finally, frank hypotension, irregular respirations, and bradycardia herald impending cardiopulmonary arrest.

Laboratory findings in shock reflect organ dysfunction (abnormal renal function tests such as an increased creatinine, elevated liver function tests) or hypoperfusion (acidosis or increased serum lactate reflecting anaerobic metabolism). Based on clinical findings, further useful laboratory investigations may include chest radiography, electrocardiography, echocardiography, serum B-type natriuretic peptide concentration, and serum myocardial enzyme profile. These investigations should be selectively applied based on clinical findings in order to be of greatest predictive value.

In addition to the general presentation described above, cardiogenic shock can be differentiated from other causes of shock through its often distinct and recognizable clinical findings. Prior symptoms such as chest pain, syncope, exercise intolerance, and palpitations may increase the suspicion of a cardiac problem. Physical signs of cardiac disease include cyanosis in the absence of significant respiratory distress, pathologic heart murmurs, nailbed clubbing, pulmonary edema, peripheral edema, hepatomegaly, differential extremity blood pressures and/or pulse amplitude, and cardiac arrhythmia. Cardiogenic shock (except for the distributive form seen with shunt lesions) can be differentiated from hypovolemic shock based on the estimated normal (or increased) atrial pressures and volume, with decreased cardiac output and a worsening (or unchanged) clinical status after an isotonic fluid bolus. Hypovolemic shock will have signs of decreased preload, and a favorable response to an isotonic fluid bolus. Distributive shock may be similar to cardiogenic shock because of shunting lesions. Historic features (e.g., fever or signs of infection, neurologic injury, or drug ingestion) and the examination (e.g., abnormal murmurs) as well as findings on echocardiography should clarify the diagnosis. Table 8-2 outlines clinical features to assess preload, afterload, and contractility. Finally, Figure 8-1 shows a combination of the differential diagnosis with clinical features as a suggested diagnostic approach.

MANAGEMENT PRIORITIES IN SHOCK

Supplemental oxygen, vascular access, hemodynamic monitoring, and frequent reassessment are the mainstays of shock management. The latter is critical, both to provide early detection of potential trends toward decompensation, as well as to guide therapeutic endpoints. The physical examination should be directed at assessing circulatory adequacy, focusing on mental status, heart rate, blood pressure, capillary refill time, arterial pulse volume centrally versus peripherally, and extremity temperature. A Foley catheter should be placed to determine urine output accurately. Monitoring catheters for central venous pressure, arterial blood pressure, and mixed venous oxygen saturation can be helpful in initial and reassessment phases of treatment. The laboratory database should serially track acid-base analysis, serum chemistries (glucose, electrolytes, ionized

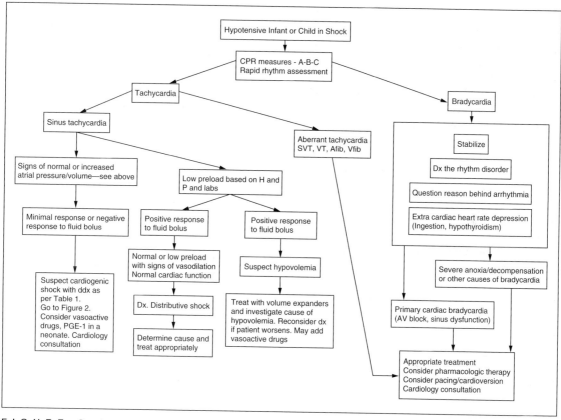

F I G U R E   8 - 1

APPROACH TO THE DIAGNOSIS AND INITIAL MANAGEMENT OF SHOCK

calcium, blood urea nitrogen [BUN] and creatinine), complete blood count, coagulation parameters, and serum lactic acid.

Within each category of shock pathophysiology (hypovolemic, distributive, cardiogenic), there are additional measures that optimize chances of recovery. The priority in hypovolemic shock is vascular access and subsequent isotonic fluid expansion of intravascular blood volume (e.g., normal saline or lactated Ringer's solution). In the case of significant hemorrhage, blood transfusion is often required. In severe cases of hypovolemic shock, addition of a vasopressor infusion may also be useful (e.g., dopamine or epinephrine). Successful treatment of septic shock is predicated on intravascular volume expansion, vasopressor and/or inotropic support, and

antibiotic therapy. Cardiogenic shock management priorities (Figure 8-2) are often contradictory to what are otherwise effective treatments in hypovolemic or distributive shock.

In cardiogenic shock, intravascular volume expansion may be deleterious when ventricular filling pressures are already elevated. Inotropic stimulants, diuretics, and/or vasodilators are likely to be more effective measures. Life-threatening cardiac arrhythmias require urgent pharmacologic or electric cardioversion into sinus rhythm (or a stable paced rhythm). Anemia can be destabilizing in cardiogenic shock, as there is limited capacity to offset the consequences of reduced oxygen-carrying capacity through increases in cardiac output. Blood transfusion to correct anemia is therefore indicated

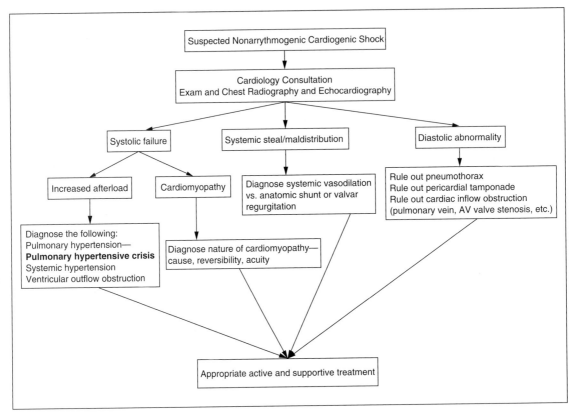

APPROACH TO THE DIAGNOSIS AND INITIAL MANAGEMENT OF CARDIOGENIC SHOCK

on this basis. Fever and pain raise peripheral oxygen consumption and therefore should be aggressively treated. In severely ill patients, sedation and neuromuscular relaxation will decrease peripheral oxygen consumption. Positive-pressure ventilation is of major benefit in cardiogenic shock, as it immediately reduces energy expenditure related to spontaneous breathing, and directly supports cardiac output by reducing the afterload of the systemic ventricle.

Compared to older children, neonates with shock present a relatively high probability of ductal-dependent cardiac malformation, especially when there are few risk factors for sepsis or hypovolemia. After obtaining vascular access, the priority in these patients should be maintaining ductal patency with prostaglandin E1 infusion until a complete echocar-

diographic assessment is obtained. When critical left heart obstruction is considered likely (e.g., hypoplastic left heart syndrome), there is added risk of steal from the systemic circulation through the ductus arteriosus if pulmonary vascular resistance is lowered or if systemic vascular resistance is raised. Thus, it is important to maintain a balance between systemic and pulmonary blood flow, and where possible, avoid treatment with supplemental oxygen, hyperventilation, and high dose vasopressor infusions. On the other hand, vasodilators are often quite beneficial, as they reduce systemic afterload and increase systemic blood flow. Clinically useful vasodilators include angiotensin-converting enzyme inhibitors (e.g., enalaprilat) and phosphodiesterase inhibitors (e.g., milrinone). Adjunctive treatment with low-dose inotropic agents (e.g., dopamine

$3-5$ μ/kg/min) can usually and sufficiently augment contractility without inducing higher vascular resistance or increased myocardial oxygen consumption on the basis of tachycardia.

Urgent referral for cardiac surgery or transcatheter intervention is indicated in infants with cardiogenic shock secondary to important congenital heart disease (e.g., coarctation of the aorta, total anomalous pulmonary venous connection, transposition of the great arteries, and certain congenital coronary anomalies). In severe or end-stage cardiac failure, mechanical support with a ventricular assist device or the extracorporeal membrane may be life-saving while awaiting recovery, or as a bridge to cardiac transplantation.

Given such inherent complexities in assessing and managing cardiogenic shock, these infants and children usually benefit from treatment in a specialized neonatal, pediatric, or cardiac intensive care unit.

SUMMARY

Although shock may begin as one of many clinically distinct clinical problems, the pathophysiology of cellular hypoxia and tissue acidosis remains the same. Early recognition of the clinical signs of compensated shock is critical if decompensated shock, end-organ dysfunction, and death are to be avoided. Hypotension must be recognized for what it is: an important but late manifestation of shock that portends an ominous and potentially imminent progression to cardiopulmonary arrest.

Although not as common as hypovolemic or septic shock, cardiogenic shock is an important problem in pediatrics, and pediatricians should be able to identify patients at risk. The most common causes of cardiogenic shock in infants and children include ductal-dependent congenital heart defects, coronary anomalies, cardiac arrhythmias, myocarditis, and primary cardiomyopathy. Management priorities in cardiogenic shock can be contrary to the usual approach to hypovolemic or septic shock, and highlight the importance of early cardiology consultation when heart disease is first suspected.

Suggested Readings

Chameides L, Hazinski MF (eds.): *Textbook of Pediatric Advanced Life Support*, 2d ed. Dallas, TX: American Heart Association, 1994.

Giroir BP, Levin DL, Perkin RM: Shock, in: *Essentials of Pediatric Intensive Care*, 2d ed. London, UK: Churchill Livingstone, 1997: 280–301.

9

FAILURE TO THRIVE

Brojendra Agarwala

Failure to thrive (FTT) in infants and in children carries a vast differential diagnosis. Primary care physicians are usually quite familiar with the definition and the differential diagnosis. It is helpful to review and understand the major pathophysiologic categories of FTT which lead to the differential diagnoses, and the manner in which congenital heart disease fits into these categories. In this short chapter, only the manner in which FTT is related to congenital heart defects (CHD) is discussed. The major categories of FTT and the general evaluation strategy are shown in Figure 9-1.

One of the major decision points is whether there is growth suppression or growth failure. Children with CHD as the cause of failure to grow usually fail to grow by body weight; however, growth in body length and head circumference is usually not affected. Growth suppression (failure to grow despite adequate caloric supplementation) is manifest by symmetric growth delay in head circumference, length, and weight. Growth failure is manifest by initial sparing of head circumference and height, with poor weight gain initially. As the physiologic derangement persists and/or progresses, growth in length followed by head circumference is also delayed. Growth failure occurs because of inadequate caloric supplementation. This can be a result of

decreased caloric intake or increased caloric expenditure. Decreased caloric intake can be a result of difficulties in feeding, emesis, or malabsorption. Increased caloric expenditure can be seen with hypermetabolic conditions, or with direct loss of calories (e.g., third space body protein loss in burn patients, urinary glucose loss in diabetic patients). Patients with CHD can fall into any of these categories.

GROWTH SUPPRESSION

Pediatricians are usually familiar with the concept that a child born with one congenital anomaly demands a search for other anomalies. This is also very appropriate for CHD. Numerous syndromes are associated with CHD. After careful evaluation of a child with CHD, it may become obvious that FTT is not primarily a result of the underlying cardiac problem; rather, it is a result of the associated syndrome (e.g., congenital rubella syndrome, fetal alcoholic syndrome, and maternal drug abuse, and so forth). In these cases, poor growth may be evident despite excellent caloric supplementation. In addition to syndromes, there may be isolated organ anomalies that can explain the FTT. An example is renal disease/failure or liver disease/failure, which may both be

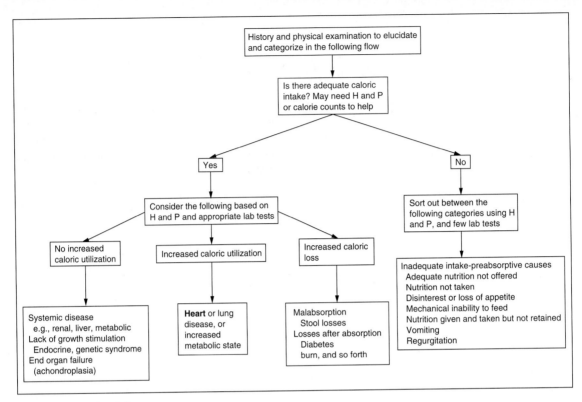

F I G U R E   9 - 1 A

WORKUP OF FTT

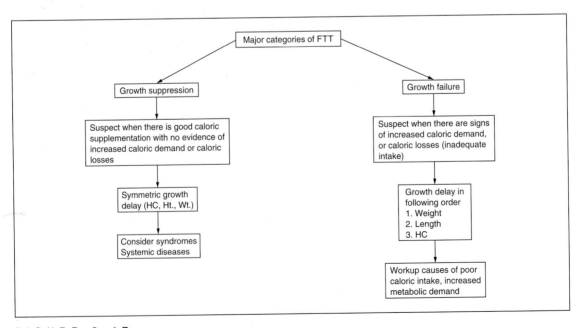

F I G U R E   9 - 1 B

MAJOR CATEGORIES OF FTT

associated with CHD and are both known to cause growth suppression by themselves. Correction of the other organ system corrects the growth disturbance despite the presence of underlying CHD. A clue that the underlying CHD is not the cause of the FTT is the lack of growth with good caloric supplementation, and improved growth when other organ system derangements are corrected. The absence of cardiac signs and symptoms is another clue. Sometimes it is impossible to isolate the cause of FTT in the face of significant CHD and failure of another organ system at the same time (e.g., liver failure in a patient with a large ventricular septal defect [VSD]).

GROWTH FAILURE

The major causes of growth failure in patients with congenital heart disease is severe cyanosis or congestive heart failure (CHF). The former can be seen with any of the cyanotic heart diseases and may itself cause growth suppression; however, tachypnea and poor feeding may also occur with significant degrees of cyanosis and contribute to the problem. Symptoms of CHF may occur with any cardiac lesion causing a large left-to-right shunt, severe obstructive or regurgitant lesions, or with myocardial dysfunction (cardiomyopathy). The symptoms of CHF owing to left-to-right shunts (VSD, patent ductus arteriosus [PDA] and common atrioventricular canal [CAVC]) have a gradual onset because of the gradual decline in pulmonary vascular resistance (PVR). Symptoms of CHF are manifest as feeding difficulties and poor calorie intake because of the increased work of breathing, irritability, and loss of appetite with subsequent FTT. In addition to poor feeding, increased respiratory effort causes increased use of energy and therefore a greater metabolic demand.

There are many other causes of FTT in these infants as described below. Of note is that children with a large atrial septal defect (ASD) frequently do not gain weight appropriately in childhood even though usually they do not develop frank signs and symptoms of CHF until adulthood. Following closure of the ASD they experience a catch-up in body weight. On the other hand, rapid onset of CHF from

critical pulmonic stenosis (PS), aortic stenosis (AS), and coarctation of the aorta (COA) is frequently a result of myocardial dysfunction, dysrhythmias, and shock, with no time to develop signs and symptoms of FTT. Children with lesser amounts of obstructive heart disease, e.g., PS, AS, and COA; and children with less severe cyanotic CHD without CHF, e.g., tetralogy of Fallot do not manifest FTT.

Other reasons for FTT in children with CHD include an increased metabolic demand of the heart itself. Patients with CHD may have increased blood volume in the heart and great vessels, which stimulates stretch receptors in the wall resulting in sympathetic stimulations and an increased catecholamine level. This will then lead to increased oxygen consumption and caloric requirement. In addition, obstructive lesions, or lesions that cause an increased afterload, will cause increased myocardial wall stress and hypertrophy. This will lead to increased myocardial oxygen consumption as well; however, it is probably not the cause of FTT. It is more likely present only in severe obstructive lesions with myocardial dysfunction in which there is an increased blood volume in the heart as well (as noted above). Increased caloric losses may occur from chronic CHF and gastrointestinal mucosal edema, which may cause protein-losing enteropathy and fat malabsorption. Deranged glucose metabolism plays an important role contributing to FTT. High catecholamine levels can cause deranged glucose metabolism. Suppression of insulin response to oral glucose load in infants with large L-R shunt has been well established. Alpha-adrenergic stimulation depresses insulin secretion by the islet cell of the pancreas. Often there is a resting hyperglycemia in this group of infants. This may interfere with tissue usage of carbohydrate.

Side effects of medications, e.g., commonly used medication such as Digitalis can cause nausea, vomiting, and lack of appetite, and is another cause for poor feeding in patients with CHD.

MANAGEMENT

Following closure of the VSD, ASD, and PDA, relief of severe obstruction causing myocardial dysfunction, correction of severe cyanosis, or optimal management of cardiac dysfunction, the growth rate usually accelerates and patients experience a catch-up to their appropriate weight. Nutritional care is very important prior to improvement or palliation of the underlying cardiac disease. Until there is an intervention to correct or palliate the CHD, intake of high calorie formula, e.g., fortified breast milk, 24–27 calorie per ounce formula feeding is recommended (see Chapter 56). Low sodium formula or salt restrictions are not recommended because they are not palatable, which may further decrease caloric intake. With the help of diuretics, the serum sodium is well controlled. A happy child with excess salt and water that cannot be controlled with diuretics is preferable to a miserable child with a poor appetite from unpalatable food. In children with carnitine deficiency and an associated dilated cardiomyopathy, replacement with L-carnitine has resulted in marked clinical improvement. Likewise, optimal medical therapy to treat symptoms of other cardiomyopathies should result in improved growth.

Primary care physicians should be prepared to handle some of the frequently asked questions from the parents of patients with CHD regarding growth and weight gain.

1. Is the child going to have a normal growth after fixing the heart defects? Unless associated with an underlying syndrome, the child should catch up with his/her body weight with time.
2. Is the FTT going to affect later stature and brain growth? Weight gain is a problem in patients with CHF because of large left-to-right shunts or cardiomyopathies. Growth in length and head circumference remain normal. Unless associated with another reason for FTT, height and brain growth will normalize following correction of the cardiac abnormality.
3. Why are defects (VSD, ASD, PDA) not closed prior to the onset of CHF and FTT? There is always a possibility of partial or complete spontaneous closure of the VSD, PDA, and ASD with time. Even though some cardiac centers are performing early closure for the above defects, there should be a reasonable indication to do so. There

is always a chance of complications with cardiac surgery and transcatheter closure of these defects. Therefore the symptoms, if any, of FTT need to be balanced against the risks of intervention or delay in intervention and the probability that spontaneous closure of a defect will occur.

SUMMARY

When dealing with FTT in children, the primary care physician should address the major categories based on clinical clues mentioned above (symptoms, symmetry of growth or growth retardation, and caloric intake). Calorie counts can further differentiate between inadequate intake and increased caloric expenditure, as can the physical examination. Using basic information from the history and physical examination, primary care physicians should be able to ascertain whether or not the underlying heart disease is the cause. In cases of FTT where there is no previously diagnosed underlying heart disease, primary care physicians should be able to diagnose the presence of an underlying CHD and understand its role as a possible contributing factor to FTT, based on a history of respiratory difficulty or findings on physical examination. Each of these presentations is discussed in other chapters in this book. Expensive testing (magnetic resonance imaging [MRI], echocardiography) without the suspicion of underlying CHD based on the history and physical examination is expensive and not cost effective.

Suggested Readings

Berman S: *Pediatric Decision Making*. St. Louis, MO, Mosby, 1996.

Green M: *Green and Richmond Pediatric Diagnoses*, 4th ed. Philadelphia, PA, WB Saunders, 1986.

Rudolph CD, et al: *Rudolph's Pediatrics*, 21st ed. New York, NY, McGraw-Hill, 2003.

Schwartz MW, et al: *The 5-minute Pediatric Consult*. Baltimore, MD, Williams & Wilkins, 1997.

10

HYPERTENSION

Donald I. Moel

INTRODUCTION

Only for the last 20–25 years have pediatricians measured and monitored blood pressure in their practices. During this time, nomograms have been developed which define normal ranges of blood pressure for age, gender, and height; however, because of its long-term implications, it is sometimes "difficult" to stigmatize an individual with the diagnosis of hypertension. The long-term effects of hypertension and its treatment as children with this diagnosis emerge into early and later adulthood are still unknown. Most children with secondary forms of hypertension have obvious hypertension, blood pressures that are greater than 10 mmHg above the 95th percentile for age, gender, and height. It is easy to justify complete evaluation and treatment of such patients; however, patients with blood pressures at or around the 95th percentile for age, gender, and height are much more problematic. Diagnostic considerations (cost/benefit) and therapeutic intervention (yes/no) are far more challenging for the clinician.

DEFINITION OF HYPERTENSION IN CHILDREN

Three major reports over the last 25 years have helped define normal blood pressure in children. These are the First and Second Task Force Reports published in 1977 and 1987, respectively[1,2] and more recently the Working Group Report[3] published in 1996. These bodies produced guidelines that define hypertension in childhood. The definition of normal and abnormal blood pressure in childhood was published in the Second Task Force Report. It used data from nine studies involving children from the United States and United Kingdom, and produced age-specific blood pressure percentile curves. Normal blood pressure was defined as systolic and diastolic blood pressure readings below the 90th percentile for age, and hypertension was defined as systolic and diastolic blood pressure greater than the 95th percentile for age. It was found that age was a primary determinant of blood pressure variability. Height was considered only a secondary contributing factor. The task force was concerned with over diagnosis of hypertension and recommended that at least three abnormal readings be obtained on three separate occasions before making the diagnosis of hypertension.

The National High Blood Pressure Education Program Working Group combined the data from the second task force with additional blood pressure data from 1988 to 1991 in the National Health and Nutrition Examination Survey (NHANES III). The Working Group Report placed greatest emphasis on height as the major variable in determining whether a child had elevated blood pressure. Tables 10-1 and 10-2 generated by the Working Group Report[3] were based on height percentiles. This working group aided in solving the problem of overdiagnosis of hypertension.

Though the working group suggested that three blood pressure determinations on three separate occasions are necessary to diagnose hypertension, there is no substitute for multiple blood pressure determinations.

METHOD OF BLOOD PRESSURE DETERMINATION

A conventional mercury column or aneroid sphygmomanometer should be used to obtain the blood pressure in school-aged children and teenagers. Although less accurate, an automated oscillometric device can be used in infants and toddlers who will not cooperate with manual blood pressure determination. The bladder of the cuff should encircle 80–100% of the circumference of the upper arm, and its width should be at 40% of the upper arm circumference. Too narrow of a cuff will falsely elevate the reading. The disappearance of the 5th Korotkoff sound is thought to best represent the diastolic blood pressure. Because of the great variability of blood pressures in an individual from one occasion to the next, it is often necessary to obtain more than three separate blood pressure determinations to diagnose hypertension. This is summarized in Table 10-3.

Because of this problem of great variability, many clinicians have used 24-h ambulatory blood pressure monitoring (ABPM). This technique has been extensively studied in adults and is now being evaluated in children. ABPM provides multiple measures using a device that is consistent over the determinations. This may well provide a "truer" picture of blood pressure in a child. The ABPM can identify white coat hypertension and patients with nocturnal hypertension (nondipers).[4] Table 10-4 demonstrates mean ABPM values in healthy children.[5]

Children who have normal blood pressure on a single reading require continued annual surveillance. Those who have high normal blood pressure (90th–95th percentile) on three consecutive measurements separated by 3 days should have three extremity blood pressures and pulses (right arm, left arm, and a leg) taken to help rule out coarctation of the aorta and urinalysis to screen for renal disease. Children with high blood pressure (>95th percentile) should be evaluated for possible treatable cause of secondary hypertension.

CAUSES OF HYPERTENSION IN CHILDREN

Several studies have investigated the prevalence of hypertension in children.[6,7,8] Using the above-described definition of hypertension, the prevalence has remained between 1% and 2%. Most studies of the causes of hypertension have come from large referral centers. Thus, there may be selection bias. Over the last 15 years a series of studies has shown a decrease in the percentage of children diagnosed with secondary hypertension and an increase in those diagnosed with the primary form of hypertension, i.e., essential hypertension.[6,7,8] In a 1988 study 84% of children with hypertension had secondary causes.[6] The most common causes of hypertension were renal disease (70%), coarctation of the aorta (15%), renovascular (7%), and endocrine (2%). In that study only 16% of children had primary hypertension.

In a 1994 study 77% of patients had secondary causes of hypertension and 23% had primary hypertension.[7] Finally, a study in 2001 found that of 146 children with confirmed hypertension, 51.4% had secondary hypertension and about 50% had primary hypertension.[8] In children with primary hypertension, a positive family history was

TABLE 10-1

BLOOD PRESSURE LEVELS FOR THE 90TH AND 95TH PERCENTILES OF BLOOD PRESSURE FOR BOYS AGE 1 TO 17 YEARS BY PERCENTILES OF HEIGHT

Age	Height Percentiles[a] BP[b]	Systolic BP (mmHg)							Diastolic BP (mmHg)						
		5%	10%	25%	50%	75%	90%	95%	5%	10%	25%	50%	75%	90%	95%
1	90th	94	95	97	98	100	102	102	50	51	52	53	54	54	55
	95th	98	99	101	102	104	106	106	55	55	56	57	58	59	59
2	90th	98	99	100	102	104	105	106	55	55	56	57	58	59	59
	95th	101	102	104	106	108	109	110	59	59	60	61	62	63	63
3	90th	100	101	103	105	107	108	109	59	59	60	61	62	63	63
	95th	104	105	107	109	111	112	113	63	63	64	65	66	67	67
4	90th	102	103	105	107	109	110	111	62	62	63	64	65	66	66
	95th	106	107	109	111	113	114	115	66	67	67	68	69	70	71
5	90th	104	105	106	108	110	112	112	65	65	66	67	68	69	69
	95th	108	109	110	112	114	115	116	69	70	70	71	72	73	74
6	90th	105	106	108	110	111	113	114	67	68	69	70	70	71	72
	95th	109	110	112	114	115	117	117	72	72	73	74	75	76	76
7	90th	106	107	109	111	113	114	115	69	70	71	72	72	73	74
	95th	110	111	113	115	116	118	119	74	74	75	76	77	78	78
8	90th	107	108	110	112	114	115	116	71	71	72	73	74	75	75
	95th	111	112	114	116	118	119	120	75	76	76	77	78	79	80
9	90th	109	110	112	113	115	117	117	72	73	73	74	75	76	77
	95th	113	114	116	117	119	121	121	76	77	78	79	80	80	81
10	90th	110	112	113	115	117	118	119	73	74	74	75	76	77	78
	95th	114	115	117	119	121	122	123	77	78	79	80	80	81	82
11	90th	112	113	115	117	119	120	121	74	74	75	76	77	78	78
	95th	116	117	119	121	123	124	125	78	79	79	80	81	82	83
12	90th	115	116	117	119	121	123	123	75	75	76	77	78	78	79
	95th	119	120	121	123	125	126	127	79	79	80	81	82	83	83
13	90th	117	118	120	122	124	125	126	75	76	76	77	78	79	80
	95th	121	122	124	126	128	129	130	79	80	81	82	83	83	84
14	90th	120	121	123	125	126	128	128	76	76	77	78	79	80	80
	95th	124	125	127	128	130	132	132	80	81	81	82	83	84	85
15	90th	123	124	125	127	129	131	131	77	77	78	79	80	81	81
	95th	127	128	129	131	133	134	135	81	82	83	83	84	85	86
16	90th	125	126	128	130	132	133	134	79	79	80	81	82	82	83
	95th	129	130	132	134	136	137	138	83	83	84	85	86	87	87
17	90th	128	129	131	133	134	136	136	81	81	82	83	84	85	85
	95th	132	133	135	136	138	140	140	85	85	86	87	88	89	89

[a]Height percentile determined by standard growth curves.
[b]Blood pressure percentile determined by a single measurement.
Source: National High Blood Pressure Education Program Working Group. Update on the 1987 Task Force Report on High Blood Pressure in Children and Adolescents: A working group report from the National High Blood Pressure Education Program. *Pediatrics* 1996; 98:649–58.

TABLE 10-2

BLOOD PRESSURE LEVELS FOR THE 90TH AND 95TH PERCENTILES OF BLOOD PRESSURE FOR GIRLS AGE 1 TO 17 YEARS BY PERCENTILES OF HEIGHT

Age	Height Percentiles[a] BP[b]	Systolic BP (mmHg)							Diastolic BP (mmHg)						
		5%	10%	25%	50%	75%	90%	95%	5%	10%	25%	50%	75%	90%	95%
1	90th	97	98	99	100	102	103	104	53	53	53	54	55	56	56
	95th	101	102	103	104	105	107	107	57	57	57	58	59	60	60
2	90th	99	99	100	102	103	104	105	57	57	58	58	59	60	61
	95th	102	103	104	105	107	108	109	61	61	62	62	63	64	65
3	90th	100	100	102	103	104	105	106	61	61	61	62	63	63	64
	95th	104	104	105	107	108	109	110	65	65	65	66	67	67	68
4	90th	101	102	103	104	106	107	108	63	63	64	65	65	66	67
	95th	105	106	107	108	109	111	111	67	67	68	69	69	70	71
5	90th	103	103	104	106	107	108	109	65	66	66	67	68	68	69
	95th	107	107	108	110	111	112	113	69	70	70	71	72	72	73
6	90th	104	105	106	107	109	110	111	67	67	68	69	69	70	71
	95th	108	109	110	111	112	114	114	71	71	72	73	73	74	75
7	90th	106	107	108	109	110	112	112	69	69	69	70	71	72	72
	95th	110	110	112	113	114	115	116	73	73	73	74	75	76	76
8	90th	108	109	110	111	112	113	114	70	70	71	71	72	73	74
	95th	112	112	113	115	116	117	118	74	74	75	75	76	77	78
9	90th	110	110	112	113	114	115	116	71	72	72	73	74	74	75
	95th	114	114	115	117	118	119	120	75	76	76	77	78	78	79
10	90th	112	112	114	115	116	117	118	73	73	73	74	75	76	76
	95th	116	116	117	119	120	121	122	77	77	77	78	79	80	80
11	90th	114	114	116	117	118	119	120	74	74	75	75	76	77	77
	95th	118	118	119	121	122	123	124	78	78	79	79	80	81	81
12	90th	116	116	118	119	120	121	122	75	75	76	76	77	78	78
	95th	120	120	121	123	124	125	126	79	79	80	80	81	82	82
13	90th	118	118	119	121	122	123	124	76	76	77	78	78	79	80
	95th	121	122	123	125	126	127	128	80	80	81	82	82	83	84
14	90th	119	120	121	122	124	125	126	77	77	78	79	79	80	81
	95th	123	124	125	126	128	129	130	81	81	82	83	83	84	85
15	90th	121	121	122	124	125	126	127	78	78	79	79	80	81	82
	95th	124	125	126	128	129	130	131	82	82	83	83	84	85	86
16	90th	122	122	123	125	126	127	128	79	79	79	80	81	82	82
	95th	125	126	127	128	130	131	132	83	83	83	84	85	86	86
17	90th	122	123	124	125	126	128	128	79	79	79	80	81	82	82
	95th	126	126	127	129	130	131	132	83	83	83	84	85	86	86

[a]Height percentile determined by standard growth curves.
[b]Blood pressure percentile determined by a single measurement.
Source: National High Blood Pressure Education Program Working Group. Update on the 1987 Task Force Report on High Blood Pressure in Children and Adolescents: A working group report from the National High Blood Pressure Education Program. *Pediatrics* 1996; 98:649–58.

EVALUATION OF HYPERTENSION

Methods
- Three separate readings
- Appropriate size cuff
  - Bladder encircles 80–90% of arm circumference
  - Width of bladder = 40% of arm circumference
- Diastolic blood pressure
  - —disappearance of 5th Korotkoff sound

Definition

Average systolic or diastolic BP > 95th percentile age, height, and gender

present in 87% of patients and a body mass index (BMI) greater than the 95th percentile for age was present in greater than 40% of patients.

Data from the NHANES III has demonstrated that the prevalence of obesity has increased for all age groups. Numerous studies[9,10,11] have demonstrated a clear association between obesity and elevated blood pressure in children. The correlation is stronger for systolic blood pressure than for diastolic blood pressure. The correlation between BMI and blood pressure remains present even for children with BMI less than 25 kg/m^2, suggesting that even mildly overweight children may be at risk of developing hypertension.

Obesity is linked not only to development of hypertension but also to other aspects of cardiovascular risk. Sinaiko[12] studied 700 children and followed them every 2 years from age 7 until

TABLE 10-4

OSCILLOMETRIC MEAN AMBULATORY BLOOD PRESSURE VALUES IN HEALTHY CHILDREN: SUMMARY FOR CLINICAL USE

Height (n) (cm)	24 hour period		Day time		Night time	
	50th	95th	50th	95th	50th	95th
Boys						
120 (33)	105/65	113/72	112/73	123/85	95/55	104/63
130 (62)	105/65	117/75	113/73	125/85	96/55	107/65
140 (102)	107/65	121/77	114/73	127/85	97/55	110/67
150 (108)	109/66	124/78	115/73	129/85	99/56	113/67
160 (115)	112/66	126/78	118/73	132/85	102/56	116/67
170 (83)	115/67	128/77	121/73	135/85	104/56	119/67
180 (69)	120/67	130/77	124/73	137/85	107/56	122/67
Girls						
120 (40)	103/65	113/73	111/72	120/84	96/55	107/66
130 (58)	105/66	117/75	112/72	124/84	97/55	109/66
140 (70)	108/66	120/76	114/72	127/84	98/55	111/66
150 (111)	110/66	122/76	115/73	129/84	99/55	112/66
160 (156)	111/66	124/76	116/73	131/84	100/55	113/66
170 (109)	112/66	124/76	118/74	131/84	101/55	113/66
180 (25)	113/66	124/76	120/74	131/84	103/55	114/66

*Daytime: 8 AM to 8 PM.
†Nighttime: midnight to 6 AM.
Source: Soergel: *J Pediatr,* Volume 130. February 1997, 178–184.

23 years of age. Weight, height, and blood pressure were measured longitudinally. Lipid and insulin levels were determined at the last follow-up visit. Weight and BMI correlated with young adult weight and BMI. Increases in weight and BMI in children also correlated with systolic blood pressure in young adulthood as well insulin levels and lipid levels in young adulthood. Increases in body mass in childhood will likely contribute to early increase in overall cardiovascular risk.

The identification of genetic determinants of essential hypertension has been challenging, even though remarkable advances have been made regarding the molecular basis of inherited Mendelian disorders. Essential hypertension does not follow simple Mendelian inheritance. Modest genetic differences become relevant only with integration of various environmental exposures.

BLOOD PRESSURE TRACKING

The establishment of normative blood pressure data has lead to the formulation of a subset of patients with intermittent blood pressure elevation or blood pressures between the 90th and 95th percentiles. To date, the data suggest that it is important to identify these patients and follow them periodically because blood pressure in childhood may predict blood pressure in adulthood. Elevated blood pressure in childhood would therefore predict that an individual may develop hypertension as an adult. This notion is called "tracking" and has been a subject of several long-term studies in children and young adults.[9,13,14,15,16] These studies generally support the hypothesis that blood pressure tracks into adulthood, especially if there is a positive family history of hypertension or other risk factors such as obesity.

The Muscatine[9] study enrolled 2445 patients aged 7–18 years in Muscatine, Iowa, and recorded family histories, blood pressures, and other measurements such as height and weight recorded between 1971 and 1978. From this cohort a subset of subjects were identified and recalled as young adults (ages 23–28 years) for repeat evaluations. Subjects with blood pressures above the 90th

percentile in childhood were four times more likely to develop adult hypertension than subjects without elevated systolic blood pressure in childhood. Children with diastolic blood pressures above the 90th percentile were twice as likely to develop adult hypertension as expected. Other factors that presupposed to adult high blood pressure were ponderosity, change in ponderosity, and a positive family history of hypertension.

Another major longitudinal blood pressure study was conducted in Bogalusa, Louisiana, between 1997 and 1983.[13] 1501 subjects aged 2–14 years were studied in 1973 and 5–24 years in 1983. As in the Muscatine study[9] the results supported the notion of blood pressure tracking, with the most significant correlations between childhood and adult blood pressure seen in children aged 10–14 years. A family history of hypertension was predictive of adult hypertension. A family history of stroke and diabetes also tended to predict higher adult blood pressure.

Longitudinal studies from the University of Pennsylvania[15] and Framingham[16] demonstrated that individuals with elevated blood pressures in early childhood were at increased risk of developing hypertension later in life.

It is therefore rational to recommend that elevated blood pressure be followed closely and monitored for the presence of other cardiovascular risks such as hyperlipidemia, stroke, or diabetes.

It has been shown in several reviews[17,18] that people who are smaller at birth tend to have higher blood pressure in later life. It is not clear whether it is fetal growth retardation or the accelerated postnatal growth that often follows that leads to higher blood pressure. A recent study found that lower birth weight and greater weight gain between 1 and 5 years of age were associated with higher systolic blood pressure in young adult life.[19] Weight gain in infancy (the first year of life) was not associated with adult systolic blood pressure; however, a more recent study did not demonstrate the inverse relationship between birth weight and adult systolic blood pressure.[20]

Another potential cause of hypertension is the role of lead exposure. There is considerable controversy originating with the initial epidemiologic study of Pirkle et al.[21] This study pointed out the linear correlation between blood lead and systolic and diastolic blood pressures in males aged 40–59, derived from NHANES II, conducted from 1976 to 1980. Staessen and colleagues,[22] in a meta-analysis of 23 such studies from the general population and 10 from occupational groups, concluded that published evidence shows only a weak positive association between blood pressure and lead exposure. At this time it cannot be concluded that elevated blood lead levels are associated with elevated blood pressure in children.

SECONDARY CAUSES OF HYPERTENSION

The incidence of secondary hypertension in children is higher than in adults. As mentioned above, the frequency of secondary hypertension in children is decreasing. Fifty percent of children with hypertension have primary hypertension. Thirty-five percent have renal parenchymal disease, 5% have renovascular disease, and 2–3% have cardiovascular disease. Endocrine and central nervous system diseases represent a very small percentage of causes of secondary hypertension. Most patients with secondary hypertension have markedly elevated blood pressures (Table 10-5). One should certainly consider searching for a secondary cause of hypertension in children with blood pressures 10 mmHg above the 95th percentile for age and height. Evaluation should focus on the three most common causes of secondary hypertension. One can detect renal parenchymal disease with a urinalysis, blood urea nitrogen (BUN)/creatinine levels, and an imaging test such as renal ultrasound. Renovascular hypertension is uncommon, but a combination of peripheral plasma renin activity and a captopril renogram provides an excellent screening combination. Doppler ultrasound studies can frequently detect turbulence across renal vessels. Because there is less perihilar fat in children, some pediatric radiologists

TABLE 10-5

DIFFERENTIATING PRIMARY FROM SECONDARY HYPERTENSION

Primary BP near the 95th Percentile	Secondary BP usually ≥ 10 mm 95th Percentile
History and Physical	History and Physical
risk factors—	Sx/SSx of systemic diseases
obesity	↑ limb BP/pulses
hyperlipidemia	Lab tests – (general screen for renal diseases)
family history	urinalysis
	BUN/Creat
	renal ultrasound
	Lab tests – specific diseases
	renovascular disease
	renal ultrasound with Doppler
	plasma renin
	coarctation of the aorta
	echocardiography/MRI
	endocrine disease
	urine and serum catecholamines

are able to identify the renal arteries more easily, and advocate that Doppler ultrasound studies are a good screening test for renovascular hypertension. Finally, coarctation of the aorta can be easily diagnosed by demonstrating pulse or blood pressure differences between the upper and lower extremities. If there are questions after the blood pressure determinations, then an echocardiogram or magnetic resonance imaging (MRI) may diagnose coarctation of the aorta. Because endocrine causes are so rare, urine collections for catecholamines and measurements of plasma and urinary steroids should be reserved for children who have very severe hypertension and symptoms such as excessive sweating, episodes of pallor and flushing, muscle cramping, or constipation.

In the newborn and during the first year of life, renovascular disease and coarctation are much more common than renal parenchymal disease. Renovascular disease in the newborn period is often related to thrombosis associated with umbilical artery catheterization.

TREATMENT OF HYPERTENSION

Table 10-6 and Figure 10-1 summarize a general approach to treatment of hypertension. Since there is

increasing literature suggesting the correlation between obesity and hypertension, the first concern in treating a child with hypertension is whether or not the patient is obese. If the BMI is greater than or equal to the 85th percentile and the patient is hypertensive, then effort is focused on weight control. This is often a frustrating exercise but clearly must be pursued.

With regard to drug therapy of childhood hypertension, there are few data available regarding antihypertensive drug efficacy and safety in children. Only captopril, enalapril, short-acting nifedipine, propanolol, methyldopa, diazoxide, hydralazine, and minoxidil have been approved for use in children.[23] The treatment of hypertension in children is based mainly on individual experience and on efficacy and safety trials in adults. The passage of the Food and Drug Administration Modernization Act in 1997 has stimulated drug industry–sponsored trials of antihypertensive agents in children; drug manufacturers benefit financially for conducting pediatric studies by receiving an additional 6 months market exclusivity. Twenty-five years ago there were few efficacious antihypertensive drugs that did not have limiting side effects. Often patients required two and three drugs given three and four times a day. The most difficult aspect of treating children and especially adolescents with antihypertensive drugs is compliance. Newer classes of drugs (Table 10-7) such as long-acting calcium channel blockers, angiolensin-converting enjyme (ACE) inhibitors, angiotensin II receptor antagonists have fewer side effects than older drugs and can often be given once or twice daily to be effective. This, of course, improves compliance considerably.

TABLE 10-6

TREATMENT OF HYPERTENSION

Appropriate Treatment of Underlying Causes
Essential hypertension—obesity
Coarctation of the aorta
Renal and renovascular disease
Endocrine disorders
Timing of Treatment/Considerations
Degree of hypertension
Reversible causes
Weight loss
Biofeedback
Pharmacologic
Nonpharmacologic

TABLE 10-7

INITIATING PHARMACOLOGIC TREATMENT OF HYPERTENSION

1. Calcium channel blockers
2. Beta-blockers
3. ACE inhibitors
4. Angiotensin II receptor antagonists

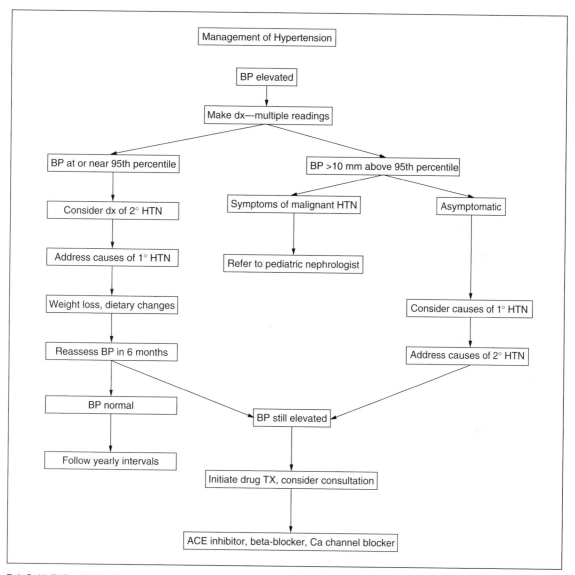

FIGURE 10-1

FLOW DIAGRAM OF INITIATION AND PHARMACOLOGIC MANAGEMENT OF HYPERTENSION

With so many antihypertensive drugs available, it is unlikely that a primary care physician has experience in pediatric patients with many of these medications. At best, one may have experience with one or two drugs in each class. Unless the primary care physician has such experience, referral to a pediatric nephrologist is recommended.

CONCLUSIONS

Elevation of blood pressure may indicate underlying renal disease or other organ disease. It may suggest future cardiovascular risk. Obesity-related hypertension is epidemic and provides a model for studying the nature of primary hypertension. Finally, with the increase in industry-sponsored pediatric antihypertensive trials, pediatricians will have better evidence-based data to guide them in treating childhood hypertension.

References

1   Task Force on Blood Pressure Control in Childhood: Report of the task force. *Pediatrics* 59:787–820, 1977.

2   Task Force on Blood Pressure Control in Children: Report of the second task force of blood pressure control in children. *Pediatrics* 79:1–25, 1987.

3   National High Blood Pressure Education Program Working Group: Update on the 1987 task force report on high blood pressure in children and adolescents: A working group report from the National High Blood Pressure Education Program. *Pediatrics* 98:649–658, 1996.

4   Ingelfinger JR: Ambulatory blood pressure monitoring as a predictive tool. *N Engl J Med* 347:778–779, 2002.

5   Soergel M, Kirschtein M, Busch C, Danne T, Gellerman J, Holl R, Krull F, Reichert H, Reusz G, Rascher W: Oscillometric twenty-four hour ambulatory blood pressure values in healthy children and adolescents: a multicenter trial including 1141 subjects. *J Pediatr* 130:178–184, 1997.

6   Feld LG, Springate: Hypertension in children. *Curr Probl Pediatr* 18:317–373, 1988.

7   Arar MY, Hogg RJ, Arant BS, Seikaly MG: Etiology of sustained hypertension in children in the southwestern United States. *Pediatr Nephrol* 8:186–189, 1994.

8   Flynn JT: Characteristics of children with primary hypertension referred to a tertiary center [abstract]. *Am J Hypertens* 239A, 2001.

9   Lauer RM, Clark WR: Childhood risk factors for high adult blood pressure: the Muscatine study. *Pediatrics* 84:633–641, 1984.

10 Luepker RV, Jacobs DR, Prineas RJ, Sinaiko AR: Secular trends of blood pressure and body size in a multi-ethnic adolescent population 1986 to 1996. *J Pediatr* 134:668–674, 1999.

11 Sorof JM, Eissa MA, Bernard L, Portman RJ: High hypertension prevalence and the relationship of body mass index to blood pressure in ethnic minority children [abstract]. *Am J Hypertens* 14:14A, 2001.

12 Sinaiko AR, Donahue RP, Jacobs Jr DR, Prineas RJ: Relation of weight and rate of increase in weight during childhood and adolescence to body size, blood pressure, fasting insulin, and lipids in young adults: the Minneapolis children's blood pressure study. *Circulation* 99:1471–1476, 1999.

13 Shear CL, Burke GL, Freedman DS, Berenson GS: Value of childhood blood pressure measurements and family history in predicting future blood pressure status: results from 8 years of follow-up in the Bogalusa Heart Study. *Pediatrics* 77:862–869.

14 Bao W, Threefoot SA, Srinivasan SR, Berenson GS: Essential hypertension predicted by tracking of elevated blood pressure from childhood to adulthood: the Bogalusa Heart Study. *Am J Hypertens* 8: 657–665, 1995.

15 Puffenbarger RS, Thorne MC, Wing AL: Chronic disease in former college students, VIII. Characteristics in youth predisposing to hypertension in later years. *Am J Epidemiol* 88:25–32, 1968.

16 Sagie A, Larson MG, Levy D: The natural history of borderline isolated systolic hypertension. *N Engl J Med* 329:1912–1917, 1993.

17 Huxley RR, Shiell AW, Law CM: The role of size at birth and postnatal catch-up growth in determining systolic blood pressure: a systematic review of the literature. *J Hypertens* 18:815–831, 2000.

18 Leon DA, Koupilova I: Birth weight, blood pressure, and hypertension: epidemiological studies, in: Barker DJP (ed): *Fetal Origins of Cardiovascular and Lung Disease.* Bethesda, MD, National Institutes of Health, 1999.

19 Law CM, Shiell AW, Syddall, ME, Shinebourne EA, Fayers PM, de Swiet M: Fetal, infant and childhood growth and adult blood pressure: a longitudinal study from birth to 22 years of age. *Circulation* 105:1088–1098, 2002.

20 Huxley R, Nell A, Collins R: Unraveling the fetal origins hypothesis: is there really an invasive association between birth weight and subsequent blood pressure? *Lancet* 360:659–665, 2002.

21 Pirkle JL, Schwartz J, Landis JR, Marland WR: The relationship between blood lead levels and blood pressure and its cardiovascular risk implications. *Am J Epidemiol* 121:246–258, 1985.

22 Staessen JA, Roels H, Lauwerys RR, Amery A: Low-level lead exposure and blood pressure. *J Hum Hypertens* 91:303–328, 1995.

23 *Physicians' Desk Reference*, 56th ed. Montvale, NJ, Medical Economics Company, 2002.

11

BASIC PATHOPHYSIOLOGY

Left-to-Right Shunts

Hitendra T. Patel

INTRODUCTION

In order to understand the abnormal, it is important first to look at the normal heart physiology and the fundamental elements of cardiac function. The physiologic purpose of the heart is to pump a specific volume of blood dictated by the metabolic demands of the body.

BASIC CARDIAC PHYSIOLOGY

The cardiac output (CO) = stroke volume (SV) × heart rate (HR). The stroke volume is determined by the preload, afterload, and contractility of the heart. Blood pressure is a product of blood flow or cardiac output and resistance. Blood flow like other fluids obeys the rules of Ohm's law, which states that electron flow or current in amperes (I) is determined by the potential difference or voltage (V) and resistance (Ω). The equation is $V = I \times \Omega$.

If we apply this equation to the blood flow circuit, the following equations are derived:

Pressure drop across the pulmonary vascular bed = pulmonary blood flow (PBF) × pulmonary vascular resistance (PVR). Or

[Mean pulmonary artery pressure (PAP) − mean left atrial pressure (LAP)] = PBF × PVR

Pressure drop across the systemic vascular bed = systemic blood flow (BF) × systemic vascular resistance (SVR). Or

[Mean aortic pressure (AoP) − mean right atrial pressure (RAP)] = SBF × SVR

(NB: For both these equations to be correct, it is assumed that no peripheral stenoses exist and the arterial pressure represents arteriolar pressure and atrial pressure represents the venous pressure of the vascular or "capacitance" bed.)

In the normal circulation with no intracardiac shunts Qp = Qs. The normal pressure drop across the pulmonary vascular bed is about 5–8 mmHg and 65–100 mmHg across the systemic vascular bed. Since Qp = Qs, the PVR has to be about 5–10% of the SVR. Normal PVR is <2 Wood's units (WU) and SVR 20–25 Wood's units. (Note the resistance units are mmHg per liter per minute or often referred to as Wood's units after Dr. Paul Wood who first introduced the concept. They can be expressed as metric units (dyn.s.cm^{-5}) by multiplying the WU resistance by 80.

The heart is divided into two components. The right side receives the deoxygenated blood, which is then pumped to the pulmonary vascular bed for gas exchange. In the pulmonary vascular capillary bed, carbon dioxide is expelled and oxygen is absorbed and bound to hemoglobin. The blood then returns from the lungs to the left side of the heart, where it is then pumped to the body tissues for metabolism. These two circulations are in series and the volume of blood coursing through the two circulations or circuits has to be equal, the input volume equals the output volume (conservation of mass). Thus, systemic venous return = pulmonary blood flow (Qp) = pulmonary venous return = systemic blood flow (Qs) which is sufficient to meet the metabolic demands of the body. Many factors, both mechanical and neuroendocrine, adjust to maintain this equality.

VENTRICULAR FUNCTION

The cardiac cycle can be divided into systole and diastole. The energy expenditure of the right ventricle (RV) is much less than the left ventricle (LV) because it has to generate a much lower pressure to overcome the PVR in order for flow to occur. Cardiac output as mentioned earlier is dependent on HR and SV. SV is dependent on the preload, contractility, and afterload on the ventricle. Myocardial wall stress and oxygen consumption are also important in understanding cardiac function.

Preload is the load present before ventricular contraction and is provided by the venous return to the atrium that empties into the ventricle.

Afterload is the load against which the ventricle has to contract. This is directly proportional to the total PVR for the RV or the SVR for the LV.

Contractility or the inotropic state is defined as the rate of change in ventricular pressure over rate of change in time. Increased contractility results in a greater velocity of contraction and the contracting ventricle reaches a greater peak tension or pressure while other influencing factors, heart rate, preload, and afterload remain constant.

Preload, contractility, and afterload are intimately linked. Starling's law of the heart states that "within physiologic limits, the larger the volume of the heart, the greater the energy of its contraction and the amount of chemical change at each contraction." Heart rate also affects contractility. A faster rate increases the force of contraction independent of preload or afterload. It is believed that repetitive Ca^{2+} entry with each depolarization leads to accumulation of cytosolic calcium. This is known as the Bowditch or Treppe phenomenon.

DETERMINANTS OF MYOCARDIAL WORK

Myocardial wall stress. This is the stress that develops during myocardial contraction and relaxation. Force (Newton: N) is the term used to describe acceleration of a moving object. Tension exists when two opposing forces are applied to an object, e.g., when a spring is pulled apart tension exists within the spring. Stress develops when tension is applied to a cross-sectional area, and obeys Laplace's law:

Ventricular wall stress (in N/m^2) = ventricular pressure × radius/2 × wall thickness.

The equation also shows how increased ventricular dilation or pressure leads to increased wall stress and compensatory wall hypertrophy will decrease wall stress. Wall stress is also helpful in understanding preload and afterload. Preload is the wall stress at the end of diastole or at the maximum

TABLE 11-1

DETERMINANTS OF MVO$_2$

Tension development, preload
Contractile state
Heart rate
Afterload
Basal metabolic cellular requirement
Electric activation, depolarization, and repolarization
Metabolic effects of catecholamine state
Uptake of nutrients for energy

TABLE 11-3

EFFECT OF MVO$_2$ FOLLOWING 50% INCREASE

Wall stress	25%
Contractility	45%
Pressure work	50%
Heart rate	50%
Volume work	4%

Source: Gould KL: *Coronary Artery Stenosis*, New York, NY, Elsevier, 1991.

resting length of the sarcomere. Afterload is the wall stress during ventricular ejection.

MYOCARDIAL OXYGEN CONSUMPTION (MVO$_2$)

The heart muscle relies almost exclusively on oxidative metabolism to meet its energy needs. It is therefore important to understand the factors that determine MVO$_2$ (see Tables 11-1 and 11-2). This can help in the understanding and management of disease states.

Tables 11-2 and 11-3 are important in showing the types of cardiac work that use the most energy and therefore are the most demanding for the cardiac muscle. It can be seen that increases in pressure work, heart rate, contractility, and wall stress all lead to substantial increase and volume work causes minimal increase in MVO$_2$.

TABLE 11-2

MVO$_2$—DISTRIBUTION AT BASAL STATE

Basal metabolic requirement	20%
Electric activity	1%
Pressure work	64%
Volume work	14%

Source: Gould KL: *Coronary Artery Stenosis*, New York, NY, Elsevier, 1991.

PRESSURE VERSUS VOLUME WORK AND MVO$_2$

The pressure volume (*P/V*) relation during ventricular contraction and relaxation is illustrated in Figure 11-1A. It shows that myocardial work is divided into internal work (IW) and external work (EW), and the *P/V* area is the sum of IW and EW. EW is quantified by the *P/V* area that represents ventricular filling and ejection or muscle shortening. IW is the energy used to generate force that occurs independent of muscle shortening. In its basic form, if the ventricle were completely empty with no pressure load, it would be at point "e" in Figure 11-1; however, even at end systole the ventricle is not empty and the resulting volume creates wall stress and therefore pressure, which requires energy. It has been shown that IW is the major determinant of MVO$_2$ compared to EW. Figure 11-1B compares the *P/V* loops of the right and left ventricles. It also shows that the total work and hence oxygen consumption of the LV is much greater than the RV.

These concepts of wall stress, IW, EW, and other factors that affect MVO$_2$, become important in a discussion of intracardiac shunts, valve stenosis, and the body's ability to compensate for these. Figure 11-1C and 11-1D illustrate the *P/V* changes that occur with a volume and pressure load on the heart. Volume load leads predominantly to an increase in EW whereas pressure work leads to an increase in IW, and therefore significantly increases in myocardial oxygen consumption. Volume load leads to increased fiber length and not pressure

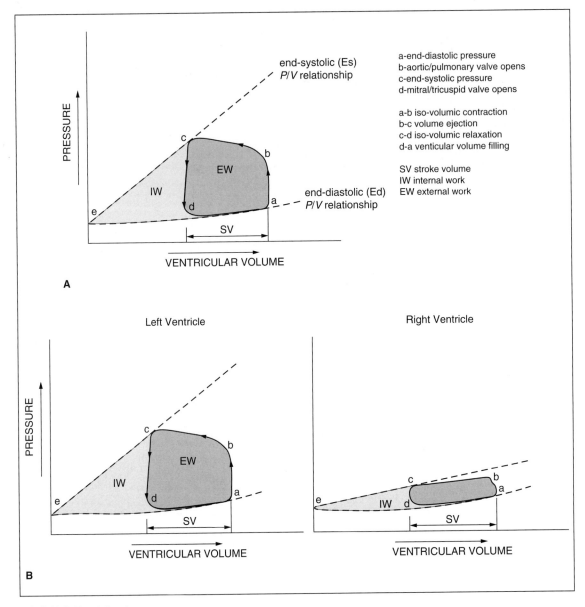

FIGURE 11-1

THE PRESSURE VOLUME RELATION DURING VENTRICULAR CONTRACTION AND RELAXATION

A. Pressure volume (*P/V*) changes during a ventricular contraction and relaxation. **B**. Right and left ventricular pressure volume (*P/V*) changes during a ventricular contraction and relaxation. **C**. *P/V* changes with volume load on ventricular work. **D**. *P/V* changes with pressure load on ventricular work. *Source:* Adapted from Opie LH. *The Heart: Physiology From Cell to Circulation*, 3rd ed. Philadelphia, PA, Lippincott-Raven, 1997.

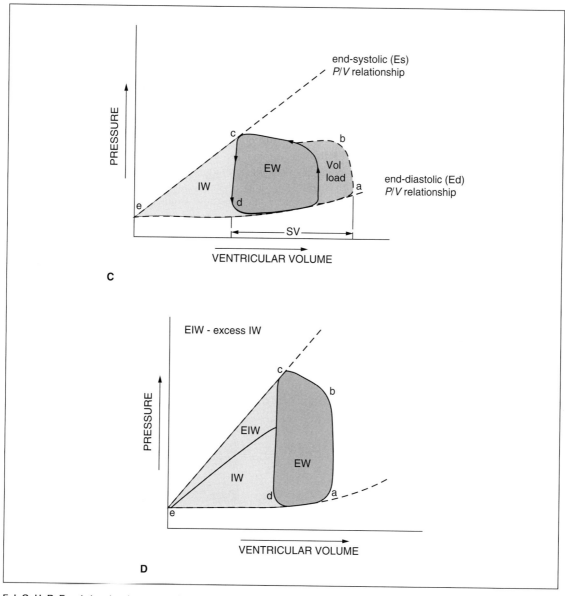

FIGURE 11-1 (continued)

increase, so the amount of EW is increased but IW stays the same, the heart is more efficient in part from the Starling principle. With a pressure load there is a significant increase in IW with an unchanged EW leading to myocardial inefficiency, higher energy expenditure for the same amount of volume ejected.

INTRACARDIAC LEFT-TO-RIGHT SHUNTS

Normally the volume of pulmonary venous return equals the left ventricular SV, which equals the volume of blood that reaches metabolizing tissues

(Figure 11-2A). The amount of blood volume required is dependent on the metabolic rate of the body. Shunts imply a "leak" or a "short circuit" in the system. A left-to-right shunt (L-R shunt) implies that not all of the pulmonary venous return reaches the metabolizing tissues and that there is a "short circuit" or pathway back to the pulmonary circulation. Blood is able to bypass one circulation and reach the other, which leads to inefficiency and increased demand on the pump. The left side of the heart is usually under higher pressures, and any communication between the right and left sides of the heart will result in blood shunting from the left to the right side. Acutely, a shunt from the left to the right side

of the heart will result in decreased flow to the body (Qs) and increased flow to the lungs (Qp) (Figure 11-2B). For the human body to continue to function and not be in shock or failure, the volume of blood reaching the metabolizing tissue has to be constant. The body therefore responds acutely with increased heart rate and contractility of the heart to acutely increase cardiac output to maintain a constant volume to the metabolizing tissues. Longer term, the body will increase the intravascular volume so that the net result will be a normal heart rate with a normal cardiac output (Figure 11-2C). The amount of any shunt is determined by the size of the hole and the net downstream resistance.

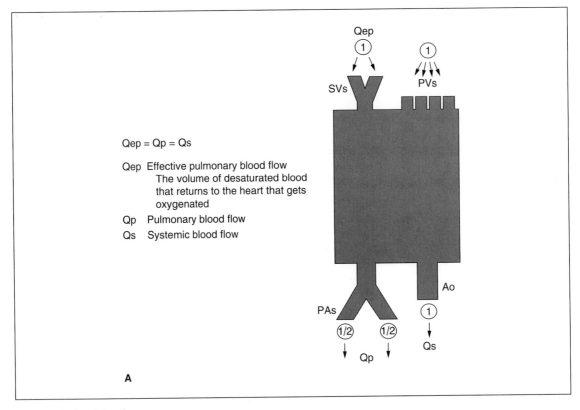

FIGURE 11-2

This figure shows a "black box" heart demonstrating that the gross effects of intracardiac shunting can be similar externally in the acute and chronic phases, but do not reveal what occurs within the heart.
A. The normal cardiac circulation. **B.** The consequence of an acute left-to-right shunt. **C.** The consequence of compensated left-to-right shunt.

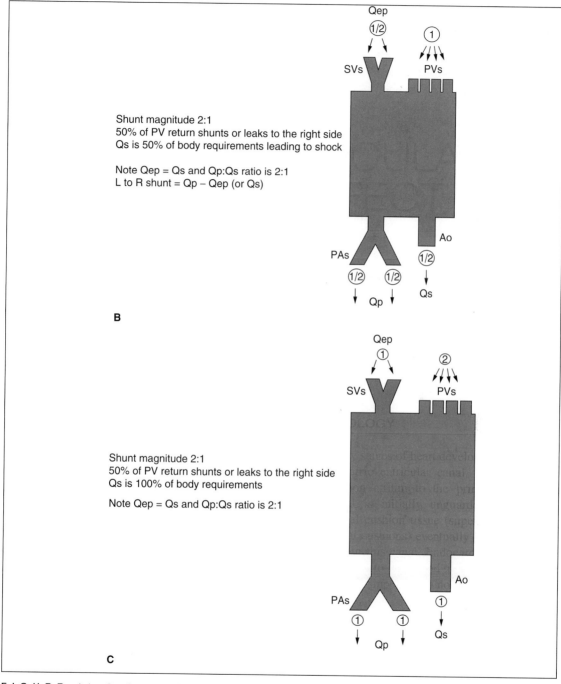

Shunt magnitude 2:1
50% of PV return shunts or leaks to the right side
Qs is 50% of body requirements leading to shock

Note Qep = Qs and Qp:Qs ratio is 2:1
L to R shunt = Qp – Qep (or Qs)

B

Shunt magnitude 2:1
50% of PV return shunts or leaks to the right side
Qs is 100% of body requirements

Note Qep = Qs and Qp:Qs ratio is 2:1

C

FIGURE 11-2 (continued)

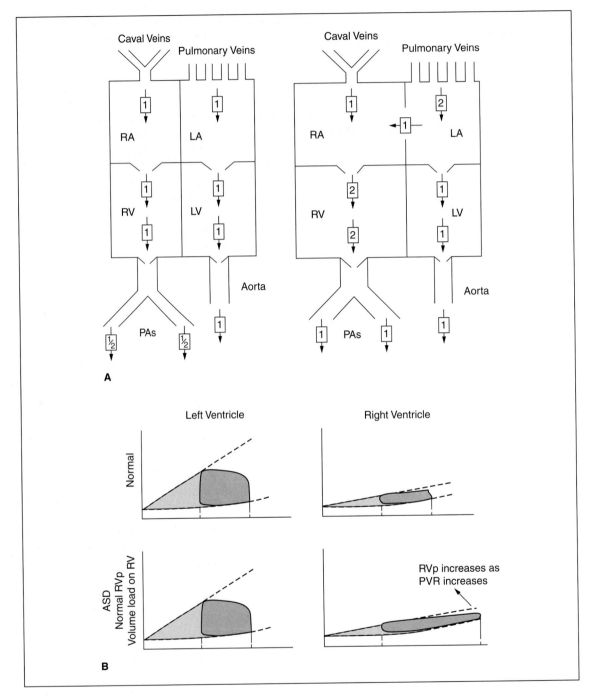

FIGURE 11-3

A. Normal heart and 2:1 atrial level (ASD) shunt. B. *P/V* changes with a large ASD.

ATRIAL LEVEL
LEFT-TO-RIGHT SHUNTS

The flow across an atrial septal defect (ASD) or other atrial level shunt occurs in diastole and its direction depends on the differences in the atrial pressures, which are determined by the amount of venous return, atrial outflow obstruction, and atrial and ventricular compliance rather than PVR or SVR (though the latter are indirect factors). The compliance of the atria is in part determined by their respective ventricular compliance. Ventricular compliance is dependent on ventricular wall thickness, which is directly proportional to ventricular pressure and the PVR in the case of the RV and SVR in the LV. As RV pressure and PVR increase the RV wall thickness increases leading to a fall in RV and RA compliance. Normally the mean LAP is 6–9 mmHg and the mean RAP is 1–4 mmHg, which favors an L-R shunt. The pressure in atria is also dependent on the compliance of the ventricles. If the ventricles are poorly compliant or stiff, then a higher atrial pressure is required for filling to occur. Unless the communicating defect is small the amount of flow is dependent on the difference in compliance of the right and left ventricles rather than the pressure since a large defect will equalize the LA and RA pressures. Normally the right ventricular compliance is much higher than the left ventricle, resulting in an L-R shunt across the ASD; its magnitude is dependent on the relative difference. At birth, because of the high PVR in utero, the RV and LV wall thickness and hence compliance are similar and the amount of flow across the ASD is minimal or even bidirectional. As soon as lung inflation occurs and PVR begins to fall, the RV compliance begins to increase relative to the LV. This leads to L-R flow across the ASD, which will continue to increase as the PVR continues to fall and the RV compliance continues to increase. LV compliance is relatively stable for the first 20–30 years of life. As aging occurs, the arteriolar elasticity decreases and SVR increases, leading to higher blood pressure (BP). This leads to higher energy expenditure by the LV to overcome increased afterload and subsequent LV hypertrophy. LV compliance decreases with a subsequent

elevation in LA pressure and further increase in L-R shunt. Figure 11-3A schematically demonstrates a 2:1 atrial level shunt. Note that since the atrial level shunt occurs in diastole there is a volume load on the RA and RV with subsequent chamber dilation. Figure 11-3B shows the *P/V* changes with an atrial level shunt. Note that myocardial work changes little from the baseline as long as the PVR and PAP remains low. This in part explains why an atrial level shunt is clinically well tolerated with minimal symptoms and signs until adulthood. The increased PBF results in a slow increase in pulmonary vascular muscularization and PVR. As PVR increases, the RV compliance decreases, reducing the L-R shunt. Rarely, usually after the fifth decade of life, right-to-left shunting may occur (see chapter on ASD).

VENTRICULAR LEVEL L-R SHUNT

The hemodynamic effects of a ventricular or great vessel level defect are similar to each other. A defect at the ventricular level allows blood in the ventricles two possible forward pathways, pulmonary or systemic. Blood will flow to the circulation with the lowest resistance, usually the pulmonary. Blood in the RV will flow to the pulmonary circulation. Blood in the LV will preferentially flow across the ventricular septal defect (VSD) into the pulmonary circulation as well as the systemic circulation. Like the ASD, the size of the defect will influence the amount of L-R flow if the defect is pressure restrictive. The size of the defect offers resistance and its hemodynamic significance can be determined by comparing RV pressure to LV pressure, as long as the PVR is normal and not affecting the baseline RV pressure. If the defect is very small the RV pressure will be near normal. In this case, the defect itself limits the amount of L-R shunting. As the defect increases in size it becomes less restrictive and PVR and SVR become more important in determining the amount of L-R flow. In a large nonrestrictive defect, the LV, RV, and PA systolic pressure are the same and the differences in PVR and SVR determines the degree of L-R shunt across the VSD.

The following equation becomes important in the ensuing discussion.

$$pressure = flow \times resistance$$

If PVR remains low, then PA and RV pressure will increase proportional to the increase in pulmonary flow secondary to the L-R shunt. Of note is that the L-R flow occurs in systole, and the shunting occurs while the right ventricle is contracting. Thus, the flow is directly to the PA and does not volume load the RV; however, the increased pulmonary blood flow returns to the left heart, creating LA and LV dilation (left-sided volume loading). There is a volume and pressure load on the pulmonary arterial circulation. The LV stroke volume is increased depending on the amount of shunt. If 50% of LV stroke volume shunts to the PA, then the LV stroke volume has to be 200% of baseline to achieve the

required systemic output. This is a 2:1 shunt; with a 3:1 shunt the LV output has to be 300% of normal Figure 11-4A. At its maximal efficiency the heart can increase cardiac output four to six times from its resting output. In a patient with a 2:1 shunt or greater the body has decreased ability to further augment the cardiac output during exercise. Typically, no ventricular level shunt occurs during diastole; however, in severe disease with LV failure and elevated LV end diastolic pressure, L-R diastolic flow may occur depending on the relative ventricular compliance. Figure 11-4B illustrates the left and right ventricular *P/V* loops for a moderate and large VSD. It shows that with a VSD the volume load on the LV leads to an increase in EW and the pressure load on the RV leads to an increase in IW and EW. Compare this to the *P/V* diagram for an ASD and it is clear that the myocardial work and

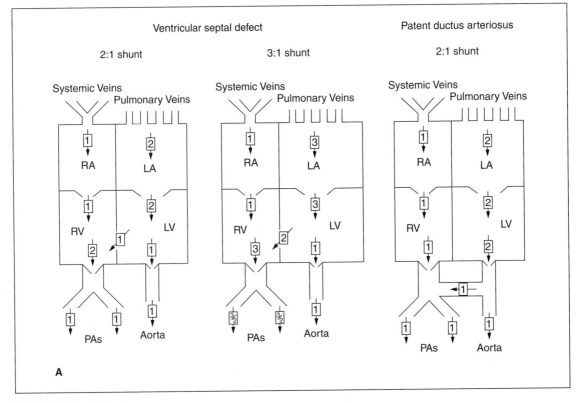

A

FIGURE 11-4

A. Ventricular and arterial level shunt. **B**. *P/V* loop changes associated with VSD.

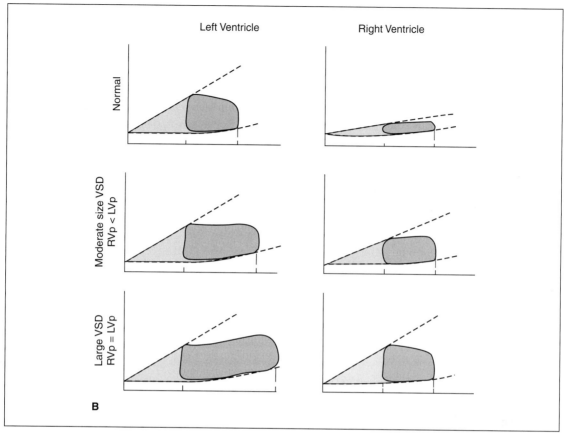

B

FIGURE 11-4 (continued)

hence oxygen consumption is significantly higher for the VSD (see chapter on VSD).

ARTERIAL LEVEL L-R SHUNT

In an arterial level shunt (Figure 11-4A), all the physiologic principles outlined above apply; however, the L-R shunt is continuous in systole and diastole. The aortic systolic and diastolic pressure and SVR are higher than the pulmonary systolic, and diastolic pressure and PVR throughout the cardiac cycle. Thus, for any given size of defect the volume load to the pulmonary vasculature, LA and LV is greater than a similar size VSD. L-R flow is determined by

the size of the communication and the difference in the PVR and SVR. Significant "aortic run off" in diastole leads to a low diastolic pressure with widened pulse pressure. This may affect coronary perfusion and myocardial oxygen supply.

Other factors that affect resistance will impact on the magnitude of the shunt. Of primary importance is blood viscosity. This is determined by the fluid composition, predominantly the hemoglobin concentration. Following birth the hemoglobin concentration falls, reaching a nadir at about 2–3 months. This coincides with the normal drop in PVR secondary to muscular atrophy of the pulmonary arterioles. Both these factors are additive in decreasing PVR and increasing the L-R shunt.

Right-to-Left Shunts

Peter Koenig

The causes of cyanosis/desaturation and the general workup have been discussed in a previous chapter. Once it has been determined that there is a cardiac cause of oxygen desaturation, a definitive cardiac diagnosis ought to be made.

Frequently, mnemonics are incorporated to arrive at a differential diagnosis such as the "four Ts and one P" meaning:

1. TGA: transposition of the great arteries
2. TOF: tetralogy of Fallot
3. Tricuspid atresia
4. Truncus arteriosus
5. TAPVC: total anomalous pulmonary venous connection
6. Pulmonary atresia

Tables have also been constructed which subgroup these "cyanotic" lesions by the relative amounts of pulmonary blood flow (as may be seen on a chest film) as follows:

1. Increased pulmonary blood flow (mixing lesions)
   a. Transposition of the great arteries
   b. Total anomalous pulmonary venous connection
   c. Truncus arteriosus
2. Normal pulmonary blood flow
   a. No lesions in this category
3. Decreased pulmonary blood flow
   a. Tetralogy of Fallot
   b. Tricuspid atresia
   c. Ebstein's anomaly
   d. Pulmonary atresia

The differential diagnosis based on key laboratory findings on electrocardiogram (ECG) and the plain chest film has also been used to arrive at the diagnosis. Key findings or clues to each of these major categories are as follows (PVM: pulmonary vascular markings; RVH: right ventricular hypertrophy; RAE: right atrial enlargement; LVH: left ventricular hypertrophy; LAD: left axis deviation; RBBB: right bundle branch block; WPW: Wolff-Parkinson-White):

Lesion	ECG	Chest x-ray (CXR)
TGA	RVH	"egg on a string" pattern, increased PVM
TAPVC	RVH, RAE	"snowman" heart—cardiomegaly, increased PVM
Truncus arteriosus	RVH	cardiomegaly with increased PVM
Tetralogy of Fallot	RVH	"Boot shaped heart," decreased PVM
Tricuspid atresia	LVH, LAD, RAE	decreased PVM
Ebsteins anomaly	RBBB, RAE, WPW	massive cardiomegaly— "wall to wall"
Pulmonary atresia		
No VSD	LVH, LAD	decreased PVM
VSD	RVH	"boot shaped heart," decreased PVM

Unfortunately, the above categories are frequently correct only a fraction of the time, and they deemphasize understanding the underlying pathophysiology. In addition, there are many variations of the above lesions, leading to more confusion. For instance, TGA may have decreased pulmonary blood flow in the face of increased pulmonary vascular resistance, and tetralogy of Fallot may have increased pulmonary blood flow and nearly normal pulmonary arteries with minimal right ventricular outflow obstruction or numerous aortopulmonary collaterals. In the variation known as tetralogy of Fallot with absent pulmonary valve, the pulmonary arteries may be massively enlarged. Therefore, the following algorithm may be more useful by emphasizing the underlying anatomic abnormality in an organized fashion followed by applying basic concepts in physiology. Each category will be discussed in general terms with reference to a more detailed discussion and diagram elsewhere in this book. Once a cardiac diagnosis of oxygen desaturation is highly suspected, the underlying diagnosis is required. This is usually performed with noninvasive imaging such as echocardiography. In general, echocardiography is definitive in sorting out the following lesions and making a definitive diagnosis. The clinical and physical features of each lesion are described in separate chapters. The following outline is a logical manner of sorting out the various lesions (Table 11-4).

TABLE 11-4

DIFFERENTIAL DIAGNOSIS OF CARDIAC CAUSES OF DESATURATION

1. Mixing lesions
   - Obligate right-to-left shunting
     - Significant obstruction to blood flow
       Right-sided obstruction
         Cortriatriatum dexter
         Tricuspid atresia
         Pulmonary atresia/critical stenosis
         PPHN
       Left-sided obstruction
         Cortriatriatum sinister
         Mitral atresia
         Aortic atresia/critical stenosis
         Critical coarctation of the aorta
     - No obstruction to blood flow
       TAPVR
       Common atrium
       Common ventricle
       Truncus arteriosus
   - Nonobligate right-to-left shunting
       ASD
       VSD
       PDA
2. Nonmixing lesion
       TGA

Mixing lesions are a cause of cyanosis or desaturation because all of them have the potential for right-to-left shunting, or mixing of desaturated blood with saturated blood. A requirement is that the mixing occur in a chamber that is connected to systemic blood flow from the heart. The net result is a level of desaturation that is proportional to the relative oxygen contents of the saturated and desaturated blood. The oxygen content is related to the amount of blood flow, the hemoglobin concentration, and the saturation. The lesions with obligate right-to-left shunting differ from those with nonobligate shunting in that the latter only have right-to-left shunting with alterations (elevation) in pulmonary vascular resistance (which may be present in utero or at birth). Obligate right-to-left shunts must mix, owing to anatomic abnormalities.

The obligate mixing lesions can be further categorized into those with obstruction and those without. The nonobstructive lesions all have in common the fact that two chambers are combined into a single mixing chamber. In TAPVR, the venous inflow "chambers" are combined into a venous mixing chamber that may be supra, infra, or intracardiac in location. In a single atrium, the two atria act as one large atrial mixing chamber. A single ventricle is similar to this. Truncus arteriosus can be thought of as a single outlet or "trunk" into which blood from both ventricles enters and mixes.

The obligate mixing lesions with obstruction can be subdivided into those with right- or left-sided obstruction. A major difference between these two categories is that the right-sided obstructive lesions require a source of pulmonary blood flow (usually a patent ductus arteriosus [PDA], with low pulmonary vascular resistance to enhance pulmonary blood flow) while the left-sided obstructive lesions require a source of systemic blood flow (usually a PDA as well, though high pulmonary vascular resistance is needed to enhance shunting to the body and minimal systemic to pulmonary artery steal). In addition, both the right-sided and left obstructive lesions require a patent foramen ovale (PFO) or VSD to decompress the chamber encountering obstruction to blood flow. This allows mixing (obligate) to occur at that location. Primary pulmonary hypertension of the newborn (PPHN) is added in the differential of obstructive, obligate mixing lesions as the elevated PVR in PPHN acts similar to an anatomic obstruction causing right-to-left shunting via the PDA. In the case of critical coarctation of the aorta, and in the presence of elevated pulmonary vascular resistance, a difference in saturation may be found between the upper and lower extremity. The amount of mixing and net oxygen saturation is determined by the relative amounts of blood flow and oxygen content. This pathophysiology is explained for each lesion in its representative chapter.

The one nonmixing lesion is transposition of the great arteries (discussed in the next chapter). Cyanosis or desaturation occurs because of a *lack of mixing*. In this lesion, the pulmonary and systemic circulations run in parallel instead of in series, resulting in nonmixing. In fact, one of the treatments is to create a large ASD (common atrium) to enhance mixing at the atrial level.

In this algorithm, the application of estimated PVR to the underlying anatomic lesion should lead to the prediction of physical findings, level of saturation, and the findings on the chest film. A detailed description of lesions is found in the respective chapters.

Physiology of Transposition of the Great Arteries

Peter Koenig

Transposition of the great arteries (TGA) is discussed separately as the physiology is different than other causes of right-to-left shunting. In other forms of cyanotic or desaturated congenital heart disease, desaturated or cyanotic blood is shunted and mixed into saturated, acyanotic blood which causes relative desaturated blood to be supplied to the body. In the case of transposition, the blood going to the body is desaturated at the start as it is the same blood returning from the body. Thus, it is a *lack of shunting or mixing* that causes cyanosis or desaturation in TGA. In a similar fashion, pulmonary blood is fully saturated as it is the same blood returning from the pulmonary veins. Both the systemic and pulmonary circulations run in parallel (Figure 31-1,) rather than in series (Figure 11-3).

Note that the type of transposition discussed in this chapter and in other chapters deals with anatomic and physiologic transposition (D-TGA). The term *transposition* merely implies that the aorta arises from the right ventricle and the pulmonary artery from the left ventricle. There are other heart lesions such as L-TGA in which the ventricles are looped abnormally and blood flows from the right atrium to the left ventricle to the pulmonary arteries. It then returns from the lungs to the left atrium, flowing to the right ventricle and out to the aorta. In this case, the aorta and pulmonary artery are transposed, but the ventricles are

switched as well. Thus, the systemic and pulmonary blood flow is in the normal direction even though the anatomy is not normal. This is also known as physiologically corrected transposition of the great arteries.

As stated, in D-TGA, the pulmonary and systemic circulations run in parallel. If there is no communication between them, systemic blood will lack oxygenation and result in death. Fortunately, the foramen ovale is usually patent (PFO) in the neonate. This allows for pulmonary venous return to mix with systemic venous return and provide oxygenation of systemic blood flow. In the absence of a foramen ovale, this will not occur. The addition of a patent ductus arteriosus (PDA) will allow augmentation of pulmonary blood flow. Shunting at the level of the ductus arteriosus is almost always from the aorta to the pulmonary artery unless there is severely elevated pulmonary vascular resistance. It is frequently and mistakenly felt that the presence of a PDA will allow highly saturated pulmonary blood to flow directly into the aorta. Contrary to this, the blood flows from the aorta to the pulmonary artery, which increases pulmonary blood flow, thereby increasing pulmonary venous return and increasing left atrial pressure. It is the latter which will increase the mixing of highly saturated blood with desaturated blood at the level of the PFO. A larger PFO or an atrial septal defect will have improved mixing.

Obstruction

Peter Koenig

OVERVIEW OF OBSTRUCTION

Physiologically, obstruction creates an increased afterload. This afterload may be dynamic (e.g., systemic or pulmonary vascular resistance) or fixed (e.g., aortic or pulmonary stenosis). In both cases, the physiologic effect is the same, with similar compensatory responses. These responses need to be sufficient to compensate for the obstruction, otherwise, heart failure occurs (inability of the cardiac system to deliver blood sufficient to the needs of the body).

ACUTE AND CHRONIC RESPONSES TO OBSTRUCTION

One general concept, the conservation of mass, prevails with any alteration in cardiac physiology. In terms of the cardiovascular system, this means that the amount of blood that leaves the heart and flows to the body (cardiac output) is the same amount of blood that returns to the heart. An acute obstruction, which overwhelms the hearts ability to compensate, will decrease the amount of blood leaving the heart and returning to it (a low-flow state or shock). With time, responses will occur to restore the heart's ability to deliver the baseline cardiac output. Depending on the reserve the heart has to overcome the obstruction, the acute decline in cardiac output may not occur at all (fully compensated obstruction), or may occur immediately (acute heart failure). It may also persist or develop over time (chronic heart failure), or may occur and disappear over time (compensated heart failure). This is shown in Figure 11-5. Even with fully compensated obstruction, if the body's demands increases, the heart may not have a reserve to compensate for the demand for an increased cardiac output in addition to the obstruction. Thus, there is the concept of heart failure as a

dynamic state, which depends on the changing demands on the heart, the underlying anatomy and pathology of the heart, and the heart's ability to compensate for any pathologic changes.

Other concepts are the general responses of the cardiovascular system when obstruction occurs. These responses are different depending on whether the obstruction occurs in the venous system, the atria, the ventricles, or the arterial system. Obstruction creates an increased afterload and wall stress on the atrial and ventricles. In general, if a chamber can reduce the wall stress, it will. This occurs via hypertrophy. Chambers able to hypertrophy will do so, such as the ventricles (Figure 11-6B), and to a much lesser extent in the atria, arteries, and veins (Figure 11-6A). Chambers unable to respond via hypertrophy become dilated. Dilation occurs in the acute setting with any chamber unable to generate a pressure sufficient to overcome the obstruction. Other than the acute setting, dilation, in general, occurs in the veins and atria.

Other effects of obstruction include dilation, which may occur as a result of the jet effect on chambers distal to the obstruction (poststenotic dilation) and is generally seen only in the arteries. Collateral formation may occur to overcome the obstruction and is seen in the arterial and venous system. Examples of this are arterial collaterals with coarctation of the aorta, and venous collaterals with obstruction of the inferior vena cava.

Obstruction, in the compensated state, also leads to pressure gradients; however, general rules apply. In order to generate a pressure gradient, there can only be one path of blood flow (no bypass of the obstruction). An example is in the pulmonary arteries. If there is obstruction in one pulmonary artery, blood may flow through the other, thus not causing an expected gradient across the area of obstruction. In addition, there is an element of time.

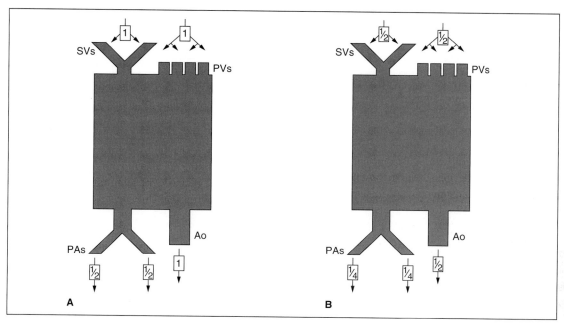

FIGURE 11-5

NORMAL HEART FLOW AND CHANGES WITH OBSTRUCTION

In this figure, the heart is represented as a "black box." Regardless of the type of obstruction, the net results shown in figures A and B are the same. The numbers inside the boxes represent relative cardiac outputs, meaning that the cardiac output is consistent with the systemic demands (a 1:1 ratio). **A** shows a heart at baseline. **B** shows a heart with acute obstruction. In this case, the heart has not yet compensated and there is a decreased cardiac output. With compensation, there is a return to the baseline state (**A**) although there are changes within the heart. These are shown in later diagrams.

An expected pressure gradient will not be seen if the blood flow can be extended over a greater period of time. An example of this is in flow across the ventricles, which have a short systolic interval, versus flow in veins, in which blood flow can be extended over a greater period during diastole. Thus, obstruction to ventricular ejection will lead to a greater gradient than will obstruction to venous blood returning to the heart.

THE PHYSICAL EXAMINATION WITH UNDERLYING OBSTRUCTION

General concepts apply to the translation of the underlying pathophysiology of obstruction to the findings on the physical examination. Hypertrophy of a ventricle leads to a ventricular tap or knock. Dilation of a ventricle will lead to the finding of a ventricular heave or lift. In each case, the location on the chest corresponds to the ventricle involved. In practice, ventricular heaves and taps may be difficult to distinguish clinically and both findings may be simply described as a hyperdynamic precordium.

Another physical finding is a pathologic murmur owing to increased turbulence across the area of obstruction. Murmurs are related to blood flow velocity. This is increased exponentially when obstruction and a pressure gradient exist. This flow velocity is greater with greater pressure gradients (higher velocities). Thus, murmurs are louder with obstructions to ventricular blood flow versus venous obstruction because of the greater pressure gradients. The murmurs will occur in the phase of the cardiac cycle in which there is turbulent blood flow. (A diastolic murmur occurs with stenosis of the mitral and tricuspid valves, a systolic murmur with stenosis

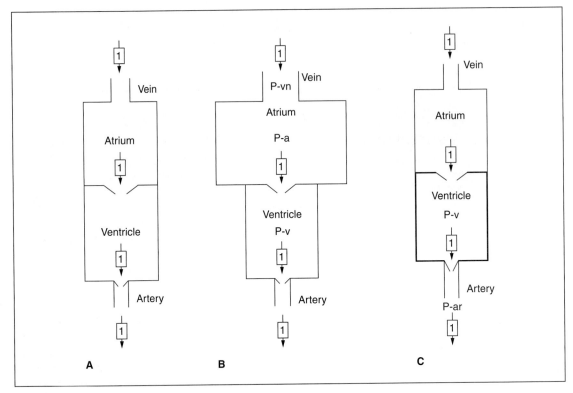

FIGURE   11-6

PATHOPHYSIOLOGY OF OBSTRUCTION

A shows a theoretical two-chamber heart. **B** shows a heart with obstruction between the proximal (atrial) and distal (ventricular) chamber. Note that the cardiac output remains the same throughout. In **B**, the atrium is enlarged and mildly hypertrophied. The pressure in the vein (P-vn) and atria (P-a) is increased in this type of obstruction. In **C**, there is an example of obstruction to outflow of the distal chamber (ventricle). There is significant hypertrophy of this chamber. The pressure in the ventricle (P-v) is increased in systole compared to the pressure in the artery (P-ar). The gradient is determined by the systolic pressure difference in each.

of the aortic and pulmonary valves, and a continuous murmur with coarctation of the aorta.)

Physical findings indirectly related to the obstruction may also be present and include signs and symptoms of heart failure if it exists, and the backward transmission of elevated pressures.

LABORATORY FINDINGS
WITH OBSTRUCTION

Laboratory findings will reflect the underlying physiologic derangements within the limits of the ability of the test to do so. Thus, the ECG may reflect hypertrophy or chamber enlargement. The chest radiograph will reflect enlargement of the ventricles in total (generally chamber enlargement rather than hypertrophy) as well as enlargement of any atria, veins, or other vessels. Echocardiography will reveal chamber enlargement and hypertrophy as well as demonstrate any areas of blood flow turbulence via Doppler. Pressure gradients may be estimated using Doppler principles as well. Finally, cardiac catheterization can directly measure pressure gradients as well as show areas of obstruction via angiography.

Regurgitation

Peter Koenig

OVERVIEW OF REGURGITATION

Physiologically, regurgitation causes an increased preload. The regurgitant blood reenters the chamber from which it came resulting in an increased volume load of that chamber. Compensatory responses in the heart need to occur when regurgitation occurs. These responses need to be sufficient to compensate for the regurgitation, otherwise, heart failure occurs (inability of the cardiac system to deliver blood sufficient to the needs of the body).

ACUTE AND CHRONIC RESPONSES TO REGURGITATION

One general concept, the conservation of mass, prevails with any alteration in cardiac physiology. In terms of the cardiovascular system, this means that the amount of blood that leaves the heart and flows to the body (cardiac output) is the same amount of blood that returns to the heart. With acute regurgitation, which overwhelms the heart's ability to compensate, there will be a decreased amount of blood leaving the heart and returning to it (a low-flow state or shock). With time, responses will occur to restore the hearts ability to deliver the baseline cardiac output. Depending on the reserve the heart has to overcome the regurgitation, the acute decline in cardiac output may not occur at all (fully compensated obstruction), or may occur immediately (acute heart failure). It may also persist or develop over time (chronic heart failure), or may occur and disappear over time (compensated heart failure). This is shown in Figure 11-7. Even with fully compensated regurgitation, if the body's demands increases the heart may not have a reserve to compensate for the regurgitation and the demand for an increased cardiac output as well.

Thus, there is the concept of heart failure as a dynamic state, which depends on the changing demands placed on the heart, the underlying anatomy and pathology of the heart, and the heart's ability to compensate for any pathological changes (Figure 11-8).

The other concepts are the general responses of the cardiovascular system when regurgitation occurs. Acutely, regurgitation is similar to a shunt, but not left to right or right to left. Rather, it can be thought of as a shunt from a distal to proximal chamber. Acute compensations include an elevated heart rate and increased contractility to increase cardiac output. Eventually, there is compensatory increased fluid retention and the stroke volume is increased with a normalizaton of the heart rate. Similar to left-to-right shunts, there will be increased blood volume, with the extra blood within the heart. Instead of a shunt volume, this extra blood is termed regurgitant volume. The amount of regurgitation depends on the size of the regurgitant orifice, the time in which regurgitation can occur, and the differences in resistance between the chamber proximal and distal to the area of regurgitation. There will be enlargement of the chambers proximal and distal to the area of regurgitation as these chambers need to accommodate both the regurgitant blood volume as well as the normal blood volume needed to generate the normal cardiac output.

In addition to blood volume changes, pressures will tend to equalize during the time of regurgitant flow (similar to pressures equalizing with an intracardiac of shunt) between the chambers proximal and distal to the area of regurgitation. There will be afterload changes as well. With atrioventricular valve regurgitation, the afterload of the ventricle is reduced, as the ventricle can pump to the lower resistance atria rather than to an arterial system. This is more important in the left ventricle.

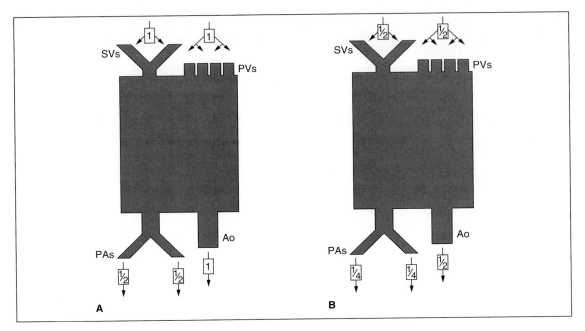

FIGURE 11-7

NORMAL HEART FLOW AND CHANGES WITH REGURGITATION

In this figure, the heart is represented as a "black box." Regardless of the type of obstruction, the net results shown in figures A and B are the same. The numbers inside the boxes represent relative cardiac outputs, meaning that the cardiac output is consistent with the systemic demands (a 1:1 ratio). **A** shows a heart at baseline. **B** shows a heart with acute regurgitation. In this case, the heart has not yet compensated and there is a decreased cardiac output. With compensation, there is a return to the baseline state (**A**) although there are changes within the heart. These are shown in later diagrams.

THE PHYSICAL EXAMINATION WITH UNDERLYING REGURGITATION

General concepts apply to the translation of the underlying pathophysiology of regurgitation to the findings on the physical examination. Dilation of a ventricle will lead to the finding of a ventricular heave or lift. The location on the chest corresponds to the ventricle involved. In practice, this may be simply described as a hyperdynamic precordium.

Another physical finding is a pathologic murmur owing to the regurgitation. This will be systolic if it involves the atrioventricular valves, and diastolic if it involves the semilunar valves. In each case, the murmur is generated by a pressure difference (gradient) during the time of regurgitation. With severe pathology and near equalization of pressures, this murmur may not be heard. In addition, there will be a murmur of functional stenosis

because of increased flow across the regurgitant valve. Since murmurs are directly related to blood flow, more blood flow will create a louder sound. Thus, the murmur across the regurgitant valve.

Another physical finding unique to systemic semilunar valve (aortic) regurgitation, is the finding of increased pulse pressures (bounding pulses). This is discussed further in Chapter 17.

Physical findings indirectly related to the regurgitation may also be present and include signs and symptoms of heart failure if it exists, and the backward transmission of elevated pressures.

LABORATORY FINDINGS WITH REGURGITATION

Laboratory findings will reflect the underlying physiological derangements within the limits of the ability of the test to do so. Thus, the ECG may

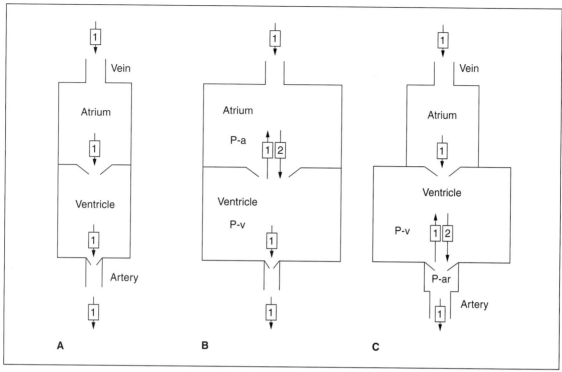

FIGURE 11-8

PATHOPHYSIOLOGY OF REGURGITATION

A shows a theoretical two-chamber heart. **B** shows a heart with regurgitation between the proximal (atrial) and distal (ventricular) chamber. This example is in the compensated state, and it is chosen to have one relative cardiac output as the regurgitant volume (other numbers can be chosen). Note that the net cardiac output remains the same as baseline, though there are now two cardiac outputs entering the atrium (one as the regurgitant volume, and one as venous return), and two cardiac outputs entering the ventricle. Of the two cardiac outputs entering the ventricle, one is pumped into the artery and one cardiac output is pumped or regurgitated back into the atrium. Since there are two cardiac outputs in the atria and ventricle, the chambers are enlarged. Furthermore, there are two cardiac outputs crossing the atrioventricular valve, which will cause a flow disturbance (functional stenosis). Finally, the pressure in the atrium (P-a) will be increased. Ventricular systolic pressure will remain the same as this is the pressure needed to pump into the arteries; however, the ventricle will have a decreased afterload as it may also pump into the atria. In **C**, there is an example of regurgitation between the ventricle and artery. Again, one relative cardiac output is chosen as the regurgitant volume. In this example, the enlarged chambers are the ventricle and the proximal artery (a theoretical chamber) since they will both contain two relative cardiac outputs. There will be increased flow across the semilunar valve; thus there will be a flow disturbance and functional stenosis. Finally, the diastolic pressure in the artery (P-ar) will be decreased as it will tend to equalize to the end-diastolic pressure of the ventricle. Systolic pressures will remain equal (or slightly increased because of the increased pulse pressure). The latter is governed by arterial resistance. The pulse pressure increases as it is the difference between systolic and diastolic arterial pressures and the diastolic pressure decreases.

reflect chamber enlargement. In addition, the ECG will reflect myocardial ischemia because of coronary artery steal in patients with aortic regurgitation. The chest radiograph will reflect enlargement of the ventricles in total (generally chamber enlargement rather than hypertrophy) as well as enlargement of

any atria, veins or other vessels. Echocardiography will reveal chamber enlargement and any areas of blood flow turbulence via Doppler. Finally, cardiac catheterization can directly measure pressure elevations and reductions as well as show areas of regurgitation via angiography.

Heart Failure and Cardiomyopathy

David J. Waight

HEART FAILURE

Heart failure is defined as the condition when the ability of the heart to generate a cardiac output is insufficient to meet the demands of the body. This denotes a dynamic process. The cardiac output can increase to a limited extent by increasing heart rate, or stroke volume. The stroke volume can increase by increasing preload and contractility or reducing the afterload. There are no limitations to the demands placed on the heart. Thus, heart failure can occur in any heart if the demands are great enough. Therefore, heart failure is a ratio of cardiac output versus demand. Healthy hearts are able to sustain a greater demand; however, abnormal hearts have a reduced ability to do so. These concepts are reflected in the New York Heart Association classification of heart failure (Table 11-5). In the most severe state,

cardiogenic shock occurs, whereby the heart fails to even sustain life.

The causes of heart failure may be due to cardiac muscle dysfunction or cardiomyopathy with resultant inability to increase the preload or contractility, or an inability to increase the heart rate (due to sinus node or conduction disturbances). Heart failure can also be due to abnormal distribution (maldistribution) of blood flow if there is a shunting lesion (systemic steal), or valvar regurgitation. The latter has a similar physiology to distributive shock in that the cardiac output is elevated, but blood flow is simply misdirected (to the lungs, back into the heart, through an arteriovenous malformation, and so forth) such that the forward systemic flow is reduced. Physiologically, the inability of the heart to fill (increase the preload) is known as diastolic dysfunction, and the inability of the heart to pump (increase the contractility) is known as systolic dysfunction. Systolic dysfunction may be a result of muscle failure (cardiomyopathy) or outflow obstruction, while diastolic dysfunction may be a result of abnormal muscle relaxation or stiffness (restrictive cardiomyopathy), pericardial disease (constrictive cardiomyopathy) or inflow obstruction. Clinically, the lack of cardiac output can be termed *forward failure*, and the congestion that occurs when accumulating blood returns to the heart can be termed *backward failure*. Both clinical findings can occur with either underlying pathophysiologic state. The signs and symptoms of low cardiac output and "forward failure" are listed in Table 11-6 and the signs and symptoms of "backward failure" and congestion are listed in Table 11-7. They can be divided into those that are owing to congestion in the lungs from left ventricular failure and those owing to congestion in the body because of right ventricular failure.

TABLE 11-5

NYHA CLASSIFICATION OF HEART FAILURE

Class	Findings
I	No limitation of physical activity. No dyspnea, fatigue, palpitation with ordinary activity
II	Slight limitation of physical activity. These patients have fatigue, dyspnea, and palpitations with ordinary physical activity but are comfortable at rest
III	Marked limitation of physical activity. Comfortable at rest. Less than ordinary physical activity causes fatigue, palpitations, dyspnea or anginal pain
IV	Symptoms are present at rest. Any physical exertion exacerbates the symptoms

TABLE 11-6

SIGNS AND SYMPTOMS OF FORWARD HEART FAILURE

Symptoms	Signs
Fatigue or decreased exercise tolerance (L, R)	Decreased exercise tolerance on testing (L, R)
Palpitations with minimal exertion (L, R)	Increased resting heart rate and with exercise (L, R)
Dyspnea with exertion (L, R)	Increased respiratory rate (L, R)
Decreased mentation (if severe) (L, R)	Decreased measured urine output (L, R)
Palpitations (L, R)	Cool extremities/poor perfusion (L, R)
Syncope (L, R)	Peripheral cyanosis (L, R)
Decreased urine output (L, R)	Arrhythmia (L, R)
Cool extremities (L, R)	
Peripheral cyanosis (L, R)	
Poor growth (L, R)	

Note: L, left heart failure; R, right heart failure.

Compensatory mechanisms in heart failure are similar to compensated shock and include tachycardia, fluid retention, and vasoconstriction; however, this fluid retention, coupled with vasoconstriction associated with heart failure, will result in further burden on the myocardium. Both will cause the diastolic ventricular pressures to increase causing a "backward" effect on the atria, causing elevation of left atrial and pulmonary venous hypertension in left heart failure. This may eventually cause right heart failure as well. Right ventricular failure causes elevation of right atrial pressure and consequently central venous pressure. Right and left atrial hypertension will also occur with diastolic dysfunction.

TABLE 11-7

SIGNS AND SYMPTOMS OF BACKWARD HEART FAILURE

Symptoms	Signs
Tachypnea/dyspnea (L)	Increased respiratory rate/distress (L)
Paroxysmal nocturnal dyspnea (L)	Rales (L)
Orthopnea (L)	Wheezing (L)
Peripheral edema (R)	Peripheral edema (R)

Note: L, left heart failure; R, right heart failure.

Left ventricular failure will lead to pulmonary edema which is worsened in the supine position when ventricular preload is increased (therefore a higher left ventricular end-diastolic pressure) and typically occurs when in bed (orthopnea) and may result in the need to sleep with additional pillows to avoid the supine position. Pulmonary edema causes dyspnea and rales on physical examination. In addition, pulmonary edema may cause airway reactivity and wheezing on examination. The latter is more common in infants and children in whom rales are seldom if ever noted. The increase in preload that occurs while sleeping supine may cause a sudden increase in airway constriction at night known as paroxysmal nocturnal dyspnea. Pulmonary edema also causes decreased lung compliance and compensatory hyperexpansion of the lungs. The latter may cause the liver to be pushed below the diaphragm and palpable. It is also the cause of hyperinflation seen on a plain chest radiograph.

Right ventricular failure leads to increased systemic venous pressures. Resultant hepatic congestion may lead to complaints of right upper abdominal pain and the finding of hepatomegaly. (The liver may also be palpable because of lung hyperexpansion without being significantly enlarged.) Bowel wall edema may lead to poor absorption and diarrhea. Distension of the jugular veins may directly reflect the increased systemic venous pressure. Peripheral edema may also occur and reflect increased systemic venous pressure as well as low oncotic pressure from hypoalbuminemia because of hepatic dysfunction and malabsorption; however, this finding is rare in children in whom hepatomegaly may be the only finding of right-sided heart failure.

In summary, backward and forward failure are clinical manifestations of underlying systolic or diastolic cardiac dysfunction. Both may occur with either type of cardiac dysfunction. The diagnosis (Table 11-8) is made after there is clinical suspicion. Clinical suspicion is raised with the finding of signs and symptoms of heart failure as described above. Testing may include an ECG, which usually demonstrates ST–T-wave abnormalities in most cardiomyopathies. In the presence of respiratory distress, a chest radiograph will typically demonstrate cardiac enlargement and pulmonary edema. Echocardiography is usually diagnostic and able to demonstrate the type of cardiomyopathy (dilated, hypertrophic, or restrictive) with an estimation of the degree of hemodynamic derangement. Cardiac catheterization will further demonstrate the hemodynamics, and allows for endomyocardial biopsy to be performed for histological examination. It should be noted, however, that the diagnosis of diastolic dysfunction is difficult and may require assessing the clinical and laboratory findings, as well as the response to clinical maneuvers. General treatment of heart failure (Table 11-8, Figure 11-9) is to treat any underlying arrhythmia and any anatomic or shunting lesion. The treatment of these may be supportive using similar treatment strategies for systolic dysfunction, but only temporarily until definitive antiarrhythmic therapy or surgical therapy is undertaken (as described in appropriate chapters in this text). General treatment strategies of systolic and diastolic dysfunction are discussed below.

CARDIOMYOPATHY

Introduction

The term *cardiomyopathy* implies heart muscle disease, cardio for heart, myo for muscle, and pathos for disease. Cardiomyopathy can occur at any age. Cardiomyopathy can be a primary disease of the myocardium without other systemic disease, or it can be secondary to systemic disorders such as glycogen storage diseases, diabetes, or AIDS. With this definition cardiomyopathy refers to structural or functional abnormalities of the myocardium, which involves the heart muscle primarily and is not secondary or compensatory to other disease processes. There are forms of secondary cardiomyopathy because of other diseases in which the muscle changes in the heart are an appropriate or physiologic response such as hypertrophy secondary to hypertension or aortic valve stenosis. This chapter deals with the physiology of cardiomyopathy as well as clinical correlates.

Cardiomyopathies are generally classified into three categories based on the pathophysiology:

1. Dilated cardiomyopathy in which the left ventricle or possibly both ventricles are enlarged and have decreased systolic function. The latter is often measured as a decreased shortening fraction or decreased ejection fraction.
2. Hypertrophic cardiomyopathy implying an abnormal thickening or hypertrophy of the heart.
3. Restrictive cardiomyopathy in which there is a decreased or impaired diastolic filling of the ventricle.

It is important to recognize that the signs and symptoms of these three classifications can be similar and overlap. The clinical history, physical examination, and cardiac testing including echocardiography, cardiac catheterization, and possibly endomyocardial biopsy help define the etiology and the severity of these diseases.

Dilated Cardiomyopathy

Dilated cardiomyopathy is characterized by an enlarged left ventricle with decreased systolic function. Decreased systolic function leads to signs and symptoms of congestive heart failure. There is an annual incidence of 2–8 cases per 100,000 in the United States. In the pediatric age group, the majority of the patients with dilated cardiomyopathy do not have a specific etiology identified. Dilated cardiomyopathy is defined as having ventricular dilation

THE DIAGNOSIS AND TREATMENT OF CARDIOMYOPATHY

Diagnosis	Pathophysiology	CXR	ECG	Echocardiogram	Treatment
Dilated cardiomyopathy	Dilated ventricles Enlarged atria—L and R Decreased systolic function Decreased cardiac output Arrhythmia Pulmonary edema respiratory distress Systemic edema-ascites Mural thrombi	Cardiomegaly ± Pulmonary edema ± Atelectasis	ST–T-wave changes Arrhythmia	Dilated LV, RV Decreased SF% Thrombi Mitral regurgitation	Afterload reduction—major form of therapy to improve forward failure Diuretics as needed for symptoms of backward failure Inotropic agents as needed to improve symptomatic forward failure
Hypertrophic cardiomyopathy	Thickened myocardium Limited cardiac output Chest pain Arrhythmia	Normal Possible PE, LAE	LVH, ± BVH Arrhythmia	Thickened myocardium Mitral valve thickening. Anterior motion of the mitral valve	Maintain fluid balance—avoid hypovolemia which will further reduce preload and increase obstruction No real role for inotropic agents or afterload reduction Role of beta blockade and calcium channel blockers under debate ICD to prevent sudden death
Restrictive cardiomyopathy	Diastolic dysfunction Limited cardiac output Pulmonary hypertension Arrhythmia	LAE PE	LAE Arrhythmia	++LAE Abnormal ventricular filling	Maintain fluid balance—avoid hypovolemia which will further reduce preload, and hypervolemia which will worsen symptoms of backward failure—use diuretics with caution No real role for inotropic agents or afterload reduction Theoretical role of beta blockade and calcium channel blockers to "relax" the muscle and improve diastolic filling Early transplant

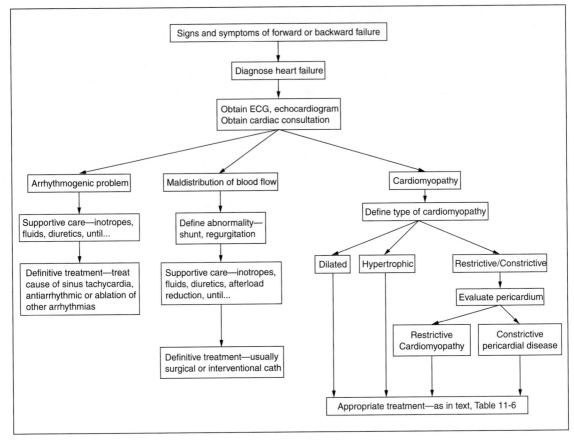

F I G U R E   1 1 - 9

DIAGNOSTIC AND THERAPEUTIC FLOW DIAGRAM OF HEART FAILURE

with gross enlargement of the heart. The heart is described as globular in shape. Despite the increased size of the ventricles, the ventricular wall thickness is usually normal. Histologic evaluation typically demonstrates myocyte hypertrophy and degeneration with evidence of interstitial fibrosis.

Pathophysiology

Dilated cardiomyopathy leads to signs and symptoms of congestive heart failure because of poor systolic function and limited cardiac output. In an effort to maintain an adequate cardiac output, the ventricles enlarge and the myocardium hypertrophies. The enlargement of the ventricle increases

the systolic wall tension within the ventricle, increases the myocardial oxygen consumption, and decreases the efficiency of the myocardial cells. Poor cardiac output diminishes renal blood flow and leads to enhancement of the renin-angiotensin system, which leads to increased fluid retention. Decreased cardiac output also leads to stimulation of the sympathetic nervous system increasing the heart rate. The increased heart rate and increased intravascular volume are physiologic mechanisms to maintain a necessary cardiac output to meet the metabolic demands of the body. Increasing metabolic demands owing to exercise will often exceed the body's physiologic ability to compensate with increasing cardiac output and lead to signs and symptoms of heart failure, which are initially noted with exercise. As the disease worsens, symptoms will become more noticeable at decreasing levels of exercise and then at rest. Mild hemodynamic abnormalities may be worsened with exercise or infections, which increase myocardial demands. Thus, symptoms may be present only with exertion. If the myocardial oxygen demands exceed the supply from the coronary arteries, ischemia (and its signs and symptoms) may occur.

In addition to other hemodynamic derangements, dilation of the heart may lead to valvar regurgitation because of dilation of the valve annulus. This leads to further myocardial oxygen demand and diminished performance.

Left ventricular enlargement can also lead to atelectasis of the lungs, most commonly in the left lung owing to compression of the lung parenchyma and the left lower lobe bronchus by the left atrium. Severe forms of systolic dysfunction will lead to diastolic dysfunction with elevation of the left ventricular end-diastolic pressure leading to an elevated left atrial pressure, pulmonary venous pressure, and the pressure in the pulmonary alveolar bed. The latter can create pulmonary edema. This can lead to decreased lung compliance and hyperexpansion of the chest with a liver pushed down below the chest. It can also lead to elevated pulmonary pressures with subsequent right ventricular failure and enlargement, and right atrial enlargement and pressure elevated. This will also cause hepatomegaly as well as distended systemic veins, and peripheral edema.

The abnormal myocytes can have significant conduction abnormalities leading to changes that can be noted on an electrocardiogram, most commonly nonspecific ST- and T-wave changes. Both atrial and ventricular arrhythmias are common in dilated cardiomyopathy. Intraventricular thrombus formation is common because of a low flow state. This may consist of microthrombi within the small trabeculations in the ventricle or large mural thrombi covering a wall, usually near the apex of the heart. These thrombi can intermittently embolize causing resultant pulmonary embolism and eventual pulmonary hypertension if they arise from the right side, or small strokes and possible

myocardial infarction if embolized from the left side. Thrombi can also embolize to any other of the systemic arteries or to the renal arteries causing renal damage. This can further complicate the poor renal function secondary to poor cardiac output because of the dilated cardiomyopathy.

Treatment

Treatment of dilated cardiomyopathies is supportive until the disease process resolves, improves, or the heart is transplanted. Afterload reduction is the main form of medical therapy. Afterload reduction, by reducing systemic vascular resistance, relieves wall stress and leads to an improved stroke volume while maintaining blood pressure. Diuretics are used mainly to reduce symptoms of backward failure (pulmonary edema, bowel wall edema with malabsorption). Inotropic agents are used to improve contractility when needed to treat symptomatic forward failure. Newer medications, and other specific treatment of the patient with dilated cardiomyopathy in heart failure is beyond the scope of this text and is undertaken in specialized heart failure centers in conjunction with consideration for transplantation.

Hypertrophic Cardiomyopathy

Hypertrophic cardiomyopathy describes a spectrum of disease of the left ventricle that features thickening of the ventricular wall. The left ventricle have symmetric hypertrophy in which both the free wall and the septum are dramatically thicker than normal, or asymmetric hypertrophy in which the ventricular septum and/or free wall is thickened to an unequal degree. Asymmetric hypertrophy can lead to left ventricular outflow tract obstruction and has been described by a multitude of terms (e.g., idiopathic hypertrophic subaortic stenosis [IHSS]) that are best reduced to the term of hypertrophic obstructive cardiomyopathy. Hypertrophic cardiomyopathy (with or without associated systemic findings such as inborn errors of metabolism) usually is an appropriate diagnosis only after other causes of left ventricular hypertrophy are excluded. These other causes include systemic hypertension, aortic valve stenosis, coarctation of the aorta, and other forms of congenital heart disease that produce obstruction to left ventricular output and compensatory ventricular thickening.

Pathology

The pathology of hypertrophic cardiomyopathy includes a hypertrophied and nondilated left ventricle. The area of hypertrophy may be symmetric or isolated. The left ventricular cavity is normal to decreased in size and there is increased left ventricular mass. The left atrium may be secondarily enlarged. The mitral valve may demonstrate thickening or fibrous changes in the septal leaflet thought to be a result of contact between the mitral valve and the intraventricular septum. There are frequently coronary abnormalities in patients with hypertrophic cardiomyopathy including hypertrophy of the walls of the small intramural coronary arteries.

Histology

Myocardial biopsy or autopsy specimens in patients with hypertrophic cardiomyopathy demonstrate fibrosis, variable myocyte hypertrophy with changes in both shape and size of the myocytes, cardiac muscle cell disorganization (often referred to as myocyte disarray), and abnormalities of the small intramural coronary arteries. These histologic changes are not seen in the enlarged myocytes present in ventricular hypertrophy secondary to hypertension or the various types of left ventricular outflow tract obstruction.

Pathophysiology

The pathophysiology of hypertrophic cardiomyopathy includes the following:

1. Systolic dysfunction and left ventricular outflow tract obstruction
2. Diastolic dysfunction
3. Coronary artery abnormalities with associated myocardial ischemia
4. Arrhythmia

1. The systolic dysfunction of hypertrophic cardiomyopathy is not the result of decreased ejection fraction, as the ejection fraction is supranormal in most patients with hypertrophic cardiomyopathy. Ventricular hypertrophy can lead to left ventricular outflow tract obstruction producing elevated pressures within the ventricular cavity. The outflow tract obstruction leads to turbulence and a pathologic murmur. In addition, the anterior leaflet of the mitral valve may be displaced into the left ventricular outflow tract, thus leading to further outflow tract obstruction. The dynamic outflow tract obstruction is increased when the ventricular preload is decreased (hypovolemia) and is the explanation for the pathologic murmur being louder with standing than with lying supine. The outflow tract obstruction can lead to changes in the mitral valve including thickening, fibrosis, and eventual mitral insufficiency. Mitral insufficiency can lead to left atrial enlargement and resulting arrhythmias. Patients with left ventricular outflow tract obstruction may have symptoms of dyspnea, chest pain, lightheadedness, or syncope. In a minority of patients, the initial hypertrophic myocardium progresses to a dilated cardiomyopathy with decreasing systolic function and enlargement of the left ventricle. This had previously been termed a "burned out hypertrophic cardiomyopathy."

2. Diastolic dysfunction is ubiquitous in patients with hypertrophic cardiomyopathy. A thick left ventricular wall demonstrates abnormal passive elasticity and decreased active elasticity because of incomplete and delayed relaxation. Myocardial relaxation is inhibited by the hypertrophy of the ventricle because of the pressure load within the left ventricle, and ischemia because of the abnormal coronary arteries typically present in hypertrophic cardiomyopathy. The left ventricle has poor compliance with decreased early diastolic filling of the left ventricle. This abnormality may be less apparent if mitral regurgitation has developed, which will increase early diastolic filling volumes but reduce the net cardiac output.

3. Myocardial ischemia is also common in hypertrophic cardiomyopathy. Ischemia results from a combination of disorders of myocardial blood flow. There is increased myocardial oxygen demand in the thickened myocardium. The coronary artery system is abnormal in the intramural portion because of both abnormally narrowed and compressed small vessels between the thickened myocytes. There is also decreased perfusion secondary to elevated myocardial wall tension with prolonged diastolic relaxation.

Ischemia presents clinically with anginal type chest pain (crushing, pressure-type left-sided chest pain which may radiate to the left arm or jaw, and is usually associated with exertion).

4. Hypertrophic myocardial cells may have abnormal electrical properties and therefore, these patients are at risk for sudden death because of ventricular arrhythmia. These abnormal rhythms may be primary or occur secondary to myocardial injury from ischemia. Atrial arrhythmias may occur in the presence of a dilated left atrium secondary to mitral regurgitation.

Treatment

The treatment for hypertrophic cardiomyopathies (Table 11-8) is supportive with attention to maintaining a normal ventricular preload and avoiding hypovolemia. There is no role for afterload reduction or inotropic support as systolic function is usually maintained. The role of beta and calcium channel blockers to decrease the outflow tract gradient and/or to reduce the incidence of sudden death is under debate; however, these medications may reduce symptoms. If there is a risk for sudden death (family history, severe hypertrophy, history of ventricular arrhythmias, or near sudden death), then placement of an implantable cardiac defibrillator is indicated.

Restrictive Cardiomyopathy

Restrictive cardiomyopathy defines a disease in which there is restriction of flow into the ventricles. This is an uncommon form of cardiomyopathy in children accounting for less than 5% of cardiomyopathies. It closely resembles constrictive pericardial disease.

Pathophysiology

Restrictive cardiomyopathy involves abnormal relaxation of the ventricular myocardium with decreased ventricular compliance. This alters the diastolic filling of the ventricle leading to increased ventricular end-diastolic pressure and elevation of atrial pressure. Elevated atrial pressure leads to enlargement of the atrium. The left ventricle and the left atrium are typically more affected than the right with severe left atrial enlargement. The left ventricular systolic function usually remains near normal and the left ventricular size does not increase. The increase in left atrial pressure and size leads to pulmonary venous congestion and eventual pulmonary hypertension. Pulmonary hypertension tends to be progressive in this disorder and becomes severe. The histology of the myocardium demonstrates myofiber hypertrophy and mild-to-moderate interstitial fibrosis.

A differentiating point is whether or not there is pericardial disease causing a similar pathophysiology as the latter can be treated with pericardial resection. Restrictive cardiomyopathy can only be treated supportively, or with cardiac transplantation.

Treatment

Medical treatment of the restrictive disease itself has had minimal success. Fluid balance is important as high atrial pressures are required to achieve an adequate ventricular preload; however, the elevated atrial pressures may lead to symptoms of congestion or "backward failure." This balance may be difficult to achieve. There is no role for inotropic or afterload reducing agents, and the role of medications to improve diastolic function is controversial. Early consideration for cardiac transplantation is usually required.

SUMMARY

Heart failure may be the result of a number of causes which disturb the heart's ability to meet the blood flow demands of the body. Heart failure may result in symptoms of forward and backward failure because of either systolic or diastolic dysfunction. Treatment of heart failure is based on the underlying pathophysiology. A diagnostic and treatment flow diagram is shown in Figure 11-7.

Causes of Heart Defects

Darrel Waggoner

INTRODUCTION

Congenital heart defects (CHD) are the most common form of birth defects in the general population and occur with a frequency of 6–8 per 1000 live births. As with most birth defects the etiology of CHD is multifactorial and includes genetic and environmental factors. The initial evaluation of a child newly diagnosed with a CHD will be quite involved, and the parents will have many questions and be inundated with medical information. In addition to the medical information, the parents will also have many questions regarding the cause, prognosis, additional complications, and possible recurrence risks associated with their child's CHD. The pediatrician will play an important role in answering some of these questions and referring the patient for appropriate evaluations to gain the information needed to provide the parents with the most complete and accurate information.

Congenital and acquired heart diseases including cardiomyopathy, atherosclerosis, arrhythmias, and others may also have a significant genetic component. Some of these disorders are a result of biochemical defects that are genetically inherited or single gene disorders that can be de novo or inherited. The most common ones, however, are a result of multifactorial inheritance, meaning there is a genetic and environmental interaction leading to the development of the condition. Understanding the genetic basis of cardiac disease is important from a scientific and clinical basis and impacts family counseling and treatment options.

ETIOLOGY
OF CONGENITAL HEART DISEASE

The genetic basis of CHD involves chromosome abnormalities including aneuploidy, submicroscopic deletions, and telomere rearrangements, recognizable syndromes, single gene defects, and teratogenic and environmental exposures. It is important to distinguish between these various causes as they impact the genetic counseling regarding the risk of recurrence for other family members, the risk of associated malformations and anomalies and the impact on growth and learning potential.

Chromosome Abnormalities

Chromosomal aneuploidy, rearrangements of chromosomes leading to loss or gain of a whole or part of a chromosome and its genetic content, is one of the most common identifiable causes of CHD. In a recent retrospective epidemiologic study of children with CHD, chromosome anomalies were reported in 14% of all patients. The most common defects were trisomy 21 followed by deletion of chromosome 22q11.2, trisomies 13 and 18, sex chromosome anomalies, and other aneuploides (see Table 11-9). The incidence of chromosome abnormality also varied when stratified by specific cardiac lesions. For example, chromosome abnormalities were seen in 63% of children with atrioventricular septal defects (mostly trisomy 21), in 50% of children with interrupted aortic arch type B (mostly 22q deletions), whereas they were only seen in 4% of children with VSD. These studies underscore the importance of chromosome anomalies contributing to CHD and potentially represent a minimal frequency as not every child with CHD has genetic studies performed nor are all of these results reported.

Submicroscopic deletion of chromosome 22q11.2 has recently been recognized to be the genetic basis of several clinical syndromes including DiGeorge syndrome and velocardiofacial syndrome. In addition, the deletion is found in approximately 50% of all children with interrupted aortic arch type

TABLE 11-9

CHROMOSOMAL DISORDERS WITH HEART ABNORMALITIES

Disorder	Extra Cardiac Features	Usual Heart Defect
Trisomy 21 (Down syndrome)	Hypotonia, characteristic facies, single palma crease, brachycephaly	Septal defects
Trisomy 13 (Patau syndrome)	Holoprosencephaly, polydactyly, defects eye, nose, lip	Ventricular septal defect
Trisomy 18 (Edwards syndrome)	Clenched hand, short sternum, small palpebral fissure	Ventricular septal defect
45,X (Turner syndrome)	Short stature, premature ovarian failure, congenital lymphoedema	Coarctation of the aorta

B. DiGeorge syndrome was originally described as a developmental field defect of the third and fourth pharyngeal pouches with conotruncal heart defects and aplasia or hypoplasia of the thymus gland and parathyroid glands leading to immune deficiency and hypoparathyroidism, respectively. Velocardiofacial syndrome was also a clinical diagnosis based on the combination of velopharyngeal incompetence, congenital heart disease (VSD and tetralogy of Fallot), characteristic dysmorphic features involving the nose, midface and fingers, and developmental delay or learning difficulties.

It is now recognized that this deletion is common in the population occurring with a frequency of 1 in 4000 live births and the clinical phenotype associated with this deletion is quite variable. The frequency of specific medical complications in these patients includes CHD the most frequent of which are the conotruncal malformations (abnormalities in the conus causing specific VSDs as seen in tetralogy of Fallot, double outlet right ventricle, interrupted aortic arch, and so forth). Congenital heart defects are seen in 74% of patients with q22 deletion. Palatal findings, including velopharyngeal incompetence and cleft lip/palate, are seen in 38%, immunodeficiency in 77%, and hypoparathyroidism in 49%. In addition, there is an increased incidence of feeding difficulties, growth deficiency, developmental delays, mental retardation, psychiatric illness, renal abnormalities, and cervical spine defects among many other possible complications. As these deletions are submicroscopic they are not detected by routine karyotype analysis and therefore specific testing is required. The deletions are detected by a FISH (fluorescent in situ hybridization) assay, which is widely available in many cytogenetic laboratories.

Telomeres mark the end of each chromosome and consist of specialized DNA sequences that ensure the integrity of the chromosome during cell division. Secondary to their size and banding characteristics, subtelomeric rearrangements leading to deletion or duplication of genetic material are difficult to recognize on routine karyotype. Multiple features of telomere structure and function lead to cryptic rearrangements of these regions. Chromosome pairing is initiated at the telomeres; subtelomeric regions are rich in pseudogenes and repeat sequences that share homology between nonhomologous chromosomes resulting in mispairing in early meiosis; and increased combination rates are observed at the telomeres. Collectively these aspects of telomeres provide the opportunity for nonhomologous pairing leading to unequal exchange events and genedosage imbalance. Genetic density at the telomeres is high and rearrangements in this region will lead to significant alterations of genetic content with the potential loss and gain of many genes. The result of this genetic imbalance, whether loss or gain of genetic material, can have a significant impact on growth and development.

As these telomeric rearrangements are not easily recognized by routine cytogenetic studies, a set of FISH probes was developed which corresponds to the most distal unique DNA segment of each human telomere. The development of these FISH probes allows for routine screening of all human telomeres and can readily detect rearrangements leading to monosomy or trisomy of these segments. Recent studies of children with mental retardation of unknown origin revealed that 5–7% of these children had telomere rearrangements, and that half were inherited from a balanced carrier parent indicating markedly increased risk of recurrence. Telomere rearrangements are associated with multiple birth defects including significant risk for CHD. One study, described in more detail below, found 36% of children with CHD, dysmorphic features and other birth defects, who did not have an identifiable syndrome or chromosome anomaly, had a telomere rearrangement which explained their features. Prior to the availability of telomere screening these children would go undiagnosed and the etiology of their CHD would remain unknown. Thus telomere screening has become another tool available to the clinician for the evaluation of mental retardation, birth defects, and CHD.

Syndromes

A syndrome is defined as a collection of anomalies, which occur in association with each other and are presumed to have a common specific etiology. Many defined and recognizable syndromes affecting patients have phenotypes that include CHD. Although many syndromes are recognized based only on the delineation of the associated clinical features, others are associated with chromosomal abnormalities, submicroscopic multiple gene rearrangements, single gene mutations and environmental teratogens. Recognition of these syndromes allows accurate counseling regarding prognosis, outcome, and recurrence risks. In addition, defining the underlying genetic basis of these syndromes has been important in defining the molecular basis of not only CHD, but normal heart development as well.

Identification of a syndrome is based on the recognition of recurrent combinations of dysmorphic features, medical complications, and the family history. Dysmorphic features may be minor: an unusual feature that has no serious medical or cosmetic consequence to the patient (e.g., ear size and shape, slanting of the eyes, palmar creases, and scalp hair patterns) and major: an unusual feature that does have serious medical or cosmetic consequence (e.g., congenital heart disease, aplasia of the kidney, and so forth), anomalies. Medical problems may be seemingly unrelated to the initially recognized defect and can include hypertension, retinitis pigmentosa, neurodevelopmental concerns, and so forth, and the family history may reveal similarly affected individuals, suggesting a specific pattern of inheritance.

Defining a specific syndrome as the cause of a CHD has several important implications for the patient and their families. Clinical benefits include access to knowledge about other medical problems associated with the specific condition (including concerns regarding anesthesia risks, bleeding diathesis, and the like) so that appropriate medical investigations and interventions can be initiated. For example, when 22q11.2 deletion is identified in a child with an interrupted aortic arch, the child should be investigated for associated problems with hypoparathyroidism, immune dysfunction, renal and cervical spine anomalies, palate abnormalities and feeding difficulties. In addition, there are multiple benefits of a syndrome diagnosis to the family including better access to developmental services, accurate counseling regarding recurrence risks for the parents and their immediate family, and referral to support groups for emotional, financial, and often medical support. Finally, the psychologic benefit of a diagnosis should not be understated. For many, the diagnosis relieves parents' own fears that they were responsible for the child's condition, enables them to stop the search for why these problems occurred, and allows them to focus their questions regarding expectations to a specific condition.

Aneuploides which lead to recognizable clinical phenotypes such as trisomy 21 (Down syndrome), trisomy 13 (Patau syndrome) and trisomy 18

(Edwards syndrome) have already been described. Multiple syndromes associated with submicroscopic deletions have now been described. These deletions are considered submicrosopic because they are not detected on routine chromosome analysis and diagnosis requires a unique FISH test specific for each syndrome. Deletion 22q (DiGeorge syndrome) was described in detail. Other submicroscopic deletion syndromes include Williams syndrome (7q11.23), Miller-Diecker syndrome (17p13.3), Wolf-Hirschorn syndrome (4p16.3), and Cri du chat syndrome (5p15.2) (Table 11-10). The deletion in each of these syndromes can affect many genes and leads to multiple features in addition to the CHD. Based on the recognition of the pattern of these clinical features, specific FISH tests can be ordered to confirm the clinical suspicion.

Many syndromes follow simple Mendelian patterns of inheritance. In these conditions, autosomal recessive, dominant, and X-linked inheritance patterns are recognized based on extensive family histories (Table 11-11). These inheritance patterns imply that the conditions are typically a result of mutations in a single gene regardless of whether the genetic basis has been identified or not. As the pathophysiology and genetic basis of these conditions is discovered, biochemical and genetic testing becomes available which assists in confirming the diagnosis, allows carrier testing, and further defines the variability of the clinical phenotype. Secondary to accurate diagnostic testing, patients who would previously not have been considered to meet the clinical criteria for a syndrome are found to have the diagnosis. Marfan syndrome, for example, is recognized based on specific skeletal features (arachnodactyly, pectus, scoliosis) ophthalmologic concerns (dislocated lens) and carries a high risk for dilation of the aortic root. The condition is caused by mutations in the fibrillin-1 gene on chromosome 15q21.1. It is now recognized that there are families with autosomal dominant segregation of fibrillin-1 gene mutations with dilated aortic root who do not have any of the other clinical features of Marfan syndrome, thus emphasizing the need for increased clinical suspicion of a genetic basis when evaluating patients with dilated aortic root or aneurysm.

Some syndromes, however, do not follow Mendelian inheritance patterns and the etiology of these conditions remains largely unknown and are referred to as "Associations" (Table 11-12). These associations are a nonrandom occurrence in two or more individuals of multiple anomalies not yet known to be a syndrome. Thus, when one or more

TABLE 11-10

MICRODELETION DISORDERS WITH HEART ABNORMALITIES

Disorder	Extra Cardiac Features	Usual Heart Defect	Inheritance
22q11 deletion (DiGeorge syndrome)	Hypocalcemia, immune dysfunction, short stature, palate abnormalities	Conotruncal defects	Autosomal dominant
Williams syndrome	Characteristic facies, short stature, hypercalcemia	Supravalvular aortic stenosis	Autosomal dominant
Miller-Diecker syndrome	Lissencephaly, polymicrogyria, characteristic facies	Variable: patent ductus arteriosus, septal defects	Autosomal dominant
Wolf-Hirschhorn syndrome	Growth deficiency, ocular hypertelorism, microcephaly, seizures	Septal defects	Autosomal dominant
Cri du chat syndrome	Cat-like-cry, microcephaly, growth deficiency, hypertelorism	Variable	Autosomal dominant

TABLE 11-11

MENDELIAN DISORDERS WITH HEART ABNORMALITIES

Disorder	Extra Cardiac Features	Usual Heart Defect	Inheritance
Holt-Oram syndrome	Upper limb defects, especially digits and radius	Atrial septal defect	Autosomal dominant
Noonan syndrome	Webbed neck, pectus excavatum, cryptorchidism	Pulmonary stenosis	Autosomal dominant
Marfan syndrome	Skeletal abnormalities, lens dislocation	Mitral valve prolapse, dilated aortic root	Autosomal dominant
Tuberous sclerosis	Hamartomas, skin nodules, seizures, phakomata, bone lesions	Intracardiac tumors	Autosomal dominant
Alagille syndrome	Cholestasis, peculiar facies, vertebral anomalies	Peripheral pulmonary artery stenosis	Autosomal dominant
Barth syndrome	Neutropenia, lipid myopathy, abnormal mitochondria, growth retardation	Dilated cardiomyopathy	X-linked
Cornelia de Lange syndrome	Synophrys, micromelia, retardation, short stature	Ventricular septal defects	Autosomal dominant
Fanconi Anemia	Radial hypoplasia, hyperpigmentation, pancytopenia	Variable	Autosomal recessive
Rubinstein Taybi syndrome	Broad thumbs and toes, slanted palpebral fissures, beaked nose	Ventricular septal defect	Autosomal dominant
Thrombocytopenia absent radius (TAR)	Bilateral absent radius, ulnar hypoplasia, thumbs present	Tetralogy of Fallot, atrial septal defect	Autosomal recessive

TABLE 11-12

NON-MENDELIAN SYNDROMES WITH HEART ABNORMALITIES

Disorder	Extra Cardiac Features	Usual Heart Defect
VATER association	Esophageal, anal, vertebral, renal, and radial limb defects	Variable
Goldenhar syndrome	Eye, ear, and facial abnormalities, first and second branchial arch syndrome	Ventricular septal defect
CHARGE association	Ocular coloboma, choanal atresia, ear and genital defects	Conotruncal defects
Kabuki syndrome	Characteristic facies, skeletal abnormalities	Coarctation of the aorta

of these anomalies is recognized in the same patient, the others in the association should be investigated. In general these conditions do not tend to recur in the same family or be passed on by the affected individual, so the exact genetic contribution to the pathogenesis remains unknown.

Taken together there are multiple genetic considerations when evaluating a child who has CHD and other birth defects or dysmorphic features. A recent study (Zackai et al., 2002) reported on the findings of a cohort of newborns with CHD and a question of dysmorphia and/or other organ system involvement. In this cohort 38% had a recognizable syndrome including 22q11.2 deletion, Noonan, CHARGE, VATER, heterotaxy and hemifacial microsomia. Of the remaining children without a recognizable syndrome but with dysmorphic features, 14% had a chromosome anomaly, and 36% had a cryptic telomere rearrangement. This information clearly indicates that genetic syndromes and chromosome abnormalities account for a significant proportion of children born with all types of CHD and therefore genetic evaluations and studies should be done in all of these children.

Single Gene Malformations

In recent years through the combined efforts of basic science research and the Human Genome project, many advances have been made in elucidating the genetic basis of cardiovascular malformations. Single genes involved in normal cardiac formation and function have been identified through a variety of mechanisms. Genetic mapping studies use families with inherited cardiac conditions to identify regions of shared homology and eventually candidate genes, which can be screened for mutations. Once a specific gene has been identified because of its ability to cause cardiac disease when mutated, then functional studies of the pathophysiology of the disease process and the normal function of the gene in cardiac development and function are undertaken. These studies reveal critical insights into the molecular basis of cardiac development and function and hold hope for the development of new and improved therapeutic approaches.

Mapping studies have been performed on patients with syndromes who have a variety of CHD

and additional anomalies. These genes facilitate the understanding of the complex developmental process of the heart in cohort with the other organ systems. Mapping of single disease traits has also been highly successful. Families with clear inheritance of cardiac anomalies including cardiomyopathy (both dilated and hypertrophic), arrhythmias, biochemical defects, and congenital anomalies have been studied to identify genes which cause isolated defects. As with syndromes, these genes can be inherited in Mendelian fashion leading to autosomal recessive and dominant, X-linked, and mitochondrial patterns of inheritance. Much of the focus of genetic research has been on identifying these genes and studying the pathogenesis of specific mutations and the role of the normal gene on heart development and function. In addition, these findings allow the development of more definitive diagnostic and carrier testing.

Most cardiovascular malformations and diseases, however, are not associated with syndromes or specific chromosome anomalies and are a result of multifactorial inheritance. It is well established that atherosclerosis, hypertension, and some congenital heart malformations, for instance, have a familial component occurring more frequently within a given family than would be predicted based on the general population risks. This implies that there is a genetic component to these conditions shared by the affected family members. The genetic basis of these more common cardiac diseases is not simple Mendelian genetics with one gene causing one disease in a predictable manner. These genes confer an increased risk for development of one of these phenotypes, but the genetic change is not solely responsible for the disease. Disease development is dependent on the specific genetic risk factors, the population genetic background, and the environment. Environmental components for example can include diet, exercise, smoking habits, and alcohol consumption. Recent advances in genetic and statistic techniques allow a rigorous approach to the identification of genes which play a role in these conditions. Identification of these risk genes and studies of how best to implement large-scale screening for these mutations are a priority as they affect a large number of individuals and thus have a large impact on public health.

TABLE 11-13
ENVIRONMENTAL CAUSES OF HEART DISEASE

Disorder	Risk of Cardiac Defect (%)	Usual Heart Defect
Maternal rubella	35	Peripheral pulmonary stenosis, septal defects
Maternal diabetes mellitus	3–5	Ventricular septal defect, coarctation of the aorta, complete transposition
Maternal phenylketonuria	25–50	Tetralogy of Fallot
Fetal alcohol syndrome	25–30	Septal defects
Hydantoin	2–3	Pulmonary and aortic stenosis, tricuspid atresia
Lithium	10–20	Ebstein's malformation, tricuspid atresia, atrial septal defect

Environmental/Teratogenic Exposures

Many environmental factors are now recognized to be associated with heart disease (Table 11-13). Environmental exposures may include infectious agents, maternal drug exposure to agents known to have teratogenic effects on heart development, and maternal disease. Some well-known teratogenic agents with a specific affect on the embryology of heart development include ecstasy, lithium, retinoic acid, and, the most common, alcohol. Teratogens do not cause birth defects in 100% of patients and the adverse outcomes are related to the timing, length, degree and combination of exposures to any given agent/s. There is little data for any given agent suggesting a safe amount or time of exposure.

Maternal diseases play a significant role in the development of heart defects in fetuses. Although the embryo does not have the disease, prolonged exposure to metabolites of the maternal disease leads to the development of congenital malformations. Maternal diabetes is by far the most common disease, and is associated with a 4% risk of CHD in the offspring. In addition to CHDs including ventricular septal defects, coarctation, and complete transposition, children may suffer from a number of other birth defects including caudal regression, femoral hypoplasia, and dysmorphic features. The risk of developing a CHD can be greatly diminished by good glucose control.

Maternal phenylketonuria (PKU) is another important contributor to the development of a CHD. PKU is a well-described inborn error of metabolism of the amino acid phenylalanine which, when untreated, leads to significant mental retardation. The importance of this condition is highlighted by the fact that all states in the United States perform newborn screening for PKU. With improved screening and treatment options most individuals affected with PKU now live long and relatively healthy lives. Children born to women with PKU have a higher incidence of CHD because of in utero exposure to high levels of phenylalanine. Careful dietary monitoring prior to conception and throughout the pregnancy can significantly lower the risks of CHD.

GENETIC EVALUATION OF PATIENTS WITH CONGENITAL HEART DEFECTS

All children recognized to have a congenital heart defect should have a genetics evaluation aimed at establishing a diagnosis and accurate recurrence risk information. A detailed three-generation family history should be obtained with specific focus on individuals with heart defects, other birth anomalies, mental retardation, miscarriages, stillbirths, or known genetic conditions. A careful examination for dysmorphic features, birth defects (e.g., cleft lip and palate, polydactyly, syndactyly, skeletal anomalies) and assessment for other organ anomalies (e.g., renal malformations, brain anomalies) should be performed. If a specific diagnosis is suggested further genetic testing specific for those conditions can be considered including chromosome analysis, FISH tests specific for microdeletion syndromes, telomere analysis, sequencing of specific genes in single gene defects, and metabolic disease testing. If a specific diagnosis is not discovered or suggested based on this initial screen, further genetic testing should still be considered including routine chromosomal analysis, and FISH studies for deletion 22q, especially in any patient with a conotruncal heart defect.

Depending on the comfort level of the primary care physician, a genetics referral is reasonable at any point in the evaluation and management of a child with newly diagnosed heart disease. A genetics referral can be helpful for recognizing subtle dysmorphic features, deciding which genetic tests would be appropriate, organizing specialized testing and interpretation of results, and providing genetic counseling for a specific diagnosis or generalized recurrence risk. Because of the multifactorial nature of heart disease and the limited nature of genetic testing, it is important to remember that negative genetic tests do not rule out a genetic cause or contribution of congenital heart defects or heart disease.

offspring and other family members including the offspring of the affected child and for the unaffected siblings. For the majority of cases the heart defect is isolated and the exact etiology cannot be established. Multiple epidemiologic studies are available and data for recurrence risks in siblings and offspring are available in general and for specific types of heart defects. The general principle used in genetic counseling for isolated, nonsyndromic heart defects is that risks to siblings fall into the 2–5% ranges and increase as more individuals in the family are affected (Table 11-14). With the advances in fetal echocardiography, and postnatal surgical and medical care, the outcome of CHD is quite good and it is reasonable to counsel in terms of the recurrence risk being small.

Prenatal testing of future children is feasible if a specific genetic etiology is discovered in the proband. Genetic tests including karyotype, FISH, and mutational analysis can all be done on samples obtained from chorionic villus sampling (CVS), amniocentesis, and cordocentesis. The increasing resolution of cardiac ultrasound imaging can now identify many structural defects in the later part of the pregnancy, when a specific etiology is unknown.

The recent advances in elucidating the genetic and molecular basis of cardiac disease are impressive, but much is still to be learned. Large-scale

RECURRENCE RISKS

As the etiology of congenital heart defects is multifactorial, the recurrence risk is dependent on the underlying cause of the malformation. Most patients will not have an obvious familial inheritance pattern, but genetic factors are likely involved in the etiology of most cases. When a chromosomal anomaly, microdeletion, specific Mendelian disorder or syndrome can be established, accurate recurrence risk information is available and often times prenatal testing options as well. In this regard genetic studies and evaluation can be very helpful in addressing the common questions and concerns about recurrence risk for future

TABLE 11-14

OVERALL RISKS OF RECURRENCE

	Risk (%)
Population incidence	0.5
Sib of isolated case	2–3
Half sibs or other second-degree relatives	1–2
Offspring of isolated case	
Father	2–3
Mother	5–6
Two affected sibs (or sib and parent)	10
More than two affected first-degree relatives	~50

accomplishments such as the Human Genome project are providing new information and tools for determining the molecular basis of normal and abnormal heart development. These scientific advances will no doubt impact diagnostic testing options and ultimately improve therapeutic approaches.

Suggested Readings

Allen HD, Gutgesell HP, Clark EB, Driscoll DJ: *Moss and Adams' Heart Disease in Infants, Children and Adolescents Including the Fetus and Young Adult*, 6th ed. Philadelphia, PA, Lippincott Williams & Wilkins, 2001.

Braunwald E, Zipes DP, Libby P: *Heart Disease: A Textbook of Cardiovascular Medicine*, 6th ed. Philadelphia, PA, WB Saunders, 2001.

Emery AEH, Rimoin DL (eds): *Principles and Practice of Medical Genetics*, 4th ed. Churchill Livingstone, Philadelphia, PA, 2002.

Garson A, Bricker JT, Fisher DJ, Neish SR: *The Science and Practice of Pediatric Cardiology*, 2nd ed. Baltimore, MD, Williams & Wilkins, 1998.

Heart disease, in: Braunwald E (ed): *A Textbook of Cardiovascular Medicine*, 5th ed. New York, NY, WB Saunders, 1997, Chap. 14:421–444.

Kloner RA: *A Guide to Cardiology*, 2nd ed. New York, NY, Le Jacq Communications 1990.

LH Opie (eds.): *The Heart: Physiology, From Cell to Circulation*, 3rd ed. Lippincott-Raven, Philadelphia, PA, 1997, Chap. 12:343–390.

Lin A, Pierpont, ME (eds): Heart developments and the genetic aspects of cardiovascular malformations. *Am J Med Genet* 97(4), 2000.

Moller JH: *Essentials of Pediatric Cardiology*, Philadelphia, PA, F.A. Davis, 1978.

Rusell, KH, Wernovsky G, Goldmuntz E, Gaynor JW, Krantz ID, Ming JE, Saitta S, McDonald-McGinn DM, Celle L, Spinner NB, Zackai EH. The utility of subtelomeric and chromosome testing in patients with congenital heart defects. *Am J Hum Genet* 71S, 983, 2002.

CHAPTER

12

ATRIAL SEPTAL DEFECTS (ASD)

Hitendra T. Patel

INTRODUCTION

An atrial septal defect is a communication between the right atrium (RA) and left atrium (LA), owing to abnormal septation. Four types are recognized:

1. Primum
2. Secundum
3. Sinus venosus (superior vena cava [SVC] type, inferior vena cava [IVC] type)
4. Coronary sinus septal defect

These are some of the most common types of congenital heart defects. To understand the different types it is important to review the embryologic development of the RA, LA, and their septation.

ANATOMY AND EMBRYOLOGY

Embryology of Atrial Septal Development

The primitive heart tube (Figure 12-1) comprises the right and left sinus horn, the sinus venosus, the primitive atrium, primitive ventricle, bulbus cordis, and the aortic sac. At about day 26 of embryonic development, the heart looping has occurred, and a common atrium, a common atrial-ventricular (AV) valve, the right and left ventricles, and a conotruncus are recognized. The common atrium is formed posteriorly by incorporation of the sinus venosus and the primitive atrium. The left sinus horn forms the left superior vena cava, which ultimately atrophies and remains as the coronary sinus. The right sinus horn remains as the SVC and the most proximal, intrahepatic portion of the IVC. At about this time, the roof of the atrium is depressed along the midline by the overlying conotruncus. This produces a crescent-shaped wedge of tissue internally called the septum primum (Figure 12-2A,A$_1$). This septum grows toward the atrioventricular canal. As septum primum grows, four tissue expansions develop around the atrioventricular valve, right, left, superior, and inferior endocardial cushions. The superior and inferior cushions grow toward each other and join, forming the septum intermedium. This divides the common AV valve into the right and left AV valves (Figure 12-2B,B$_1$). The septum primum grows to fuse with the septum intermedium closing the ostium primum and dividing the atrium into right and left. As this occurs perforations develop in the superior part of the septum

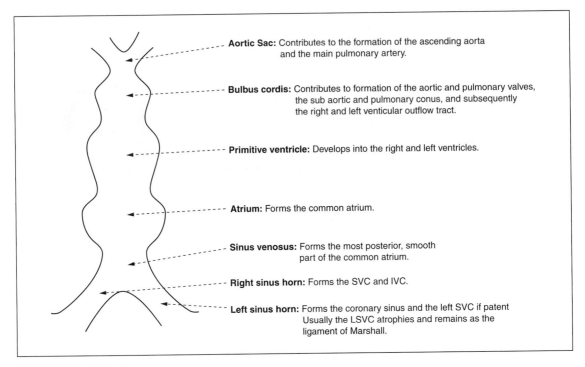

Aortic Sac: Contributes to the formation of the ascending aorta and the main pulmonary artery.

Bulbus cordis: Contributes to formation of the aortic and pulmonary valves, the sub aortic and pulmonary conus, and subsequently the right and left venticular outflow tract.

Primitive ventricle: Develops into the right and left ventricles.

Atrium: Forms the common atrium.

Sinus venosus: Forms the most posterior, smooth part of the common atrium.

Right sinus horn: Forms the SVC and IVC.

Left sinus horn: Forms the coronary sinus and the left SVC if patent Usually the LSVC atrophies and remains as the ligament of Marshall.

FIGURE 12-1

SCHEMATIC REPRESENTATION OF THE PRIMITIVE HEART TUBE AND ULTIMATE CONTRIBUTIONS TO THE FULLY DEVELOPED HEART

primum, which coalesce to form the ostium secundum (Figure 12-2C,C_1). A new ridge of tissue grows adjacent and to the right of septum primum superiorly. This septum secundum (Figure 12-D,D_1) is crescent shaped and grows toward septum intermedium but does not fuse with it (Figure 12-2E,E_1). This leaves an opening between septum secundum and septum primum through the ostium secundum into the left atrium called the foramen ovale (Figure 12-2F,F_1). The most posterior part of the septum is formed by contribution from the sinus venosus and the primitive SVC and IVC valves. The relation of the SVC and IVC to the atrial septum is shown in Figure 12-2H,H_1.

Anatomy of and Embryology of Specific Atrial Septal Defects (ASDs)

Primum ASD

This is an abnormality in the attachment of septum primum with the endocardial cushion. If septum primum does not fuse with septum intermedium or if the superior and inferior endocardial cushions do not fuse, then a primum atrial septal defect will exist. It is closely associated with the tricuspid and mitral valves. The heart has morphologic features that are identical to a common complete canal defect but there is no ventricular component. (See also Chapter 14) This defect is shown in Figures 12-2C,C_1 and 12-3.

Secundum Atrial Septal Defect

This is a defect or deficiency of the septum primum and leads to incomplete overlap of septum primum by septum secundum. The defects are bordered superiorly by the C-shaped septum secundum or the superior limbic band. It comprises 7% of congenital heart defects, and is twice as common in females. This defect is shown in Figure 12-3.

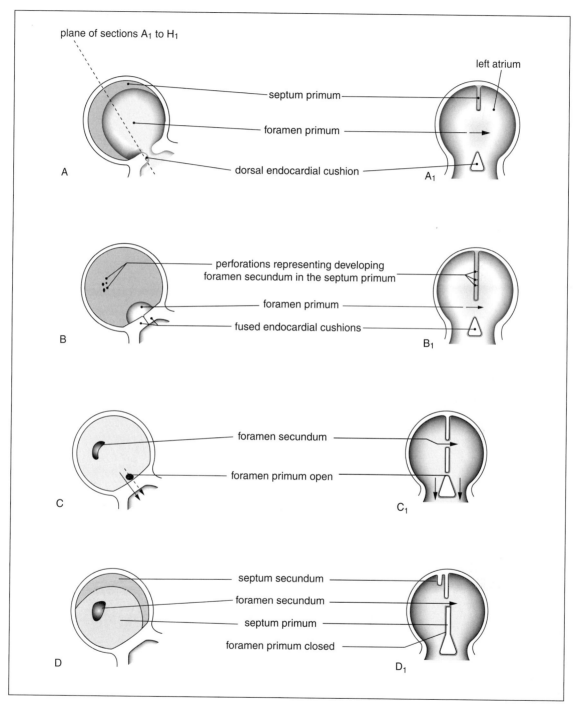

FIGURE 12-2

EMBRYOLOGY OF THE INTERATRIAL SEPTUM

Source: Moore KL. *The Developing Human. Clinically Oriented Embryology*. 4th ed. Philadelphia: WB Saunders, 1988.

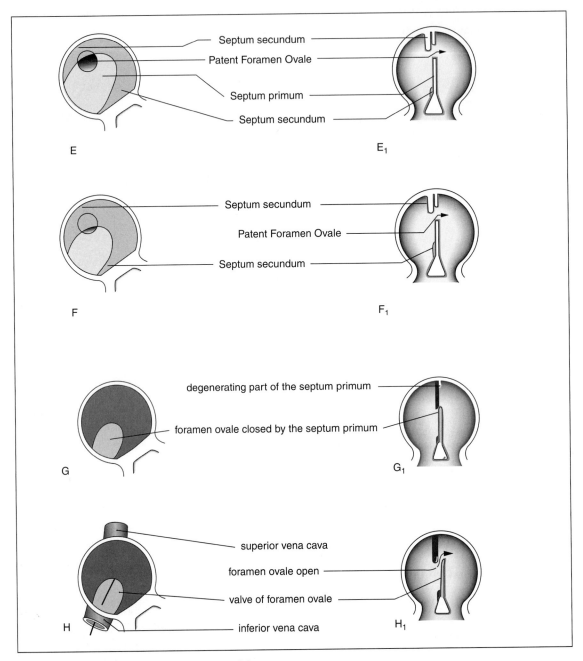

FIGURE 12-2 (continued)

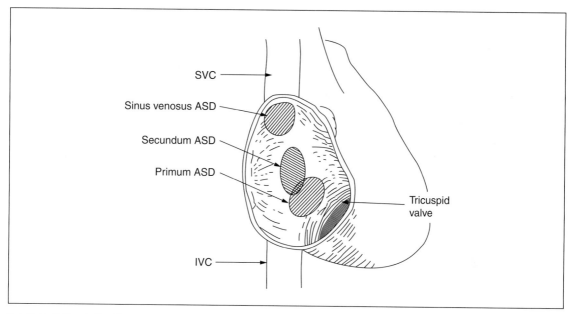

FIGURE 12-3

LOCATION OF THE DIFFERENT TYPES OF ATRIAL SEPTAL DEFECTS

Source: Park MK. *Pediatric Cardiology for General Practitioners.* 2nd ed. Chicago: Year Book, 1988.

Sinus Venosus ASD

This is a defect in the sinus venosus portion of the atrial septum. The defect may occur superiorly near the SVC/right upper pulmonary vein (RUPV) junction or inferiorly at the IVC/right lower pulmonary vein (RLPV) junction. By definition, superior defects have anomalous drainage of the RUPV to the RA; however, there may be true anomalous insertion of the right upper pulmonary vein into the SVC. Inferior defects may be associated with anomalous RLPV drainage to the RA. This defect is shown in Figure 12-3.

Coronary Sinus Septal Defect or Unroofed Coronary Sinus

Coronary sinus septal defects result from abnormal development of the left sinus horn and coronary sinus. The coronary sinus roof, which separates it from the left atrium, does not form and so a communication exists. The left sinus horn usually persists as the left superior vena cava in these defects.

There may or may not be a bridging vein connecting the left SVC to the right SVC.

GENETICS OF ATRIAL SEPTAL DEFECTS

There is no known direct genetic cause of ASDs as most are sporadic. Primum ASDs are associated with trisomy 21. Holt-Oram syndrome, an autosomal dominant disorder characterized by upper limb skeletal abnormalities; absent or hypoplastic radii and conduction defects of cardiac rhythm (especially first-degree heart block and isolated first-degree heart block) is associated with secundum ASDs. Complete absence of the atrial septum is associated with Ellis von Creveld. Associated anatomic lesions include mitral valve prolapse, partial anomalous pulmonary venous return, and complex congenital heart defects.

PATHOPHYSIOLOGY

The basic pathophysiology is the same for all the atrial septal defects despite the anatomic variation. This is discussed in the chapter on left-to-right shunts. The left-to-right shunt at the atrial level results in right-sided volume loading. Thus, the right atrium, right ventricle (RV), pulmonary arteries, and pulmonary vascular bed are enlarged because of the increased volume of the shunt. There is increased flow across an otherwise normal tricuspid and pulmonary valve, leading to increased turbulence or a flow-related gradient across these valves.

CLINICAL FINDINGS

Natural History

Small defects, usually less than 5 mm without right-side volume overload, have no effect on the natural history of the individual. Some of these defects may close spontaneously. Patients with moderate to large defects are usually asymptomatic until the second decade of life. Rarely, patients can present with congestive heart failure or pulmonary vascular disease (<<1%) in infancy or childhood. Children with significant defects are often smaller than expected but true failure to thrive is rare. The physiologic impact of the left-to-right shunt increases with age. Initially it manifests with decreased exercise tolerance and can lead to overt congestive heart failure. There is a progressive increase in symptoms in the second to third decade of life. Platypnea-orthodeoxia is a rare pattern of dyspnea with arterial hypoxemia usually presenting in the fifth to sixth decade of life. Platypnea is defined as dyspnea induced by upright posture and it is relieved by the recumbent position. Orthodeoxia refers to arterial desaturation resulting from assuming an erect or upright position. It has been shown that posture affects intracardiac streaming of blood. In patients with platypnea-orthodeoxia the IVC flow is directed preferentially across the atrial septal defect or patent foramen ovale in the upright posture. This is not evident in the recumbent position. Patients with significant shunts and therefore enlarged atria are prone to atrial arrhythmias

including atrial flutter, atrial fibrillation, and automatic (ectopic) atrial tachycardia. These arrhythmias are rare in childhood and usually present after the second decade of life. Pulmonary vascular disease may develop in 5–10% of patients with significant defects. It predominantly affects women in a ratio much higher than 2:1. Paradoxic cerebral or systemic emboli may occur. Infective endocarditis is very uncommon and prophylaxis is not recommended for atrial septal defects without other associated defects, such as cleft mitral valve with a primum ASD or mitral valve prolapse.

Physical Examination

In large defects with a large left-to-right shunt, the height and weight may be normal to slightly below normal. Associated defects such as limb anomalies or features of Down syndrome may be seen if there is an underlying genetic abnormality. The heart rate is usually normal. Occasionally a low-grade tachycardia can be seen. The blood pressure is normal. There may be a prominent precordial bulge or right ventricular heave in some patients with a volume loaded enlarged RV. The auscultatory findings reflect the physiology. An atrial septal defect results in an increased volume load on the RA and RV. This can produce a split S1 with loud second component because of forceful and late closure of the tricuspid valve. The classical finding is a wide fixed splitting of S2. The wide split results from the late closure of the pulmonary valve. Late closure occurs because of the increased volume load that is ejected by the RV. The late closure is accentuated by increased capacitance of the pulmonary bed. In patients with a dilated RV the time required for depolarization is increased. This is manifest by the incomplete right bundle branch block observed on the surface ECG in these patients. This further prolongs right ventricular ejection time delaying pulmonary valve closure, compared to the left ventricle. Normal physiologic splitting of S2 results from respiratory variations in loading of the right and left side of the heart (i.e., increased venous return to the RV with inspiration and increased venous return to the left ventricle with expiration). In the presence of an atrial septal communication, these changes are transmitted to both sides and respiratory variation of S2 splitting cannot occur. An ejection systolic murmur, usually grade 2-3/6, results from relative pulmonary valve stenosis produced by increased blood flow across it. Occasionally, a middiastolic flow murmur can be heard secondary to increased flow across tricuspid valve.

LABORATORY FINDINGS

Chest Radiography

Cardiomegaly, mild to moderate, is seen secondary to a dilated RA and RV. There are increased pulmonary vascular markings in patients with large left-to-right shunts.

Electrocardiogram (ECG)

Typically, there is normal sinus rhythm with right-axis deviation, intraventricular conduction delay with deep S wave in lead 1 and an RSR′ in V1 and V3R. The ECG may demonstrate an atrial arrhythmia, defects of conduction and sinus node dysfunction, especially after the second decade. A counter-clockwise loop, with left-axis deviation and Q waves in lead 1 and AVL is usually seen in patients with primum ASDs or other endocardial cushion defects.

Echocardiograpy

ASDs can be seen with transthoracic echocardiography in infants and children, or transesophageal echocardiography in older patients. The location of the atrial septal defect can usually be identified via echocardiography. A dilated RA and RV are noted as well as paradoxic interventricular septal motion secondary to a volume loaded RV. Flow acceleration across the tricuspid and pulmonary valves is seen because of the increased volume across these valves. It is important to demonstrate normal pulmonary venous return, and this can usually be performed with echocardiography.

Cardiac Catheterization

This is usually not required for diagnosis. It may be required to assess the severity and reversibility of pulmonary vascular resistance in patients suspected of having pulmonary vascular disease. It also may be indicated in the case of a sinus venosus ASD to demonstrate pulmonary venous return (help exclude anomalous pulmonary venous return. Catheterization may be used for intervention as described below.

MANAGEMENT

A hemodynamically significant ASD requiring closure is said to exist if there is RA and RV volume overload. There is no real role for medical management of a hemodynamically significant atrial septal defect. In rare circumstances, a diuretic may be used to decrease pulmonary congestion, and afterload reducing agents have a theoretical role in decreasing systemic relative to pulmonary vascular resistance (thereby decreasing the left-to-right shunt).

Secundum ASD

Surgical closure is usually performed at 4–5 years of age prior to entering first grade at school. Most centers are now reporting a near 0% mortality with surgical closure. Surgical closure is performed using standard cardiopulmonary bypass techniques. A brief period of cardioplegic cardiac arrest allows a small defect to be closed primarily (suture only). With larger defects, a pericardial (autologous) or Gore-Tex patch is used to prevent atrial distortion. There is rarely a need for inotropic support. Although postoperative management and results vary amongst institutions, the patient is usually extubated on the operating room table or shortly after arrival to the ICU. The ICU stay is usually 24 h and the hospital stay is usually 3–4 days. Some surgeons use minimally invasive techniques to perform ASD closures. These techniques result in shorter incisions and/or avoidance of a full sternotomy (ministernotomy). In adults, ASDs have been closed using robotic techniques without the need for a sternotomy.

Closure before 10 years of age is advised as later closure is associated with increased incidence of atrial arrhythmias. Closure before 25 years is associated with a normal life expectancy.

This is not the case if repaired after 25 years of age. This is even more dramatic if repaired after 40 years of age. Atrial arrhythmias or sinus node dysfunction continues to be a problem in some postoperative patients. It is not clear if this is related to surgery or residua from the ASD; however, postmortem findings in patients with sudden death following surgery demonstrated surgical damage to the sinus node and fibrosis of the conduction tissue. Postpericardiotomy syndrome and patch dehiscences are other complications associated with surgical closure.

Transcatheter device closure is a relatively new method and only applicable for secundum ASDs. Many devices have been developed but the Amplatzer septal occluder (ASO) device (AGA Medical, Minneapolis, MN, USA) is the only FDA approved device. The results of closure with ASO device are similar to surgical closure; however, complications are fewer and hospital stay is shorter for device closure. An early increase in the frequency of atrial arrhythmias may be observed by both surgical and catheter closure and usually resolve by 6 months. Rarely, complete heart block is noted but this may be avoided with careful patient selection. Headaches, which resolve by 6 months, have been observed in 5%. No significant late complications have been observed to date.

Management Controversies

The debate of surgical versus device closure is active. Device closure is only possible for secundum defects. The patient's size, and indirectly the atrial size, will determine the largest device size that can be accommodated. Large devices alter the flexibility of the atrial septum. The long-term results (greater than 6 years) for device closure are not known; however, one study comparing the neuropsychologic outcomes of patients who underwent surgical closure versus transcatheter device closure of their ASDs, showed a small but significant decrease in Full-Scale IQ and Performance IQ in the surgical group.

Sinus Venosus ASD

Surgical closure is the only accepted method of treatment of a sinus venosus ASD. The surgical approach is complicated by pulmonary venous anatomy. Sometimes the SVC needs to be augmented anteriorly to accommodate the RUPV baffle to the LA. This can lead to sinus node dysfunction. Transsection and reimplantation of superior vena cava to the right atrial appendage is another surgical option. Transcatheter closure of sinus venosus ASDs with devices is not possible at this time.

Coronary Sinus Type ASD

Surgery consists of patch closure of the coronary sinus ostium. This will result in coronary venous blood draining to the left atrium. If there is a left SVC with a large bridging vein (communicating vein between the right and left SVC) the left SVC can be ligated. If there is a small or absent bridging vein, the left SVC can usually be reimplanted into the right atrial appendage.

Primum ASD

Surgical closure is the only treatment option of a primum ASD as well. Details of the procedure are described as part of the management of endocardial cushion defects in the chapter on AV canals.

Suggested Readings

Bichell DP, Geva T, Bacha EA, Mayer JE, Jonas RA, del Nido PJ: Minimal access approach for the repair of atrial septal defect: the initial 135 patients. *Ann Thorac Surg* 70:115–118, 2000.

Emmanoulides GC, Allen HD, Riemenschneider TA, Gutgesell HP (eds.), *Moss and Adams' Heart Disease in Infants, Children, and Adolescents: Including the Fetus and Young Adult*, 5th ed. Baltimore, Williams & Wilkins, 1995, Chap. 51–52, pp. 687–723.

Garson A, Bricker JT, Fisher DJ, Neish SR (eds.), *The Science and Practice of Pediatric Cardiology*, 2nd ed. Baltimore, Williams & Wilkins, 1998, Chap. 51, pp. 1141–1140.

Visconti KJ, Bichell DP, Jonas RA, Newburger JW, Bellinger DC: Developmental outcome after surgical versus interventional closure of secundum atrial septal defect in children. *Circulation* 100(19):145–150, 1999.

C H A P T E R

13

VENTRICULAR SEPTAL DEFECT

David J. Waight

INTRODUCTION

Ventricular septal defects (VSD) are the most common significant form of congenital heart disease. They are only surpassed in frequency by a bicuspid aortic valve. VSDs account for approximately 20% of all congenital heart defects. Ventricular septal defects are also the most common lesion in chromosomal syndromes. Despite the high frequency in chromosomal syndromes, more than 95% of the patients with a ventricular septal defect have normal chromosomes.

ANATOMY

The intraventricular septum is a complex structure separating the left ventricle from the right ventricle, and in the most superior portion, the left ventricle from the inferior right atrium. The ventricular septum is primarily made up of contractile muscle. This constitutes the inferior, anterior, and posterior portions of the ventricular septum. The most superior portion of the ventricular septum is called the membranous septum. It is just below the aortic and

pulmonary valves and extends into the inlet portion of the ventricles under the mitral and tricuspid valves. This most superior portion in the inlet portion separates the right atrium from the left ventricle. A VSD in this location leads to shunting of blood from the left ventricle to right atrium. VSDs can occur in both the muscular and the membranous, or what is often termed the perimembranous, portion of the ventricular septum. This portion is near the membranous septum and in the area of the membranous-to-muscular septum transition. Muscular ventricular septal defects can occur in the mid-muscular (which are most common), anterior muscular, posterior muscular, or apical muscular septum. There may also be more than one ventricular septal defect, or multiple VSDs known as a "Swiss cheese" septum. VSDs range in size from very small (1 mm), to very large defects, which may include nearly the entire ventricular septum.

PATHOPHYSIOLOGY

Ventricular septal defects lead to left-to-right shunting secondary to the increased pressure in the left ventricle versus the right ventricle and pulmonary artery and the increased compliance (decreased resistance) of the pulmonary arterial bed versus the systemic arterial bed. A left-to-right shunt occurs during systole when both the right and left ventricles are contracting and the aorta and pulmonary valves are open. This leads to the majority of the shunt going from the left ventricle through the ventricular septum into the right ventricular outflow tract and into the pulmonary artery bed. The increased flow into the pulmonary arterial bed leads to volume overloading of the pulmonary arteries, pulmonary veins, left atrium, and left ventricle.

The physiology of all VSDs is similar, but the natural history varies. The size and location of the defect alter the risk of volume loading, heart failure, aortic valve changes, and progression to pulmonary hypertension. Volume overload leads to left atrial and left ventricular enlargement and can lead to congestive heart failure. This heart failure is a result of volume overload of the pulmonary venous bed, left atrium, and left ventricle with resulting increased left ventricular end-diastolic pressure, and increased left atrial mean pressure leading to pulmonary congestion. Pulmonary congestion can lead to respiratory symptoms, frequent respiratory infections, and eventually to pulmonary edema. Large left-to-right shunts may also cause a relative decrease in the systemic cardiac output as a majority of the left ventricular stroke volume goes to the lungs instead of the body (Figure 13-1). This can lead to signs of poor output with exercise intolerance noted in older children. Similar findings are noted in infants and small children with difficulty eating, diaphoresis with feeds or with other activities, poor feeding, failure to thrive, and frequent infections. Some of these symptoms may be a result of pulmonary congestion rather than systemic cardiac output insufficient to meet systemic demands (the definition of heart failure). Thus, the concepts of heart failure and pulmonary overcirculation are frequently (and perhaps mistakenly) used interchangeably.

With large ventricular septal defects, there may be equalization of ventricular pressure with no pressure gradient from the left ventricle to the right

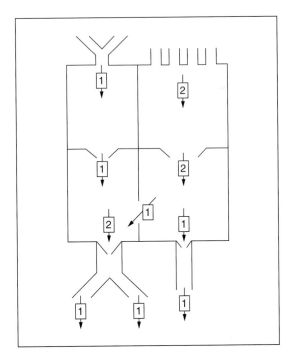

FIGURE 13-1

PHYSIOLOGY OF VENTRICULAR SEPTAL DEFECT

A single blood volume enters the right atrium from the IVC and SVC. In the right ventricle an additional blood volume enters from the left ventricle across the VSD. This volume flows to the pulmonary artery, pulmonary veins, left atrium, and left ventricle. The pulmonary blood flow (Qp) in this example is now twice the systemic blood flow (Qs). Qp/Qs = 2, a 2:1 left-to-right shunt.

ventricle and right ventricular hypertension or pressure overload of the right ventricle. Pressure overload leads to right ventricular hypertrophy. Patients with unrestrictive ventricular septal defects leading to right ventricular hypertension will develop alterations of their pulmonary vasculature and irreversible pulmonary hypertension (pulmonary vascular disease) if they remain unrepaired. Irreversible pulmonary hypertension in the setting of a ventricular septal defect is termed Eisenmenger syndrome. This degree of pulmonary hypertension eventually leads to reversal of the shunting with a net right-to-left shunt causing decreased systemic arterial saturation or cyanosis. This occurs as the pulmonary vascular resistance exceeds the systemic vascular resistance causing reversal of the shunting from left-to-right to right-to-left.

CLINICAL FINDINGS

History

The natural history of patients with ventricular septal defects varies with the size of the ventricular septal defect and the degree of left-to-right shunting. The most common presentation for patients with VSD is a pathologic murmur noted on physical examination shortly after birth. Newborn infants, in the first few hours to days after birth, may not have a VSD murmur because the right ventricular pressure and the pulmonary artery pressure are elevated and there is no pressure gradient to cause turbulent flow across the VSD and produce the typical holosystolic murmur of a VSD. These newborns may be discharged from the nursery with no pathologic murmur noted. They may then have a loud holosystolic murmur heard best at the left lower sternal border when evaluated in the first few weeks to months of life. The patients may also present with diaphoresis, poor feeding, failure to thrive, and frequent respiratory infections.

The degree of symptoms varies with the size of the left-to-right shunt. Small ventricular septal defects with minimal shunting and a Qp:Qs ratio of less than 1.5 are generally asymptomatic. Patients with larger shunts with a Qp:Qs of 1.5–2 may show some signs of pulmonary overcirculation but generally do well. Patients with a Qp:Qs greater than 2 often have significant symptoms or failure to thrive. The size of the shunt varies directly with the size of the ventricular septal defect and the pulmonary vascular resistance. Many newborns with ventricular septal defects will be asymptomatic in the first 1–2 months of life. As the pulmonary vascular resistance falls, the degree of left-to-right shunting increases and they will typically develop symptoms by 3 months of age if they are going to develop symptoms. Patients with any ventricular septal defect are at risk for endocarditis and only rarely will have acute bacterial endocarditis as the initial presentation.

Spontaneous closure of ventricular septal defects varies directly with their size and location. Small VSDs will close spontaneously up to 75% of the time or greater. These defects are generally less than 3–4 mm in size. Moderate-size defects have a significant chance of closure of up to 30–50%. Large ventricular septal defects often will decrease in relative size as the patient grows but have a low spontaneous closure rate. Muscular ventricular septal defects that are small to moderate in size have a higher incidence of closure than perimembranous defects. Perimembranous VSDs often achieve partial closure with a layer of tissue underneath the tricuspid valve that forms over the perimembranous ventricular septal defect. This is termed a tricuspid valve aneurysmal pouch. Echocardiographically, it often appears as a sock-like formation of thin tissue with a smaller residual VSD shunt.

Ventricular septal defects may be complicated by bacterial endocarditis. This is felt to be a result of the high velocity jet lesion across the ventricular septal defect that alters the endocardial tissue in the right ventricle and at the area of the septum. These patients require SBE prophylaxis for life or until the VSD has completely closed. In defects near the aortic valve, there is a risk of aortic valve regurgitation developing because of the negative pressure formed by rapid flow across the ventricular septal defect that may cause the right aortic valve leaflet to prolapse into the ventricular septal defect. This aortic regurgitation can occur at any time with this type of VSD and may progress if left untreated producing left ventricular enlargement and left heart failure. Some defects can cause the right aortic cusp to prolapse owing to lack of support structure. Long-term complications also include left atrial and left ventricular dilation, which may produce atrial or ventricular arrhythmia (Table 13-1).

Physical Examination

The most prominent physical examination feature of VSDs is a holosystolic murmur heard at the left lower sternal border. This may be a 2-5/6 harsh murmur that may radiate throughout the chest wall. Very small ventricular septal defects in the muscular septum may have an early high-pitched systolic

TABLE 13-1

VENTRICULAR SEPTAL DEFECTS

VSD Type	Clinical	History	Therapy
Muscular			
Small	Short systolic murmur, nl ECG/CXR	Spontaneous closure— no failure	Clinical observation
Moderate	Holosystolic murmur, abnl ECG/CXR	Possible spontaneous closure— possible heart failure Possible pulmonary hypertension	Clinical observation— possible anticongestive therapy, VSD closure
Large	Holosystolic murmur, diastolic rumble, abnl ECG/CXR	Spontaneous closure unlikely— heart failure Pulmonary hypertension	Anticongestive therapy, VSD closure—variable timing. possible pulmonary banding
Multiple	Holosystolic murmur, diastolic rumble	Spontaneous closure unlikely— heart failure, possibly severe Probable pulmonary hypertension	Anticongestive therapy, VSD closure—variable timing, technique possible pulmonary banding
Perimembranous			
Small	Holosystolic murmur, nl ECG/CXR	Possible spontaneous closure with tricuspid aneurismal pouch—possible heart failure Possible aortic regurgitation	Clinical observation— possible anticongestive therapy, VSD closure definite if aortic valve regurgitation develops
Larger	Holosystolic murmur, diastolic rumble, abnl ECG/CXR	Possible reduction in size or spontaneous closure with tricuspid aneurismal pouch— heart failure Possible aortic regurgitation Possible pulmonary hypertension	Possible anticongestive therapy, VSD closure
Inlet	Holosystolic murmur, abnl ECG/CXR	Does not close spontaneously Possible pulmonary hypertension	Possible anticongestive therapy, surgical VSD closure
Outlet/supracristal/ subaortic/ subpulmonary	Holosystolic murmur— possible early diastolic murmur	Does not close spontaneously Induces aortic regurgitation Possible pulmonary hypertension	Surgical VSD closure

CXR = Chest x-ray.

mild aortic regurgitation in the presence of a VSD does not clearly support the need for surgical closure of these VSDs; however, many physicians recommend closure of membranous or perimembranous VSDs that appear to alter the aortic valve to prevent the risk or progression of any aortic regurgitation.

The use of pulmonary artery banding has decreased significantly over the last few decades. It is now used only in cases in which the VSD cannot be closed due to a "Swiss cheese" septum, or other anatomic or medical conditions precluding closure. This procedure can produce permanent alteration in the pulmonary artery anatomy with main pulmonary artery and branch pulmonary artery stenosis. This requires additional surgical correction at the time of VSD closure and may require subsequent therapy with balloon dilation or stenting during cardiac catheterization.

Suggested Readings

Graham TP, Gutgesell HP: Ventricular septal defects, in: Emmanoulides GC, Riemenschneider TA, Allen HD, Gutgesell HP (eds.): *Moss and Adams Heart Disease in Infants, Children, and Adolescents*, 5th ed. Baltimore, MD, Williams & Wilkins, 1995.

Gumbiner CH, Takao A: Ventricular septal defect, in: Garson A, Bricker JT, Fisher DJ, Neish SR (eds): *The Science and Practice of Pediatric Cardiology*, 2nd ed. Baltimore, MD, Williams & Wilkins, 1998.

McNamara DG, Latson LA: Long-term follow-up of patients with malformations for which definitive surgical repair has been available for 25 years or more. *Am J Cardiol* 50:560–568, 1982.

Nicholson IA, Bichell DP, Bacha EA, del Nido PJ: Minimal sternotomy approach for congenital heart operations. *Ann Thorac Surg* 71:469–472, 2001.

Weidman WH: Second natural history study of congenital heart defects. *Circulation* 87(Suppl 2):I1–3, 1993.

14

ATRIOVENTRICULAR CANAL DEFECT

Ra-id Abdulla

INTRODUCTION

There are many forms of atrioventricular canal defect (AVCD). In its extreme form, it includes an atrial septal defect which is in continuity with a ventricular septal defect with lack of septation of the common atrioventricular canal into a mitral and tricuspid valve, leading to the formation of only one (common) atrioventricular valve. This is referred to as complete AVCD or CAVC. In many instances AVCD is not complete; instead it may include abnormalities of the atrial septum, AV valves, and ventricular septum in a spectrum of abnormal development of the endocardial cushions.

INCIDENCE

Sixty-nine percent of all patients with AVCD have Down syndrome. On the other hand, 40% of all patients with Down syndrome have congenital heart disease, one-half of which is AV canal defect. Children with Down syndrome may manifest a unique combination of two congenital heart diseases (AVCD and tetralogy of Fallot), which is not known to occur in non-Down children. Common atrium is a characteristic lesion of Ellis-Van-Creveled syndrome. Ivemark syndrome (asplenia) common AV canal defect.

EMBRYOLOGY

In the early stages of heart development, there is a common atrioventricular canal, which connects the common atrium to the primitive ventricle. This canal is initially unguarded by a valve. Endocardial cushion tissue (superior and inferior endocardial cushions) eventually forms valve-like structures in this canal. Endocardial cushions are not precursors to mitral and tricuspid valves; however, they are important in normal development of these valves.

The superior and inferior endocardial cushions grow toward each other, then fuse in the middle to separate the common AV canal into left and right passages. The left passage connects the left side of the common atrium to the left ventricle and the right passage connects the right side of the common atrium to the right ventricle. The atrial and ventricular septa then grow toward the fused area of the two endocardial cushions. This then separates the AV canal into the two atria and ventricles. Therefore, failure of the superior and inferior endocardial cushions to meet will lead to failure of the atrial and ventricular septa to completely separate the right and left atria and ventricles, leading to AVCD. Incomplete fusion leads to the variations of AVCD described below.

ANATOMY

The spectrum of lesions in AVCD varies. It does not always involve all defects (atrial septal defect [ASD], ventricular septal defect [VSD], and a common AV valve). The various pathologic forms are as follows:

1. Complete AV canal (CAVC). This consists of a primum ASD, an inlet VSD, and a common AV valve.
2. Transitional AV canal, also known as intermediate AV canal. This consists of a primum ASD, an inlet VSD, and a common AV valve with fusion of the anterior and posterior bridging leaflets. The latter can lead to restriction of the ventricular septal defect.

3. Partial AV canal (more commonly known as a primum ASD). This consists of a primum ASD and almost always, a cleft in the anterior leaflet of the mitral valve. There is no ventricular septal defect.
4. Incomplete AV canal. This is an uncommonly used term. It refers to cleft mitral valve without other abnormalities.

Complete AV canal defect is categorized into A, B, or C according to the anatomy of the common AV valve leaflets to the right and left ventricles. These types are as follows:

*   Type A: The anterior leaflet is divided and attached to the crest of the VSD.
*   Type B: Anterior leaflet is divided and chordae from left-sided leaflet cross and insert in the right ventricle.
*   Type C: Anterior leaflet is bridging (single) with no chordal attachment (free floating).

Because of the displacement of the right- and left-sided portions of the common AV valve (compared to the normal location of the tricuspid and mitral valves) to the midportion of the heart, there may be obstruction to left ventricular outflow seen as "goosenecking" on angiography (Figure 14-1).

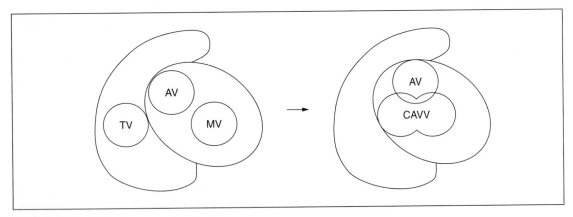

FIGURE 14-1

DISPLACEMENT OF ATRIOVENTRICULAR VALVES

Diagram showing the displacement of the atrioventricular valves toward the middle of the heart causing obstruction to the left ventricular outflow tract. TV: tricuspid valve; MV: mitral valve; AV: aortic valve; CAVV: common AV valve. Note the encroachment of the CAVV near the aortic valve.

PATHOPHYSIOLOGY

The pathophysiology of an AVCD is similar to that described for ASDs and VSDs. In addition, there may be the superimposed pathophysiology of mitral or tricuspid valve regurgitation as well as left ventricular outflow tract obstruction or right ventricular outflow obstruction (tetralogy of Fallot variant) as described in those respective chapters.

The atrial and ventricular septal defects cause left-to-right shunting leading to increased pulmonary blood flow (PBF) (Figure 14-2). This increase in PBF will cause congestion of the pulmonary circulation leading to shortness of breath and subsequently limitation of the child's ability to exercise or feed, resulting in failure to thrive. Furthermore, the cardiac output through the left ventricle to the body may be reduced, owing to excessive pulmonary blood flow, causing symptoms of poor cardiac output, such as easy fatigability.

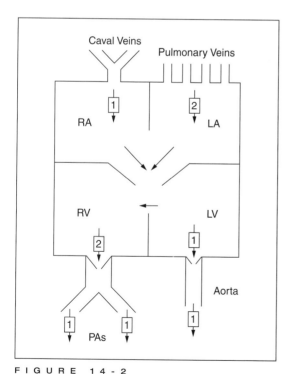

FIGURE 14-2

DIAGRAM REPRESENTING A COMPLETE AV CANAL DEFECT

Because of the large VSD, the right ventricular pressure will be systemic. The increased pulmonary blood flow and elevated pressures will eventually cause pathologic changes in the pulmonary vasculature, causing pulmonary vascular resistance to be elevated. Initially, these changes are reversible; however, if untreated the abnormal pulmonary vascular resistance will be permanent, leading to irreversible pulmonary hypertension. Children with Down syndrome tend to develop pulmonary vascular resistance elevation earlier than normal children.

CLINICAL FINDINGS

Patients with an isolated primum ASD and/or cleft mitral valve will have clinical and laboratory findings typical of those respective lesions.

Patients with AVCD develop symptoms of congestive heart failure because of increased pulmonary blood flow as a result of the atrial and ventricular septal defects. Occasionally, particularly in patients with large ventricular septal defects, mixing of oxygenated and deoxygenated bloods leads to a mild drop in oxygen saturation when measured by pulse oximetry. This does not manifest as visible cyanosis. If cyanosis is seen in a patient with Down syndrome, then associated tetralogy of Fallot should be suspected. Congestive heart failure symptoms will include easy fatigability, shortness of breath, and failure to thrive. Infants will feed poorly and develop tachypnea, tachycardia, sweating, pallor, and diaphoresis with exercise such as feeding.

The physical examination will usually reveal an increase in heart and respiratory rate and possibly mild to moderate respiratory distress. The capillary refill may be delayed because of poor cardiac output as a result of left-to-right shunting of blood (systemic steal) and myocardial fatigue from the increased pulmonary blood flow. There may be hepatomegaly (owing to hyperexpansion of the lungs from pulmonary congestion with decreased lung compliance), but splenomegaly is rare. The precordium is hyperactive with increased right and left ventricular impulses.

On auscultation, the lungs will continue to be clear, even with pulmonary edema, since respiratory sounds in children are typically bronchial and not alveolar. Therefore, alveolar pathology such as pulmonary edema is not as audible as bronchial pathology such as reactive airway disease.

Cardiac auscultation reveals a long, harsh systolic murmur at the left mid-to-upper sternal border owing to left-to-right shunting and blood flow across the pulmonary valve. This is best heard over the left lower sternal border. If the VSD is small or restrictive, a more typical harsh holosystolic murmur is noted at the left mid-sternal border. A holosystolic murmur at the apex may also be heard secondary to mitral regurgitation. A diastolic rumble indicative of increased mitral flow may be heard between the left lower sternal border and the apex.

LABORATORY FINDINGS

Electrocardiography

The ECG shows a "northeast QRS axis: 180-270°" owing to displacement of the normal position of the atrioventricular node. There may also be right ventricular hypertrophy and left ventricular hypertrophy. In an isolated primum ASD, superior axis deviation may also be seen, with or without incomplete right bundle branch, which reflects right-sided volume loading.

Chest Radiography

The heart is enlarged (biventricular enlargement) with increased pulmonary blood flow. With a primum ASD, cardiomegaly with increased pulmonary blood flow is typically seen. Cardiomegaly may be out of proportion to left-to-right shunting secondary to mitral insufficiency.

Echocardiography

The cardiac anatomy of an AVCD and shunting of blood flow will be seen well with echocardiography. The type of AVC defect, and the size of the ASD and VSD can be determined. In addition, the common atrioventricular valve anatomy, its

alignment to the ventricles, leaflet attachments, and spacing of the papillary muscles can be seen. Valvar regurgitation is easily identified. In addition to the cardiac anatomy, ventricular size and function can be assessed. Echocardiography can provide enough information needed for surgical repair. Therefore, in typical cases of AVCD, when pulmonary vascular obstructive disease is not suspected, echocardiography will suffice in preparation for surgery.

In patients with an isolated primum ASD, echocardiography shows the primum ASD as well as a cleft mitral valve and mitral insufficiency. Mitral regurgitation may be directed to the right atrium through the atrial septal defect. This may explain the lack of a dilated left atrium.

In addition to the primary lesion, echocardiography can demonstrate associated lesions such as tetralogy of Fallot, hypoplasia of the ventricles or arteries, and a left superior vena cava.

Cardiac Catheterization

Cardiac catheterization is indicated when there is evidence of elevated pulmonary vascular resistance. Angiography should be performed in special planar views (the hepatoclavicular view) to demonstrate the VSD as well as mitral regurgitation. An aortogram is also performed to evaluate for a patent ductus arteriosus, which is a common finding in patients with AV canal and Down syndrome. The primum ASD and inlet VSD are not amenable to device closure in the catheterization laboratory.

MANAGEMENT

Surgical repair will be necessary in all patients with a complete AV canal. This is performed at 6–12 months of age, because the likelihood of developing irreversible pulmonary vascular obstructive disease is higher after 1 year of age. Standard cardiopulmonary bypass techniques with moderate hypothermia are usually employed. Intraoperative transesophageal echocardiography (TEE) is performed to confirm the preoperative anatomy, and to assess the repair postoperatively prior to decannulation from cardiopulmonary bypass. The procedure is performed during a brief period of cardioplegic cardiac arrest, in which the defect is exposed through a right atrial incision, and the anatomy examined. There are three techniques described to repair a CAVC. All consist of closure of the ASD and VSD using one or two patches. The common AV valve is then reconstructed to make two functional (mitral and tricuspid) AV valves.

1. The double patch technique: A patch of Goretex, Dacron, or pericardium is used to close the VSD component while another patch is used to close the ASD component. The cleft of the left-sided AV valve is usually closed.
2. The single patch technique: The common AV valve is divided in a plane parallel to the septum and a single patch is used to close both the VSD and ASD components. The valve leaflets are then reattached to the patch. The cleft of the left-sided AV valve is usually closed.
3. Single patch technique without a VSD patch: The VSD is closed primarily by approximating it to the undersurface of the AV valve. This is mainly used when the VSD component is small. The cleft of the left-sided AV valve is usually closed.

Pulmonary artery banding is no longer performed as a temporizing procedure, since complete repair is possible, even in the neonatal period; however, in unstable neonates, pulmonary artery banding may be performed to reduce pulmonary blood flow until the child is older and more stable. Pulmonary artery banding may be associated with increased AV valve insufficiency and should be avoided if possible.

Postoperatively, support depends on the severity of the underlying lesions. There is rarely a need for significant postoperative inotropic support for a complete AV canal repair. The postoperative course is often dependent on the adequacy of the repair, mainly the amount of residual mitral regurgitation. In trisomy 21 patients especially (80% of all CAVC repairs), the presence of pulmonary dysfunction, pulmonary vascular disease or tracheomalacia can result in a protracted postoperative course; however, provided the repair is adequate, the vast majority of patients survive the operation and do well. Potential complications that are specific to CAVC surgery include AV block (5%), residual mitral or tricuspid regurgitation, or residual septal defects (unusual). Long-term results of surgery are good, and depend to a great extent on the amount of residual or recurrent MR. Approximately 10–20% of patients will require repeated mitral surgery for regurgitation.

Suggested Readings

Casteneda AR, Jonas JA, Mayer JE, Hanley FL: *Cardiac Surgery of the Neonate and Infant.* Philadelphia, PA, WB Saunders, 1994.

Crawford FA, Stroud MR: Surgical repair of complete atrioventricular septal defect. *Ann Thorac Surg* 72:1621–1629, 2001.

Fyker DC: *Nadas' Pediatric Cardiology.* Chicago, IL, Mosby Year Book, 1992.

Garson A, Bricker JT, Fisher DJ, Neish SR: *The Science and Practice of Pediatric Cardiology*, 2nd ed. Baltimore, MD, Williams & Wilkins, 1998.

Laks H: Atrioventricular canal. *Semin Thorac Cardiovasc Surg* 9(1):1–55, 1979.

Perloff JK: *Clinical Recognition of Congenital Heart Disease*, 5th ed. WB Saunders, 2003.

Snider AR, Serwer GA: *Echocardiography in Pediatric Heart Disease*, 2nd ed. Chicago, IL, Mosby Year Book, 1998.

15

PATENT DUCTUS ARTERIOSUS

David G. Ruschhaupt

ANATOMY AND EMBRYOLOGY

The ductus arteriosus is a muscular artery with circular arranged smooth muscle cells. The origin of this vessel is from the embryonic sixth aortic arch and it connects the very proximal left pulmonary artery (LPA) to the upper descending aorta approximately 2–10 mm from the origin of the left subclavian artery. In the patients with a right aortic arch, the majority have a left ductus arteriosus. The origin of the ductus arteriosus will then be from the innominate artery or the proximal left subclavian artery. It then joins the LPA. Rarely, a right-sided ductus arteriosus will join a right-sided descending aorta (mirror image) and very rarely bilateral ducti will occur with a left ductus from the aorta to LPA, and a right ductus connecting the innominate artery to the right pulmonary artery (RPA).

The ductus arteriosus is critical to the parallel circuit function of the fetal circulation (described in the chapter on fetal cardiology). It allows the fetal right ventricle to bypass the pulmonary circulation and pump blood to the descending aorta and the placental circulation.

Closure of the ductus occurs in two stages. During the first 10–15 hours there is contraction of the smooth muscle with shortening of the structure and thickening of the wall. Approximation of intimal cushions assists in the closure process. Complete closure occurs over the next 2–3 weeks with diffuse fibrous proliferation of the intima. Complete closure may take as long as 8 weeks, ending with a fibrous ligament known as the ligamentum arteriosum.

PATHOPHYSIOLOGY

Cardiac pathology associated with an isolated patent ductus arteriosus (PDA) depends on the size of the ductus and the relative systemic and pulmonary vascular resistances (PVR). The ductus itself has a larger aortic opening and a more restrictive orifice on the pulmonary arterial side. Because resistance to blood flow is usually higher in the aortic circulation than in the pulmonary arterial circulation, blood flows into the lungs from the aorta, increasing pulmonary blood flow. The increased pulmonary blood flow increases the volume of venous return to the left atrium as well as increasing the volume of flow across the mitral valve and the left ventricular stroke volume. The degree of enlargement that occurs to the left heart structures is a reflection of how much extra blood volume is accommodated or "shunted" through the PDA (Figure 15-1). The ascending aorta and the aortic arch up to the level of the PDA will also be enlarged.

Physiologically, a PDA can be thought of as small, moderate, or large. The advent of echo and Doppler echocardiography has created a fourth category of PDA, the "silent ductus." A silent PDA is seen by color flow Doppler but not heard clinically.

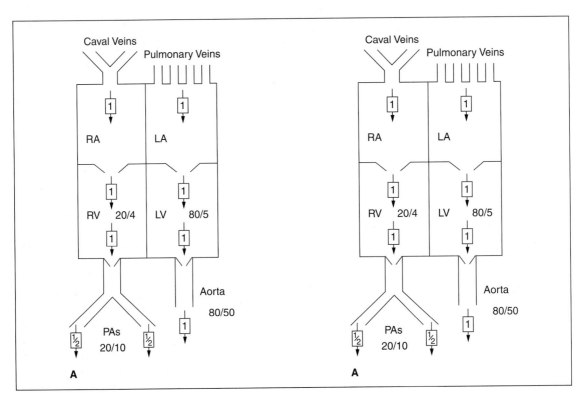

FIGURE 15-1

VENTRICULAR AND ARTERIAL PRESSURE

Part **A** shows a diagram of a normal heart with associated ventricular and arterial pressures. A diagram of a moderate to large size PDA is shown in part **B**. A left-to-right shunt of 1 relative cardiac output was chosen for this example. Note the left atrial and ventricular enlargement. This is because the left atrium and ventricle contain 2 relative cardiac outputs. This will not be present with a small or "silent" PDA. Note also the increased flow across the mitral and aortic valves. This increased flow will cause increased turbulence and a murmur of functional stenosis. This may not be clinically apparent as the continuous murmur of flow through the ductus arteriosus may be more prominent. The murmur of the ductus arteriosus is continuous because of the persistent gradient in both systole and diastole. In this example, the gradient is from 85 to 30 mmHg in systole and 40 to 10 mmHg in diastole. Note also that the systolic pressure in the aorta and pulmonary arteries has risen from baseline (**A**) and the diastolic pressure in the aorta has decreased. The latter reflects the diastolic runoff or systemic steal. Clinically, this is seen with an increased pulse pressure and bounding pulses. Although there is a tendency for equalization between the systolic and diastolic pressures in the aorta and pulmonary artery, the diastolic pressure in the pulmonary artery may increase minimally as long as the pulmonary vascular resistance (PVR) is low. In a large PDA, there will be equalization of the systolic pressures with a slower equalization of diastolic pressures until PVR is elevated, at which point it may be irreversible (Eisenmenger's physiology).

TABLE 15-1

SUMMARY OF PATHOLOGY FOUND IN PATENT DUCTUS ARTERIOSUS

Type of PDA	Silent	Small	Moderate[a]	Large
Pathology	Normal heart		LAE LVH	LAE BVH
History	Normal development		Tachypnea possible FTT	Tachypnea sweating FTT
Examination	Normal	Machinery murmur	Machinery murmur Tachypnea; diastolic Rumble; precordial hyperactivity	Short mid-systolic murmur; Tachypnea Precordial hyperactivity

[a]LAE: left atrial enlargement; LVH: left ventricular hypertrophy; BVH: biventricular hypertrophy; FTT: failure to thrive.

These categories are outlined in Table 15-1 with corresponding clinical and laboratory findings. A small PDA will have typical clinical findings without cardiac enlargement or symptoms. A moderate PDA will be associated with a volume of pulmonary blood flow that approximates twice the volume of systemic blood flow with corresponding enlargement of the left atrium and left ventricle. A large PDA is associated with unrestricted shunting into the pulmonary arteries and significant elevation of the pulmonary arterial pressure. The presence of pulmonary hypertension will cause additional hypertrophy of the right ventricle. The actual amount of shunting will be determined by the pulmonary vascular resistance. If the resistance is low, there will be a very large shunt. If the vascular resistance is high, the amount of shunting may be minimal or there may even be shunting from the pulmonary artery to the aorta (Eisenmenger's physiology). Pressure is the product of volume flow and vascular resistance (pressure = flow × resistance). The large, unrestricted PDA will have either high flow/low resistance pulmonary hypertension or low flow/high resistance pulmonary hypertension. With larger shunts there is increasing diastolic flow into the pulmonary arteries and decreasing aortic diastolic pressure known as "diastolic runoff" (Figure 15-1).

CLINICAL HISTORY

The signs and symptoms of a patient with a PDA are directly related to the volume of increased pulmonary blood flow. At birth, a significant PDA may go undetected because the pulmonary vascular resistance is high. Similar to ventricular septal defect physiology, the amount of blood flow through the shunt may be minimal at birth and increase over the first 3 months of life, when the pulmonary vascular resistance reaches its lowest level. Once the pulmonary resistance has decreased, clinical presentation will depend on the volume of the shunt. A "silent PDA" will leave the patient symptom free throughout life. The risk of endarteritis or other complications is unknown at this time. Small PDAs also leave the patient totally asymptomatic, although there is a small risk of endarteritis. The larger PDAs will result in progressively more symptoms, depending on the volume of pulmonary blood flow. In the face of a large shunt, pulmonary compliance decreases producing an increased work of breathing. Tachypnea, poor feeding, sweating with feeds and failure to thrive are additional symptoms of chronic left ventricular volume overload and heart failure. In larger shunts, pulmonary vascular disease with Eisenmenger's physiology may occur, but usually not before the second birthday.

Adult patients may develop aneurysmal dilatation, calcifications, and/or rupture of the ductus.

CLINICAL EXAMINATION

The classic clinical finding for a patient with a patent ductus arteriosus is described as a "machinery" murmur, so called because of its continuous systolic and diastolic components. This murmur occurs because of the pressure differential that exists between the aorta and pulmonary artery throughout the cardiac cycle. The murmur is heard best at the left upper sternal border, in the left infraclavicular area. As the pulmonary blood flow approaches a volume that is approximately twice the systemic cardiac output, a separate diastolic rumble murmur can be heard toward the apex of the heart. This murmur is created by the turbulence of increased diastolic blood flow across the mitral valve. Tachypnea and tachycardia will be present in cases of pulmonary over-circulation (large shunts) or myocardial dysfunction. Increasing amounts of pulmonary vascular resistance, which leads to less shunt flow, eliminates the diastolic murmur and shortens the systolic portion of the murmur. If the murmur disappears, the PDA either has closed or pulmonary vascular resistance has become severely elevated. The newborn presents a special circumstance. Usually, in the newborn period, the pulmonary vascular resistance remains high enough that only a relatively short systolic murmur will be heard. If a typical "machinery" murmur of a patent ductus is observed in the newborn, the clinician should ascertain why the pulmonary vascular resistance is so low that this murmur is heard. It is possible that there is a ductal-dependent congenital heart defect such as pulmonary valve or tricuspid valve atresia. Suspicion of this possibility ought to prompt an appropriate evaluation.

LABORATORY FINDINGS

Chest Radiography

The radiographic findings in PDA are very nonspecific. Depending on the amount of pulmonary blood flow, the chest radiograph may demonstrate left ventricular and left atrial enlargement. The lung vascular markings may also be increased. In the case of pulmonary hypertension with increased vascular resistance, cardiomegaly will be replaced by a large, dilated main pulmonary artery.

Electrocardiogram

The electrocardiogram may be normal, or reflect left ventricular and left atrial enlargement depending on the amount of the shunt. The T waves are normal unless there is very severe left ventricular enlargement with possible ischemia or the patient is receiving lanoxin for management of the congestive heart failure.

Echocardiography

The echocardiogram should demonstrate the anatomic structure of a PDA as well as blood flow through it via Doppler. Estimations of pulmonary artery pressures may also be made with Doppler. Chamber size may be measured and compared to normal, indirectly demonstrating the amount of volume overload. Other associated congenital heart lesions are also seen. Echocardiography is diagnostic.

Cardiac Catheterization and Angiography

Catheterization can also confirm the presence of a patent ductus by showing an increase in oxygen saturation in the pulmonary artery. Catheter measurement of pulmonary artery pressure, along with calculation of pulmonary artery blood flow leads to an estimation of pulmonary vascular resistance. Finally, the catheter may actually pass from the pulmonary artery to the aorta (or from the aorta to the pulmonary artery), proving the presence of the ductus. An aortogram, injection of contrast medium in the aorta at the level of the left subclavian artery, will outline the diameter and length of the ductus. Catheterization is not currently used as the primary means of diagnosis. Rather, it is used only if there are diagnostic dilemmas or for treatment.

TREATMENT

Timing of Treatment

Clinical detection of a persistently patent ductus arteriosus is an indication for its closure. Timing and the type of procedure depend on symptoms. If congestive heart failure is present, immediate closure is indicated. This is true for premature infants, neonates, and children. Adult patients will rarely present with signs of congestive heart failure. In the absence of heart failure, a PDA may be closed electively at the convenience of the family and physician. In the asymptomatic full-term or premature infant, allowing time for spontaneous closure (up to a few months) may be prudent.

Types of Treatment

In the premature infant, an initial trial of indomethacin is usually undertaken in the absence of contraindications for its use. Failure of medical closure is usually recognized after two or three attempts.

Unless there is another illness prohibiting closure, there is little if any role for long-term medical management of a symptomatic patient with a PDA. Heart failure has traditionally been managed by the combined use of digitalis and diuretics along with the restriction of fluid, though the use of these medications is controversial. Successful surgical ligation of a ductus arteriosus was first accomplished in 1938 by Dr. Robert Gross. Since then, surgical ligation through a lateral thoracotomy has been the standard management. Newer surgical techniques have allowed the procedure to be performed via thorascopy with a minimal surgical incision. Recanalization of a ductus ateriosus closed with simple ligation has been observed. Thus, it may be best to both ligate and divide the ductus. Risks of division include bleeding and injury to surrounding

structures. Currently, it has become routine to perform percutaneous coil embolization of the ductus arteriosus in the cardiac catheterization laboratory. Other occlusion devices may soon be approved, making it feasible to close even a very large ductus, one that is too large for coil embolization. There are patient size limitations which make percutaneous closure prohibitive in small or premature infants; however, newer types of devices are being designed and tested that most likely will make it feasible to close all PDAs in the catheterization laboratory. SBE prophylaxis is recommended for 6 months after the complete closure of a PDA.

CONTROVERSIES

The silent ductus arteriosus: The broad availability of ultrasound not infrequently demonstrates the presence of a small ductal shunt that is not otherwise detectable. It is unclear if such a shunt should be closed. If surgery is the only option, then the answer is probably no; however, with the availability of coil or device closure in the cardiac catheterization lab, the answer is probably yes. The risk/benefit ratio of elective closure of a "silent" ductus arteriosus is unknown. Whether or not these require SBE prophylaxis is also unknown.

Suggested Readings

Allen HD, Gutgesell HP, Clark EB, Driscoll DJ: *Moss and Adams' Heart Disease in Infants, Children, and Adolescents Including the Fetus and Young Adult*, 6th ed. Philadelphia, PA, Lippincott Williams & Wilkins, 2001.

Garson A, Bricker JT, Fisher DJ, Neish SR: *The Science and Practice of Pediatric Cardiology*, 2nd ed. Baltimore, MD, Williams & Wilkins, 1998.

16

OTHER LEFT-TO-RIGHT SHUNT LESIONS

Hitendra T. Patel

INTRODUCTION

There are a number of other rare anatomic cardiac abnormalities causing left-to-right shunts, which have not been discussed in the previous chapters. Much of the pathophysiology of these lesions is similar to those already discussed; however, for completeness, a brief list and description, although not exhaustive, of these lesions is provided in this chapter. The lesions will be subdivided based on the underlying pathophysiology.

ATRIAL LEVEL LEFT-TO-RIGHT SHUNTS

Atrial level shunts that are not atrial septal defects include unobstructed total anomalous pulmonary venous connection and return (TAPVC) and partial anomalous pulmonary venous connection (PAPVC). In each of these lesions, there will be increased volume loading of the right atrium and subsequent volume loading of the right ventricle in diastole. TAPVC is discussed in a separate chapter. PAPVC has many anatomic variations in which the connections of the various pulmonary veins to the systemic

veins have been reported. The right pulmonary veins usually connect anomalously to derivatives of the right cardinal venous system (i.e., the SVC, IVC, or right atrium). The left anomalous pulmonary veins connect to the left cardinal venous system (i.e., the coronary sinus, persistent LSVC, and the innominate vein). Scimitar syndrome is a rare and variable congenital malformation of the right lung. In its complete form it comprises PAPVC of all the right-sided pulmonary veins to the IVC, an intact atrial septum, hypoplasia of the right lung with dextrocardia, and hypoplasia of the right pulmonary artery. The latter does not supply all lung segments (usually no supply of the right lower lobes). These segments are supplied by aorto-pulmonary vessels arising from the subdiaphragmatic aorta, and are referred to as sequestrated lung segments. The Scimitar syndrome derives its name from the Turkish sword as the anomalous pulmonary veins have a C-shaped appearance on the right side of the radiographic cardiac silhouette. The pathophysiology of PAPVC is virtually identical to an atrial septal defect (ASD) as is the clinical presentation and physical examination. The overall presentation is determined by: (1) the number of anomalously draining pulmonary veins, (2) the site of connection, and (3) the presence or absence of an associated atrial septal defect. As in all patients with a shunt, pulmonary vascular resistance (PVR) is another factor in clinical presentation. In patients with an intact atrial septum and no associated pulmonary artery abnormalities, a greater percentage of total pulmonary blood flow (PBF) and pulmonary venous return will be toward the direction of the anomalously draining pulmonary vein. This is a result of the higher compliance of the right atrium compared to the left atrium. In patients with Scimitar syndrome or its variation, the amount of anomalous flow is dependent on the resistance to flow offered by the abnormal pulmonary artery vasculature. It is interesting to note that development of pulmonary vascular disease has not been reported in PAPVC and intact atrial septum without associated anomalies. The physiology of PAPVC and associated ASD is identical to that of a large ASD. The left-to-right shunt is large as it is the combined flow of the systemic venous return, the anomalous venous return, and the left-to-right flow of blood across the ASD from the normally draining pulmonary veins. The finding of an enlarged right atrium and ventricle should always include an evaluation for an atrial level shunt. If this is not present then alternative causes for right-side volume overload should be sought.

Clinical abnormalities are noted when the predominant venous flow of one lung drains anomalously. The clinical presentation is similar to patients with an ASD. Most are asymptomatic or complain of mild exertional dyspnea. Cyanosis is absent if the atrial septum is intact. In patients with an ASD, cyanosis may be a presenting feature after the third decade of life. This is associated with changes in right atrial compliance and a right-to-left shunt. In patients with Scimitar syndrome and abnormal lung parenchyma, frequent pulmonary infections are common. Finding of dextrocardia on the chest x-ray may be the presenting complaint.

PAPVC is associated with an ASD (see also chapter on sinus venosus ASD). Heterotaxia syndrome, particularly the asplenia type, has a high association with PAPVC. The polysplenia type has a higher association with TAPVC. A higher incidence of PAPVC is noted in patients with Turner and Noonan syndrome.

Laboratory testing should reveal an enlarged right atrium and ventricle (via chest radiograph, echocardiography, or other imaging modality) if the shunt is hemodynamically significant. The abnormally draining pulmonary vein may be seen with noninvasive imaging (e.g., chest radiograph in Scimitar syndrome, echocardiography, or magnetic resonance imaging (MRI)); however, these are not definitive studies. When there is sufficient suspicion, cardiac catheterization and angiography should be performed to make the definitive diagnosis.

Treatment of TAPVC is without controversy and consists of surgical correction. Treatment of PAPVC is indicated if there is significant volume loading of the right heart. Surgery usually directs the anomalous pulmonary venous blood to the left atrium using a baffle fashioned from pericardium or Dacron. Direct reimplantation of the pulmonary vein is usually not performed because of the high risk of scarring and stenosis. Depending on the nature of the baffle there is a long-term risk of baffle stenosis especially if it is long or tube-like. This can be a difficult problem to address, ultimately requiring resection of the lung to manage the obstructed pulmonary vein.

ARTERIAL LEVEL LEFT-TO-RIGHT SHUNTS

There are a number of lesions with pathophysiology similar to a patent ductus arteriosus (PDA).

Aorto-Pulmonary (AP) Window

This is a direct connection between the aorta and pulmonary artery, usually the ascending aorta with the main pulmonary artery. The defect is typically large (essentially no length) and therefore little resistance to flow. Shunting is determined entirely by the relative resistances of the systemic and pulmonary vascular beds. Similar to a PDA, there will be continuous flow between the aorta and pulmonary artery with volume loading of the pulmonary vascular bed, the left atrium, and the left ventricle. If the diastolic "run-off" is large with very low aortic diastolic pressure (<20 mmHg), there is risk of myocardial ischemia because of reduced coronary perfusion pressure and an increased myocardial oxygen demand secondary to the loading conditions.

The clinical history will be similar to a large PDA, and symptoms may be absent during the neonatal period if the PVR is elevated. Physical findings may also be minimal during this period, and may be more reflective of a right-to-left shunt with cyanosis or desaturation rather than signs and symptoms of a large left-to-right shunt. Once the PVR decreases, the latter should occur. If the left-to-right shunt is large enough, there will be systemic to pulmonary artery steal, with a clinical presentation of "shock."

The diagnosis is made noninvasively with echocardiography. The electrocardiogram (ECG) may show right ventricular or biventricular hypertrophy, right atrial enlargement, and rarely, ST- and T-wave changes of myocardial ischemia. The chest radiograph may show findings of a large left-to-right shunt (LA and LV enlargement, with increased pulmonary vascular markings).

Treatment is surgical closure of the defect, usually with a Dacron or pericardial patch.

Other Shunts Between the Aorta and Pulmonary Artery

A number of shunts between the aorta and pulmonary artery are recognized. Their pathophysiology is also similar to a PDA. These consist of: (1) systemic to pulmonary artery collaterals, which may be seen in association with chronic lung disease, cyanotic heart defects, or isolated findings, and (2) iatrogenic or surgical systemic to pulmonary artery shunts such as the central Potts or Waterston shunts, classical or modified BT shunts, or their modifications (see figure in surgical chapter).

The surgical shunts are fashioned to augment PBF in lesions with restricted PBF (tetralogy of Fallot with severe right ventricular outflow tract obstruction) or ductal-dependant PBF (pulmonary atresia/critical pulmonary stenosis). The shunt is created in lieu of the ductus arteriosus. The surgical shunt offers controlled (restrictive) PBF allowing for a lower pulmonary artery pressure. The classical Blalock-Taussig shunt consists of division and ligation of the distal subclavian artery and anastomosis of the proximal end to the corresponding branch pulmonary artery in an end to side manner. It is associated with poor limb growth and the subclavian artery steal phenomenon. This has been replaced by the modified Blalock-Taussig shunt, which uses a Gore-Tex interposition graft between the subclavian artery and the corresponding branch pulmonary artery. In the newborn period, the diameter of the Gore-Tex tube graft used is 3.5–4 mm. This size provides adequate pulmonary blood flow until the infant is 5–6 months old, at which time the shunt is usually "outgrown" (the amount of PBF through the shunt is not adequate to keep up with body growth). These shunts are palliative, allowing for growth of the infant and a fall in pulmonary vascular resistance until more definitive surgery can be attempted. The classical central shunts, Waterston-Cooley and Potts, are no longer performed. They are direct connections from the aorta to the right and left pulmonary arteries, respectively, with no length to cause resistance to blood flow. Thus, it is difficult to control the amount of PBF and therefore these shunts are associated with the development of pulmonary vascular disease. The Potts shunt is also technically difficult to take down from a surgical standpoint. In the current era, if a central shunt (direct aortic rather than aortic branch to pulmonary artery connection) is used, it is in a modified form. Usually, a Gore-Tex tube of specified diameter (offering length and hence resistance) connects the ascending aorta to the main, right, or left pulmonary artery. Clinical findings are proportional to the amount of L-R shunt across the shunt and those from the underlying heart defect. The amount of shunting is determined by the size and length of the tube as well as pulmonary vascular resistance.

Treatment of all these other left-to-right shunts is either surgical closure or transcatheter occlusion of the communicating channels or shunts using coils or devices and surgical repair of the underlying heart defect in the case of surgically created palliative shunt.

MIXED PHYSIOLOGY SHUNTS

There are a number of cardiac and vascular abnormalities of mixed physiology (atrial, ventricular, or arterial level shunts). These include systemic arteriovenous malformations (AVMs), arteriovenous fistulae (AVF), coronary artery fistulae (CAF), and left ventricular to right atrial (LV-RA) shunts.

Systemic Arteriovenous Malformation and Fistula

Anatomy

Systemic AVMs and AVFs are either congenital or acquired. The congenital defects can occur at any site. The most common site of symptomatic AVMs in infancy are the intracranial communications between the carotid arterial system and jugular venous systems, such as the Vein of Galen (the majority) and the cerebral, cerebellar, and dural locations. Other common sites are the liver, skin, lungs, limb extremities, and airway, especially the upper airway and kidney. Intracranial AVMs have a 2:1 male:female ratio, but all other AVMs have an equal gender distribution. The acquired lesions can result from trauma, (penetrating injuries and from vascular access), arterial dysplasia (as seen with neurofibromatosis), hemorrhagic hereditary telangiectasia, Klippel-Trenaunay-Weber syndrome, atherosclerosis, Wilm's tumor, syphilis, and surgically created peripheral fistulae used for renal dialysis.

Both congenital and acquired AVMs consist of an abnormal vessel formation (or synthetic tube) resulting in a connection from the systemic arterial to the systemic venous system. The congenital AVMs have multiple afferent arterioles arising from a systemic artery, which then drain via efferent venules into single or multiple systemic vein(s). The congenital fistulae have a single large vessel, which connects the systemic artery to the systemic vein. These lesions differ from hemangiomas in that the arterial and venous vessels are very abnormal with a disorganized vessel wall. They also have no potential for cellular proliferation or involution.

Pathophysiology

The physiologic consequences are the result of a direct communication from a high pressure, high resistance system to a low pressure, low resistance system. Fluid dynamics dictate that the amount of flow is proportional to the resistance offered by the malformed communicating blood vessels. The amount of flow, which may be massive, creates a volume load on the circulation. It may also "steal" blood from the systemic circulation. If this "steal" is massive, it may lead to shock and end organ failure. These lesions may also produce local effects such as compression or obstruction.

The pathophysiology in the newborn is unique. Newborns have a high PVR with the ability to shunt at the atrial (patent foramen ovale [PFO]) and the arterial (ductus ateriosus) level. The hypertrophied right ventricle is also poorly compliant. The AVM significantly reduces the systemic vascular resistance and the left-to-right shunt leads to an increased venous return to the right atrium. The decreased right ventricular compliance combined with the increased volume of venous return lead to an elevation in right atrial pressure and a right-to-left shunt across the PFO. High PVR with low SVR also promotes decreased left-to-right or even right-to-left shunting across the ductus arteriosus with resulting reduced PBF. This leads to a decrease in left atrial pressure, which will further increase the atrial level right-to-left shunt.

The pathophysiology of AVMs in the fetal and transition into the neonatal period is also unique. Because of the low resistance in the placenta, the relative systemic steal of the AVM is minimized. Removal of the placental circulation (other source of low resistance) after birth results in significantly increased shunting through the AVM. Thus, symptoms usually are absent in the fetus and begin in the neonatal period. Placental AVMs or chorioangiomas may result in a significant shunt from the maternal to fetal circulation producing hydrops fetalis.

Clinical Findings

The clinical manifestation of an AVM depends on the location and size of the AVM or AVF and the patient's age. As discussed above, placental AVMs may present with fetal congestive heart failure (CHF) or hydrops fetalis. This is associated with a very high mortality; however, symptoms in other AVMs may not be present until after birth. Neonatal presentation is associated with large defects, which cause severe congestive heart failure, cyanosis, and possibly local effects. The defects are usually cranial, hepatic, or thoracic. The neonate typically appears ill and lethargic. Bruits over the lesion may be heard, especially with cranial lesions. The arterial pulses are usually bounding with a wide pulse pressure in vessels proximal to the AVM and diminished with low blood pressure in arteries distal to the AVM. The precordium is hyperdynamic. The pulmonary component of the second sound is loud and the second heart sound may appear single. An S3 or S4 gallop may be present. A pansystolic murmur from AV valve regurgitation or murmurs from increased flow across the semilunar or AV valves (relative stenosis) produce an ejection systolic murmur or mid-diastolic rumble, respectively.

Patients with smaller lesions tend to present later in life. These patients have a compensated high output state. They may have exercise intolerance or show poor weight gain. Bounding pulses with a wide pulse pressure are usually present. Bruits may be noted on auscultation (cranial, abdominal, and so forth). Signs and symptoms secondary to local effects, such as increased head circumference, seizures, intracranial hemorrhage, neurologic deficits, stridor, or hematuria are more common. Symptoms of CHF are less prominent.

Laboratory Findings

Chest radiography: The chest radiograph may show cardiomegaly with increased pulmonary vascular markings, pulmonary edema, and pleural effusions. In those with a right-to-left shunt and cyanosis, the pulmonary vascular markings may be normal or reduced. In addition, a wide mediastinum may be seen because of dilation of the SVC (with intracranial AVMs) and aorta. This reflects increased flow in those areas. In older patients the chest radiograph may be normal or show mild cardiomegaly.

Electrocardiography: The ECG may show non-specific findings which may reflect chamber size such as right-axis deviation, right atrial enlargement, RVH, or biventricular hypertrophy. ST- and T-wave changes from myocardial ischemia may be present.

Echocardiography: The echocardiogram will demonstrate normal intracardiac anatomy with chamber enlargement and abnormal flow patterns. The SVC or IVC may be enlarged with increased flow depending on the location of the AVM.

Ultrasound: An ultrasound of the site of interest should demonstrate the abnormal vessels, especially using color Doppler imaging. Cranial ultrasound may be used in neonates.

Noninvasive imaging: A CT scan with contrast or MRI may be helpful in localizing and determining the size of the lesion, especially in an intracranial location.

Cardiac catheterization and angiography: Cardiac catheterization and angiography are usually not required for the diagnosis; however, vascular angiography remains the gold standard for determining the nature of arterial feeder vessels and venous drainage.

Management

Medical management of CHF and shock is difficult. Rapidity in the diagnosis and treatment of the underlying AVM is paramount. Supportive management consists of mechanical ventilation, anticongestive, and inotropic therapies. These measures are usually unnecessary for the older, less symptomatic child.

Catheter-directed embolization is becoming the therapy of choice. It is more selective and can therefore preserve normal adjacent vessels. Multiple procedures may be needed. Total (usually only possible in a well localized superficial lesion) or subtotal surgical excision or ligation of the afferent arterial vessel carry significant morbidity and mortality. The morbidity is related to the destruction of adjacent normal structures and disruption of blood flow within normal vital vessels. Surgical therapy usually results in significant neurologic deficits in the case of a cerebral AVM.

Short- and Long-Term Outlook

The prognosis for large AVMs presenting in the newborn is very poor despite treatment. Long-term outlook is good in successfully treated patients, essentially a cure. SBE prophylaxis is not required if there are no residual abnormities.

Coronary Arteriovenous and Coronary Cameral Fistulae

Anatomy

Coronary arteriovenous and coronary cameral fistulae are rare anomalies. They consist of a connection between the coronary artery and a cardiac chamber (coronary cameral fistula) or a connection to the coronary sinus, SVC, IVC, or PA (coronary arteriovenous fistula). The majority (55–60%) arise from the right coronary artery. The most common site of drainage is the right ventricle, followed by the right atrium and the pulmonary artery. The fistulous connection varies greatly in size. It can be a single channel or a plexiform lesion with multiple efferent channels entering the cardiac chambers or pulmonary artery. The lesions can have aneurysmal dilatations or areas of stenosis.

Etiology

Coronary arteriovenous and coronary cameral fistulae are usually congenital in origin in children; however, they may also be acquired secondary to trauma (penetrating injury from a knife or projectile) or from cardiac interventions such as pacemaker implantation, endomyocardial biopsy, coronary angiography, or cardiac surgery.

Pathophysiology

Small fistulae are hemodynamically insignificant. Large lesions lead to a significant volume load on the chamber or vessel in which they terminate and the structures distal to this. Large lesions with significant flow may steal blood from the normal coronaries leading to myocardial ischemia. When the fistulae enter systemic venous channels, right-sided heart chambers, the pulmonary arteries, or left atrium, the shunt flow is continuous. The latter is due to the persistent gradient in systole and diastole between the coronary artery (aortic pressures) and the terminal chamber/vessel. If the fistula enters the left ventricle, then flow occurs only during diastole, as there should be no gradient between the systolic pressures in the left ventricle and the aorta.

Clinical Presentation

Patients with small fistulae are asymptomatic. Large lesions produce congenital heart failure in the neonate or infant. Patients with small to moderate size shunts usually become symptomatic in the second to third decade of life. They may present with atrial arrhythmia (especially atrial fibrillation), exercise intolerance, exertional dyspnea or angina. Infective endocarditis can also be a presenting feature.

The natural history is variable. Small lesions may never be hemodynamically significant or may close spontaneously. Large symptomatic lesions lead to the features described above. Rarely does myocardial infarction or rupture occur.

Physical findings depend on the location of the fistulous connection. A continuous murmur is heard in lesions associated with continuous flow, and a diastolic murmur alone is noted in lesions entering the left ventricle. The murmur is best heard over the right or left sternal border. Signs of a large left-to-right shunt can mimic those of an ASD, ventricular septal defect (VSD), or PDA depending on the drainage site. The presentation of a coronary artery to left ventricular fistula is similar to aortic regurgitation.

Laboratory Tests

Chest radiography: The chest radiograph may show cardiomegaly with increased pulmonary vascular markings. Specific chamber enlargement may also be seen.

ECG: The ECG may show changes that reflect chamber enlargement and hypertrophy, especially with large lesions. ST- and T-wave changes indicative of myocardial ischemia may also be seen, especially with exercise.

Echocardiography: Echocardiography has been very useful for diagnosis. It can usually demonstrate the fistula anatomy and its physiologic impact. Stress echocardiography may demonstrate regional wall motion abnormalities suggesting ischemia in patients with significant steal from coronary artery blood flow.

Cardiac catheterization and angiography: This remains the gold standard for demonstrating coronary artery lesions. In addition, embolization can be performed at the same time as diagnosis.

Management

Except for very small lesions, most should be closed to prevent infective endocarditis (or more appropriately, endarteritis), or the other sequelae described above. Current therapy is usually initiated with transcatheter embolization using coils or devices. It is important to ensure that the normal coronary artery blood flow is preserved. The alternative to transcatheter therapy is surgical ligation. Surgical ligation can usually be performed without cardiopulmonary bypass by identifying the fistula on the epicardial surface. Cardiac bypass is required if a cardiac chamber requires opening in order to ligate the termination points of the fistula.

Left Ventricular to Right Atrial Shunts

The Gerbode defect is a rare ventricular septal defect, which connects the left ventricle to the right atrium. This is possible as the tricuspid valve is normally more apically located than the mitral valve. A ventricular septal defect in the part of the septum that separates the two AV valves produces a left ventricular to right atrial defect and shunt. This type of shunt can exist with a common AV canal defect. It can also be produced iatrogenically following surgical repair of a canal-type VSD or common complete AV canal defect. The importance of this defect is its hemodynamic impact. The systemic pressures in the left ventricle transmit directly to the low pressure and compliant right atrium. This will produce a significant shunt even if the defect is small in size. Large defects will lead to right atrial hypertension. The signs and symptoms reflect right side volume overload as seen with ASD. Unlike an ASD, there is right atrial hypertension, producing symptoms and signs of right-sided congestive heart failure. This is a poorly tolerated defect. The diagnosis is made by echocardiography and surgical closure is indicated.

Suggested Readings

Emmanoulides GC, Allen HD, Riemenschneider TA, Gutgesell HP (eds). *Moss and Adams' Heart Disease in Infants, Children, and Adolescents: Including the Fetus and Young Adult*, 5th ed. Baltimore, MD, Williams & Wilkins, 1995, Chapters 57–52, pp. 791–810; 59, pp. 838–874.

Garson A, Bricker JT, Fisher DJ, Neish SR (eds). *The Science and Practice of Pediatric Cardiology*, 2nd ed. Baltimore, MD, Williams & Wilkins, 1998, Chapters 74, pp. 1677–1688, 63, pp. 1431–1441.

Spray TL, Bridges ND: Surgical management of congenital and acquired pulmonary vein stenosis. *Semin Thorac Cardiovasc Surg* 2:177–188, 1999.

17

NONCRITICAL VALVE LESIONS

David J. Waight

TRICUSPID VALVE ABNORMALITIES

Introduction

The tricuspid valve (TV) is a three leaflet valve that separates the right atrium from the right ventricle. Systemic venous blood returns via the superior vena cava, inferior vena cava and coronary sinus into the right atrium. Blood collects in the right atrium during ventricular systole when the tricuspid valve is closed. At the end of systole, the tricuspid valve opens in early diastole and the majority of blood flow enters the right ventricle. At end diastole, after the P wave is noted on electrocardiogram (ECG), there is atrial systole and additional blood is pumped from the right atrium to the right ventricle through the tricuspid valve.

The tricuspid valve is supported by multiple chordae tendonae connected to small papillary muscles that insert into the intraventricular septum, the apex of the right ventricle and the right ventricular (RV) free wall. With normal physiology, the tricuspid valve produces no obstruction and has minimal, or what is termed *physiologic*, tricuspid regurgitation.

The tricuspid valve is the least common of the four major heart valves to demonstrate pathology. Tricuspid stenosis and tricuspid regurgitation can be congenital or acquired. Tricuspid valve sounds are auscultated at the left lower sternal border where the flow into the right ventricle or regurgitation into the right atrium is heard.

Tricuspid Stenosis

Congenital stenosis of the tricuspid valve is extremely rare. Critical stenosis of the tricuspid valve or tricuspid valve atresia (Chapter 20) is more common than mild or moderate degrees of tricuspid valve stenosis. Acquired tricuspid stenosis is most commonly noted with rheumatic heart disease. Approximately 5–10% of patients with rheumatic heart disease complicating rheumatic fever will develop some degree of tricuspid stenosis. This stenosis is a result of thickening and alteration of the tricuspid valve because of the rheumatic disease process. Typically these patients have more severe mitral valve disease and the stenosis and regurgitation of the tricuspid valve is not the primary clinical problem for these patients. Tricuspid

TABLE 17-1

TRICUSPID STENOSIS

History	Testing	PE	Pathophysiology
Limited exercise tolerance	ECG—right atrial enlargement (RAE), atrial arrhythmia	Hepatomegaly, ascites, systemic edema	Elevated RA pressure Decreased cardiac output
Complaints of swelling	Chest x-ray (CXR)—RAE	Soft diastolic murmur	
Rheumatic fever	Echocardiography—increased velocity across TV, right atrial enlargement		
Previous TV surgery			

stenosis may also result from a postsurgical procedure including repair of AV canal or repair of an abnormal tricuspid valve associated with Ebstein anomaly (Chapter 23).

Pathophysiology

Tricuspid stenosis presents as an obstructive lesion on the right side of the heart, which decreases the forward flow through the tricuspid valve into the right ventricle (Figure 17-1**B**). This increases the pressure in the right atrium and subsequently in the superior vena cava, inferior vena cava, and the hepatic venous system. This increased pressure can lead to right atrial enlargement, hepatomegaly, systemic edema and severe tricuspid valve disease can lead to ascites. A fixed obstruction across the tricuspid valve can lead to a limited cardiac output and exercise intolerance.

Clinical and Laboratory Findings

The diagnosis of tricuspid stenosis is suspected on the clinical history and the exam which may demonstrate an abnormal murmur with findings of elevated right atrial pressure as described above (Table 17-1). The diagnosis of tricuspid stenosis is confirmed through echocardiography, which demonstrates an increased flow velocity across the tricuspid valve into the right ventricle. A gradient from the right atrium to the right ventricle may also be noted during catheterization where direct measurement of the right ventricular pressure and right atrial pressure during the different phases of the cardiac cycle

reveal a higher pressure in the right atrium than the right ventricle throughout diastole.

Treatment

Treatment of tricuspid stenosis may include anticongestive therapy with diuretics although significant tricuspid stenosis is likely to require a surgical intervention. This typically involves open-heart surgery, with various valve repair techniques beyond the scope of this book. Mechanical valve replacement is not an option in the low-pressure right-sided circulation. Bioprosthetic valves are available, including the use of pulmonary valve homografts. The latter have long-term complications such as stenosis or regurgitation.

Tricuspid Regurgitation

The tricuspid valve typically has a very mild degree of regurgitation during ventricular systole. This is physiologic regurgitation and is present in a large number of healthy individuals. This physiologic regurgitation is not noted on auscultation and causes no hemodynamic instability. In the field of pediatric cardiology, physiologic tricuspid regurgitation is useful in the echocardiographic assessment of the heart as it allows a Doppler estimate of the right ventricular pressure by measuring the velocity of the tricuspid regurgitation jet. This allows a reliable assessment for pulmonary hypertension or elevated right ventricular pressures. More than this trivial regurgitation is felt to be pathologic.

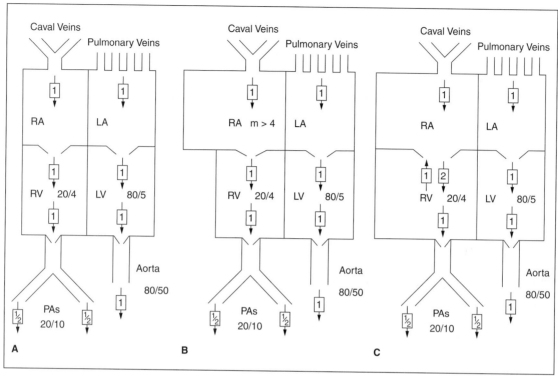

FIGURE 17-1

CHANGES IN CARDIAC OUTPUTS AND PRESSURES

Part **A** shows a schematic of a hypothetical heart with relative cardiac outputs (numbers in boxes) and pressures. Part **B** shows the hemodynamic changes with tricuspid stenosis, namely, RA dilation and an elevated mean atrial pressure, greater than the RV end-diastolic pressure of 5 (m > 5). Part **C** shows the changes with tricuspid regurgitation, namely, RA and RV dilation. Note the regurgitant volume is 1 relative cardiac output in this example, thus, 2 cardiac outputs cross the tricuspid valve so that the net to the pulmonary circulation is 1 cardiac output.

Pathologic tricuspid regurgitation may be congenital or acquired. Congenital tricuspid regurgitation is often described as a variation of Ebstein anomaly of the tricuspid valve. Acquired tricuspid regurgitation may be the result of rheumatic fever or endocarditis in intravenous drug users. Tricuspid insufficiency may also be noted postoperatively after repair of an atrioventricular canal type defect or any procedure performed through the tricuspid valve. This surgical approach carries some potential of damage to the chordal apparatus of the tricuspid valve. A flail tricuspid valve leaflet following surgical damage of the support apparatus of the tricuspid valve usually requires repeat surgical intervention. The tricuspid valve can also be damaged during right ventricular endomyocardial biopsy following cardiac transplantation or during the evaluation of a patient with cardiomyopathy. This is a very rare complication of cardiac catheterization and endomyocardial biopsy.

Pathophysiology

Pathologic tricuspid regurgitation ranges from a mild tricuspid abnormality with mild regurgitation that generally does not cause any systemic illness to severe tricuspid regurgitation associated with Ebstein's anomaly that can present with severe cyanosis, poor cardiac output, and heart failure. With more severe forms of tricuspid insufficiency,

TABLE 17-2

TRICUSPID REGURGITATION

History	Labs	Exam	Pathophysiology
None—murmur, limited exercise tolerance	ECG—RAE, RVH atrial arrhythmia	Hepatomegaly, ascites, systemic edema	Elevated RA pressure
Palpitations	CXR—RAE	Soft systolic murmur left lower sternal border	RA dilation
Previous TV surgery	ECHO—tricuspid regurgitation, right atrial and right ventricular enlargement		Limited cardiac output
S/P endocardial biopsy			RV enlargement

there is a large proportion of the right ventricular volume that is ejected back into the right atrium with each cardiac cycle (Figure 17-1C). This causes increased volume loading of the right atrium and the right ventricle with right atrial and right ventricular enlargement. Right atrial enlargement also increases the incidence of atrial arrhythmias including atrial flutter or atrial fibrillation.

Clinical Findings

Patients with tricuspid regurgitation can present with signs and symptoms of right-sided heart failure with exercise intolerance including feeding intolerance in infants (Table 17-2).

The murmur of tricuspid insufficiency is heard at the left lower sternal border, is pansystolic and typically less high-pitched than the murmur of mitral insufficiency. Because of increased right atrial pressures and volumes, patients with tricuspid regurgitation may develop hepatomegaly, ascites, and even jugular venous distention. Jugular venous distention is very difficult to assess in infants and small children but may be visible in older children and teens. A third heart sound may also be audible in tricuspid regurgitation because of the increased volume load in the right atrium and right ventricle.

Laboratory Findings

The chest radiograph typically shows right atrial enlargement, manifest by a more lateral position of the right heart border in the anterior posterior

(AP) projection (Table 17-2). The ECG typically shows right atrial enlargement and right ventricular hypertrophy. Right atrial enlargement is diagnosed via the tall P waves in the right precordial leads, V1, V2, and V3.

A diagnosis of tricuspid regurgitation may be suspected by the clinical picture with an enlarged liver, enlarged right atrium on chest radiography, right atrial enlargement on the ECG, atrial arrhythmias, or auscultation. It is generally confirmed by echocardiography, which easily demonstrates a regurgitant jet across the tricuspid valve. The severity of the tricuspid regurgitation is graded indirectly by the degree of enlargement of the right atrium and right ventricle. It is also graded by the width of the tricuspid regurgitation jet in comparison to the tricuspid valve annulus.

Treatment

The need for treatment of tricuspid regurgitation depends on severity. Mild to moderate forms of tricuspid regurgitation are generally well tolerated unless atrial arrhythmias develop. Anticongestive therapy with diuretics may improve the clinical symptoms, but definitive therapy entails surgical repair of the tricuspid valve. Tricuspid valve repair is not as well established as mitral valve repair and is less frequently necessary. Tricuspid valve replacement is rarely necessary and is generally avoided in small children because of the high incidence of morbidity and mortality following tricuspid valve replacement early in life.

PULMONARY VALVE ABNORMALITIES

Pulmonary Stenosis

The pulmonary valve is a trileaflet valve separating the right ventricle and the main pulmonary artery. A normal pulmonary valve has no obstruction to flow from the right ventricle to the pulmonary artery (PA) and has only minimal (physiologic) pulmonary insufficiency.

Pathophysiology

A thickened or stenotic pulmonary valve produces a pressure gradient from the right ventricle to the main pulmonary artery (Figure 17-2A). This pressure gradient causes right ventricular hypertension, which leads to right ventricular hypertrophy. Right ventricular hypertrophy produces decreased compliance of the right ventricle, which can lead to right atrial enlargement and atrial arrhythmias. If the pulmonary valve stenosis is critical, hypoxia will be noted in the newborn period (Chapter 22). Mild to moderate, or even severe pulmonary stenosis can be a result of congenital abnormalities of the pulmonary valve including pulmonary valve dysplasia, fusion of the pulmonary valve leaflets, and thickening of the pulmonary valve tissue. The pulmonary valve may be structurally normal with a small annulus creating the same physiology of obstruction.

Clinical Findings

Presentation of pulmonary valve stenosis is determined by the severity of the stenosis (Table 17-3). Usually, pulmonary stenosis will present with a pathologic murmur noted during auscultation. The majority of patients are asymptomatic unless they have resultant right ventricular dysfunction or shunting across a septal defect. Severe pulmonary stenosis can cause cyanosis in the newborn or congestive heart failure in older patients. Less severe forms may present with exercise intolerance or fatigue owing to the inability of the patient to increase cardiac output because of fixed obstruction across the pulmonary valve. If significant right ventricular hypertrophy develops with resultant right atrial enlargement, signs of right-sided congestive heart failure may be present with arrhythmia, hepatic enlargement, or jugular venous distention.

The natural history of pulmonary stenosis also varies with severity. Mild pulmonary stenosis most commonly remains mild or becomes insignificant with time. Moderate stenosis has a small incidence of progression to more severe pulmonary stenosis requiring therapy, but a significant portion of patients with moderate stenosis have a stable gradient across

TABLE 17-3

PULMONARY STENOSIS

History	Labs	Exam	Pathophysiology
Murmur	ECG—normal, RVH, RAE, atrial or ventricular arrhythmia	SEM at left upper sternal border	Increased right ventricular pressure
Newborn cyanosis		Parasternal heave	Limited cardiac output
Exercise intolerance	CXR—normal, main pulmonary artery (MPA) enlargement	Ejection click	Decreased right ventricular compliance and right atrial enlargement
	ECHO—increased flow velocity across PV, RVH, thickened PV leaflets, MPA post-stenotic enlargement	Widely split second heart sound	
		Loud P2 (mild-severe)	
		Decreased P2 (immobile valve with severe PS)	

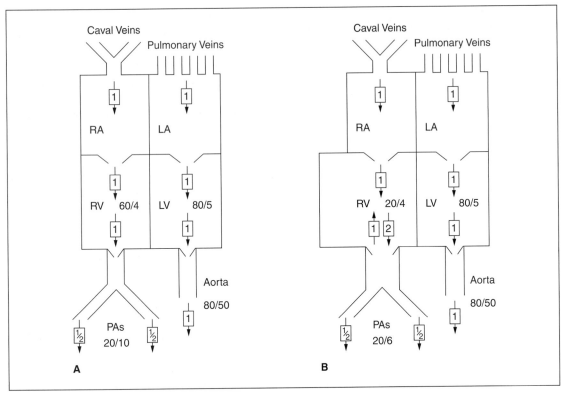

FIGURE 17-2

CHANGES IN CARDIAC OUTPUT AND PRESSURE WITH PULMONARY STENOSIS AND PULMONARY REGURGITATION

Part **A** is based on the hypothetical diagram in Figure 17-1**A**, showing the changes with pulmonary stenosis. Note the elevated systolic pressure. The systolic gradient is 40 mmHg in this example. Part **B** shows the changes with pulmonary regurgitation, namely, RV and proximal PA enlargement. The diastolic pressure in the PA is decreased. In this example, the regurgitant volume is 1 relative cardiac output, thus two cardiac outputs cross the pulmonary valve in order to yield one net cardiac output to the pulmonary circulation.

the pulmonary valve. Less commonly, patients with moderate gradient will have a decreasing gradient over time with eventual mild pulmonary stenosis. Severe pulmonary stenosis invariably requires treatment or will result in right ventricular dysfunction, arrythmia, and a shortened lifespan.

The physical exam of patients with pulmonary stenosis demonstrates a systolic ejection murmur at the left upper sternal border. It is also often audible in the suprasternal notch or the left infrascapular border and may radiate to the lung fields and the back. If the pulmonary valve is thickened, an ejection systolic click may be noted at the left upper sternal border. If right ventricular hypertrophy has

developed, a parasternal tap will be noted during systole. With significant pulmonary stenosis, the second heart sound is widely split owing to delayed ejection of the right ventricle across a stenotic pulmonary valve. The pulmonary component of the second heart sound may also be diminished because of the immobility of the pulmonary valve when it is severely thickened.

Laboratory Findings

The chest radiograph will demonstrate a normal heart size unless the patient has significant congestive heart failure. If the heart is enlarged, a prominent right atrium signifying right atrial enlargement would be seen. There may also be poststenotic dilatation of the main pulmonary artery in patients with significant valvar pulmonary stenosis (not seen with sub or supravalvar pulmonary stenosis). Pulmonary vascular markings are normal unless the patient has critical pulmonary stenosis, in which case they are decreased due right-to-left shunting at the ventricular or atrial level through a septal defect.

ECG findings are normal in up to 50% of patients with mild to moderate pulmonary stenosis. If the stenosis is more severe, right ventricular hypertrophy may be present with an RSR' pattern most notably seen in lead V1. Right atrial enlargement with a tall P wave may also be seen. Right-axis deviation owing to right ventricular enlargement may also be noted. Significant right ventricular hypertrophy may be diagnosed with a positive T wave in V1 in infants and children up to midadolescence (normally the T wave becomes inverted somewhere around day 3 to day 10 of life and remains so until mid-to-late childhood or adolescence).

An echocardiogram is a diagnostic or confirmatory test in patients with pulmonary stenosis and will demonstrate thickened or dysplastic pulmonary valve leaflets with decreased motion and an abnormal opening pattern referred to as doming of the pulmonary valve. Doppler evaluation demonstrates increased flow velocity across the pulmonary valve. The severity of pulmonary stenosis is graded by the flow velocity, which estimates the pressure gradient across the pulmonary valve. Mild pulmonary stenosis is defined as a gradient of 1–40 mmHg. Moderate pulmonary stenosis is 40–80 mmHg. Severe stenosis is greater than 80 mm Hg. It should be noted that these evaluations may be inaccurate in neonatal patient with other routes of blood flow (e.g., patent foramen ovale).

The diagnosis and evaluation of pulmonary stenosis can also be defined during cardiac catheterization where direct pressure measurements of the right ventricle, main pulmonary artery, and branch pulmonary arteries are recorded. This defines the true gradient in mmHg from the right ventricle to the pulmonary arteries. The gradient measured at catheterization is often similar to the mean gradient estimated by echocardiography.

Treatment

Mild pulmonary stenosis should be treated conservatively (no intervention) with SBE prophylaxis for indicated dental and surgical procedures. Follow-up with a pediatric cardiologist is infrequent. Moderate to severe pulmonary stenosis is generally treated with transcatheter balloon valvuloplasty as a first therapy. This is the procedure of choice for pulmonary stenosis and is very effective. Patients with dysplastic pulmonary valves and severe pulmonary stenosis have a small incidence of recurrent pulmonary stenosis following balloon valvuloplasty. There is a small incidence of induced pulmonary insufficiency following balloon valvuloplasty. This incidence is increased in patients with a severely dysplastic monocusp (unicuspid) pulmonary valve. Severe pulmonary stenosis may also require surgical intervention if balloon angioplasty fails to achieve a long-term resolution of the gradient across the pulmonary valve. Patients with pulmonary stenosis require SBE prophylaxis for life.

Pulmonary stenosis can also be associated with supravalvar pulmonary stenosis. The differentiation between valvar and supravalvar stenosis can be suggested by the absence of a systolic ejection click indicating a normal pulmonary valve and the likelihood of supravalvar pulmonary stenosis. The murmur and physiology of these anomalies are not distinguishable. Echocardiography evaluation can differentiate pulmonary valve stenosis from supravalvar stenosis unless the supravalvar stenosis is very close to the pulmonary valve annulus. Balloon angioplasty is usually not successful in treating supravalvar pulmonary stenosis, which may require surgical repair if it is moderate to severe.

Pulmonary Regurgitation

Pulmonary regurgitation occurs when the pulmonary valve fails to seal completely during ventricular diastole. During this period, the pulmonary artery pressure is higher than the diastolic pressure in the right ventricle. If the valve is incompetent, blood will return to the right ventricle from the main pulmonary artery and the branch pulmonary arteries. Congenital pulmonary regurgitation of a moderate to severe form is very uncommon with the exception being the absence of the pulmonary valve that can be associated with tetralogy of Fallot (known as "tetralogy of Fallot with absent pulmonary valve" or more correctly "ventricular septal defect [VSD] with absent pulmonary valve"). Acquired pulmonary regurgitation is much more common and is typically the sequelae of previous transcatheter or surgical therapy for some form of pulmonary stenosis. Pulmonary regurgitation secondary to balloon angioplasty of the pulmonary valve for pulmonary stenosis is usually mild and well tolerated but can be more severe and require further therapy.

The most common form of pulmonary regurgitation is postsurgical after repair of pulmonary atresia or tetralogy of Fallot with a transannular pulmonary artery patch. This involves an incision across the right ventricular outflow tract and the pulmonary valve with a patch placed that produces an open area with no pulmonary valve tissue. Surgical variations including a monocusp pulmonary valve may prove to be competent early postoperatively but generally develop significant pulmonary regurgitation after several months.

Pathophysiology

Pulmonary regurgitation leads to volume overload of the right ventricle and the proximal pulmonary artery bed (Figure 17-2B). The increased blood volume ejected by the right ventricle (the normal stroke volume plus the additional volume of regurgitant blood) leads to increased flow across the pulmonary valve and functional pulmonary stenosis. Right atrial enlargement can develop secondary to right ventricular enlargement and tricuspid annulus enlargement with resultant tricuspid regurgitation.

These patients may develop atrial or ventricular arrhythmias as their presenting sign.

Clinical Findings

The physical examination typically reveals a diastolic murmur heard at the right lower sternal border and also at the mid-to-left upper sternal border (Table 17-4). There may be an associated systolic ejection murmur at the left upper sternal border because of the increased volume flow across the pulmonary valve leading to a relative pulmonary valve stenosis. It is sometimes described as a "to and fro" murmur. A right ventricular heave may also be noted because of right ventricular enlargement.

The chest plain film demonstrates right ventricular enlargement and main pulmonary artery enlargement proportional to the amount of regurgitation.

The ECG may demonstrate right ventricular enlargement or hypertrophy.

The diagnosis of pulmonary regurgitation is generally made by physical exam but is confirmed by echocardiography demonstrating reversal of flow across the pulmonary valve via color Doppler. A trivial or very mild degree of pulmonary regurgitation is termed physiologic pulmonary regurgitation and is found in many otherwise healthy patients and is not a clinical problem. The severity of pulmonary regurgitation is evaluated by the degree of right ventricular enlargement and the width of the pulmonary regurgitation jet in comparison to the pulmonary valve annulus.

Catheterization is not required for evaluation of pulmonary regurgitation. If a catheterization is performed for a separate indication, angiography in the main pulmonary artery will demonstrate the

TABLE 17-4

PULMONARY REGURGITATION

History	Labs	Exam	Pathophysiology
Murmur	ECG—Normal, RVE	Diastolic murmur at right lower sternal border. Systolic ejection murmur at left upper sternal border "to and fro" murmur	Volume overload of RV with RVE
Palpitations	CXR—Normal, RVE		Limited cardiac output if severe
	ECHO—diastolic flow from MPA to RV, RVE		

insufficiency and the severity can be graded from mild to severe.

Treatment

Therapy for pulmonary regurgitation varies with the severity. Historically, pulmonary regurgitation is well tolerated and has been followed expectantly, especially in patients who have undergone tetralogy of Fallot repair. Therapy may include medical management with diuretics and digoxin as treatment for right-sided congestive heart failure. Definitive management of pulmonary regurgitation requires surgical intervention with placement of a competent pulmonary valve. Recent studies have indicated that significant right ventricular dysfunction and right ventricular arrhythmias owing to the right ventricular enlargement from pulmonary regurgitation cause significant morbidity and mortality in the postsurgical population of tetralogy of Fallot patients. Earlier surgical intervention to prevent or reduce the degree of right ventricular enlargement by placing a competent pulmonary valve is becoming a common clinical practice in pediatric cardiology.

MITRAL VALVE ABNORMALITIES

Mitral Stenosis

Mitral stenosis is defined as a narrowing of the mitral valve orifice. Mitral stenosis is a relatively rare form of congenital heart disease, with congenital mitral stenosis accounting for only 0.5% of congenital heart disease. Mitral stenosis is most commonly associated with other forms of congenital heart disease, most prominently other left-sided obstructive lesions. Most mitral valve stenosis seen in the pediatric population is acquired.

Acquired mitral stenosis is more frequently diagnosed than congenital stenosis. Acquired mitral valve stenosis includes postsurgical procedures on the mitral valve, most commonly complete AV canal repair or repair of a cleft mitral valve. Endocarditis can produce significant thickening and myxomatous changes of the mitral valve that can produce stenosis. Rheumatic fever is the most common source of acquired mitral stenosis in the pediatric age group but is still a rare phenomenon except in areas where

rheumatic fever is highly prevalent. Infiltration disorders including glycogen storage diseases can produce mitral stenosis. Neoplasms that cause masses within the left atrium or in the area of the mitral valve apparatus in the left ventricle can cause abnormal motion of the mitral valve and obstruction. They may encase the mitral valve within the tumor mass, producing severe mitral stenosis.

There are five types of mitral stenoses that all produce obstruction of left atrial flow to the left ventricle. They are:

1. Supravalvar stenosing ring.
2. Hypoplastic mitral valve apparatus with a small mitral valve annulus.
3. Abnormal mitral valve (parachute mitral valve, double orifice mitral valve).
4. Abnormal papillary muscle/apparatus.
5. Severe mitral valve narrowing or a form of mitral atresia/critical mitral stenosis that is part of the hypoplastic left heart syndrome.

A supravalvar stenosing ring or supravalvar mitral membrane partially obstructs flow into the mitral valve orifice producing an elevated left atrial pressure and a gradient between the left atrium and the left ventricle without any significant abnormality of the mitral valve itself.

A hypoplastic mitral valve apparatus generally implies a small mitral valve annulus but also can be associated with forms of a parachute mitral valve which implies the presence of thickened leaflets and absent or abnormal chordal insertions, referred to as mitral arcade. There can be papillary muscle hypoplasia or fused papillary muscles. Thickened valve or short chordae are seen with acute rheumatic fever (ARF), but the annulus is normal or even enlarged.

A double orifice mitral valve is the result of fusion of the anterior and posterior mitral valve leaflets at some point along the opposing surfaces of the mitral valve. This can be, but is not necessarily, associated with any mitral valve obstruction. A parachute mitral valve has the form of a funnel or "parachute" with multiple small holes in the sides of the tissue. There is no central orifice and functional obstruction is present. A single papillary muscle is usually present.

Pathophysiology

The pathophysiology of mitral stenosis and similar lesions consists of a pressure gradient from the left atrium to the left ventricle (Figure 17-3A). In normal physiology during ventricular diastole, the left atrium empties rapidly into the left ventricle with no significant pressure gradient from the left atrium to the left ventricle. At end diastole, the left atrial pressure is equal to the left ventricular pressure and, as the left ventricular pressure rises, the mitral valve closes with no regurgitation. In patients with mitral stenosis, the left atrial pressure is always higher than the left ventricular pressure throughout diastole. This results in left atrial dilation, pulmonary venous dilation, and a backward transmission of elevated pressures to the pulmonary arteries, right ventricle, right atrium, and eventually the systemic veins.

Clinical Findings

Mitral stenosis presents with signs and symptoms related to pulmonary venous congestion or increasing pressure load in the left atrium (Table 17-5). Infants often present with tachypnea, feeding intolerance, and diaphoresis, most commonly with feedings. Older children will present with dyspnea with activity, tachypnea, and exercise intolerance.

An opening snap, which is a sharp high-pitched sound occurring after S2 corresponding to the mitral valve opening and left atrial flow into the left ventricle, may be audible. The murmur associated with mitral stenosis is heard at the apex and is a low-frequency, mid-to-late diastolic murmur. This murmur increases in intensity, with expiration secondary to increased pulmonary venous return causing increased flow across the mitral valve. In patients who have developed pulmonary hypertension, they will have an increase in the intensity of the P2 portion of the second heart sound.

Patients with moderate to severe mitral stenosis will have a chest radiograph demonstrating pulmonary venous congestion and left atrial enlargement. The latter produces the following findings: a straight upper left heart border, a double atrial shadow, an elevated left mainstem bronchus, and posterior displacement of the cardiac silhouette.

Left atrial enlargement and possibly increased right ventricular forces and right-axis deviation owing to resultant pulmonary hypertension are seen in the ECG. Arrhythmias can also be noted on the ECG, Holter, or event monitor in patients with significant atrial enlargement, including atrial flutter and atrial fibrillation.

Echocardiography, including Doppler flow studies across the mitral valve, can demonstrate both an abnormal mitral valve and mitral valve apparatus and measure the flow gradient from the left atrium to the left ventricle. Left atrial enlargement is easily seen with transthoracic echocardiography. The severity of mitral stenosis correlates with the degree of left atrial enlargement and the

TABLE 17-5

MITRAL STENOSIS

History	Labs	Exam	Pathophysiology
Tachypnea Feeding intolerance Diaphoresis Dyspnea with exertion	ECG—LAE, RVH, atrial arrhythmia CXR—cardiomegaly with LAE and pulmonary edema, elevated left mainstem bronchus ECHO—increased flow velocity across MV and LAE	Opening snap Low frequency murmur at apex	Increased LA pressure transmits to the pulmonary veins and cause pulmonaryedema Decreased cardiac output owing to fixed obstruction across MV

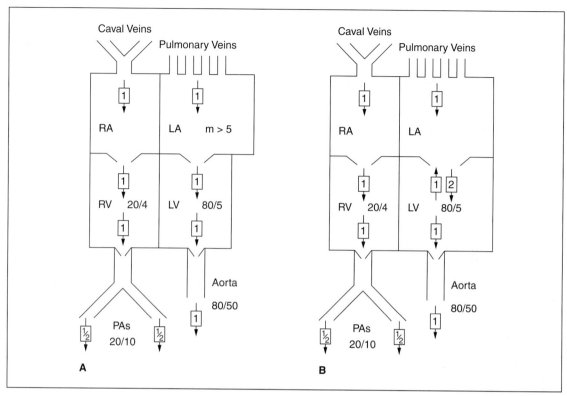

FIGURE 17-3

CHANGES IN CARDIAC OUTPUT AND PRESSURE WITH MITRAL STENOSIS AND MITRAL REGURGITATION

Part **A** is based on diagram 1a and shows changes with mitral stenosis. Note the dilated LA and elevated atrial pressure with a mean greater than the RV end-diastolic pressure (m > 5). Part **B** shows changes with mitral regurgitation, namely, LA and LV dilation. Note that if there is a regurgitant volume of one relative cardiac output, two cardiac outputs are required to cross the mitral valve in order to yield one net cardiac output to the systemic circulation.

gradient across the mitral valve. A common method of evaluating the severity of mitral stenosis is to measure the mitral valve area. The mitral valve area is the area the blood flows across—it is the functional size of the mitral valve orifice. Normals, as related to body surface area, have been defined for both children and adults. Echocardiography may be adequate in many patients with mitral stenosis to define severity and progression of the mitral valve obstruction but in some patients additional information is required and cardiac catheterization is performed.

During cardiac catherization for the evaluation of mitral stenosis, catheters are advanced from the descending aorta across the aortic valve into the left ventricle. A separate catheter is advanced

across a patent foramen ovale, atrial septal defect or placed in the left atrium via a transseptal puncture. The left atrial and left ventricular pressures are measured simultaneously and the gradient across the mitral valve is definitively measured. This gradient can also be estimated by positioning a catheter in the pulmonary artery, occluding the antegrade flow through the pulmonary artery via a balloon, and measuring the pressure distal to the balloon (known as a pulmonary artery wedge pressure). This pressure should be equal to the left atrial pressure. Although this method is not the gold standard for measuring degrees of mitral stenosis, it is very useful to rule out significant mitral stenosis. If the wedge pressure and the left atrial, or left ventricular diastolic pressures are equal during diastole, mitral stenosis is not present. The mitral valve area can also be calculated from cardiac catheterization data using the Gorlin equation: mitral valve area = (cardiac index/heart rate × diastolic filling period)/(37.7 × square root of the mean gradient across the mitral valve).

Treatment

Therapy for mitral stenosis varies with the severity of the obstruction. Mild mitral stenosis is often followed clinically with serial echocardiograms to evaluate any left atrial enlargement and the progression of the gradient across the mitral valve. These patients are often asymptomatic and the stenosis may or may not progress. Moderate degrees of mitral stenosis produce pulmonary venous obstruction and pulmonary venous congestion that can be palliated with diuretics. This may decrease the symptoms by reducing the degree of pulmonary edema.

Medical management for mitral stenosis is a temporizing measure but may be useful to delay intervention until the patient is larger and less likely to require mitral valve replacement. Patients with mitral stenosis are at risk for endocarditis and are at increased risk for severe respiratory illnesses. These patients may be more ill than the normal population with common respiratory viruses, including respiratory syncytial virus (RSV). Patients with severe mitral stenosis require early intervention. Balloon valvuloplasty in the cardiac catheterization lab is the most common initial therapy for mitral stenosis in adults and has been used in children. The low incidence of mitral stenosis has limited any large experience with balloon mitral valvuloplasty in smaller children.

Surgical intervention for mitral stenosis can entail repair or replacement of the mitral valve. Mitral valve replacement most commonly requires a mechanical (prosthetic) valve with the resultant need for anticoagulation. A prosthetic mitral valve placed in childhood eventually requires replacement as the child outgrows it.

Mitral Regurgitation

Congenital mitral regurgitation is a rare form of congenital heart disease that is usually associated with other forms of congenital heart disease, particularly complete AV canal, isolated mitral valve cleft or mitral valve prolapse. Secondary mitral regurgitation is most commonly a postoperative finding. It may occur with myocardial or papillary muscle infarction or significant ischemia. This may be seen in patients with ischemic cardiomyopathy, which may be secondary to coronary artery abnormalities such as anomalous origin of the left coronary artery from the pulmonary artery. Acquired mitral regurgitation can also occur with inflammatory diseases and infectious agents causing myocarditis, endocarditis, Kawasaki disease, or rheumatic fever.

Pathophysiology

Mitral regurgitation produces an increased left atrial volume, which leads to left atrial enlargement owing to the high left atrial compliance (Figure 17-3B). This can lead to an increased left atrial pressure. An enlarged left atrium can produce arrhythmias and possible airway compression owing to compression of the left mainstem bronchus from the dilated left atrium. The regurgitation and increased left atrial volume load cause an increased left ventricular preload. This leads to dilation of the left ventricle and enlargement of the mitral valve annulus, producing progressive mitral valve insufficiency with increased volume loading and increasing left atrial enlargement. Furthermore, mitral regurgitation leads to reduced left ventricular afterload, since the left ventricle can pump into the lower-resistance left atrium versus the higher-resistance aorta.

Clinical Findings

Trivial mitral regurgitation may be present in normal individuals, though this is less common than tricuspid and pulmonary regurgitation (Table 17-6). Patients with mitral regurgitation are often asymptomatic for long periods of time and develop symptoms only if the regurgitation worsens. The initial presentation may include an increased heart rate and tachypnea that is increased with activity. With increased severity, patients develop exercise intolerance and dyspnea with exercise. Infants with significant regurgitation will have diaphoresis with feedings, respiratory distress or dyspnea, poor feeding and failure to thrive.

TABLE 17-6

MITRAL REGURGITATION

History	Labs	Exam	Pathophysiology
Murmur	ECG—LAE, LVH Atrial arrhythmia	Holosystolic high frequency murmur at the apex, diastolic rumble, S3	Increased LA volume and pressure leading to left atrial enlargement and pulmonary edema
Tachycardia and tachypnea	CXR—cardiomegaly with LAE, LVE and pulmonary edema		
Feeding intolerance			
Diaphoresis	ECHO—regurgitant jet across mitral valve in systole		Increased stroke volume of the left ventricle but with decreased forward flow, limited cardiac output
Dyspnea with exertion			

Findings on physical examination include a hyperactive precordium and a left ventricular impulse that is displaced laterally. The second heart sound may be increased because of an increased P2 component from pulmonary hypertension. The murmur of mitral regurgitation is heard at the apex of the heart and radiates to the left axilla as a high frequency holosystolic (blowing) murmur. With worsening mitral regurgitation, a diastolic rumble can be heard secondary to the increased volume crossing the mitral valve with each heartbeat. A third heart sound can also be audible with severe mitral regurgitation, and represents the rapid ventricular filling phase during early diastole.

The chest radiograph may demonstrate cardiomegaly with left atrial enlargement and left ventricular enlargement. The findings are similar to those of mitral stenosis with a double atrial shadow, an elevated left mainstem bronchus, and increased pulmonary vascular markings with pulmonary edema indicating more severe mitral regurgitation. The presence of these findings correlate with the severity of mitral regurgitation.

The electrocardiogram demonstrates left atrial enlargement, left ventricular hypertrophy, and possible arrhythmias such as atrial flutter or atrial fibrillation.

Echocardiography can make the diagnosis of mitral insufficiency and is a very sensitive test, often recording very minimal or trivial mitral regurgitation.

Mitral regurgitation is generally graded as mild, moderate, or severe by echocardiography. This is a useful test to noninvasively follow the progression of mitral regurgitation and assess for left atrial and left ventricular enlargement changes over time. In older patients and patients with poor acoustic windows, a transesophageal echocardiogram will give excellent imaging of the mitral valve and defines the mitral regurgitation.

Left ventricular angiography is used to define the severity of mitral regurgitation and is combined with hemodynamic evaluation during cardiac catheterization to rule out mitral stenosis in patients with an abnormal mitral valve and regurgitation. Mitral regurgitation is graded on a scale of 1+ to 4+ as assessed by left ventricular angiography (1+ indicates a faint jet of opacification, 2+ indicates faint opacification in the left atrium, 3+ indicates that the left atrium and left ventricle have similar densities of opacification, and 4+ indicates the left atrium is more densely opacified than the left ventricle).

Treatment

Therapy of mitral regurgitation varies with the severity of the regurgitation. Mild to moderate regurgitation is often treated with anticongestive therapy such as diuretics and afterload reduction such as ACE inhibitors. Digitalis has also been used in combination with diuretics, though its role is unclear. Surgical intervention is indicated before left ventricular dysfunction occurs. Attempts at repair after long-standing regurgitation of moderate or greater degrees can result in poor left ventricular function because of the higher afterload resulting from a competent mitral valve. Severe mitral regurgitation requires early surgical intervention with mitral valve repair or mitral valve replacement.

Mitral Valve Prolapse

Mitral valve prolapse is defined as the mitral valve leaflets "prolapsing," or moving back across the mitral valve annulus into the left atrium during ventricular systole. Mitral valve prolapse has been reported in 3–8% of people over 15 years of age. It is very commonly diagnosed in adults and is also commonly overdiagnosed in children when echocardiograms are performed and interpreted by individuals not trained in pediatric echocardiography and congenital heart disease.

Mitral valve prolapse has variable severity and can be associated with primary leaflet abnormalities or result from abnormalities of the mitral valve apparatus. Mitral valve prolapse is associated with other pathology of the heart, including endocarditis, Marfan syndrome, connective tissue disorders, myocarditis, cardiomyopathy, congenital heart disease, ruptured chordae tendonae, left ventricular aneurysm, left atrial myxomas, hyperthyroidism, systemic lupus erythematosus, polyarteritis nodosa, trauma, inherited metabolic disorders, and coronary artery disease. Mitral valve prolapse has also been described as part of an autosomal dominant trait with variable penetrance. It is strongly associated with connective tissue disorders, such as Ehlers-Danlos syndrome, pseudoxanthoma elasticum, osteogenesis imperfecta, and is almost always present in patients with a diagnosis of Marfan syndrome, which is an autosomal dominant disorder.

Mitral valve prolapse has been described as a common feature of connective tissue disorders in a continuum of severity. Clinical Marfan syndrome is at one end of severity and isolated or minor abnormalities similar to the clinical features of Marfan syndrome are at the mild end of this continuum. Patients with mitral valve prolapse often

are described as thin with an increased height to weight ratio. They generally have a narrow AP chest diameter, a long arm span, and commonly abnormalities of the chest including pectus excavatum, pectus carinatum, and scoliosis or straight back syndrome. Because of these associations, any patients with these clinical findings, mitral valve prolapse should be evaluated for possible. It is important that any patient with the physical habitus consistent with the diagnosis of Marfan syndrome have a cardiac evaluation including evaluation of the ascending aorta and aortic root for dilation, which is associated with that disease.

Mitral valve prolapse is also associated with congenital heart diseases including secundum atrial septal defect, aneurysm of the atrial septum, aortic valve prolapse, Ebstein anomaly, Uh anomaly, corrected transposition, accessory AV pathways, cystic medial necrosis of the aorta, and coronary anomalies.

Pathophysiology

The pathophysiology of mitral valve prolapse is a result of the amount of mitral valve regurgitation. The hemodynamic changes are as discussed above.

Clinical Findings

Many patients with mitral valve prolapse are asymptomatic and are diagnosed secondary to a click or a pathologic murmur. The common presentations include palpitations, chest pain, dyspnea without orthopnea, decreased exercise tolerance, fatigue, syncopal or near syncopal episodes, and postural orthostasis. The most common complaint is palpitations. These may be secondary to premature atrial contractions or premature ventricular contractions. The second most common complaint is atypical and nonspecific chest pain. This type of chest pain is not produced during an exercise stress test and is of variable severity. Additional complaints associated with mitral valve prolapse include anxiety or panic attacks and migraine headaches. Patients also have a significant incidence of supraventricular tachycardia, ventricular arrhythmias, and some incidence of bradycardia secondary to sinus node dysfunction or variable atrioventricular block. Despite the above associations, clinical studies have shown that the presence and severity of complaints do not seem to correlate well with the presence or severity of mitral valve prolapse.

The physical exam findings in mitral valve prolapse often can make the diagnosis without any additional testing. Patients with significant mitral valve prolapse will have a mid-systolic click with or without a late systolic murmur (felt because of regurgitation). The click is a high-pitched sound of short duration. The murmur is heard best at the apex and is a medium to high-pitched systolic crescendo murmur that is audible until S2. The quality of the murmur has been described as "honking" or "whooping." The most important feature of the murmur and the click in mitral valve prolapse is its variability with maneuvers designed to increase or decrease the left ventricular systolic volume. With maneuvers that decrease the left ventricular systolic volume, the click and murmur occur earlier in systole. This includes anything that decreases venous return, decreases restriction of the left ventricular outflow, increases contractility, or increases heart rate. The common maneuvers are changing from a supine to a sitting position, from a sitting to a standing position, moving from a squat to a standing position, Valsalva, and during inspiration. Giving amyl nitrate also causes an earlier click and murmur.

Based on the same principle, maneuvers that increase left ventricular systolic volume will cause the click and following murmur to occur later in systole. This includes going from a sitting to a supine position, standing to a sitting position, or standing to a squatting position. A passive leg raise with increase of venous return and isometric exercise will also move the murmur later in systole. Administration of phenylephrine raises the systolic pressure and will also move the second heart sound later in systole.

The timing of the click and murmur also varies with severity. A later click and murmur are usually associated with milder prolapse, and as the prolapse and regurgitation become more significant, the click will move earlier in systole.

Echocardiographic evaluation of the mitral valve is used to confirm the diagnosis and evaluate the severity of the prolapse and the mitral regurgi-

tation at presentation. The diagnosis of mitral valve prolapse requires visualization of the mitral valve moving back into the left atrium across the plane of the mitral valve in two planes on two-dimensional echocardiography. Mitral valve regurgitation can be seen in any of the two-dimensional views but is most commonly graded on an apical four-chamber view.

Treatment

The natural history of mitral valve prolapse is excellent for patients with mild prolapse and mild degrees of mitral regurgitation. They are at risk for endocarditis and do require SBE prophylaxis if regurgitation is present. The group of patients at significant risk of arrhythmia owing to mitral valve prolapse include those with moderate to severe mitral regurgitation who have developed left atrial enlargement and left ventricular enlargement. There is an increased incidence of complications in males and individuals greater than 50 years of age.

Arrhythmias are relatively common in patients who have developed left atrial enlargement and left ventricular enlargement but there is a poor correlation between patient's symptoms of palpitations and the severity of their arrhythmia. Surgical repair or replacement of the mitral valve is reserved for those patients with moderate to severe mitral regurgitation with significant arrhythmias and left atrial and left ventricular enlargement.

AORTIC VALVE ABNORMALITIES

Aortic Stenosis

Aortic stenosis is a narrowing or abnormality of the aortic valve or the aortic annulus that causes obstruction of the left ventricular outflow to the ascending aorta. This obstruction produces a pressure gradient from the left ventricle to the ascending aorta and increased left ventricular pressure. Aortic stenosis constitutes approximately 3.5% of congenital heart disease. Left ventricular outflow tract (LVOT) obstruction is also caused by subaortic stenosis, which is stenosis occurring below the level of the aortic valve, and supravalvar aortic stenosis

TABLE 17-7

AORTIC STENOSIS

History	Labs	PE	Pathophysiology
Murmur	ECG—LVH, ST-T-wave changes	Systolic ejection murmur at right upper sternal border, radiating to carotids	Increased LV pressure
Chest pain with exertion	Ventricular arrhythmia		LVH
Syncope	CXR—normal, dilated ascending aorta		Limited cardiac output owing to fixed obstruction across AV
Exercise intolerance	ECHO—increased flow velocity across the AV, LVH, post stenotic dilation of AAO	Narrow pulse pressure	
Dyspnea on exertion		Loud A2, fixed or paradoxically split	Subendocardial scarring owing to deceased perfusion to thickened myocardium at increased LV diastolic pressure
		Apical heave	
		Active precordium	
		Ejection click	LV failure

occurring just above the aortic valve. These abnormalities produce similar presentations, clinical findings, and pathophysiology (Table 17-7).

Valvar aortic stenosis is the most common form of left ventricular outflow tract obstruction and involves an abnormal aortic valve. The aortic valve morphology is normally a trileaflet valve that is completely unobstructed. There is no pressure gradient across a normal aortic valve.

The most common abnormality of the aortic valve is a bicuspid aortic valve, which is the most common form of any congenital heart disease with up to 5% of the population having a bicuspid aortic valve. This may be the most common congenital heart lesion, although it is usually of minimal, if any hemodynamic significance. Only a small percentage of these bicuspid valves are stenotic and produce any significant obstruction. The stenosis often occurs when these two abnormal leaflets fuse and create a narrowed orifice.

An aortic valve that is tricuspid but develops stenosis is the most commonly acquired form of valvar stenosis with thickening of abnormal valve leaflets. A unicuspid aortic valve with a small effective orifice is the most severe form of aortic valvar stenosis and presents early in life. Unicuspid valves do not respond well to therapy and often require replacement.

Subvalvar aortic obstruction can be a result of increased ventricular septal thickening, which produces a muscular ridge underneath the aortic valve causing obstruction, or a membrane that develops beneath the aortic valve in the left ventricular outflow tract. A third form is a fibrous or tunnel type obstruction in the left ventricular outflow tract.

Supravalvar aortic stenosis can be a result of a membrane just above the aortic valve, typically at the sino-tubular ridge above the coronary sinuses. It can also result from an hourglass narrowing of the proximal ascending aorta, as is frequently seen in William's syndrome. A hypoplastic ascending aorta also results in supravalvar obstruction but is most commonly associated with hypoplastic left heart syndrome or critical aortic valve stenosis.

Pathophysiology

Left ventricular outflow tract obstruction produces a pressure gradient between the left ventricle and

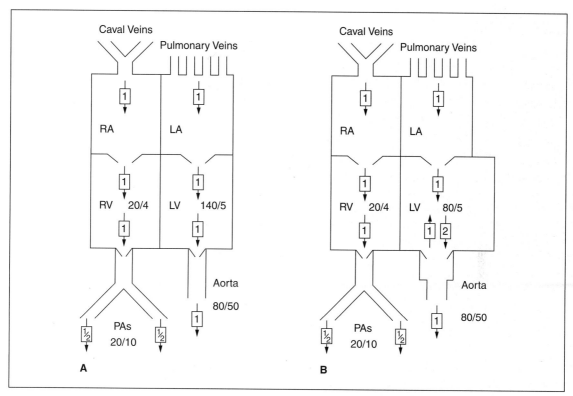

FIGURE 17-4

CHANGES IN CARDIAC OUTPUT AND PRESSURE WITH AORTIC STENOSIS AND AORTIC REGURGITATION

Part **A** is based on figure 1a and shows the changes with aortic stenosis. Note the elevated systolic pressure. In this example, the systolic gradient is 60 mmHg. Part **B** shows the changes with aortic regurgitation, namely, LV and proximal aortic dilation. Note the decreased aortic diastolic pressure (widened pulse pressure). In this example, with a regurgitant volume of one cardiac output, two cardiac outputs cross the aortic valve during systole in order to yield a net cardiac output of 1 to the systemic circulation.

the distal ascending aorta (Figure 17-4A). A pressure gradient results in increased left ventricular pressure which progresses with increasing degrees of obstruction. The left ventricular muscular wall thickens (i.e., left ventricular hypertrophy develops). As the left ventricle hypertrophies it becomes less compliant and the left ventricular end-diastolic pressure also increases. This transmits a higher pressure to the left atrium and can lead to left atrial enlargement.

With significant left ventricular hypertrophy and increased left ventricular end-diastolic pressure, the diastolic gradient from the ascending aorta through the coronary arteries to the left ven-

tricle decreases. This produces a lower perfusion pressure to a thickened myocardium. Since the myocardium is perfused from the outer to the inner portions, the subendocardium of the left ventricle is perfused from the most distal portion of the coronary vasculature, which is of the smallest caliber. With an increasing left ventricular end-diastolic pressure, and because of the increased perfusion distance owing to the hypertrophied left ventricle, this tissue can develop chronic ischemia. This chronic ischemia leads to scarring of the subendocardium and subendocardial fibroelastosis develops. This produces an even less compliant left ventricle, which further elevates the left ventricular end-diastolic pressure. Left ventricular function may decrease because of ischemia and limit the ability of the heart to increase its cardiac output. This limited cardiac output can lead to clinical signs of left ventricular failure, meaning that the left ventricle is unable to supply the body with sufficient blood flow to meet its metabolic demands.

Clinical Findings

The presentation of valvar aortic stenosis is dependent on the severity of the obstruction. Neonates with severe aortic stenosis or critical aortic stenosis present with congestive heart failure, shock, feeding intolerance, acidosis, and hypotension. Outside of the neonatal period, symptoms of aortic stenosis are similar to that with patients with left ventricular outflow tract obstruction from subaortic or supraaortic stenosis. These patients may have chest pain that is increased during increased metabolic demand that occurs with vigorous exercise. They can also present with syncopal events or near syncopal events. These symptoms may also occur during or immediately following exercise. Exercise intolerance is also common, with dyspnea on exertion being a frequent symptom. In mild forms of left ventricular outflow tract obstruction, the patients may be completely asymptomatic.

With significant left ventricular outflow tract obstruction and ventricular dysfunction, there is a limited stroke volume for each heartbeat, producing a narrow pulse pressure measured by direct arterial measurements or cuff blood pressure. In severe obstruction, pulses may be decreased and the physical findings of decreased cardiac output with poor perfusion, including a capillary refill time greater than 2 s. The point of maximum impulse of the heart is normal unless significant heart failure has developed and the left ventricle has started to dilate. There is often an apical tap with an active precordium. The second heart sound may be narrowly split, single, or paradoxically split with S2 occurring at the same time as P2 or after P2. There is a systolic ejection murmur most commonly audible at the right upper sternal border and the suprasternal notch that radiates to the carotid arteries. An end-diastolic murmur (S4) may be heard at the left lower sternal border because of decreased compliance of the thickened left ventricle, with increased reliance on active atrial contraction to fill the left ventricle. In valvar aortic stenosis, an ejection systolic click heard at the left lower sternal border and at the right upper sternal border is audible. This click will be absent in supravalvar or subvalvar stenosis.

The chest radiograph may demonstrate a prominent ascending aorta because of the poststenotic dilatation of the ascending aorta and is seen in valvar aortic stenosis but will not be present in subaortic or supravalvar aortic stenosis. The heart size is generally normal unless there is left ventricular failure.

The ECG demonstrates left ventricular hypertrophy, and with progressive left ventricular hypertrophy, there may be ST and T-wave changes with ST depression and T-wave inversion in the lateral precordial leads (V5, V6). With an elevated left ventricular end-diastolic pressure, left atrial enlargement may be noted on ECG. In mild forms, the ECG will be normal.

Two-dimensional echocardiographic imaging can diagnose the site of the left ventricular outflow tract obstruction and make an accurate evaluation of the anatomy. In valvar aortic stenosis, the number of aortic valve leaflets can be defined and abnormal leaflets with restrictive motion are noted if present. The annulus can be directly measured and compared to a normal population. Doppler evaluation is used to evaluate the severity of the obstruction by estimating the gradient. This estimation will not be accurate if there is significant left ventricular failure, as the ventricle will not generate a high gradient despite severe aortic stenosis, owing to poor systolic function.

Direct hemodynamic measurement is useful in the evaluation and management of left ventricular outflow tract obstruction and is still considered the gold standard for measurement of a gradient from the left ventricle to the ascending aorta. In valvar aortic stenosis, a gradient of 1–40 mmHg is considered mild; 40–75 mmHg, moderate; and severe is greater than 75 mmHg. Cardiac catheterization is also useful for therapy of valvar aortic stenosis, which usually responds well to balloon valvuloplasty.

Treatment

The therapy of aortic stenosis and left ventricular outflow tract obstruction is dependent on the form and severity of the obstruction. Valvar aortic stenosis requires SBE prophylaxis for life, as the valve is always considered to be abnormal. Mild forms of valvar aortic stenosis generally require no significant therapy. All patients are followed clinically and with serial echocardiograms to evaluate for progression of their stenosis.

Balloon aortic valvuloplasty is generally very effective for moderate and severe valvar aortic stenosis. It has limited effectiveness in patients with unicuspid aortic valves. Balloon valvuloplasty can be used in any patient, at any age and can be repeated if necessary. The major risk of balloon valvuloplasty is the development of significant aortic regurgitation. Patients with only mild aortic regurgitation are generally treated with balloon valvuloplasty, but those with more severe regurgitation are referred for surgical intervention owing to the risk of increasing the amount of regurgitation with further balloon valvuloplasty.

Surgical treatment of critical neonatal aortic stenosis involves open commissurotomy, whereby the fused commissures are opened with a scalpel, or closed commissurotomy with a dilator via the LV apex or retrograde. Closed commissurotomy is rarely performed.

Treatment of aortic valve stenosis in the older child depends on whether there is associated significant aortic annular hypoplasia. If the aortic annulus is near normal in size, it is usually treated by aortic valve sparing procedures. Prosthetic valve implantation is usually a last resort. Aortic valve repair procedures involve commissurotomies, cusp extensions with pericardial patches, and other maneuvers. Aortic valve repair is mainly indicated in patients whose main pathology is aortic regurgitation, whether in a tricuspid or bicuspid aortic valve. Mild aortic stenosis can also be dealt with at repair. Repair techniques involve a variety of maneuvers aimed at increasing the coaptation surface of the individual cusps such as pericardial patch extension of a deficient or "rolled up" cusp, resuspension of the cuspal commissure to the aortic wall or "tightening" of commissural edges to

each other, debridement of any fibrous material, shaving of the cusps to give them further pliability, and so forth. Aortic valve replacement is carried out if repair is not feasible. The younger the child, the less duration biological prostheses such as homografts or pericardial valves will have. Mechanical prostheses can last a lifetime if one can implant an adult-size prosthesis, but require life-long anticoagulation with warfarin with its associated complications (bleeding) in a growing, active child. The pulmonary autograft procedure (Ross operation) is an alternative treatment in growing children and involves harvesting the native pulmonary artery and valve and implanting it into the left ventricular outflow tract after removal of the diseased aortic valve. This involves reimplantation of the coronaries, and the placement of an RV to PA homograft. Survival after the Ross operation is greater than 95%, and immediate complications include bleeding, coronary malperfusion, and temporary myocardial dysfunction from prolonged cardioplegic arrest. Long-term results are gratifying. Long-term complications include the need for RV-PA conduit replacements, and progressive autograft root dilation leading to neoaortic valve regurgitation. Contraindications to the Ross procedure include connective tissue disease such as Marfan syndrome, and rheumatic heart disease. Relative contraindications include an older age (>45 years). In the past, aortoannular ectasia, isolated aortic valve regurgitation (AR), bicuspid aortic valves, and ascending aortic aneurysms were considered relative contraindications because of reports of progressive autograft dilation and neoaortic valve regurgitation; however, most surgeons performing a Ross for these indications now fix the aortic annulus at a prechosen (normal) size with a strip of either native pericardium or felt. Recent reports indicate that this may offer a solution to the problem of autograft failure.

Membranous subaortic stenosis may be conservatively managed with observation for increasing stenosis or resulting aortic insufficiency in its mild stages. The natural history of membranous subaortic stenosis is variable but this is commonly treated at the time of diagnosis with surgical resection. Subaortic obstruction because of a membrane is treated by resection and septal myomectomy. The LVOT is approached via an aortotomy. While carefully protecting the aortic valve cusps, the membrane is completely excised. Any associated septal hypertrophy causing obstruction may be treated by resecting a trench of septal muscle underneath the right-left aortic valve commissure. Subaortic obstruction because of a muscular tunnel-like lesion is treated by an aggressive myomectomy or the so-called "modified Konno" operation. This involves an incision into the subaortic septum, essentially creating a VSD, and then patching the defect. The aortic valve remains intact (thus the addition "modified").

Supra valvar aortic stenosis is usually repaired using patch augmentation of the ascending aorta. The patch is usually made of Dacron or Gore-Tex (PTFE).

Patients with any form of left ventricular outflow tract obstruction that produces turbulent flow are at risk for bacterial endocarditis and should receive SBE prophylaxis. All three forms of left ventricular outflow tract obstruction can produce turbulence at, below, or above the aortic valve that can lead to significant aortic insufficiency. Moderate to severe forms of left ventricular outflow tract obstruction can lead to decreased cardiac output and a significant decrease in the ability to increase the cardiac output with exercise. This can lead to exercise intolerance and congestive heart failure. The risk of sudden death owing to valvar aortic stenosis is increased if the gradient across the aortic valve exceeds 40 mmHg.

Aortic Regurgitation

Aortic valve regurgitation (AR) occurs when the aortic valve fails to seal completely during ventricular diastole. During this period, the aortic artery pressure is higher than the diastolic pressure in the left ventricle. If the valve is incompetent, blood will return to the left ventricle from the aorta. Congenital aortic regurgitation is uncommon and usually associated with a morphologically abnormal valve (bicuspid or unicuspid). Acquired aortic regurgitation is much more common and is associated with other forms of congenital or acquired heart disease. Aortic regurgitation secondary to balloon angioplasty of the aortic valve for aortic valve stenosis is usually mild but can be more severe and require further therapy. Acquired AR can also occur with rheumatic heart disease or endocarditis (Table 17-8).

Pathophysiology

Aortic regurgitation leads to volume overload of the left ventricle and can lead to left heart failure (Figure 17-4B). This can be a result of poor forward flow to the systemic circulation or poor left ventricular function as the left ventricle dilates. Low diastolic blood pressure and flow from the aortic root back into LV lead to poor coronary perfusion, causing a worsening of the heart failure.

TABLE 17-8

AORTIC REGURGITATION

History	Labs	Exam	Pathophysiology
Murmur	ECG—LVH, ST-T-wave changes	Diastolic murmur at left lower sternal border, mid-sternal border	Left ventricular volume overload and LV dilation
Chest pain with exertion	Ventricular arrhythmia		
Syncope	CXR—normal, LVE	Wide pulse pressure, bounding pulses	Limited cardiac output owing to decreased forward flow in aorta
Exercise intolerance	ECHO—Diastolic flow across AV to LV, LV dilation, retrograde flow in DAO	Laterally and inferiorly displaced PMI	LV failure
Dyspnea on exertion			Poor coronary perfusion

The stroke volume is increased, as it is the volume of blood needed for a normal cardiac output plus the regurgitant volume. Thus, there is increased blood flow across the aortic valve.

Clinical Findings

Patients with significant aortic regurgitation can develop signs of left heart failure with left ventricular enlargement. Mild to moderate aortic valve regurgitation results in a diastolic heart murmur at the left lower sternal border and also at the mid-to-right upper sternal border. There may be an associated systolic ejection murmur at the right upper sternal border because of the increased volume flow across the aortic valve. Moderate to severe AR presents with a pathologic murmur, signs of left heart failure with exercise intolerance, chest pain during exertion, arrhythmia, and possibly sudden death. The point of maximal impulse (PMI) may be displaced laterally and inferior, owing to left ventricular enlargement. Left atrial enlargement can develop secondary to left ventricular enlargement and mitral annulus enlargement with resultant mitral regurgitation and a systolic murmur. The AR lowers the effective diastolic blood pressure producing a wide pulse pressure and bounding pulses.

The chest plain film demonstrates left ventricular enlargement.

The ECG may demonstrate left ventricular enlargement or hypertrophy.

The diagnosis of aortic insufficiency is generally made by physical exam but is confirmed by echocardiography demonstrating color Doppler reversal of flow across the aortic valve. A normal aortic valve does not demonstrate any regurgitation. The severity of AR is evaluated by the degree of left ventricular enlargement and the width of the aortic insufficiency jet in comparison to the aortic valve annulus. Severe AR causes reversal of flow in the proximal descending aorta because of a large volume of blood flowing back into the left ventricle.

Catheterization is not usually required for the evaluation of aortic regurgitation. Angiography in the proximal ascending aorta or aortic root will demonstrate the regurgitation, and the severity can be graded from mild to severe. This is usually done during the evaluation of aortic valve stenosis.

Treatment

Therapy for aortic regurgitation varies with the severity. Historically, AR is not well tolerated and is often progressive. Therapy may include medical management with diuretics and afterload reducing agents to decrease any pulmonary edema and promote forward flow in the aorta. Trivial to mild AR may not require management other than frequent evaluation for progression. Moderate to severe AR requires surgical intervention. If repair of the valve is not possible, then the valve can be replaced with a homograft valve, a mechanical valve, a tissue valve, or a pulmonary autograft (Ross procedure), as discussed above.

Suggested Readings

Bacha EA, Satou GM, Moran AM, Zurakowski D, Marx GR, Keane JF, Jonas RA: Valve-sparing operation for balloon-induced aortic regurgitation in congenital aortic stenosis. *J Thorac Cardiovasc Surg* 122:162–168, 2001.

Elkins RC, Knott-Craig CJ, McCue C, Lane MM: Congenital aortic valve disease. Improved survival and quality of life. *Ann Surg* 225:503–511, 1997.

Emmanoulides GC, Riemenschneider TA, Allen HD, Gutgesell, HP (eds.): *Moss and Adams Heart Disease in Infants, Children, and Adolescents*, 5th ed. Baltimore, MD, Williams & Wilkins, 1995, Chapters 61, 62, 63, 69, 70, 71, 72.

Garson A, Bricker JT, Fisher DJ, Neish SR (eds): *The Science and Practice of Pediatric Cardiology*, 2nd ed. Baltimore, MD, Williams & Wilkins, 1998, Chapters 54, 55, 56.

Stamm C, Friehs I, Zurakowski D, Bacha E, Moran A, Mayer JE, Jonas RA, del Nido PJ: Surgery for bilateral outflow tract obstruction in elastin arteriopathy. *J Thorac Cardiovasc Surg* 120:755–763, 2000.

C H A P T E R

18

ARTERIAL ABNORMALITIES

Hitendra T. Patel

INTRODUCTION

Aside from the intracardiac lesions listed in the prior chapters, and the lesions causing obstruction or regurgitation, there are a number of other cardiac abnormalities that involve the arteries. These may involve individual or combinations of the aorta, pulmonary and coronary arteries. This chapter details the physiology and physical findings of these lesions.

ANOMALIES OF THE AORTIC ARCH—VASCULAR RINGS AND SLINGS

Aortic arch anomalies result from abnormalities of branching, arch position, supernumerary arches, interruption of the aortic arch, and anomalous origin of the pulmonary artery (PA).

Embryology

The normal development of the aorta and the pulmonary artery is complicated. Structures are derived from the primitive trunco-aortic sac (TA sac), which divides to form the ascending aorta and the main pulmonary artery as shown in Figure 18-1. The paired dorsal aortae fuse to form the descending aorta. The aortic arch, which connects the ascending aorta to the descending aorta, is formed by contributions from six paired branchial arches (BAr). These early aortic arches form by cellular differentiation of cells derived from the branchial pouches. These arches (I–VI) form at different times and regress by apoptosis as the mature circulation forms. In the fully differentiated state, the left aortic arch is derived from BAr IV. The right and left carotid arteries are derived from the right and left BAr III, and the right and left subclavian arteries from the seventh right and left intersegmental arteries. The usual left ductus arteriosus is derived from the left BAr VI. The distal pulmonary arteries derive from the respective lung buds and grow to join the main pulmonary artery that differentiates from the TA sac. The right and left aortic arch refers to the bronchus that is crossed by the aortic arch and not which side of the midline the aortic arch ascends. The normal left aortic arches over the left main bronchus.

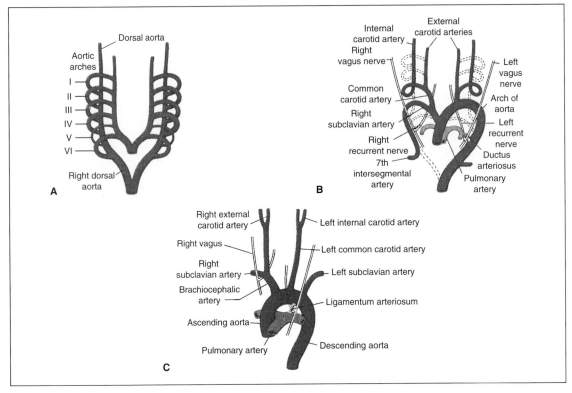

FIGURE 18-1

SCHEMATIC DIAGRAM OF THE TOTIPOTENTIAL AORTIC ARCH

Source: Sadler TW. *Langman's Medical Embryology*. 7th ed. Baltimore: Williams & Wilkins, 1995.

Abnormal development or failure to regress at appropriate times, of the many vascular structures that contribute to the development of the aortic arch and the pulmonary arteries during embryonic development, result in many types of vascular abnormalities. This becomes clinically important when the trachea and esophagus are encircled by vascular structures, causing compression known as a vascular ring.

Clinical Presentation of Vascular Rings

Compression of the esophagus results in dysphagia and airway compression leads to stridor. Stridor is usually the predominant finding in the neonate or infant. Symptoms may include "noisy breathing" with the onset at birth. The severity can change with position or with the presence of an intercurrent respiratory infection. Unusual presentations in infants include reflex apnea with feeding and

hyperextension of the neck. Toddlers and older patients present with dysphagia or choking on food. Incidental discovery is also common following imaging for another problem. Tables 18-1 and 18-2 summarize the findings.

Complete Vascular Rings

Double Aortic Arch

A double aortic arch is an anomaly in which there is persistence of the right and left fourth branchial arches. Usually the right arch is larger and more superior than the left. Rarely the left arch is dominant or both arches are equal in size (least common). Both arches may be patent, or one arch, usually the left, is hypoplastic or atretic. All double arches form a ring; however, symptoms depend on the tightness of the ring. If both arches are widely patent, the ring is usually tight with presentation

TABLE 18-1

RIGHT AORTIC ARCH ABNORMALITIES

Abnormality	Type of Presentation	Diagnostic Test	Treatment
Right aortic arch with retroesophageal diverticulum of Kommerell. This is the last branch of the right arch and gives rise to the left ductus arteriosus and the left subclavian artery	Vascular ring	ECHO Angiography MRI/CT scan	Division of the ductus or the entire diverticulum
Right aortic arch with left descending aorta and left ductus arteriosus	Vascular ring	CXR Ba. Swallow ECHO Angiography MRI/CT scan	
Right aortic arch with retroesophageal innominate artery	Rare. Tracheal compression		Ligation, division, and reimplantation

usually in the newborn period. As with other vascular rings, late presentation is associated with dysphagia or respiratory symptoms.

The diagnosis of a double aortic arch is suggested by chest radiography (CXR). The tracheal air column is indented on the right side superiorly by the right arch and inferiorly on the left by the left arch. A right aortic arch that descends on the left side at the level of the diaphragm is very suggestive of this anatomy. A barium esophagogram will show similar findings with a superior right and posterior indentation by the right arch and inferior left side indentation by the left arch. If both aortic arches are patent, the diagnosis can be confirmed by transthoracic echocardiography; however, both MRI or CT scans have now become the "gold standard" for the diagnosis and may yield information about the severity of the tracheoesophageal compression. Angiography is rarely required given the current era of noninvasive imaging.

Surgical ligation and division of the diminutive or atretic arch is indicated in symptomatic patients. A left posterolateral thoracotomy is the usual approach.

TABLE 18-2

LEFT AORTIC ARCH ABNORMALITIES

Abnormality	Presentation	Diagnostic Test	Management
Left aortic arch with retroesophageal right subclavian artery	Although not a vascular ring, it can present with dysphagia	Barium swallow. Posterior indentation	Ligation and division or reimplantation of the subclavian artery
Left aortic arch with right descending aorta and right ductus or ligamentum	Vascular ring	CXR Ba. Swallow MRI/CT scan Angiography	Ligation and division of the right ductus. Note a right thoracotomy or midline approach

Right Aortic Arch Abnormalities

Right aortic arch with retroesophageal diverticulum of Kommerell: In this lesion there is persistence of the right fourth branchial arch with disappearance of the left fourth arch. The left dorsal aorta forms the retroesophageal diverticulum of Kommerell, which connects to the left seventh intersegmental artery to form the left subclavian artery and the left sixth branchial arch. The sixth branchial arch forms the left ductus arteriosus, which connects the left dorsal aorta to the left pulmonary artery (LPA), thus completing the vascular ring.

In a symptomatic child, this anomaly should be suspected in the presence of a right aortic arch on a CXR. Barium esophagogram should reveal a large posterior esophageal indentation. To make a definitive diagnosis in the presence of a ductal ligament, a retroesophageal diverticulum (from which the left subclavian artery arises) needs to be demonstrated. This can be achieved with an MRI/CT scan (spiral is best) or aortic angiography. The presence of a left ductal ligament can then be inferred.

The management consists of surgical ligation and division of the left ductal ligament using a left posterolateral thoracotomy or median sternotomy.

Right aortic arch with left descending aorta and left ductus arteriosus: Embryologically, in this lesion, there is persistence of the right fourth branchial arch and disappearance of the left. The right arch courses behind the esophagus to connect to the left dorsal aorta. A left ligamentum from the left sixth branchial arch completes the vascular ring.

The diagnostic findings are similar to the anomaly discussed above, right aortic arch with retroesophageal diverticulum of Kommerell; however, the left subclavian is not aberrant.

In symptomatic patients, surgical ligation and division of the ligamentum arteriosus is indicated.

Left Aortic Arch Anomalies

Left aortic arch with right descending aorta and right ductus or ligamentum: This lesion is the mirror image anatomy of a right aortic arch with a left descending aorta and a left ductus arteriosus.

The chest radiograph may show evidence for a left aortic arch and a right-sided descending aorta at the level of the diaphragm. A barium esophagogram

will show a posterior indentation. The diagnosis is made by an MRI/CT scan or angiography.

This rare anomaly requires ligation and division of the ductus/ligamentum arteriosus. This is best performed via a *right* posterolateral thoracotomy or mid-line sternotomy.

Partial Vascular Rings

Left Aortic Arch Anomalies

Left aortic arch with retroesophageal right subclavian artery: Although not a true vascular ring this anomaly is associated with stridor and dysphagia. The diagnosis can be made with transthoracic echocardiography, which shows the absence of an innominate artery and the first branch off the aortic arch as the right carotid artery. The origin of the left subclavian and it retroesophageal course may be difficult to visualize by transthoracic echocardiography. Barium esophagography can be useful. It demonstrates a small posterior indentation slanting upward toward the right. The filling defect is smaller than those produced by indentation from the right arch in a double aortic arch or diverticulum of Kommerell (see below). The definitive diagnosis is made by a CT or MRI scan. 3D reconstruction can be very useful to demonstrate the spatial anatomy.

Significant symptoms requiring surgical intervention is rare. Repair consists of a left thoracotomy with mobilization, division and reimplantation of the retroesophageal right subclavian artery.

Other Great Artery Anomalies Presenting With Stridor or Dysphagia

Cervical aortic arch: This is a rare anomaly. The arch is located superiorly above the level of the clavicles. Presentation may be a pulsatile mass in the supraclavicular fossa, or tracheal compression with stridor, dyspnea, or frequent respiratory tract infections. In adults dysphagia is common. Surgical repair depends on other associated arch anomalies and can be challenging. The main objective is to connect the ascending aorta to the descending aorta, either directly or with an interposition graft.

Anomalous origin of the left pulmonary artery from the right pulmonary artery or the pulmonary artery sling: In this lesion, the left pulmonary artery arises from the right pulmonary artery and courses behind the trachea and in front of the esophagus to reach the left hilum. There is a high association of associated cardiac defects and abnormal tracheal development. Specifically, this abnormality is associated with complete cartilaginous rings in the trachea.

The usual presentation of patients with a pulmonary artery sling is respiratory difficulty and stridor.

Laboratory findings include an abnormal lateral plain film of the chest, which leads to suspicion of this abnormality. Usually the trachea and the esophagus are close to one another at the level of the carina. If the LPA courses between them, a soft tissue space is noted. A barium esophagogram will reveal the presence of anterior compression on the esophagus. This is the only lesion with these findings on the barium swallow. Echocardiography, MRI, or angiography can all make the definitive diagnosis.

Treatment is indicated if symptoms and signs of airway obstruction are present. The LPA is divided and surgically reimplanted onto the MPA with the aim to leave the LPA course anterior to the trachea and esophagus. Presence of obstructing tracheal rings is a difficult problem to correct and should be evaluated by bronchoscopy at the time of surgery.

Innominate artery compression of the trachea: This is a rare and poorly understood lesion. There is anterior compression of the trachea by the innominate artery. It presents with stridor usually in early infancy. MRI with 3D reconstruction is the best method for diagnosis. If symptoms persist then surgical fixation of the innominate artery to the sternum may relieve the compression.

Many other rare aortic arch variations exist that are beyond the scope of this book. It is important to suspect this type of vascular abnormality if a patient presents with stridor and/or dysphagia.

Anomalous origin of a pulmonary artery branch from the ascending aorta: Unlike the other arterial lesions described thus far, this is a lesion not associated with airway compression, but rather, a left-to-right shunt. In this lesion, it is usually the right pulmonary artery with an anomalous origin. It can be associated with other congenital cardiac defects. If the left pulmonary artery origin is anomalous, then there is usually a right aortic arch and a high incidence of tetralogy of Fallot.

The clinical presentation of patients with this lesion usually occurs during infancy with symptoms and signs of a large arterial level left-to-right shunt (congestive heart failure or pulmonary overcirculation). Similar to a ventricular septal defect (VSD) or large patent ductus arteriosus (PDA), symptoms may include difficulty feeding and poor growth with an increased work of breathing. Physical findings may show tachypnea with respiratory distress. The pulse pressure may be increased if the pulmonary vascular resistance (PVR) is low because of the diastolic runoff from the aorta into the anomalous pulmonary artery. There may be a left ventricular heave due to left sided volume loading. Auscultation may reveal a continuous murmur similar to PDA. A murmur of increased flow across the mitral valve (diastolic rumble) may be difficult to distinguish from the continuous murmur of the shunt itself. Similar to a large VSD or PDA, patients may develop pulmonary vascular disease in the affected lung, though it may occur more rapidly, as soon as 6 months.

Laboratory findings include an abnormal chest radiograph, which may show asymmetric pulmonary vascular markings. This suggests differential pulmonary blood flow (greater to one lung). Echocardiography should demonstrate the abnormality definitively. Cardiac catheterization is performed to assess the hemodynamics prior to repair, especially if there is a question of irreversible vascular disease in the affected lung, which may be inoperable. Angiography of the ascending aorta will outline the abnormal anatomy.

Management consists of surgical division and reimplantation of the anomalous pulmonary artery into the main pulmonary artery. This is performed prior to the development of irreversible pulmonary vascular disease (Eisenmenger syndrome).

ANOMALIES OF THE CORONARY ARTERY ORIGIN

Introduction

Abnormalities of coronary artery origin include those in which the coronary artery arises from a vessel other than the aorta, and abnormalities in which one or more of the coronary arteries arise from an abnormal location of the aorta.

Incidence

The incidence of isolated coronary artery anomalies is not precisely known. These anomalies are noted in approximately 0.5% of pediatric autopsies.

Embryology

Understanding of the coronary artery development is still poor. It is thought that sinusoids in the primitive myocardium coalesce and develop into intramural vessels. A network of cells, possibly derived from the primordial liver, spread over the epicardium and develop into coronary vessels. These vessels join the intramural vessels and grow toward and penetrate the aortic sinuses. The signaling mechanisms and local controlling factors are not known. Abnormalities in these signals are thought to result in coronary artery anomalies.

Common anomalies are discussed but many variations exist. In patients who present with acute onset of left ventricular dysfunction, especially with mitral regurgitation and symptoms and signs of myocardial ischemia or syncope with exercise, it is essential to consider variations of coronary artery anatomy as part of the differential diagnosis. These diagnoses ought to be made urgently since there may be a higher association of sudden cardiac death, which may be preventable with surgical intervention.

Anomalous Origin of a Coronary Artery From the Pulmonary Artery

All possible variations of anomalous origin of the coronary arteries from the pulmonary artery have been described. These are rare but important defects to recognize.

The most common abnormality is the anomalous origin of the left main coronary artery from the pulmonary artery (ALCAPA, also known as Bland-White-Garland syndrome). The incidence is approximately 1:300,000 live births. It is usually an isolated defect but may be associated with other congenital heart defects, especially conotruncal abnormalities such as tetralogy of Fallot and Truncus arteriosus. As it is the most common of these types of lesions, it will be discussed, though similar lesions (e.g., anomalous origin of the right coronary artery (RCA) from the pulmonary artery) have the same pathophysiology.

Anatomy: The left main coronary artery (LCA) usually originates from the posterior or left sinus of the pulmonary artery root. It then courses in its usual distribution.

Pathophysiology: In the newborn period, when the PVR is elevated, antegrade flow occurs into the LCA from the PA. Although the blood is desaturated, myocardial ischemia is not present. Problems begin to occur when the PVR falls with a subsequent fall in LCA perfusion pressure. Flow to the LCA distribution is then dependent on the presence of collaterals from the RCA to the LCA. If no collaterals are present, myocardial ischemia will occur early, as soon as PVR decreases. With coronary artery collaterals, as PVR continues to decrease, flow will preferentially pass (from the RCA via collaterals) retrograde through the LCA into the PA and thereby "steal" blood from the myocardium normally supplied by the LCA (and to a lesser extent the RCA). Myocardial ischemia will occur early if collateral supply to the LCA is inadequate or later if "steal" phenomenon occurs.

Clinical findings: The symptoms and signs are secondary to myocardial ischemia. This results in left ventricular dysfunction and mitral regurgitation secondary to papillary muscle ischemia or infarction. This is compounded by a dilated mitral valve annulus from left ventricular dilatation. Most patients with ALCAPA present during infancy. Failure to thrive, symptoms of congestive heart failure, and irritability because of angina are the primary symptoms. Angina in infancy should be suspected when acute discomfort with intense crying occurs with exertion such as feeding. Presentation may occur later in life in patients with an extensive collateral coronary supply from the right coronary artery. In this case, the presentation may be for the evaluation of exercise-induced chest pain or syncope, or for evaluation of a continuous murmur. Unfortunately, the first signs or symptoms of this entity may be sudden death.

Examination of a symptomatic infant usually reveals a sick infant with signs of congestive heart failure. On auscultation, the second heart sound may be loud and single with a pansystolic murmur of mitral regurgitation, with an associated diastolic rumble of functional mitral stenosis if the mitral regurgitation is severe. Examination of an older child or adolescent with extensive collaterals may either reveal no obvious abnormalities, or subtle signs of congestive heart failure. Auscultation may demonstrate a continuous murmur from the coronary artery collaterals, or the murmur of mitral regurgitation.

Laboratory findings

Electrocardiography: The ECG typically shows lateral ischemia or infarction with pathologic q waves and inverted T waves in the lateral limb and precordial leads (I/avL/V5/V6).

Chest radiography: The plain film of the chest typically shows cardiomegaly (enlarged LV and LA) and pulmonary edema.

Echocardiography: The echocardiogram typically shows a dilated LV with poor function. Any associated mitral regurgitation is easily demonstrated via Doppler echocardiography with a secondarily dilated left atrium if it is significant. The anomalous origin of the LCA usually may be visualized with 2D and color flow Doppler imaging.

Cardiac catheterization with angiography remains the gold standard for demonstrating the anatomy and hemodynamics of this lesion. Typically, there is an elevated right ventricular and pulmonary artery pressure secondary to elevated left ventricular end-diastolic pressure (the physiologic hallmark of ventricular dysfunction). An aortic root angiogram shows a dilated right coronary artery with absence of the left coronary system. Collateral supply to the left coronary artery system with flow into the pulmonary artery may be seen with prolonged viewing (levophase). This is better demonstrated with a selective right coronary angiogram. Injection of contrast into the main pulmonary artery may delineate the origin of the left coronary artery.

Management: Patient stabilization and early consideration of the differential diagnosis is the first priority in a patient with signs and symptoms of shock. After the diagnosis is confirmed, surgical intervention is undertaken without significant delay. Surgical techniques include: (1) ligation of the LCA if there is good collateral network from the RCA; (2) creation of an intrapulmonary artery tunnel from the aortic root to the LCA (Takeuchi procedure); and (3) reestablishment of a two coronary artery system via removal of the anomalous coronary artery from the PA and reimplantation into the aorta. The latter is the preferred option, and has replaced the first two options in most cardiac centers. Rarely is cardiac transplantation the only option.

Long-term outlook: The long-term outcome in patients with this lesion is variable and depends partly on the degree of myocardial injury prior to intervention. In infants, ventricular function may recover significantly (to a normal or near normal range), especially if the coronary artery reimplantation is performed early in life. In all patients with congenital cardiac defects it is important to define the coronary artery anatomy, especially in those defects where pulmonary artery pressure is systemic. If unrecognized, left ventricular infarction or ischemia may occur following surgical repair with a sudden decrease in pulmonary artery pressure.

Origin of a Coronary Artery From the Inappropriate Sinus of Valsalva

Aside from the coronary artery arising from the incorrect artery, coronary arteries may also arise from the inappropriate sinus of valsalva. One of the well described lesions is the origin of the left main or left anterior descending coronary artery from the right coronary artery.

Anatomy: This is a rare abnormality in which the left coronary distribution remains the same. In order to supply the normal distribution of the left coronary artery, the anomalous coronary artery has a course posterior (behind) the aorta or between the aorta and pulmonary artery, which necessitates an acute angle at its origin. This course between the great vessels is associated with sudden cardiac death or exercise-induced syncope, near syncope, or chest pain. It is thought that with exercise and increased cardiac output there is dilation of the aortic and pulmonary roots. This causes extrinsic compression of the left coronary artery, as well as a further increase in the acute angle at its origin. This subsequently leads to decreased blood flow and myocardial ischemia, and/or sudden death. The other theory is that the acute angle of origin causes narrowing and is the reason for sudden death with exercise.

Clinical findings: This may be an incidental finding in an asymptomatic patient. Otherwise, there may be exercise-induced syncope, near syncope, or chest pain. The most feared presentation is sudden death. There are typically no abnormal physical findings.

Laboratory findings

Electrocardiography: The ECG is usually normal at rest. ST elevation and T-wave axis changes with exercise are indicators of coronary ischemia.

Nuclear imaging: Myocardial perfusion imaging with radioactive thallium or technetium at rest and immediately following exercise can be useful in locating areas of hypoperfusion.

Chest radiography: The plain film of the chest typically will show no abnormalities.

Echocardiography: Improved technology has enabled excellent resolution of coronary artery anatomy, which may demonstrate the abnormality.

MRI: This can be a valuable additional investigation to confirm the echocardiographic diagnosis and visualize the course of the coronary artery between the great vessels.

Cardiac catheterization and angiography: This is rarely needed for diagnosis, though remains the gold standard for imaging coronary artery anatomy. It may be difficult to demonstrate the course of the coronary arteries and their relation to other structures in 3D space.

Management: Surgical intervention is warranted in the symptomatic patient. It is also probably prudent in the asymptomatic patient who is at significant risk of sudden death. The exact surgical approach is less certain. Techniques include enlargement of the narrowed ostium of the left coronary artery and aorto-coronary bypass graft using saphenous vein or internal mammary artery grafts. The long-term patency of the graft remains the limiting factor. Some surgeons have proposed division of the main pulmonary artery near its bifurcation and reimplantation in a more leftward position on the left pulmonary artery. This potentially increases the space between the great vessels and may prevent coronary artery compression. Another approach is to incise a portion of the anomalous left coronary from the origin along its length and anastomose this open section of the coronary artery to a corresponding incision along the aorta. This essentially "marsupializes" the coronary artery to the aorta. The long-term success of these operations is not yet known.

Other Rare Coronary Anomalies

There are many other rare coronary artery abnormalities that include intramural and intramuscular coronary arteries, myocardial bridges, coronary atresia or stenosis, and single coronary artery. These are important to consider in patients presenting with symptoms and signs of myocardial ischemia, in particular chest pain or syncope with exercise. Appropriate evaluation of these signs and symptoms should lead to the correct diagnosis. Further discussion of these rare coronary artery abnormalities is beyond the scope of this book.

Suggested Readings

Allen HD, Gutgesell HP, Clark EB, Driscoll DJ: *Moss and Adams' Heart Disease in Infants, Children and Adolescents Including the Fetus and Young Adult*, 6th ed. Philadelphia, PA, Lippincott Williams & Wilkins, 2001.

Garson A, Bricker JT, Fisher DJ, Neish SR: *The Science and Practice of Pediatric Cardiology*, 2nd ed. Baltimore, MD, Williams & Wilkins, 1998.

19

HETEROTAXY

Joel T. Hardin

INTRODUCTION

In the spectrum of congenital heart malformation, cardiac malposition and heterotaxia syndromes are arguably the most complex. There is an equally complex and often confusing nomenclature involved in describing these defects. Levocardia versus dextrocardia, levoposition versus dextroposition, situs solitus versus situs inversus, and asplenia versus polysplenia are some examples of the pediatric cardiology lexicon that are not intuitively clear to other clinicians. In this chapter, a practical approach to evaluating "other than normal" cardiac position is presented, including a detailed discussion of heterotaxia.

TERMINOLOGY DEFINED

With the physical examination, and subsequent analysis of the chest radiograph and echocardiogram, cardiac position within (or rarely outside of) the thorax is usually readily apparent. Normal cardiac position is within the left hemithorax, and the appropriate designation is cardiac *levoposition*. The majority of cardiac malformations occur with cardiac levoposition. When the heart is largely in

the right hemithorax, the appropriate designation is cardiac *dextroposition*. Although finding a right-sided heart on exam or chest radiography should prompt consideration of associated intracardiac disease, it is important to emphasize that entirely normal intracardiac anatomy can coexist with cardiac dextroposition (e.g., left tension pneumothorax or left diaphragmatic hernia). Occasionally the heart is midline, and designated as cardiac *mesoposition*. In the most unusual of cardiac malposition, *ectopia cordis*, the heart protrudes through a sternal deformity to lie largely outside the thorax. In summary, for this gross cardiac anatomic description, nothing other than the heart's position within or outside of the thorax is implied by the designation levo-, dextro-, or mesoposition.

The next component of anatomic description relates to the orientation of the cardiac base-apex axis. One can define the base-apex axis as either normal (*levocardia*) or abnormal (*dextrocardia* or *mesocardia*). Note that the designation of normal or abnormal base-apex axis is completely independent of cardiac position within the thorax, and likewise does not necessarily imply associated cardiac malformation. A patient with situs inversus (see below), for example, can have entirely normal intracardiac anatomy with cardiac dextroposition and dextrocardia. In the previous example of a patient with left tension pneumothorax, one would potentially find abnormal cardiac dextroposition and normal levocardia. It should be apparent that defining base-apex axis in this fashion requires intracardiac imaging, which in clinical practice is generally predicated on results of echocardiography (although MRI and cardiac angiography can also be used).

After defining cardiac position and orientation of the base-apex axis, one should systematically analyze all three embryonic cardiac segments: (1) viscero-atrial situs, (2) atrioventricular connection, and (3) ventriculo-arterial connection. In this chapter, the focus will be on variations of viscero-atrial situs, with the other connections described elsewhere within this text.

Lastly, there may be anatomic variations of the caval veins and aortic arch, once again independent of cardiac position, base-apex axis, or cardiac segmental relationships. Important venous anomalies (e.g., persistent left superior vena cava, interrupted inferior vena cava) are discussed below, while conditions such as right aortic arch, double-aortic arch, and other aortic arch anomalies are discussed in Chapter 18.

VISCERO-ATRIAL SITUS

All vertebrates exhibit normal lateral asymmetry of the thoracic and abdominal organs, under control of multiple genes (Hox genes) that define antero-posterior relationship and laterality during embryonic development. Altered Hox gene expression in mice, for example, can lead to various cardiac malposition syndromes, pulmonary isomerism, and splenic abnormalities in patterns similar to the human heterotaxia syndromes.[1]

There are three fundamental relationships between atria and thoraco-abdominal viscera (i.e., viscero-atrial situs). In the usual pattern, *situs solitus,* the anatomic right atrium connects to right-sided caval veins. The major lobe of the liver is on the right, while the stomach, spleen, and descending aorta lie to the left. The right-sided lung has three lobes and an eparterial bronchus. Normal viscero-atrial situs

solitus can coexist with cardiac levoposition, cardiac dextroposition, or cardiac mesoposition; and likewise with levocardia, dextrocardia, or mesocardia.

Situs inversus is the mirror image of situs solitus. The major lobe of the liver is on the left, the stomach and spleen are on the right, and the left lung has three lobes with an eparterial bronchus. Left-sided caval veins connect with the anatomic right atrium. As mentioned above, situs inversus is most commonly (but not exclusively) associated with cardiac dextroposition and dextrocardia. Furthermore, a finding of situs inversus may have noncardiac diagnostic implications, including potential Kartagener's syndrome.

Situs ambiguus, or heterotaxia, represents viscero-atrial arrangements other than situs solitus or situs inversus. Heterotaxia is derived from Greek roots meaning 'other than normal arrangement or order.' In heterotaxia, the normal pattern of visceral asymmetry is absent and somewhat unpredictable, although two general tendencies are observed. In the *asplenia* syndrome, the spleen is absent with typically bilateral right-sided structures elsewhere (e.g., bilateral trilobed lungs each with eparterial bronchi; transverse liver with symmetric major lobes; and bilateral right atrial appendages). In the *polysplenia* syndrome, multiple splenic masses are present bilaterally with typically bilateral left-sidedness with respect to characteristics of the lungs, bronchi, and atrial appendages.

SELECTED SYNDROMES OF CARDIAC MALPOSITION

The most common anatomic variations involve instances of *cardiac dextroposition with situs solitus.* This includes conditions extrinsic to the heart that simply shift cardiac position rightward (e.g., left diaphragmatic hernia). Most of these patients do not have associated intracardiac malformation, but there are important exceptions. In complex forms of transposition of the great arteries, for example, the heart can lie in the left or right hemithorax, while still retaining normal viscero-atrial relationships (i.e., situs solitus). Other conditions that can coexist with dextroposition and situs solitus include ASDs, VSDs, atrioventricular septal defects, coarctation of the aorta, double-outlet right ventricle, and tetralogy of Fallot.

Another important consideration in patients with cardiac dextroposition and situs solitus is the *Scimitar syndrome*. In this condition, there can be levocardia or dextrocardia. The right lung and right pulmonary artery are usually hypoplastic, and the right pulmonary veins connect anomalously to the inferior vena cava. In addition, there is an anomalous systemic arterial supply to the right lung from the descending aorta. The clinical presentation varies, but symptomatic infants with Scimitar syndrome incur high mortality secondary to pulmonary hypertension and congestive heart failure. Although not universally present on frontal views of the chest x-ray, the anomalous right pulmonary veins can form the shape of a scimitar along the right side of the heart. For severely symptomatic infants, treatment can be problematic. A staged approach may be feasible, first involving transcatheter embolization of the aortopulmonary collateral(s), followed by surgical diversion of the anomalous right pulmonary vein to the left atrium, along with repair of associated intracardiac defects. Some cases of Scimitar syndrome, however, are best treated with right pneumonectomy along with any required intracardiac repair.[2]

Cardiac malposition with situs inversus occurs most often with significant additional malformations (e.g., ASD, VSD, double-outlet right ventricle). When it occurs with concordant or normal atrioventricular connection, normally-related great arteries, and no intracardiac anomaly, there may be no outward clinical manifestations (although heart sounds should be detected loudest on the right). This is the so-called mirror-image dextrocardia that coexists in Kartagener's syndrome. This familial syndrome encompasses findings of situs inversus, chronic sinusitis, and bronchiectasis, all secondary to ciliary dyskinesia.[3]

HETEROTAXIA

As mentioned above, the heterotaxia syndromes of asplenia and polysplenia result from disordered embryogenesis related to thoraco-abdominal visceral, right-left asymmetry. There is a male predominance with familial inheritance patterns also observed. Asplenia (also known as Ivemark syndrome) generally encompasses more severe cardiac and gastrointestinal malformation, and is often referred to as "bilateral right-sidedness." Polysplenia syndrome usually includes a right-sided stomach with multiple small splenic masses along the stomach's greater curvature. Associated heart disease is generally less severe. The hepatic portion of the inferior vena cava is frequently absent, such that venous drainage of the abdomen and lower extremities continues to the superior vena cava via the azygous system. Polysplenia is often referred to as "bilateral left-sidedness."

Heterotaxia is associated with complex congenital heart disease. Atrioventricular septal defects, pulmonary atresia or stenosis, transposition of the great vessels, anomalous pulmonary venous connection, univentricular heart disease, and double-outlet right ventricle are typical examples. Cyanotic heart defects are more common in asplenia, whereas acyanotic defects are more common in polysplenia. Univentricular heart disease in heterotaxia carries a very poor prognosis, with greater perioperative morbidity and higher surgical mortality relative to palliation of other univentricular heart defects.[4] When there is an associated anomalous pulmonary venous connection, survival rates after neonatal heart surgery are lower, approximately 45% at 1 year of age.[5] Thus, some institutions do favor cardiac transplantation for selected cases of complex congenital heart disease in heterotaxia.[6]

Comprehensive evaluation of a patient with suspected heterotaxia should include examination of the peripheral blood smear for Howell-Jolly bodies (abnormal if present in neonates older than 7 days). Their presence is consistent with asplenia or functional asplenia. Abdominal ultrasound may identify the presence or absence of splenic tissue; however, a technetium-99m radionuclide scan provides a better assessment of splenic function.

The asplenic patient who survives infancy encounters higher mortality rates (in addition to the risk associated with congenital heart disease) because of serious bacterial infection. Measures to mitigate infectious complications include routine vaccination against H influenzae type b, pneumococcus, and meningococcus. Antibiotic prophylaxis against these and other bacteria is equally important, although there is no consensus on the duration of prophylaxis. Many cardiologists and infectious disease experts recommend oral amoxicillin 125 mg BID for children younger than 2 years, and oral penicillin 250 mg BID thereafter. Erythromycin is a suitable alternative for those who are allergic to penicillin. Finally, when dental procedures or other indications for endocarditis prophylaxis occur in a patient already taking prophylactic antibiotics for asplenia, temporary substitution of a different class antibiotic will minimize the risk of endocarditis secondary to penicillin-resistant oral streptococci. Even with these measures, asplenic patients can present with fulminant sepsis after a trivial appearing clinical prodrome.

Upper gastrointestinal radiographic series should be conducted to diagnose intestinal malrotation, which places affected patients at risk for midgut volvulus. If malrotation is present, pediatric surgical consultation is recommended to help identify patients who are candidates for an elective Ladd's procedure.[7] Other gastrointestinal problems in heterotaxia include biliary atresia, duodenal web or membrane presenting with intestinal obstruction, and pancreatic hypoplasia or agenesis.

Less common heterotaxia associations include central nervous system malformation (e.g., holoprosencephaly) and renal (e.g., multicystic kidney) and adrenal anomalies.

SUMMARY

Cardiac malposition encompasses a broad spectrum of clinical presentation from simply a radiographic curiosity to severe and complex congenital heart disease with poor survival rates. When confronted with apparent cardiac malposition on the basis of exam or chest radiograph, primary care providers should enlist the aid of a pediatric cardiologist consultant to systematically evaluate potential congenital heart disease. Patients with cardiac malposition, most importantly those with heterotaxia, often have noncardiac malformations in addition to heart disease, emphasizing the need for a multidisciplinary approach to evaluation and management.

References

1   Oh SP, Li E: The signaling pathway mediated by the type IIB activin receptor controls axial patterning and lateral asymmetry in the mouse. *Genes Dev* 11(14):1812–1826, 1997.

2   Huddleston CB, Exil V, Canter CE, Mendeloff EN: Scimitar syndrome presenting in infancy. *Ann Thorac Surg* 67(1):154–159, 1999.

3   Kartagener M. Zur Pathogenese der Bronchiektasian: Bronchiektasian bei Situs Viscerum Inversus. *Beitr Klin Tuberk Spezif Tuberkuloseforsch* 83:489, 1933.

4   Stamm C, Friehs I, Duebener LF, Zurakowski D, Mayer JE Jr, Jonas RA, del Nido PJ: Improving results of the modified Fontan operation in patients with heterotaxy syndrome. *Ann Thorac Surg* 74(6):1967–1977, 2002.

5   Gaynor JW, Collins MH, Rychik J, Gaughan JP, Spray TL: Long-term outcome of infants with single ventricle and total anomalous pulmonary venous connection. *J Thorac Cardiovasc Surg* 117(3):506–513, 1999.

6   Larsen RL, Eguchi JH, Mulla NF, Johnston JK, Fitts J, Kuhn MA, Razzouk AJ, Chinnock RE, Bailey LL: Usefulness of cardiac transplantation in children with visceral heterotaxy (asplenic and polysplenic syndromes and single right-sided spleen with levocardia) and comparison of results with cardiac transplantation in children with dilated cardiomyopathy. *Am J Cardiol* 89(11):1275–1279, 2002.

7   Lessin MS, Luks FI: Laparoscopic appendectomy and duodenocolonic dissociation (LADD) procedure for malrotation. *Pediatr Surg Int* 13(23):184–185, 1998.

20

TRICUSPID ATRESIA

Brojendra Agarwala

ANATOMY AND PATHOPHYSIOLOGY

In tricuspid atresia (TA), the tricuspid valve is absent without any direct communication between the right atrium (RA) and the right ventricle (RV) (Figure 20-1A). Therefore, the infant born with TA should have associated cardiac defects such as atrial septal defect (ASD) to decompress the right atrium and allow blood to flow from the RA to the left atrium (LA) to maintain adequate cardiac output. A patent ductus arteriosus (PDA) is usually necessary to provide pulmonary blood flow (PBF) for blood oxygenation. A frequently associated lesion is a ventricular septal defect (VSD) (Figure 20-2). The presence of a VSD and its size also determine the amount of PBF, possibly making the PDA unnecessary as the only source of PBF. In patients with a PDA with or without a VSD, or with a VSD alone, pulmonary blood flow will also be influenced by pulmonary vascular resistance (PVR) and will probably be decreased in the neonate with high PVR despite the size of the PDA or VSD. In an infant with TA without a VSD, the RV is atretic and therefore the pulmonic valve is also atretic. In infants with TA and a VSD, the RV size varies and the PV may be either normal or stenotic.

In 70% of patients, TA is associated with normally related great arteries (NGA). In 30% of patients, there is transposition of the great arteries (TGA) meaning the ascending aorta arises from the right ventricle and the pulmonary artery from the left ventricle (LV) (Figures 20-1B and 20-3). In both groups (NGA and TGA), the size of the VSD plays a major role in clinical presentation and management in the future. In TA with NGA, the larger the VSD, the more the PBF, and the less cyanotic the infant will be. With TA and TGA, a small VSD may result in decreased systemic blood flow (SBF). The latter may also occur with TA, TGA, and a large VSD as the PVR decreases. The latter is also known as "systemic steal."

HISTORY AND PHYSICAL EXAMINATION

The clinical presentation varies with the combination of VSD size, status of the pulmonary valve (presence or absence of stenosis) or right ventricular outflow tract, the origin of the great arteries, and the PVR. For the purpose of discussion they can be grouped as follows:

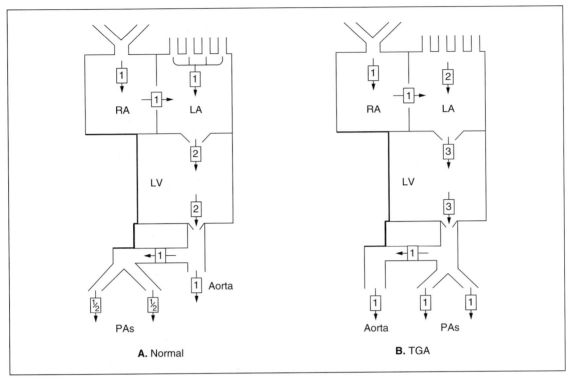

A. Normal

B. TGA

FIGURE 20-1

TRICUSPID ATRESIA WITH NO VSD

Group 1: Normally Related Great Arteries and no VSD (Figure 20-1A)

Infants in this group usually present with severe cyanosis, with the degree of cyanosis varying with the size of the PDA and PVR. A PDA murmur may or may not be audible. The second heart sound is single. Closure of the PDA will lead to severe cyanosis and shock.

Group 2: Normally Related Great Arteries and Small VSD, or a Large VSD with PS (Figure 20-2A)

Cyanosis and a heart murmur from the PS are the usual presentation in the newborn nursery. The VSD murmur is not usually noted (as is typical of small VSDs), as there is usually significant pulmonary stenosis and the murmur from blood flow across the pulmonary valve is much louder than the left-to-right shunt across the VSD. The degree of cyanosis may be less marked than in group 1, and oxygen saturation may be in the high 80s depending on the size of the defect, the degree of pulmonary stenosis, and pulmonary vascular resistance. Initial presentation in the neonate may be the same as in group 1 when the PVR is very high. Both a small VSD and increasing degrees of pulmonary stenosis will lead to decreased pulmonary blood flow and thus increased cyanosis. Over weeks to months, the VSD may become smaller and the PS may worsen, leading to progressive cyanosis over time. Unlike patients in group 1, closure of the PDA will not necessarily lead to severe cyanosis and shock unless the VSD is very small or the PS severe.

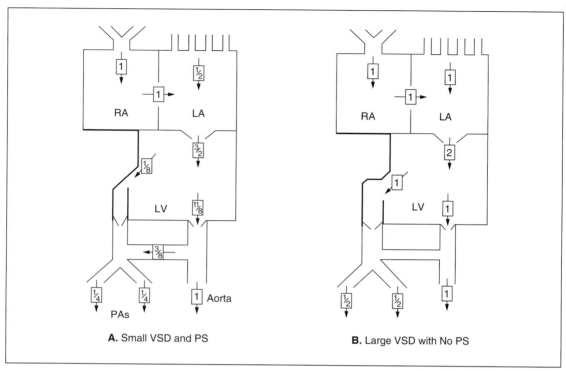

A. Small VSD and PS   **B.** Large VSD with No PS

FIGURE 20-2

TRICUSPID ATRESIA WITH A VSD

Group 3: Normally Related Great Arteries, Large VSD, and no PS (Figure 20-2B)

In the newborn nursery, cyanosis may not be clinically appreciated; however, the pulse oxymeter may show saturations of 90–94% and a heart murmur from flow across the VSD and the right ventricular outflow tract is heard. At 3–4 weeks of age, when the pulmonary vascular resistance decreases, the infant will present with signs and symptoms of congestive heart failure (CHF).

Group 4A: Infants with TGA, a Small VSD and/or Pulmonary Atresia (PA)/Stenosis (Figure 20-3A)

These infants will present with cyanosis and a systolic heart murmur from PS or the VSD. The

pulmonary blood flow and oxygen saturation are ductal dependent if there is significant pulmonary stenosis or atresia. In the absence of the latter, the *systemic blood flow* is ductal dependent. This is because the systemic blood flow is dependent on flow from the left ventricle through the VSD and to the aorta. If the VSD is small, blood will flow preferentially from the LV to the pulmonary artery rather than through the VSD to the aorta. Therefore, when the ductus closes the infant may develop shock.

Group 4B: TGA, Large VSD, and No PS (Figure 20-3B)

The usual presentation is CHF with mild cyanosis. The cyanosis may be clinically difficult to detect. As the PVR decreases, there may be steal from the systemic circulation into the pulmonary circulation,

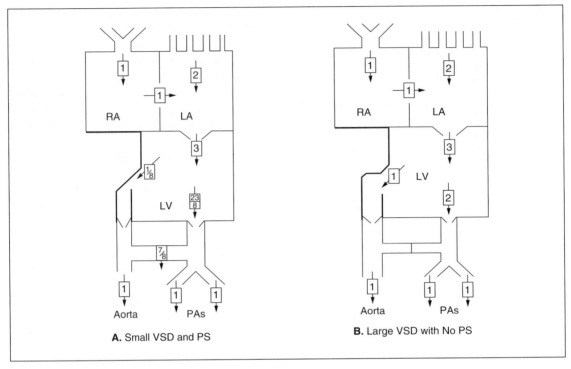

A. Small VSD and PS

B. Large VSD with No PS

FIGURE 20-3

TRICUSPID ATRESIA, TGA, AND A VSD

and signs and symptoms of low cardiac output and systemic perfusion may occur.

LABORATORY FINDINGS

Electrocardiogram

In **Group 1 Through 4A**

Left-axis deviation (QRS axis between 0 to −90°), lack of RV force and left ventricular dominant voltage (LVH) and right atrial hypertrophy are classical findings; however, with TGA, only 50% of the infants will have left-axis deviation.

Chest Radiograph

The heart size and shape are usually normal. The pulmonary vascularity may be diminished bilaterally.

In infants with a large VSD and no PS with or without TGA, the heart size may be enlarged with increased pulmonary vascularity.

2D Doppler Echocardiogram: The echocardiogram clearly defines the anatomy and the relative size of the ASD, VSD, and PDA and the direction of shunts.

Cardiac Catheterization

Cardiac catheterization is not needed to confirm the echocardiographic diagnosis. Balloon atrial septostomy may be required to enlarge a restrictive ASD or patent foramen ovale to provide an unrestricted RA to LA shunt; however, future cardiac catheterizations are usually needed following different types of palliative surgery that are discussed below.

MANAGEMENT

Medical

Groups with Diminished Pulmonary Blood Flow

Tricuspid atresia with or without VSD and pulmonary atresia/PS. A prostaglandin E1 infusion is given to keep the PDA open to maintain adequate oxygenation until a palliative procedure is performed.

Groups with Increased Pulmonary Blood Flow

Tricuspid atresia, NGA, or TGA with large VSD and no PS. This group of infants usually presents with pulmonary edema (CHF), which is medically managed with diuretics. Use of digoxin is controversial. These patients require clinical observation for cyanosis because the VSD may close spontaneously with time, resulting in diminished PBF (or systemic blood flow in the case of TGA).

Surgical

Because of the single ventricle physiology (LV), a univentricular repair is needed. Usually a Glenn anastomosis is performed at approximately 6 months of age followed by a Fontan type of surgery at 2 years of age (Chapter 49).

1. **With diminished pulmonary blood flow:** A Blalock-Taussig shunt is performed in the neonatal period followed by a Glenn shunt. The latter is an anastomosis of the superior vena cava to the right pulmonary artery, also known as a bidirectional cavo-pulmonary shunt. This is usually performed around 6 months of age, when the pulmonary vascular resistance is low. Following this surgery, the oxygen saturation is expected to be about 85% in room air.

2. **With increased pulmonary blood flow:** Very rarely, pulmonary artery banding is needed. This is performed in order to protect the pulmonary vasculature from developing irreversible elevated vascular resistance (i.e., pulmonary vascular disease) prohibiting future surgery (e.g., Glenn

and Fontan procedures, which require very low pulmonary vascular resistance). The pulmonary artery band decreases the pressure in the pulmonary arteries (a major determinant in the development of pulmonary vascular disease) by creating a pressure gradient and reducing blood flow. Frequently the VSD becomes smaller or closes spontaneously with time so PA banding is not always necessary.

3. **With diminished systemic blood flow:** Transposition of the great arteries and restrictive VSD, the main pulmonary artery is transected and the proximal end is anastomosed with the ascending aorta in order to maintain adequate systemic blood flow bypassing the restrictive (small) VSD. This surgery is known as the Damus-Kaye-Stansel procedure. In addition a Blalock-Taussig shunt to the transected distal end of the pulmonary artery is required to maintain pulmonary blood flow. Around 6 months of age, a Glenn procedure is performed.

Fontan Type of Surgery

This surgery is usually performed between 2 and 3 years of age. In this procedure the inferior vena cava and the hepatic venous blood are directed to the right pulmonary artery through a tunnel. There are various ways of doing this procedure.

1. A tunnel is created within the RA draining the inferior vena cava and hepatic venous blood to the right pulmonary artery (frequently termed the "lateral tunnel" operation). At the time of this surgery a small (3–4 mm) fenestration (a "pop off") is frequently created. This is to allow more rapid recovery and fewer complications in the immediate postoperative period by "popping off" and reducing systemic venous, and therefore, pulmonary arterial pressure. Forty percent of the time the fenestration closes spontaneously in a few months; if closure does not occur, a transcatheter device may be placed to close the fenestration.

2. An external conduit is created (frequently termed "extra cardiac conduit Fontan") to connect the inferior vena cava and the hepatic venous blood

outside the heart to the right pulmonary artery. This conduit can be made from autologous pericardial tissue, a homograft, or a Gore-Tex tube.

Important Physiologic and Anatomic Considerations Prior to Glenn and Fontan Procedure

1. The pulmonary vascular resistance and the pulmonary arterial pressure must be normal otherwise the systemic venous blood will not flow to the pulmonary artery.
2. Pulmonary artery anatomy must be normal, e.g., peripheral pulmonary artery stenosis should not be present, or if present they should be removed surgically or via angioplasty during catheterization.
3. Left ventricular function must be normal.
4. Mitral valve anatomy and function should be normal.

The above four parameters are evaluated with echocardiography and cardiac catheterization prior to each surgical procedure.

FREQUENTLY ASKED QUESTIONS FROM THE PARENTS

In the newborn nursery following the diagnosis, frequently asked questions during family discussions arise. The primary care physician should also be aware of these questions and answers as they may also arise during routine well child-care visits.

1. Is a Fontan surgery all that the child requires? The conservative answer is probably not. The Fontan anastomosis may need to be revised in the future because of various reasons, e.g., prolonged chylothorax, ascites, protein-losing enteropathy, and so forth. Very rarely the child may need heart transplant if severe LV dysfunction develops in the future.
2. After Fontan surgery will the child be normal and be able to play competitive football, basketball, or other sports? The conservative answer is most likely no. Functional capacity is usually not as good as in a healthy child. Thus, the child

who has had a Fontan procedure may not be able to compete normally. Recreational physical activities, however, are encouraged. Parents are encouraged to motivate the child toward arts, music, and theater, in which physical competition and possible failure will not be a problem.

3. What are the long-term problems? Following Fontan surgery the complications or problems are as follows:
   a. Chylous pleural effusion. The incidence is relatively low following fenestration of the conduit or tunnel. It usually occurs a day or two after operation and is most likely due to injury of the thoracic duct or lymphatic channels during the operation, though may also be aggravated by elevations in central venous (the same as pulmonary artery pressure) from elevated pulmonary vascular resistance. A chest tube may need to be placed to drain the fluid and a period of (4–6 weeks) fat-free diet is required.
   b. Ascites may be a long-term problem requiring a meticulous medical therapy and possible revision of the Fontan surgery. This is also a result of elevations in central venous pressure.
   c. Protein-losing enteropathy. More likely in child with elevated systemic venous pressure in the inferior vena cava, thereby increasing hepatic and intestinal congestion and malabsorption and decreasing hepatic production of albumin.
   d. Atrial tachyarrhythmias such as ectopic atrial tachycardia, atrial flutter, and atrial fibrillation may require revision of the Fontan surgery as well as a Maize procedure at the same time. These arrhythmias are a result of the combination of scarring created by surgery in the atria and altered hemodynamics.
   e. Left ventricular dysfunction.
   f. Sudden death.
   g. Arteriovenous fistula, e.g., pulmonary AV fistula, systemic veno-venous fistula. The former are felt to be a result of the lack of a "hepatic factor" delivered to the lungs when the hepatic venous drainage does not go to the lungs (as seen after a Glenn anastomosis

or if the Fontan anastomosis does not incorporate the hepatic veins in the conduit or tunnel to the lungs). The latter is seen in cases with altered hemodynamics, namely, elevated central venous pressure.

In this era of insurance referrals from primary physicians, and for the general knowledge of the primary care physician and families, it is important to understand the nature and reason for long-term follow-up. The following can be expected:

LABORATORY TESTING

1. Multiple (serial) echocardiograms (both transthoracic and transesophageal) for objective evaluation of the anatomy and function.
2. Serial Holter monitor or event recordings to help screen for and diagnose different types of arrhythmias.
3. Serial exercise stress testing to assess functional capability.
4. Cardiac catheterization for further evaluation of cardiac anatomy, function, and pressures. This is usually performed when abnormalities or suspicion of these arises from the history, physical examination, or noninvasive testing.

LONG-TERM MEDICATIONS

Most children with tricuspid atresia who have had Fontan surgery will be on medications indefinitely. To support the left ventricle and maintain adequate function, the following medications may be needed for life:

1. Diuretics (furosemide or others). These are used in cases of pulmonary or systemic venous congestion if mechanical means are unsuccessful to reduce the pressure (e.g., obstruction). Examples where these would be used include AV valve regurgitation and ventricular dysfunction.
2. After load-reducing agents such as angiotersin-converting enzyme (ACE) inhibitors. These are used to reduce the wall stress of the ventricle and improve function. Their use in dilated cardiomyopathies has been shown to be beneficial. The data regarding their use in single ventricular physiology (Fontan patients) is unclear. ACE inhibitors are teratogenic, and this ought to be discussed by the primary care physician during discussions of adolescent sexuality.
3. Inotropic agents (Digoxin). These are used to improved ventricular function. Data showing a clear benefit from long-term use is not clear.
4. Anticoagulant or antithrombotic agents (aspirin or coumadin). Because of the single ventricle physiology and sluggish (passive) blood flow to the lungs, patients who have had Fontan surgery are known to develop thrombi and emboli to various organs (strokes if a fenestration is present with a right-to-left shunt). Although the data are unclear as to whether, or what type, of medication to use, most Fontan patients receive aspirin, coumadin, or another type of medication to prevent thrombi. An adolescent female taking coumadin needs to be aware of the teratogenicity of this drug and this ought to be discussed during discussions of adolescent sexuality.
5. Bacterial endocarditis (SBE) prophylaxis. Required for appropriate dental, GI and GU procedures for life.

LONG-TERM QUALITY OF LIFE

With intensive care, dedication of the parents, and technical advances, infants with this heart defect are living to adulthood with the opportunity of education becoming self-supporting. This ought to be known by the primary care physician who then may also be able to offer hope and guidance to families during child-care visits.

Suggested Readings

Allen HD, Gutgesell HP, Clark EB, Driscoll DJ: *Moss and Adams' Heart Disease in Infants, Children, and Adolescents Including the Fetus and Young Adult*, 6th ed. Philadelphia, PA, Lippincott Williams & Wilkins, 2001.

Garson A, Bricker JT, Fisher DJ, Neish SR: *The Science and Practice of Pediatric Cardiology*, 2nd ed. Baltimore, MD, Williams & Wilkins, 1998.

21

TETRALOGY OF FALLOT

Ra-id Abdulla

INTRODUCTION

Tetralogy of Fallot (TOF) is the result of anterior deviation of the ventricular outflow septum toward the right ventricular outflow tract (RVOT) resulting in narrowing (stenosis) of the pulmonary valve and the RVOT. This deviation of the ventricular outflow septum will result in a ventricular septal defect (VSD) referred to as malalignment type VSD. The deviation of the ventricular outflow septum with the resulting VSD underneath it exposes the aorta to the right ventricle, giving the appearance of the aortic valve straddling or "overriding" the VSD. There is right ventricular hypertension, which results in right ventricular hypertrophy. The four components of the "tetralogy" are: (1) ventricular septal defect; (2) pulmonary stenosis; (3) overriding aorta; (4) right ventricular hypertrophy.

INCIDENCE

This occurs in about 0.19–0.26/1000 live births. It constitutes 8% of all congenital heart diseases. It is the most common cyanotic congenital heart disease beyond 1 week of age.

EMBRYOLOGY

The single embryologic ventricle divides into two at about 40 days of gestation. At the same time of ventricular septation, the outflow tract, also known as the bulbus cordis, is divided by the in-growth of endocardial tissue. This results in an anterior right ventricular outflow tract and a posterior left ventricular outflow tract. Abnormal development of the outflow tract septation process, such as anterior displacement of the conal septum, will cause the RVOT and pulmonary valves to become small. Furthermore, the abnormally developing outflow tract will become interiorly malaligned, resulting in failure to fuse with the remainder of the developing ventricular septum. This will cause a ventricular septal defect.

ANATOMY

The ventricular septal defect is located in the membranous region of the ventricular septum. It is subaortic and sometimes extends to the subpulmonic valve area. The VSD is large causing equalization of left ventricular (LV) and right ventricular

(RV) pressures. These defects do not usually get smaller and are not known to close spontaneously. The right ventricular outflow tract is hypoplastic and almost always obstructive. Occasionally at birth, the RVOT shows no significant obstruction and results in the so-called pink tetralogy of Fallot. Mild hypertrophy of the moderator band and ventricular septal defect should be distinguished from tetralogy of Fallot, as the prognosis is different. The pulmonary valve annulus is typically small and the leaflets deformed in tetralogy of Fallot. The main pulmonary arteries (MPA) are small, in contrast to pulmonary stenosis with an intact ventricular septum, in which they are normal in size or enlarged because of poststenotic dilation. Branch pulmonary artery stenosis may also be present. Bronchial arterial collaterals are sometimes present, which connect to the peripheral pulmonary arteries. The main pulmonary artery is occasionally atretic, and the pulmonary arteries are fed either by a patent ductus arteriosus or collateral vessels. This is sometimes referred to as tetralogy of Fallot with pulmonary atresia, or pulmonary atresia with a VSD. The aortic valve is typically large.

PATHOPHYSIOLOGY

The underlying physiology is depicted in Figure 21-1. Significant stenosis of the RVOT and pulmonary valve will cause portions of the blood ejected from the right ventricle to shunt across the VSD into the aorta. The greater the stenosis, the more right ventricular blood will shunt into the aorta. Since right ventricular blood is deoxygenated, this will result in cyanosis. Cyanosis increases in severity as the RVOT and pulmonary valve stenosis worsens. Unlike most other congenital heart diseases, the pulmonary blood flow will be reduced. Therefore, pulmonary overcirculation (congestive heart failure) does not typically occur.

Turbulence will occur across the area of narrowing and will be proportional to the amount of blood crossing the area and indirectly proportional to the diameter of the right ventricular outflow. This is consistent with the pathophysiology of murmurs as discussed in Chapter 2. Thus, a murmur of pulmonary stenosis will exist. Unlike the murmur of pulmonary stenosis, the worse the RVOT obstruction in tetralogy Fallot, the softer the murmur (as blood is shunted across the VSD instead).

CLINICAL FINDINGS

The right ventricular outflow tract obstruction may be minimal in the early neonatal period, leading to significant left-to-right shunting at the VSD with symptoms and signs of congestive heart failure; however, this tends to be transient, if it occurs at all. As the right ventricular outflow tract becomes progressively more obstructive, the resistance of blood flow into the pulmonary circulation exceeds the systemic vascular resistance, resulting in right-to-left shunting. Cyanosis, caused by right-to-left shunting, induces an increase in hemoglobin concentration because of increased erythropoietin production.

Cyanosis may be minimal in some patients with tetralogy of Fallot despite severe pulmonary stenosis. This is seen in patients with large or multiple collaterals from the systemic arterial circulation to the pulmonary arterial circulation causing increased pulmonary blood flow. This counters the decreased pulmonary blood flow from the right ventricular outflow tract obstruction. If there are few collaterals, the cyanosis will not be improved. If there are many large collaterals (with low pulmonary vascular resistance), the cyanosis will be less marked.

Patients with tetralogy of Fallot are typically mildly cyanotic with no other symptoms. Hypercyanotic spells (as described below) do not typically occur in early infancy. Increasing cyanosis occurs with age, associated with clubbing of the digits. Grunting and crying cause a transient increase in cyanosis.

On examination, patients are mildly to moderately cyanotic. The capillary refill is brisk. There is no hepatomegaly. The precordium is typically hyperactive with an increased right ventricular impulse (at the left lower sternal border) because of right ventricular hypertrophy. A palpable thrill in

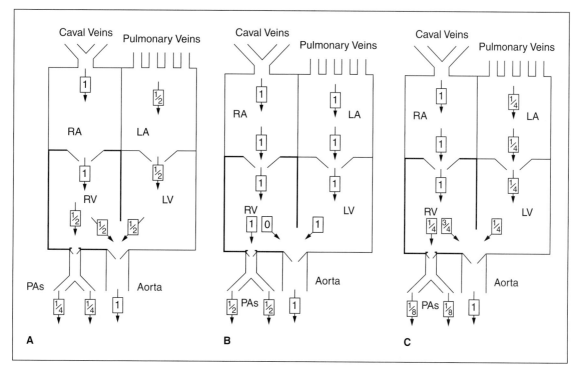

FIGURE 21-1

PATHOPHYSIOLOGY OF TETRALOGY OF FALLOT

A. The flow to the lungs via the pulmonary arteries is one-half of the systemic cardiac output to the body. The pressure in the RV equals the LV since the VSD is large and nonrestrictive. Thus, there is no pathologic flow murmur heard from flow across the VSD. The gradient from the RV to the PAs depends in part on the pulmonary vascular resistance. If the pulmonary vascular resistance (PVR), thus pulmonary pressure is elevated (pressure = flow multiplied by resistance), there will be no significant gradient across the pulmonary valve. As the PVR falls, the pressure gradient will increase if there is any significant pulmonary or subpulmonary valve stenosis. There will then be a murmur across this area of obstruction. If there is minimal obstruction, then the systolic pressures in the RV will be similar to the PAs and no gradient or signifi-cant murmur will be noted. The other extreme is severe or critical pulmonary/subpulmonary stenosis. In this case, there will be minimal flow across the pulmonary valve and the murmur of pulmonary stenosis will be absent, however, if there were narrowing to this degree, the systemic venous return would shunt mainly right to left at the ventricular level and cyanosis would be apparent. The net saturation in example A is proportional to the amount of pulmonary blood flow (1/2 relative cardiac output in this case) mixed in the left ventricle with the amount of systemic venous return which crosses the VSD into the left ventricle (1/2 relative cardiac output in this case).

Diagram B depicts tetralogy of Fallot with a balanced circulation (pulmonary blood flow = systemic blood flow). It Is balanced because the degree of RVOT obstruction is equal to the obstruction to systemic outflow because of systemic vascular resistance. This example shows a scenario in which the obstruction or the pulmonary vascular resistance is less than in A. If the anatomic obstruction remains the same, then A reflects the physiology in the neonate, and B after a few days to weeks of age when PVR falls.

Diagram C demonstrates the physiology of very high PVR or severe RVOT obstruction which may occur after months or years. A noted, pulmonary blood flow is one-fourth of the systemic blood flow. The net saturation in this case is a mix-ture of one-fourth relative cardiac outputs of highly saturated pulmonary venous return, mixing with three-fourth relative cardiac outputs of desaturated systemic venous return which is shunted from the RV to the LV across the VSD. Thus, the RVOT narrowing has caused a decrease in pulmonary blood flow and more desaturation than in A and B. The decreased flow across the RVOT causes a shortening of the systolic murmur.

the region of the RVOT may be present because of the turbulence in this area. On auscultation, the second heart sound may appear to be single with a harsh 3-4/6 (or louder) systolic ejection murmur noted at the left to left upper sternal border. Typically there is no diastolic murmur. Patients with associated systemic to pulmonary arterial collaterals have continuous murmurs.

Hypercyanosis, or "tetralogy spells," are transient episodes of severely increased cyanosis in patients with tetralogy of Fallot. There are a number of theories of their cause. In one theory, it is felt that these episodes are caused by a transient increase in RVOT stenosis resulting in increased right-to-left shunting at the VSD and significant reduction of pulmonary blood flow. It is felt that the RVOT obstruction is worsened with increasing acidosis. Thus, if there is increasing cyanosis leading to acidosis, then the RVOT obstruction will worsen, again leading to increased cyanosis in a vicious cycle. In another theory (perhaps better supported by data), it is felt that the cause of hypercyanosis is an increased systemic venous return (as would be noted with crying or increased ventilation, the latter occurring with acidosis). The increased systemic venous return encounters a fixed obstruction in the RVOT and thus shunts right to left. This causes increased cyanosis leading to acidosis and increased ventilation. Therefore, a vicious cycle occurs with this theory of hypercyanosis as well. Spells of hypercyanosis are uncommon in the first six months of life. They are most common in infants and toddlers. They again become rare in children after 4 years of age.

Patients with tetralogy of Fallot, particularly older children, tend to squat. Squatting helps to relieve cyanosis, as it increases pulmonary blood flow by increasing systemic vascular resistance and therefore systolic pressures in the LV and RV.

LABORATORY FINDINGS

Electrocardiography

The typical ECG shows right ventricular hypertrophy with right-axis deviation. Severe axis deviation is seen in patients with tetralogy of Fallot and AV canal defect. Right ventricular hypertrophy and left ventricular hypertrophy are seen in acyanotic infants with left-to-right shunting causing congestive heart failure.

Chest Radiography

In tetralogy of Fallot, a boot-shaped (Coeur en sabot) heart is the classically described finding on the chest radiograph. This is caused by the small main pulmonary artery, which results in a narrow mediastinum. The boot shape is also achieved by uplifting of the cardiac apex because of right ventricular hypertrophy.

Echocardiography

Echocardiography details the cardiac defect including the VSD, right ventricle, ventricular outflow tract (obstruction), and pulmonary stenosis. The peripheral branch pulmonary arteries are not well appreciated by echocardiography. Flow across patent ductus arteriosus and collaterals may be detected by echocardiography; however, the extent and origin of collaterals may not be fully appreciated. The side of the aortic arch and coronary artery origins are usually well seen with echocardiography as well.

CARDIAC CATHETERIZATION

In typical cases of tetralogy of Fallot there is no need for cardiac catheterization. Details of pulmonary arteries and collaterals require cardiac catheterization.

Management

Medical Management

Cyanotic spells: These typically occur when babies or toddlers are upset, leading to an increase in circulating catecholamines, which result in increased right ventricular outflow tract obstruction and right-to-left shunting at the ventricular septal defect level. Alternatively, the crying results in increased systemic venous return, which results in right-to-left shunting, and an increase in cyanosis. A simple intervention is to ask a parent to hold and comfort the child, which may terminate the hypercyanotic episode. When holding the child it is best to place him/her in the knee-chest position to increase the systemic vascular resistance. If this fails, then one or more of the following measures can be attempted:

1. Morphine: subcutaneously or intravenously to relax the RVOT and calm the child.
2. Beta-blockers such as an esmolol drip or intravenous inderal; negative inotropic agents which cause the RVOT to relax.
3. Vasoconstrictors such as a epinephrine or phenylephrine hydrochloride which will cause vasoconstriction and elevation of the systemic vascular resistance with less right-to-left shunting.
4. A fluid intravenous fluid bolus which will increase systemic venous return (leading to increased cyanosis) and increase systemic pressure (leading to decreased cyanosis). Usually, a fluid bolus will help increase pulmonary blood flow.

Surgical Management

Surgical repair of tetralogy of Fallot is performed at 6–12 months of age.

Standard cardiopulmonary bypass techniques with moderate hypothermia are usually employed. Intraoperative TEE is usually performed to assess the anatomy and adequacy of the repair. Using cardioplegic cardiac arrest, the MPA or the RVOT are opened. The pulmonary valve is inspected and sized. Based on the diameter of the pulmonary annulus and its anatomy, a decision is made whether to preserve the annulus or perform a transannular patch. The VSD is exposed either through the MPA, the infundibular incision, or a right atrial incision. The VSD is usually patched with a synthetic patch such as Dacron. The MPA or RVOT incisions are patched, usually using autologous pericardium. Any atrial communication, unless it is large, is left patent to provide a pop-off mechanism for postoperative right ventricular dysfunction. Inotropic support

(dopamine 3–10 μg/kg/h) is usually required perioperatively. Once the VSD is adequately closed, the postoperative course depends on the degree of RV dysfunction (usually temporary; 24–48 h) and the status of the RVOT with respect to pulmonary regurgitation (usually very well tolerated) or residual pulmonary stenosis (usually less well tolerated). Tetralogy of Fallot surgery has a wide range of individual variability. Some surgeons are reluctant to make any incisions into the RVOT, preferring to always close the VSD and resect muscle via the right atrium. Other surgeons prefer to make a large incision in the RVOT (with resection of any obstruction), close the VSD through this infundibular incision, and then close this incision with a large transannular patch (thus leaving a widely patent RVOT). Associated pulmonary artery narrowing is addressed during the same operation. Mortality for standard TOF surgery is very low (<5%). Potential complications that are specific to TOF surgery include RV dysfunction (usually limited), AV block (<5%), junctional ectopic tachycardia (JET) (<5%), patch dehiscence, and residual RVOT obstruction. It is increasingly common to require pulmonary valve replacement in older patients with residual pulmonary regurgitation.

Tetralogy of Fallot with pulmonary atresia has a wide range of variability with respect to the size of the pulmonary vasculature. TOF/PA with short-segment atresia and mild branch PA hypoplasia can be repaired (VSD closure and RV-PA conduit placement) during the neonatal age with good results. Some surgeons prefer to delay the repair and place an initial BT shunt. TOF/PA with major aortopulmonary collateral arteries (MAPCAs) is often approached by unifocalization of the MAPCAs (combining them as one), either through a midline sternotomy approach or by sequential thoracotomies. The unifocalized PAs are then connected to native branch PAs and then anastomosed to an RV-PA conduit. The VSD can be closed if the pulmonary vasculature is adequate (low enough resistance such that the RV can support an entire cardiac output). If this is not the case, the VSD closure may be required during another procedure. Difficulty in surgical repair of this lesion is due to multiple and repeated stenoses of the intra and extra-parenchymal pulmonary arteries.

Suggested Readings

Allen HD, Gutgesell HP, Clark EB, Driscoll DJ: *Moss and Adams' Heart Disease in Infants, Children, and Adolescents Including the Fetus and Young Adult*, 6th ed. Philadelphia, PA, Lippincott Williams & Wilkins, 2001.

Bacha EA, Scheule AM, Zurakowski D, Erickson LC, Hung J, Lang P, del Nido PJ, Mayer JE Jr, Jonas RA: Long-term results after early primary repair of tetralogy of Fallot. *J Thorac Cardiovasc Surg* 122:154–161, 2001.

Garson A, Bricker JT, Fisher DJ, Neish SR: *The Science and Practice of Pediatric Cardiology*, 2nd ed. Baltimore, MD, Williams & Wilkins, 1998.

Guntheroth WG, Mortan BC, Mullins GL, Baum D: Venous return with knee-chest position and squatting in tetralogy of Fallot. *Am Heart J* 75(3):313–318, 1968.

Morgan BC, Dillard DH, Guntheroth WG: Effect of cardiac and respiratory cycle on pulmonary vein flow, pressure, and diameter. *J Appl Physiol* 21(4): 1276–1280, 1966.

Reddy VM, McElhinney DB, Amin Z, Moore P, Parry AJ, Teitel DF, Hanley FL: Early and intermediate outcomes after repair of pulmonary atresia with ventricular septal defect and major aortopulmonary collateral arteries. *Circulation* 101:1826–1832, 2000.

22

PULMONARY ATRESIA, INTACT VENTRICULAR SEPTUM

Ra-id Abdulla

INTRODUCTION

Pulmonary atresia is lack of communication between the right ventricle (RV) and the pulmonary artery because of abnormal development of the pulmonary valve. This may be as simple as fusion of the pulmonary valve cusps, forming a membrane between the right ventricular outflow tract and the main pulmonary artery, with reasonably well developed main and branch pulmonary arteries. The other extreme of pulmonary atresia is when the pulmonary valve and entire main pulmonary artery are atretic with small branch pulmonary arteries.

INCIDENCE

This is the tenth most common congenital heart disease among neonates. It is the 23rd most common congenital heart disease. It occurs in 0.07/1000 live births.

EMBRYOLOGY

The following facts support that this is most probably an acquired disease in utero rather than an aberration of development:

- Well-formed pulmonary valve leaflets in some instances
- Near-normal size of the pulmonary arteries
- Variable RV size
- Rarity of associated lesions

ANATOMY

The pulmonary valve annulus is usually small but not hypoplastic. The pulmonary valve leaflets are well formed but fused. The main pulmonary artery is small but rarely is atretic as seen with pulmonary atresia and ventricular septal defect (sometimes referred to as tetralogy of Fallot with pulmonary atresia). The patent ductus arteriosus is usually

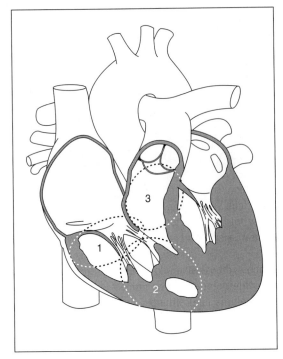

F I G U R E   2 2 - 1

THE COMPONENTS OF A TRIPARTITE RIGHT VENTRICLE

The inflow portion (area number 1) is the area which contains the tricuspid valve apparatus. The trabecular portion (area number 2) contains the portion of the right ventricle between the inflow and the outflow tract. The outflow tract (area number 3) is separated from the trabecular portion of the right ventricle by a semicircular arch composed of 4 muscle bands (parietal band, infundibular septum, septal band, and moderator band).

small because it carries blood from the aorta to the pulmonary arteries in utero and not from the pulmonary arteries to the aorta, as is normal in fetal cardiovascular circulation. The right ventricle, which can be described in terms of three (tripartite) components (Figure 22-1) may be of several types:

- Type I is tripartite (an inflow, trabecular and outflow portions)
- Type II bipartite (atretic body or trabecular portion).
- Type III unipartite (atretic body or trabecular portion and atretic infundibulum or outflow portion).

- The tricuspid valve might be deformed and stenotic in any of these, though this is more likely in types II and III.

Sinusoids (primitive embryologic connections) from the right ventricular cavity to the myocardium and from the myocardium to the coronary arteries may be present.

PATHOPHYSIOLOGY

In pulmonary atresia, desaturated (blue) blood returning to the right atrium encounters resistance of flow into the right ventricle as the right ventricle is typically hypertrophied (noncompliant), and may be small. In addition, there may be associated tricuspid stenosis or severe tricuspid regurgitation. In either condition, blood in the right atrium travels the path of least resistance and will cross an atrial communication (patent foramen ovale [PFO] or atrial septal defect [ASD]) into the left atrium. This will cause cyanosis as desaturated blood coming from the right atrium will "contaminate" or mix with the well-oxygenated blood from the left atrium. As blood cannot get to the pulmonary circulation through the pulmonary valve, it will reach the pulmonary circulation through a patent ductus arteriosus (PDA) instead. Life cannot be maintained without these two communications (PFO or ASD, and PDA). The ductus arteriosus allows blood to flow to the lungs, thus oxygenation, and the PFO allows blood to return from the body. In the absence of the former, there will be no oxygenation. In the absence of the latter, there will be cessation of blood flow (shock). If the PFO is restrictive, right atrial pressure will be elevated and this pressure will be transmitted to other organ systems (hepatic congestion, peripheral edema). Figure 22-2 demonstrates the underlying physiology.

With increasing tricuspid regurgitation, the right ventricle and atrial sizes will become larger with a physiology similar to Ebstein anomaly (see Chapter 23).

The pathophysiology of sinusoids is an important consideration. In utero and at birth these RV to

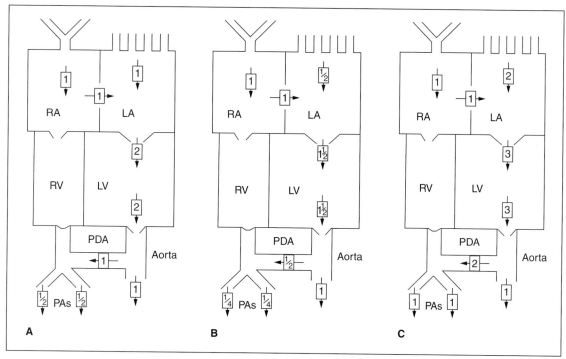

FIGURE 22-2

PATHOPHYSIOLOGY OF PULMONARY ATRESIA

In this diagram, 1 cardiac output goes to the body and returns to the right atrium. This entire cardiac output crosses the atrial septum via a PFO or ASD and mixes with blood returning from the lungs via the pulmonary veins. Therefore, the left atrium contains 2 cardiac outputs (thus LA enlargement), which cross the mitral valve (increased flow across the mitral valve), and enters the left ventricle, which also contains 2 cardiac outputs (thus LV enlargement). The equivalent of 2 cardiac outputs cross the aortic valve and enter the aorta. This flow then divides into the PDA and distal aorta (equally in this example) so that 1 cardiac output flows to the lungs, and one to the body. The net oxygen saturation is determined by the ratio of pulmonary venous return mixing with systemic venous return.

Elevated pulmonary vascular resistance (PVR) or a very small PDA, (**B**) will result in less pulmonary venous return and the saturations will be lower (the ratio of pulmonary venous return to systemic venous return is $1/2$ to 1). Low PVR with a large PDA, (**C**) will result in increased pulmonary venous return and higher net saturations (the ratio of pulmonary venous return to systemic venous return is now 2 to 1).

coronary sinusoids do not pose a problem as the RV cavity pressure is excessively high and blood from within the RV travels across the sinusoids into the right coronary arterial circulation. This will cause reduced blood flow across the right coronary artery ostium, which may result in stenosis of this orifice. If the RV pressure is reduced, blood flow will reverse from the right coronary artery to the RV cavity through the sinusoids, causing steal of blood from the coronary circulation and possible myocardial ischemia. Thus, if the obstruction (pulmonary

atresia) is relieved, the right ventricular pressure will be lowered and blood will flow from the coronary arteries to the right ventricle (rather than to the myocardium) if the RV systolic pressure is less than systemic.

CLINICAL MANIFESTATIONS

At birth the ductus arteriosus provides pulmonary blood flow and there may or may not be cyanosis evident in the immediate neonatal period. As the ductus arteriosus closes, there will be less pulmonary blood flow, causing cyanosis.

On examination, the patient will appear to be cyanotic; however, if the PDA is large and the PVR low, the patient may be minimally cyanotic or not at all (oxygen saturation above 85%). In the latter case, patients will be noticeably short of breath because of pulmonary edema secondary to increased pulmonary blood flow. Peripheral pulses and perfusion are typically normal. There usually is no associated hepatomegaly, unless the atrial communication is restrictive. The RV impulse will be reduced with a normal or increased LV impulse. A thrill is not usually present. A continuous murmur from a PDA may be heard throughout systole and most of diastole. This is heard best in the left subclavicular region. The second heart sound is single. Patients with severe tricuspid regurgitation will have a holosystolic murmur heard best at the left lower sternal border.

Electrocardiography

The ECG typically shows a leftward axis. Seventy-seven percent of patients will have a QRS axis of 0–90°. This is a result of absence of right ventricular predominance, as is normally seen. Right-axis deviation is seen in patients with pulmonary atresia, with severe TR causing the RV to be dilated. In tricuspid atresia, 16% of patients have a QRS axis less than 0°, while with pulmonary atresia and a ventricular septal defect, 70% will have a QRS axis of more than 90°.

Chest Radiography

The chest radiograph shows a small cardiac silhouette; however, in the presence of severe tricuspid regurgitation there will be severe cardiomegaly, which may lead to poor lung development as in patients with diaphragmatic hernias.

Echocardiography

Echocardiography shows that pulmonary blood flow is supplied through the patent ductus arteriosus. The pulmonary valve leaflets are fused and there is variable hypoplasia of the right ventricle. The main pulmonary artery tends to be well developed and the PDA is usually tortuous and siphon shaped. The diameter of the tricuspid regurgitation jet obtained by color Doppler and the size of the right atrium are good indicators of the severity of tricuspid regurgitation.

Cardiac Catheterization

A Rashkind atrial septostomy may be required to allow right-to-left shunting across the atrial septum. Cardiac catheterization is indicated in all cases to assess pulmonary arterial anatomy as well as coronary arterial to RV fistula or sinusoids.

TREATMENT

Prostaglandin infusion is started to keep the ductus arteriosus open to provide pulmonary blood flow. A surgical pulmonary valvotomy (or valvuloplasty via interventional cardiac catheterization) is required. A systemic to pulmonary arterial shunt may also be required depending on the RV size and anterograde blood flow across the pulmonary valve. If the RV is small, a systemic to pulmonary arterial shunt will be necessary to provide pulmonary blood flow until antegrade flow through the pulmonary valve is adequate; however, if the pulmonary arteries are not too small, with a good-sized right ventricle, then pulmonary valvotomy alone may be adequate.

Decompression of the right ventricle by pulmonary valvotomy may cause reversal of flow in the coronary artery to right ventricular sinusoids, thus blood may then flow from the coronary artery to RV cavity (via coronary sinusoids) instead of the myocardium, leading to poor myocardial perfusion. This is especially true with coronary artery ostial stenosis, which may be present with this congenital heart disease. Therefore, right ventricular decompression should not be performed in the presence of significant coronary sinusoids, especially if coronary artery ostial stenosis is noted.

In patients with small pulmonary arteries, pulmonary valve intervention with placement of a systemic to pulmonary arterial shunt may be an initial procedure. If the RV continues to be small (inadequate) then a Glenn procedure (superior vena cava to right pulmonary artery shunt) may be performed at a later time to divert some of the systemic venous blood return directly into the pulmonary arterial circulation, thus bypassing the small right ventricle. If the right ventricle grows, then the Glenn shunt can be taken down. If not, future interventions proceed toward a Fontan circulation. Patients with severe coronary to RV fistulae may require cardiac transplantation. Sinusoids are typically not present in patients with severe tricuspid insufficiency and a normal right ventricular size; however, in patients with significant tricuspid insufficiency and low RV pressure, valvotomy may not result in effective forward flow through the right ventricle because of the tricuspid insufficiency (similar to the physiology of Ebstein anomaly with "functional" pulmonary atresia).

CONTROVERSIES IN MANAGEMENT

Most of the principles of management of pulmonary atresia with intact septum are agreed on. The exact technique of intervention (surgical vs. interventional catheterization) varies from institution to institution. Controversies surround the quantification of RV size and decision making over what constitutes an RV that is too small to accept a full cardiac output, when to place a systemic to pulmonary artery shunt, and whether or not to pursue a univentricular repair (Glenn and Fontan operations). Controversy surrounds RV sinusoids and whether they are significant enough to preclude intervention on the pulmonary valve and proceed with cardiac transplantation.

Suggested Readings

Allen HD, Gutgesell HP, Clark EB, Driscoll DJ: *Moss and Adams' Heart Disease in Infants, Children and Adolescents Including the Fetus and Young Adult*, 6th ed. Philadelphia, PA, Lippincott Williams & Wilkins, 2001.

Garson A, Bricker JT, Fisher DJ, Neish SR: *The Science and Practice of Pediatric Cardiology*, 2nd ed. Baltimore, MD, Williams & Wilkins, 1998.

23

EBSTEIN ANOMALY

Peter Koenig

ANATOMY

Ebstein anomaly is an abnormality of the tricuspid valve first described by Wilhelm Ebstein in 1866. The pathologic finding is the displacement of the attachments of the septal and posterior leaflets of the tricuspid valve toward the right ventricular apex. Thus, the functional annulus of the tricuspid valve is displaced into the right ventricle. This has the effect of "repartitioning" the right atrium and right ventricle such that the right atrium becomes larger (atrialization of the right ventricle) and the right ventricle becomes smaller. The anterior leaflet is often large, redundant, and resembles a sail. Rarely, the redundancy creates an imperforate membrane and anatomic tricuspid atresia; however, this membrane may have perforations in it, creating tricuspid stenosis. The right ventricle is thin at the atrialized portion, with a normal thickness in the functional portion of the right ventricle. Commonly associated lesions include an interatrial communication (patent foramen ovale or atrial septal defect [ASD]). Less commonly, a ventricular septal defect, pulmonary valve stenosis, or atresia is present.

In addition to anatomic abnormalities, there are associated abnormalities of electrical conduction. The atrialized portion of the right ventricle is nevertheless a right ventricle with right ventricular electrical depolarization and repolarization. The latter may cause an unusual appearance of the mechanical contraction of the right ventricle. There is associated preexcitation (Wolff-Parkinson-White) in 20–30% of patients, and a right bundle branch block pattern in those without preexcitation.

The embryology of this abnormality is felt to be a lack of normal undermining of the ventricular wall, which normally forms the tricuspid valve leaflets and chordae. The genetics and exact mechanism of Ebstein anomaly are unclear though there is an association with maternal lithium use during pregnancy.

PATHOPHYSIOLOGY

The major hemodynamic abnormality in Ebstein anomaly is the degree of tricuspid regurgitation. The degree of tricuspid valve regurgitation is directly related to the degree of right atrial and ventricular dilation (in addition to the atrial enlargement intrinsic to the abnormality), as seen in Figure 23-1B. With severe or free tricuspid regurgitation, the net blood flow across the pulmonary valve will be in part determined by the difference in right

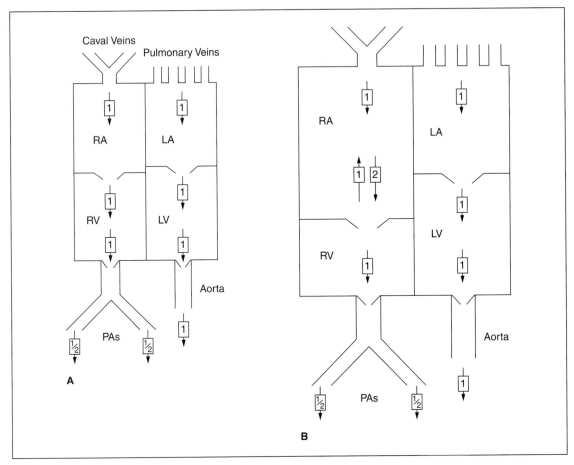

FIGURE 23-1

PATHOPHYSIOLOGY OF EBSTEIN ANOMALY

(**A**) Normal heart. This shows a normal heart with a normal cardiac output (the 1 in a box). RA: right atrium, RV: right ventricle, LA: left atrium, LV: left ventricle PAs: pulmonary arteries. Note the minimal apical displacement of the tricuspid valve annulus compared to the mitral valve annulus. (**B**) Mild Ebstein abnormality. Note the lack of an atrial level shunt in this example and the maintenance of a normal cardiac output (represented by the 1 in a box). There is a regurgitant volume of one cardiac output (arrow) with two cardiac outputs flowing in a normal direction across the tricuspid valve. This will cause a murmur of functional tricuspid stenosis in addition to the tricuspid regurgitation murmur. Systemic oxygen saturations would be normal in this example. (**C**) In this example, there is severe tricuspid valve regurgitation in the presence of increased pulmonary vascular resistance (or pulmonary valve stenosis). In either case, the resistance of right ventricular outflow is much greater than is the resistance to blood flow back into the right atrium. Thus, there is no anterograde pulmonary blood flow and a ductus arteriosus or other source of pulmonary blood flow is required. In addition to the volume of blood flow, there will be systemic desaturation as the pulmonary venous return will mix with the amount of blood shunted right to left across the PFO/ASD (both one cardiac output in this example) in the left atrium. (**D**) Severe Ebstein anomaly with low PVR. Noted the change from C. There is now forward flow across the pulmonary valve, the PDA is closed, and there is no flow across the PFO/ASD. The latter can again recur if PVR rises or any other type of obstruction to pulmonary blood flow. In this case, the amount of right-to-left shunting across the PFO/ASD will be equal to a decrease in pulmonary blood flow. The net result is that a decreased amount of pulmonary venous return will mix with the shunted blood to cause systemic desaturation.

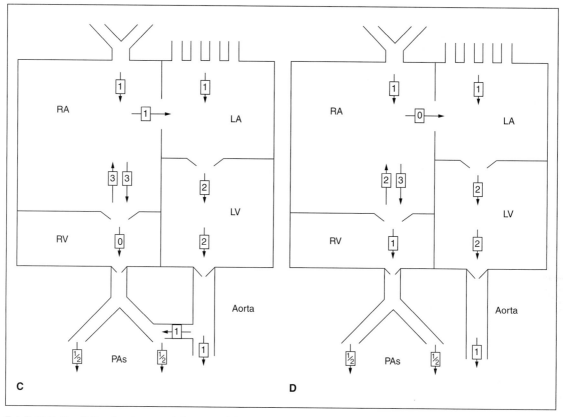

FIGURE 23-1 (continued)

ventricular afterload (pulmonary vascular resistance or any anatomic obstruction) and the resistance to regurgitant flow (resistance offered by the right atrium). Blood will move in the path of least resistance. In a neonate with high pulmonary vascular resistance and severe tricuspid regurgitation, little or no blood will move forward across the pulmonary valve creating functional pulmonary atresia (Figure 23-1C). In the presence of an ASD or patent foramen ovale (PFO) (necessary if there is functional pulmonary atresia), desaturated blood will cross from the right atrium to the left atrium and cause cyanosis (a right-to-left shunt). In addition to the tricuspid regurgitation, a small right ventricle may not serve as a sufficient pump to handle an adequate blood volume to generate a normal cardiac output. This may result in compensatory

tachycardia, or the need for blood to bypass the right ventricle via an ASD or PFO (right-to-left shunt) as if there were functional tricuspid stenosis. Physiologically, this is a diastolic right ventricular filling abnormality because of a small RV size. In addition, right ventricular inflow may be impeded by the abnormal contraction pattern of the atrialized portion of the right ventricle. All of the above physiologic derangements vary in severity, which is partly dependent on the degree of the anatomic abnormality. Thus, a very mild amount of tricuspid valve displacement may result in very mild regurgitation, which will result in little if any cyanosis, atrial or ventricular dilation or dysfunction. A severe tricuspid valve abnormality will result in severe regurgitation with significant cyanosis and right atrial dilation.

CLINICAL HISTORY AND PHYSICAL FINDINGS

The clinical presentation varies, as does the degree of the anatomic abnormality. In the mildest form, there may be no clinical symptoms or physical findings and the abnormality will be an incidental finding postmortem. In the most severe form, the presentation will be in the neonatal period and will consist of cyanosis and respiratory distress. As the pulmonary vascular resistance is elevated in the neonatal period, there may be little pulmonary blood flow with severe tricuspid regurgitation. As long as the neonatal ductus arteriosus is patent, enough pulmonary blood flow may be achieved for adequate oxygenation. In addition to the lack of pulmonary blood flow, right atrial dilation will occur in proportion to the degree of tricuspid regurgitation. The dilation may be to such a degree that the lung volume may be decreased, leading to inadequate ventilation. This may further increase pulmonary vascular resistance (rising PCO_2) and lead to a further decrease in pulmonary blood flow and tricuspid regurgitation. This will in turn lead to increasing right atrial dilation in a vicious cycle.

In the absence of an adequate interatrial communication (ASD or PFO) and severe tricuspid regurgitation, cyanosis will not occur. Instead, respiratory distress and shock will occur as blood accumulates in an increasingly dilated right atrium with no route of escape. With less severe tricuspid regurgitation and lack of an interatrial communication, right atrial dilation and right atrial hypertension will occur. The amount of the latter will depend on the degree of tricuspid regurgitation. The increased right atrial pressures will be transmitted to the systemic veins and organs, causing venous distension (JVD), organ distension (hepatomegaly), and edema.

The physical examination will reflect the degree of the underlying physiologic derangement. With very mild tricuspid regurgitation, no overt findings may be present or multiple systolic and diastolic clicks may be noted and may be a result of widened S2 splitting, an S3 and S4. A systolic or holosystolic murmur of tricuspid regurgitation may be present along the left sternal border. With increasing severity of tricuspid regurgitation, a right ventricular heave or lift (signifying right ventricular enlargement) may be present along with cyanosis, decreased perfusion, peripheral edema, hepatomegaly, and jugular venous distension (JVD).

LABORATORY FINDINGS

ECG: The ECG and rhythm strip may show rhythm abnormalities, which are common in patients with more severe tricuspid regurgitation. These mainly consist of atrial tachycardias (ectopic atrial tachycardia and atrial flutter) as well as AV reentry tachycardia in the presence of Wolff-Parkinson White (WPW). As stated previously, right bundle branch block and a delta wave of preexcitation may be present. A tall P wave in the right precordial leads (V1–V3) is consistent with right atrial enlargement.

Chest radiograph: The chest radiograph may correlate with the degree of tricuspid regurgitation and right atrial enlargement. With severe tricuspid regurgitation, the heart may be "wall to wall" and resemble a balloon such as that seen with a large pericardial effusion. The convexities of the right and left heart borders produce a characteristic globular appearance. Pulmonary vascularity may be decreased in the presence of severe tricuspid regurgitation and elevated pulmonary vascular resistance or with pulmonary stenosis or atresia.

TREATMENT

Treatment of Ebstein anomaly depends on the degree of tricuspid regurgitation and symptoms. The natural history of the very mild form of the abnormality is one of a normal life without symptoms. With increasing severity of tricuspid regurgitation, cyanosis, and a decreased cardiac output and its symptoms will significantly affect a normal life. In the neonatal period, mortality is high with severe Ebstein anomaly, though improvement generally occurs if the infant survives. This is probably a result of the decreasing pulmonary vascular resistance allowing increased pulmonary blood flow, decreased tricuspid regurgitation, and cyanosis.

Sometimes, a period of supportive care is required until pulmonary vascular resistance decreases. This supportive care may include the use of prostaglandins to keep the ductus arteriosus patent, oxygen, and nitric oxide to lower pulmonary vascular resistance, mechanical ventilation, or even extracorporeal membrane oxygenation (ECMO).

In rare neonatal patients with severe regurgitation, surgical management is required as a life-saving maneuver. Surgical options are few and can consist of tricuspid valvuloplasty, or conversion into single ventricle. The latter consists of closure of the tricuspid valve and pulmonary artery and the insertion of an aorto-pulmonary shunt. The surgical mortality of neonates with Ebstein anomaly is greater than 50%.

After the neonatal period, management is mainly observation. Diuretics may have a role in reducing symptoms of right atrial hypertension. In general, however, management consists of observation for untoward complications of the disease (arrhythmias, decreasing exercise tolerance, increasing tricuspid regurgitation). These will help determine the timing of surgical intervention. The latter is the main mode of treatment if symptoms develop.

Children presenting with symptomatic Ebstein anomaly require tricuspid valvuloplasty. Tricuspid valve replacement is rare in this age group. The older the patient, the more likely it is that the tricuspid valve has to be replaced. Valvuloplasty techniques have been developed by Drs. Carpentier (Hôpital Broussais, Paris) and Danielson (Mayo clinic). They consist of plication of the atrialized ventricular tissue (in order to bring the valve closer to the normal level of the annulus), and repositioning (rotation) of the posterior and anterior leaflets to cover the deficient septal leaflet. Any associated cardiac malformation (i.e., ASD) is repaired concomitantly. Survival in children and adults is excellent. Complications are unusual but include heart block and residual or recurrent tricuspid insufficiency. Bioprosthetic valves or homografts are usually used as replacements.

CONTROVERSIES IN THE MANAGEMENT OF EBSTEIN ANOMALY

Controversies in the management of Ebstein anomaly remain. One is in the neonatal period and whether to continue aggressive medical management including ECMO (to maintain patient stability while allowing the pulmonary vascular resistance to decrease) or proceed with surgical intervention. The former has been shown to allow a delay or avoidance of surgical intervention with its associated high mortality; however, both have high mortality rates.

Another controversy is whether and when to intervene in a patient with significant tricuspid valve regurgitation without symptoms. In a similar fashion, in patients with lesser degrees of tricuspid valve regurgitation, it is unclear whether and when to intervene. In general, it is common to intervene when there is significant tricuspid regurgitation associated with right atrial enlargement. The indication has been to try to prevent the development of future atrial dysrhythmias. Again, the question remains as to what constitutes significant enough atrial enlargement to pose a risk for future dysrhythmia.

Intervention in mild, asymptomatic Ebstein anomaly is not clearly indicated and poses no significant controversy.

Suggested Readings

Allen HD, Gutgesell HP, Clark EB, Driscoll DJ: *Moss and Adams' Heart Disease in Infants, Children, and Adolescents Including the Fetus and Young Adult*, 6th ed. Philadelphia, PA, Lippincott Williams & Wilkins, 2001.

Danielson GK, Driscoll DJ, Mair DD, Warnes CA, Oliver WC Jr: Operative treatment of Ebstein's anomaly. *J Thorac Cardiovasc Surg* 104:1195–1202, 1992.

Garson A, Bricker JT, Fisher DJ, Neish SR: *The Science and Practice of Pediatric Cardiology*, 2nd ed. Baltimore, MD, Williams & Wilkins, 1998.

24

PERIPHERAL PULMONARY STENOSIS

David J. Waight

INTRODUCTION

Branch pulmonary artery (PA) stenosis or peripheral pulmonary stenosis (PPS) describes a variety of lesions that involve narrowing of the left, right, or both pulmonary arteries beyond the main pulmonary artery. It constitutes approximately 3% of congenital heart disease. There may be a single site of narrowing or multiple sites. PPS may be an isolated congenital anomaly or associated with complex lesions. Sixty-six percent of patients with PPS have additional congenital heart disease, with pulmonary valve stenosis and ventricular septal defect occurring most frequently. Patent ductus arteriosus and atrial septal defect are also commonly associated with PPS and often occur in patients with Rubella syndrome (Figure 24-1).

PPS often occurs after surgical procedures that involve patching or an anastomosis of the pulmonary artery that extends onto the branch PAs. This is most commonly seen following repair of tetralogy of Fallot. PPS is also a complication after the arterial switch procedure for transposition of the great arteries. This can occur owing to stretching of the branch PAs when the main PA is transferred

anterior to the aorta (known as the LeCompt maneuver). PPS is frequently present in patients with pulmonary atresia who have had unifocalization of collateral vessels to form central pulmonary arteries.

Mild PPS is often seen in newborns and is more prominent in premature infants. This mild form of PPS is not clinically significant and resolves with normal growth and development of the pulmonary arteries.

Pulmonary artery hypoplasia is a severe form of PPS, with extremely small branch pulmonary arteries. These patients have severe proximal PA and RV hypertension and may have severe cyanosis because of very limited pulmonary blood flow. If the PAs cannot be enlarged surgically or with interventional techniques these patients may require lung transplantation as primary therapy.

SYNDROMES ASSOCIATED WITH PPS

Several syndromes have PPS as a component of associated congenital abnormalities.

Williams syndrome patients often have both PPS and supravalvar aortic stenosis. They may also have renal artery stenosis. Hypocalcemia is a prominent feature of this disorder. Patients with Williams syndrome and severe PPS have a significant risk of arrhythmia and sudden death at the time of cardiac catheterization. The PPS may improve and the supravalvar AS usually progresses with time. These patients have mental disabilities, peculiar facial features, and tend to be abnormally friendly. Most patients with Williams syndrome have a deletion on chromosome no. 7. This can be confirmed with fluorescent in situ hybridization (FISH) chromosomal testing.

Alagille syndrome (arteriohepatic dysplasia) patients have intrahepatic cholestasis and often have PPS that can be severe. These patients often require liver transplantation and may require intervention to relieve the PPS prior to liver transplantation to avoid high RV and RA pressures. High RA pressure may compromise the perfusion of the transplanted liver.

Congenital rubella syndrome may occur when a pregnant mother becomes infected with rubella in the first trimester and it is transmitted to the fetus.

These patients have a high incidence of CHD including PDA, PPS, VSD, and ASD.

Connective tissue disorders including Ehlers-Danlos Syndrome and Cutis Laxa may have PPS. Noonan Syndrome often includes pulmonary stenosis and may additionally include PPS.

PATHOPHYSIOLOGY

PPS produces a pressure gradient from the main pulmonary artery to the distal pulmonary arteries (Figure 24-1). This pressure gradient causes main pulmonary artery and right ventricular hypertension, which leads to right ventricular hypertrophy. Right ventricular hypertrophy produces decreased compliance of the right ventricle, which can lead to right atrial enlargement and atrial arrhythmias. Stenosis in only one PA will lead to overcirculation and potential pulmonary vascular disease in the normal contralateral lung. Isolated focal PPS can produce poststenotic dilation of the pulmonary artery segment distal to the narrowing.

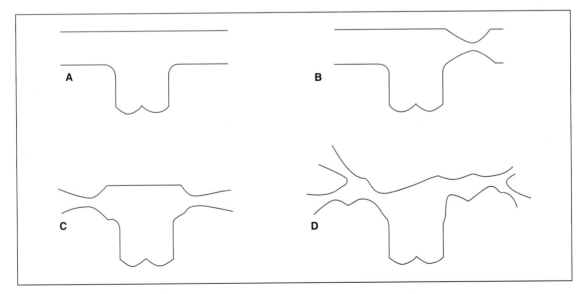

FIGURE   24-1

PATHOPHYSIOLOGY OF PERIPHERAL PULMONARY STENOSIS

(**A**) Normal main and branch pulmonary arteries. (**B**) Isolated proximal left pulmonary stenosis. (**C**) Bilateral branch pulmonary artery stenosis. (**D**) Multiple areas of stenosis throughout the pulmonary arteries.

PRESENTATION

The presentation of PPS is determined by the severity of the stenosis. Most commonly, PPS will present with a murmur noted by auscultation. The majority of patients are asymptomatic unless they have severe PPS. Severe PPS can cause cyanosis in the newborn because of right-to-left shunting in the presence of an atrial or ventricular septal communication. In older individuals, congestive heart failure may occur. Less severe forms may present with exercise intolerance or fatigue because of the inability of the patient to increase cardiac output owing to fixed obstruction across the pulmonary arteries. Right ventricular hypertrophy with resultant right atrial enlargement may present with signs of right-sided congestive heart failure including arrhythmia, hepatic enlargement, or jugular venous distention.

The natural history of PPS varies with severity and etiology. Mild to moderate PPS may remain mild or becomes insignificant with time. Severe pulmonary stenosis usually requires treatment. The exception to this may be patients with Williams syndrome in which the PPS may improve with growth.

PHYSICAL EXAM

Patients with PPS have a soft systolic ejection murmur. This can be heard at the left upper sternal border if the lesion is located at the proximal branch pulmonary arteries or is in the left pulmonary artery. The murmur may be heard at the right upper sternal border if the lesion is more distal in the RPA. These murmurs are also audible and may be louder in the back over the distribution of the affected PA. There may be radiation to the axilla. The murmur may become continuous if there are multiple tight lesions with a significant diastolic gradient from the proximal PA to the distal PA. If the affected PA is severely hypoplastic or absent, the murmur may be over the contralateral lung field because of increased flow to that lung. The first heart sound is normal. The second heart sound frequently has a normal P2 but is widely split with normal respiratory variation. The

split widens during inspiration. If the PPS is severe and there is an elevated main pulmonary artery pressure the second heart sound will be louder than normal. This is similar to pulmonary hypertension from other causes, but there is absence of distal pulmonary hypertension (pulmonary vascular disease). A systolic ejection systolic click will not be noted if the pulmonary valve is normal. If right ventricular hypertrophy has developed, a parasternal heave will be noted during systole.

LABORATORY STUDIES

Chest Radiography

The chest radiograph generally demonstrates a normal heart size unless the patient has significant congestive heart failure. If the heart is enlarged, a prominent right atrium signifying right atrial enlargement would be seen. There is no poststenotic dilatation of the main pulmonary. Pulmonary vascular markings are normal if there is balanced, bilateral obstruction. If there is unbalanced perfusion owing to stenosis of only one branch pulmonary artery, there will be decreased pulmonary vascular markings in the affected lung field.

Electrocardiography

ECG findings are normal in many patients with mild to moderate PPS. If the stenosis is more severe, right ventricular hypertrophy may be present with an RSR' pattern most notably seen in lead V1. Right atrial enlargement with a tall P wave may also be seen. Right-axis deviation owing to right ventricular enlargement may also be noted. Significant right ventricular hypertrophy may be diagnosed with a positive T wave in V1 in infants and children up to midadolescence. Patients with congenital rubella syndrome and Noonan syndrome have left-axis deviation.

Echocardiography

An echocardiogram is a diagnostic or confirmatory test in patients with PPS and will demonstrate the narrowed segment of the branch PA if the stenosis is proximal. Distal stenoses will not be well imaged or missed entirely by 2D imaging because of the surrounding lung tissue. Doppler evaluation demonstrates increased flow velocity across the branch PAs and may suggest a distal stenosis that was not imaged directly; however, of note is that distal stenoses may be undetected by the both 2D and Doppler imaging. This may hold true for distal pulmonary artery hypoplasia.

Cardiac Catheterization and Angiography

The diagnosis and evaluation of PPS can also be defined during cardiac catheterization where direct pressure measurements of the right ventricle, main pulmonary, and distal branch pulmonary arteries are measured. This defines the true gradient in mmHg across the branch PA stenosis. PAs with multiple areas of stenosis may have several small changes in pressure across the length of the vessel or may have a gradient across the most proximal stenosis without a pressure change across more distal severe stenosis. Angiography is the most accurate way to assess the branch PA anatomy as it can demonstrate multiple areas of stenosis throughout the entire PA. Angiography will also image very distal or small subsegment stenosis. The renal arteries should be imaged with angiography or with renal ultrasound in all patients with Williams syndrome.

MRI

Magnetic resonance imaging may provide excellent imaging of the branch PAs if performed in a center with experience in imaging children. Magnetic resonance angiography (MRA) is useful for evaluation of complex lesions.

Radionuclide Perfusion Scan

A nuclear medicine perfusion/ventilation scan can be used to determine how the PPS affects the distribution of the pulmonary flow to each lung. Radiolabeled albumin is administered through a peripheral vein and becomes entrapped in the pulmonary capillary bed. A quantitative evaluation of the radioactivity provides an accurate measure of segmental and global pulmonary flow. These are reported as a percent of the total flow with a normal range of 50–60% of flow to the right lung. This is a useful test to evaluate the results of balloon or surgical angioplasty if performed pre and postprocedure. The results will be inaccurate if any shunting is present.

TREATMENT

SBE prophylaxis for appropriate dental and surgical procedures is indicated. Moderate to severe PPS can be treated with surgery or transcatheter balloon angioplasty or angioplasty with stenting. Distal PPS that is beyond the hilum of the lung is not approachable with surgical techniques and requires transcatheter therapy. Unifocalized collateral vessels in patients with pulmonary atresia often require multiple interventional procedures for "rehabilitation" of these abnormal vessels. Stents implantated in the branch PAs during childhood will require further evaluation and subsequent balloon expansion as the child grows.

Patients with Williams syndrome may have severe PPS at birth that becomes less significant as the child grows. These patients may not require any therapy for their PPS if they have an adequate oxygen saturation. They are likely to eventually require therapy for their progressive supravalvar aortic stenosis.

CONTROVERSIES IN DIAGNOSIS AND MANAGEMENT

The treatment for patients with Williams syndrome and PPS often creates debate among cardiologists and surgeons. The severe RV hypertension can cause significant symptoms in infants and can be improved with intervention, but RV HTN is often well tolerated in infants and the PPS may improve spontaneously.

The controversy of surgical versus transcatheter therapy for PPS continues to be the major issue. Balloon angioplasty has a limited effectiveness in

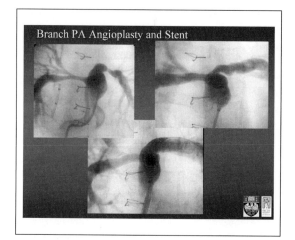

Branch PA Angioplasty and Stent

FIGURE 24-2

ANGIOGRAM OF PULMONARY ARTERIES WITH BILATERAL PPS

(1) Upper left, demonstrates severe proximal stenosis of right and left pulmonary arteries. (2) Upper right, after stent placement in proximal RPA demonstrating improved RPA size and LPA stenosis. (3) Lower, after LPA stent with excellent expansion of the proximal LPA.

native PPS with a success rate of approximately 50–60% and a restenosis rate of up to 20%. Surgical patch angioplasty is only effective for proximal PPS and has a significant restenosis rate. Stent implantation and balloon expansion is very effective, but this requires additional catheteriza-

tions and reexpansion of the stents (Figure 24-2). There is limited data on long-term follow-up of stents in branch pulmonary arteries in children. A combined approach of surgery and interventional therapy of PPS appears to be best for this complex lesion.

Suggested Readings

Bacha EA, Kreutzer J: Comprehensive management of branch pulmonary artery stenosis. *J Interv Cardiol* 14(3):367–375, 2001.

Cheatham JP: Pulmonary Stenosis, in: Garson A, Bricker JT, Fisher DJ, Neish SR (eds), *The Science and Practice of Pediatric Cardiology*, 2nd ed. Baltimore, MD, Williams & Wilkins, 1998.

Giddens NG, Finley JP, Nanton MA, Roy DL: The natural course of supravalvar aortic stenosis and peripheral pulmonary artery stenosis in Williams syndrome. *Br Heart J* 62:315–319, 1989.

Ing FF, Grifka RG, Nihill MR, Mullins CE: Repeat dilation of intravascular stents in congenital heart defects. *Circulation* 92(4):893–897, 1995.

Rothman A, Perry SB, Keane JF, Lock JE: Balloon dilation of branch pulmonary artery stenosis. *Semin Thorac Cardiovasc Surg* 2(1):46–54, 1990.

Rocchini AP, Emmanouilides GC: Pulmonary Stenosis, in: Emmanoulides GC, Riemenschneider TA, Allen HD, Gutgesell HP (eds), *Moss and Adams Heart Disease in Infants, Children, and Adolescents*, 5th ed. Baltimore, MD, Williams & Wilkins, 1995.

25

CORTRIATRIATUM

Brojendra Agarwala

INTRODUCTION

Cortriatriatum is a congenital cardiac anomaly in which an atrium is divided into two chambers by a fibromuscular membrane. Thus, the term implying three atrial chambers. This lesion can exist in both the right atrium (RA) (cortriatriatum dexter) and the left atrium (LA) (cortriatriatum sinister).

ANATOMY

In cortriatriatum sinister, the three chambers, or "atria," are proximal and distal chambers in the LA and the RA. The pulmonary veins enter a proximal accessory chamber which communicate with the distal portion of the LA, or "true LA," through an opening in the fibromuscular membrane. The left atrial appendage communicates with the distal chamber, thus defining the true left atrium and differentiating this lesion from a supravalvar mitral ring. The size of the opening between the proximal and distal chambers of the LA determines the clinical manifestations as described below. There are variations in the sites of pulmonary venous drainage, and the proximal chamber may communicate with the RA directly (Figure 25-1). There

may be a vertical vein draining the proximal chamber to another site or other variations of pulmonary venous return similar to total anomalous pulmonary venous connection as described in Chapter 28.

In cortriatriatum dexter, the systemic veins, including the coronary sinus, enter a proximal chamber that is partitioned from the distal right atrial chamber by a membrane that incorporates the eustachian valve tissue, the thebesian valve (of the coronary sinus), and the crista terminalis (valve of the superior vena cava). There can be variations in the manner in which the systemic veins return to the heart. This includes direct entry of the superior or inferior vena cava to the left atrium. The clinical manifestations are dependent on the size of the communication between the proximal and distal chambers of the right atrium. There may be an obligatory right-to-left shunt.

EMBRYOLOGY

The LA has two sources of origin. The proximal part originates from the common pulmonary vein and the distal part (which includes the LA appendage) originates from the primitive cardiac tube. Normal

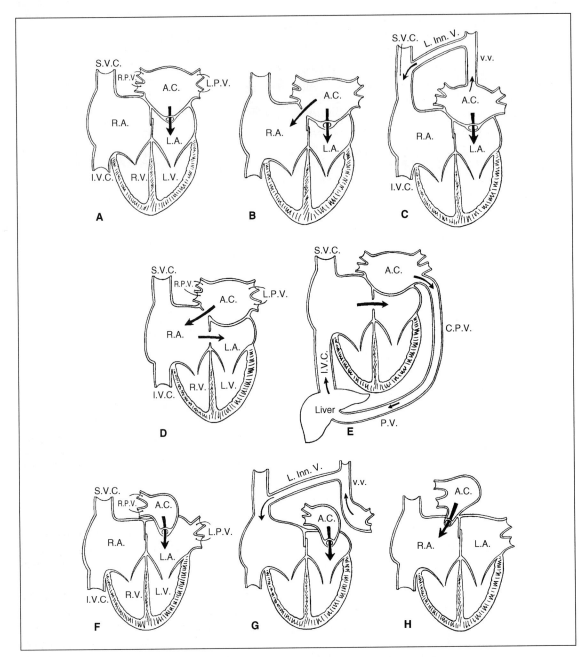

FIGURE 25-1

VARIATIONS IN DRAINAGE WITH CORTRIATRIATUM SINISTER

RPV = right pulmonary vein; LPV = left pulmonary vein; CPV = common pulmonary vein; PV = pulmonary vein; AC = accessory chamber (e.g. proximal chamber); SVC = superior vena cava; IVC = inferior vena cava; L inn V = left innominate vein; VV = vertical vein.

Source: Moss' Heart Disease in Infants, Children, and Adults. 4th ed. Baltimore: Williams & Wilkins, 1989.

embryologic development requires incorporation of the common pulmonary vein into the cardiac tube (see Chapter 28). When there is a failure of incorporation of the common pulmonary venous connection with the LA, the membrane between the common pulmonary vein and the cardiac tube persists and cortriatriatum sinister develops. With complete failure of incorporation of the common pulmonary vein into the cardiac tube, total anomalous pulmonary venous connection develops. The difference between these two lesions is that there is a communication between the proximal and distal chambers in the former lesion.

The right atrium also originates from the cardiac tube and includes the right atrial appendage. Similar to LA embryology, the RA consists of incorporation of the primitive venous system into it. The veins include the coronary sinus, from the cardinal veins, the inferior vena cava, and the superior vena cava from the right horn of the sinus venosus. In normal embryologic development, the veins are completely incorporated into the right atrium with remnants of the primitive veins remaining as the valve of the inferior vena cava (eustachian valve), valve of the coronary sinus (thebesian valve), and valve of the superior vena cava (crista terminalis). Failure to completely incorporate these primitive veins results in various amounts of primitive membranes remaining, which may cause these valves to remain attached to one another in various combinations and to various degrees. Lesser degrees of persistence of these attachments are termed Chiari network. The latter is nonobstructive.

PATHOPHYSIOLOGY

The pathophysiology of this lesion is demonstrated in Figure 25-2. Unless there is anomalous pulmonary venous drainage, there will be no shunting. There will be pressure elevation in the proximal left atrial chamber (PC), which will be transmitted to the pulmonary veins, pulmonary arteries, and the right ventricle. The pressure overload of the proximal chamber will be proportional to the size of the communication between it and the distal chamber. There will be compensatory dilation of this chamber.

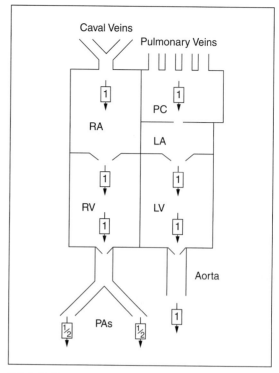

FIGURE 25-2

CORTRIATRIATUM SINISTER WITH NO VEIN DRAINING THE PROXIMAL CHAMBER (PC)

Note that there is 1 relative cardiac output leaving and entering the heart. The pressure in the PC will be elevated as a result of the obstruction. The distal chamber is the true left atrium (LA).

The pressure elevation in the pulmonary veins may cause pulmonary edema. The pulmonary arterial hypertension and right ventricular hypertension will eventually lead to right ventricular hypertrophy.

In the presence of near total obstruction of the communical between the proximal and distal LA chambers, routes for blood flow to bypass this obstruction are required. These include an anomalous pulmonary venous drainage and a communication between the RA and the distal LA chamber. The former will lead to a left-to-right shunt and pulmonary overcirculation. The latter will lead to a right-to-left shunt and varying degrees of cyanosis. The amount of cyanosis, or desaturation, is dependent on the net ratio of pulmonary venous return and systemic venous return mixing and entering the distal left atrial chamber. The amount of pulmonary venous return to the distal chamber is dependent on the size of the communication between the proximal and distal LA chambers, as well as the pulmonary vascular resistance. An increased pulmonary vascular resistance will lead to decreased pulmonary blood flow, decreased pulmonary venous return, and a greater degree of desaturated blood entering the distal LA chamber (Figure 25-3). The amount of blood entering the distal LA chamber is also somewhat dependent on the size of the communication between it and the RA.

In the presence of low pulmonary vascular resistance (PVR) and anomalous pulmonary venous connection, there will be increased pulmonary blood flow (Figure 25-4). If the communication between the proximal and distal LA chambers is restrictive, this increased pulmonary blood flow will return mainly to the RA and cause RA enlargement. The ratio of pulmonary venous return to systemic venous return will increase and cause the net saturation of the mixed venous blood to increase. Depending on the size of the communication between the RA and proximal LA chamber with the distal LA chamber, the amount of shunting to the distal LA chamber will vary.

The pathophysiology of cortriatriatum dexter is similar. The partition between the proximal and distal RA chambers will cause the pressure in the proximal RA chamber to be elevated and transmitted to the systemic veins and organs. There is usually a connection between the proximal RA chamber and the LA causing desaturated blood to shunt right to left and mix with pulmonary venous return in the LA. The amount of desaturation (cyanosis) will depend on the ratio of the amount of right-to-left shunt and pulmonary venous return. In the presence of a connection between the RA and the LA, the pulmonary venous return is dependent on pulmonary blood flow, which is in turn dependent on PVR and the size of the communication between the proximal and distal RA chambers. It will be increased with low PVR and a large communication, and decreased with high PVR and a small communication. If the communication between the proximal and distal RA chambers is

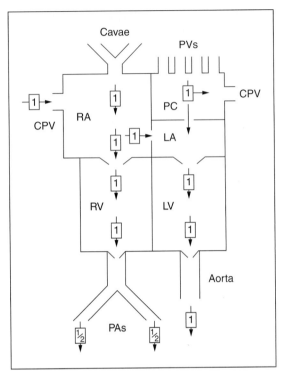

FIGURE 25-3

CORTRIATRIATUM SINISTER WITH ANOMALOUS PULMONARY VENOUS CONNECTION, AN ATRIAL COMMUNICATION, AND ELEVATED PULMONARY VASCULAR RESISTANCE

Note that the net cardiac output is still 1 (the number represented in the box). Minimal blood flow crosses the membrane partitioning the proximal chamber (PC) and the left atrium (LA); 2 cardiac outputs return to the right atrium (1 via the anomalous pulmonary venous connection or common pulmonary vein [CPV], and another from the caval veins); 1 cardiac output crosses an atrial septal defect, and 1 cardiac output flows to the lungs. In this example, 1 cardiac output of desaturated blood mixes with 1 cardiac output of saturated blood to yield the net saturation. With further elevations of PVR, pulmonary blood flow and return via the anomalous pulmonary connection will be decreased, with a stable return from the caval veins. The net result is a decreased ratio of saturated to desaturated blood in the right atrium which crosses the atrial septal defect.

very restrictive, no pulmonary blood flow will occur, and the lesion will be physiologically similar to tricuspid atresia and require the presence of a patent ductus arteriosus.

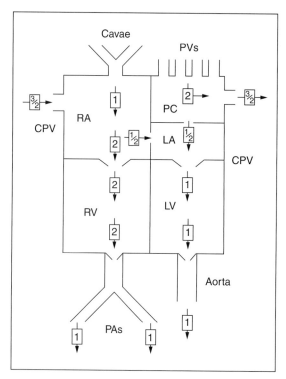

FIGURE 25-4

CORTRIATRIATUM SINISTER WITH LOW PULMONARY VASCULAR RESISTANCE

Compared to Figure 2, note the increased return to the right atrium via the anomalous pulmonary venous connection. Note the increased blood flow to the right atrium and right ventricle. In this example, the right atrium receives $2^{1}/_{2}$ relative cardiac outputs (1 from systemic venous return via the caval veins and $1^{1}/_{2}$ from the common pulmonary vein (CPV) draining the proximal chamber); $^{1}/_{2}$ cardiac output crosses an atrial septal defect of patent foramen ovale; 2 cardiac outputs enter the right atrium and the pulmonary arteries. The systemic cardiac output remains constant. The saturation of systemic blood will be high, as the mixed blood in the RA is from 2 cardiac outputs of highly saturated pulmonary venous return mixed with 1 cardiac output of systemic venous return.

Based on the above pathophysiology, the differential diagnosis of cortriatriatum sinister includes mitral stenosis, total anomalous pulmonary venous return, left atrial tumor (myxoma), LA thrombus and persistent fetal circulation in neonates. The differential of cortriatriatum dexter includes tricuspid stenosis, and a right atrial tumor/thrombus.

CLINICAL FINDINGS

Classic cortriatriatum, where all the pulmonary veins are draining into the common pulmonary venous chamber and this proximal chamber is communicating with the distal chamber with variable size opening, can be divided into two categories.

Group I: Small or restrictive communication. This group of infants is sick soon after birth because of pulmonary venous obstruction. The presentation consists of severe respiratory distress and cyanosis (owing to pulmonary edema and/or a right-to-left shunt between the RA and distal chamber). Clinically, this mimics neonates with respiratory distress syndrome and persistent fetal circulation, or total anomalous pulmonary venous connection with obstruction. In addition to respiratory distress and cyanosis, poor cardiac output and shock may occur. The physical examination is significant for cyanosis and respiratory distress with signs of shock. There are no clear findings on auscultation to define this lesion.

Group II: Mild to moderately restrictive communication. The usual clinical presentation begins in the first few months of life, and rarely in later child or adulthood. The usual signs and symptoms are respiratory infection including pneumonia, shortness of breath, and wheezing, which is frequently diagnosed and treated as reactive airway disease (asthma). Signs and symptoms may mimic primary pulmonary hypertension. The physical examination follows the pathophysiology of pulmonary hypertension and may reveal a right ventricular heave, a loud and single second heart sound, and a soft ejection systolic murmur with an ejection systolic click from pulmonary hypertension. Examination of the chest may reveal wheezing and rales. An enlarged liver may be present because of long-standing right ventricular failure or overexpansion of the lungs. With very mild restriction of the communication, few, if any, signs or symptoms may be present.

In cortriatriatum with anomalous pulmonary venous connection, the clinical findings are similar to those of total or partial anomalous venous connection. This will vary with the size of the communications between the RA and proximal chambers with the distal LA chamber as well as the pulmonary vascular resistance. The connection between the RA and LA is usually not restrictive. These can also be grouped into two categories.

Group I: Small or restrictive communication between the proximal and distal LA. In this group, the initial presentation will be in the neonatal period when PVR is elevated. This will result in decreased pulmonary blood flow and cyanosis, as described above. As the PVR decreases, the cyanosis will decrease and be replaced with signs and symptoms of pulmonary overcirculation. This will include tachypnea and possibly respiratory distress with failure to thrive. The physical findings of pulmonary overcirculation include a right ventricular lift, a wide split S2, and murmurs of functional tricuspid and pulmonary stenosis (similar to an atrial septal defect).

Group II: Mild to moderately restrictive communication between proximal and distal LA. With very mild restriction, the clinical findings will essentially be the same as an atrial septal defect and described in that chapter. Total anomalous pulmonary venous connection does not usually occur in this setting of minimal restriction, though partial anomalous venous connection does. There will be signs and symptoms of pulmonary overcirculation. These will be minimal with an elevated PVR, and increased as the PVR decreases. The physical findings may include an RV lift, a wide split S2, and murmurs of functional tricuspid and pulmonary stenosis.

In cortriatriatum dexter, the clinical findings will be of cyanosis if there is a right-to-left shunt at the atrial level and right-sided obstruction. The latter will include hepatomegaly, peripheral edema (rare in children), jugular venous distention, and poor perfusion if the obstruction is severe with no atrial level communication.

LABORATORY FINDINGS

Chest Radiography

The chest radiograph in cortriatriatum sinister may reveal a prominent RA and RV with a dilated MPA and pulmonary edema. Kerley B lines may be present. The shadow of an anomalously draining pulmonary vein ("snowman") may be seen. There are typically no significant findings with cortriatriatum dexter.

Electrocardiography

The ECG in cortriatriatum sinister usually reveals right atrial and right ventricular hypertrophy. There may be no significant findings with cortriatriatum dexter.

Echocardiography

2D echocardiography is usually diagnostic. In cortriatriatum sinister, the membrane within the LA is usually clearly visible. The size and amount of restriction of the left atrial communication can be seen with 2D echocardiography and further assessed with Doppler echocardiography. The pulmonary veins and return (including abnormal connections) can be seen with 2D and Doppler echocardiography as well. In a similar fashion, echocardiography may demonstrate the anatomy and hemodynamics of cortriatriatum dexter.

Cardiac Catheterization and Angiography

This invasive procedure is not usually required in the current era; however, hemodynamic may be more fully evaluated and angiography may better demonstrate abnormalities of pulmonary venous drainage. This is used if questions remain prior to surgical intervention.

Other imaging modalities such as an MRI are usually not needed.

MANAGEMENT

Once the diagnosis is confirmed, surgical intervention is the only form of treatment at this time in which the membrane of either form of cortriatriatum can be removed. In addition, any venous abnormalities may also be connected. The surgical result is excellent (essentially curative), as is the long-term prognosis. The pulmonary hypertension (as seen with cortriatriatum sinister) disappears within a short time after the operation. Long-term problems consist of atrial dysrhythmias owing to atrial scarring, and sinus node dysfunction if there was any intervention near the sinus node.

Commonly asked questions include whether the membrane can grow back after removal and whether there are any long-term restrictions. Once the membrane is removed, it does not recur, unlike a subaortic membrane. Usually, there are no restrictions in athletic activities with a nonrestrictive membrane or after successful surgical intervention. SBE prophylaxis is still recommended, though it is not clear if there is an increased risk of endocarditis to justify this practice.

The one controversy in management is whether or not all membranes need to be removed. In general, it is felt that those with no significant obstruction do not cause any long-term risks and do not require intervention.

Suggested Readings

Allen HD, Gutgesell HP, Clark EB, Driscoll DJ: *Moss and Adams' Heart Disease in Infants, Children, and Adolescents Including the Fetus and Young Adult*, 6th ed. Philadelphia, PA, Lippincott Williams & Wilkins, 2001.

Garson A, Bricker JT, Fisher DJ, Neish SR: *The Science and Practice of Pediatric Cardiology*, 2nd ed. Baltimore, MD, Williams & Wilkins, 1998.

26

HYPOPLASTIC LEFT HEART SYNDROME (MITRAL ATRESIA)

Ra-id Abdulla

INTRODUCTION

The lack of development of several components of the left heart, such as the mitral valve, left ventricle, aortic valve, and ascending aorta, is referred to as the hypoplastic left heart syndrome (HLHS). The extent of hypoplasia of the various components may vary. In HLHS the left ventricle is typically too small to sustain systemic cardiac output.

INCIDENCE

This is the 13th most common congenital heart disease. It occurs in 0.05–0.25/1000 live births (1.5% of all congenital heart disease at all ages).

EMBRYOLOGY

The embryology of HLHS is not entirely clear. One theory is that the primary problem is a restrictive patent foramen ovale (PFO) in utero, leading to decreased flow to the left atrium and thus decreased flow to all distal structures. It is felt that the decreased blood flow to these structures leads to decreased growth and hypoplasia. Another theory is that the primary problem is an abnormality of the mitral valve (dysplasia, stenosis, or atresia), leading to decreased blood flow to the left ventricle and distal structures, therefore leading to distal hypoplasia. The "no flow, no grow" theory is supported by the finding of hypoplasia of all structures distal to the primary obstruction. It may be possible that any point of obstruction may lead to the same outcome, thus, a restrictive PFO or mitral valve abnormality may both cause the hypoplastic left heart syndrome. The degree of blood flow to the left ventricle appears to determine the degree of hypoplasia.

ANATOMY

The most severe form of HLHS consists of mitral atresia, an extremely hypoplastic left ventricle (essentially nonexistent), aortic valve atresia, and a hypoplastic ascending aorta. The ascending aorta may be as small as 2 mm but large enough to supply coronary arteries in a retrograde fashion. The transverse aorta is as large as or larger than the ascending aorta (the opposite of normal). Coarctation of the isthmus portion of the aorta is felt to be present in many if not all patients with hypoplastic left heart syndrome. It may not be evident at birth, but is noted thereafter. It may also be difficult to ascertain in the presence of aortic arch hypoplasia and a large PDA. The latter is present at birth in all patients. There may be an ASD or a small patent foramen ovale. Occasionally, the latter is restrictive or not patent. When the interatrial septum is intact (no PFO), there is usually a venous pathway decompressing the left atrium. This may be a vertical vein from the left atrium to the innominate vein (a persistent embryologic connection during the formation of the pulmonary venous system).

In the absence of mitral atresia, the left ventricle size varies, usually proportional to the degree of mitral valve stenosis (annular hypoplasia, dysplastic leaflets, or papillary muscle pathology). The presence of a ventricular septal defect may be associated with an increased LV size (suggesting increased blood flow to the left ventricle in utero). In the absence of mitral valve pathology, the left ventricular growth may be nearly normal. This is seen with isolated aortic valve atresia or stenosis. (See Chapter 17.) However, aortic valve atresia is frequently associated with mitral valve pathology and varying degrees of left ventricular hypoplasia (similar to pulmonary valve atresia with an intact septum).

The atrial septum is thick, which may be a result of the increased left atrial pressure in utero, leading to LA hypertrophy, or this may be the primary pathology causing decreased right-to-left shunting in utero at the PFO level, leading to hypoplasia of the left heart.

In addition to the above findings in HLHS, there may be anomalies of pulmonary venous return, and coronary artery abnormalities. Total anomalous pulmonary venous connection may cause a small LV

because of underfilling, and this should not be confused with HLHS.

PATHOPHYSIOLOGY

Although a hypoplastic left heart is the most lethal congenital heart disease, the cardiac anatomy is adequate for intrauterine life where the PVR is elevated. In utero, and immediately after birth, the right ventricle provides blood to the pulmonary arterial circulation and to the aorta through the PDA. Pulmonary blood flow is dependent on pulmonary vascular resistance, which in turn is partially dependent on the level of restriction of the patent foramen ovale. When the patent foramen ovale is restrictive, left atrial pressure will be elevated causing increased pulmonary vascular resistance and less pulmonary blood flow. The greater the pulmonary blood flow, the greater the systemic oxygen saturation; however, this is not desirable, because increased pulmonary blood flow will steal blood from the systemic circulation and cause a low output state (shock). These findings are outlined in Figures 26–1A–C.

Blood flow to the head and coronary arteries is completely dependent on retrograde blood flow through the PDA. This may be decreased after birth because of coarctation of the aorta secondary to constriction of ductal tissue in the aortic arch. This will prevent retrograde blood flow to the head and neck as well as the coronary arteries.

Maneuvers that are usually used to treat shock (oxygen therapy, vasoconstrictive agents, bicarbonate infusion, intubation, and hyperventilation) will decrease pulmonary vascular resistance and change the ratio of systemic to pulmonary blood and cause systemic to pulmonary steal. The end result is a vicious cycle and worsening shock. If the PFO is restrictive, these maneuvers will cause worsening pulmonary edema. In the scenario of a restrictive or absent PFO, blood will flow to the lungs and severe pulmonary venous congestion will result. Oxygen saturations will be severely decreased since there is no pulmonary venous return to mix with systemic venous return. In

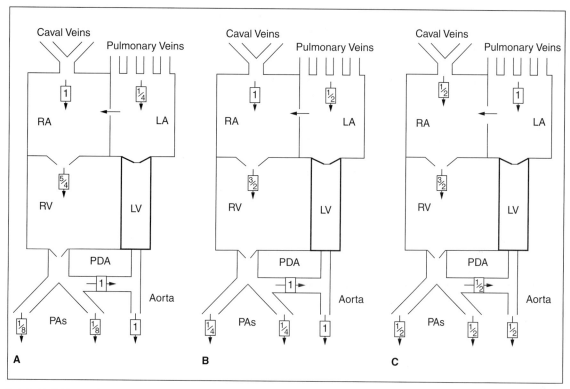

FIGURE 26-1

HYPOPLASTIC LEFT HEART SYNDROME

In these figures, there is a small LV with aortic and mitral atresia vs. severe or critical stenosis. The physiology demonstrated in these figures is similar for any lesion resulting in the lack of blood flow from the left ventricle to the aorta (aortic atresia, mitral atresia, critical mitral or aortic stenosis, or the complete lack of a left ventricle with the hypoplastic left heart syndrome). **(A)** Condition with elevated PVR is demonstrated. The elevated PVR leads to a greater amount of blood flow to the aorta than to the pulmonary arteries (1 vs. $1/4$ relative cardiac outputs); however, only $1/4$ cardiac output returns via the pulmonary veins to mix in the right atrium (after flowing through a PFO) with 1 relative cardiac output returning from the superior and inferior vena cava. Thus, the ratio of saturated to desaturated blood is $1/4$ to 1, and the net blood will be saturated. The end result will be a patient with cyanosis and good aortic (systemic) blood flow. **(B)** PVR has decreased, resulting in increased pulmonary blood flow. The systemic blood flow has remained constant in this scenario (which would be a result of an increased total body blood volume, $3/2$ vs. $5/4$ relative cardiac outputs). In this example, $1/2$ relative cardiac outputs of highly saturated blood returning from pulmonary veins mix in the right atrium with 1 relative cardiac output of desaturated blood returning from the superior and inferior vena cava. The ratio of saturated to desaturated blood mixing in the right atrium is $1/2$ to 1, thus the net oxygen saturation will be increased compared the example given in **A**. In **C**, an example is given with low PVR and a nonrestrictive ASD. The blood volume is the same as in **B** ($3/2$ total relative cardiac outputs), which assumes that the acute change in PVR did not allow the body to retain more fluid (as would be seen with maneuvers to lower PVR such as treatment with oxygen, and hyperventilation). As noted, the blood flow to the pulmonary arteries is increased and the blood flow to the aorta is decreased (1 vs. $1/2$ relative cardiac outputs). The net saturation is increased, since the ratio of highly saturated blood returning from the pulmonary veins to the desaturated blood returning from the caval veins and mixing in the right atrium is (1 to $1/2$ relative cardiac outputs). The end result in the example given in **C** is a patient with less cyanosis, but shock. The body will respond to the decreased cardiac output with tachycardia, and reflexes to increase blood flow to vital organs (e.g., brain), which will increase systemic vascular resistance; however, an increased systemic vascular resistance will increase blood flow to the lungs and may decrease cardiac function because of the increased afterload. Thus, shock may progress. Note the presence of a PDA in all these examples, as well as a PFO. Occlusion of either one of these will interrupt blood flow and result in death.

this scenario, there will be severe desaturation and shock.

CLINICAL MANIFESTATIONS

Initially, children with HLHS may be asymptomatic. This will continue as long as there is a PDA and the PVR is elevated. Usually, the PVR will remain elevated but the PDA will close. Closure of the PDA will lead to decreasing systemic output and early signs of shock. These may consist of tachypnea, poor perfusion, and poor feeding. The resulting acidosis may tend to keep the ductus arteriosus patent; however, the PDA will eventually narrow or close to a critical diameter in which there is inadequate cardiac output to sustain life. At this point, there will be clear signs and symptoms of shock. The initial response of caretakers is to treat shock and impending cardiopulmonary arrest using standard techniques of CPR; however, the treatment with oxygen and hyperventilation will lower PVR and decrease systemic blood flow if the ductus arteriosus is still patent. If the ductus arteriosus is closed, all efforts at resuscitation will fail. It is the early recognition of the lack of clinical improvement with resuscitation, which will lead to the consideration of underlying critical heart disease rather than the usual causes of shock in the neonate (see Chapters 5, 6, 8). Alternatively, if the PVR is elevated and the ductus arteriosus patent, the initial presentation may be cyanosis (Figure 26-1B). (See Chapter 5.) Prior to the development of frank shock, there is dyspnea (see Chapter 6) or tachycardia (see Chapters 8 and 36) which may prompt further workup with the eventual suspicion of a cardiac cause.

Poor cardiac output after birth will lead to poor renal perfusion and an increase in intravenous volume as well as in hyperkalemia. These children will develop poor appetite leading to hypoglycemia. The increase in intravascular volume, hyperkalemia, and hypoglycemia, coupled with decreased coronary blood flow owing to the restriction of the PDA, will lead to myocardial injury. Children are asymptomatic at birth, but as the ductus arteriosus starts to close, manifestations of poor cardiac output, eventually leading to cardiogenic shock, ensue.

On examination children with hypoplastic left heart syndrome are cyanotic with a grey ashen skin color. The capillary refill is poor. Peripheral pulses are week. The precordium is hyperactive with an increased RV impulse and a reduced or absent LV impulse. Typically, there is no palpable thrill. On auscultation, the second heart sound is single because of absent aortic component. There may be a nonspecific systolic flow murmur owing to increase blood flow across the pulmonary valve; however, in the state of shock (low flow) no flow murmurs will be typically heard. A PDA murmur is not typically audible, as it shunts right to left without a significant pressure gradient.

In summary, the historical and physical findings are of unexplained cyanosis, dyspnea or respiratory distress, or shock. Appropriate, logical evaluation should lead to the suspicion of a cardiac cause and the correct diagnosis.

LABORATORY FINDINGS

Electrocardiography

Because of RV predominance, there are signs of RVH and poor R-wave progression, indicating reduced LV forces owing to hypoplasia of the left ventricle; however, since the RV is dominant in the neonate, the finding of the lack of LV voltage is more difficult in the neonate with HLHS.

Chest Radiography

The chest radiograph typically shows a narrow mediastinum, cardiomegaly because of RV dilation, and increased pulmonary blood flow.

Echocardiography

The details of left heart hypoplasia can be seen by 2D echocardiography. The extent of mitral and aortic valve atresia is noted. Color and Doppler flow will determine flow across the mitral and aortic valves. Assessment of the patency of the ductus arteriosus is important, as is an assessment of the relative amount and direction of blood flow. The aortic arch is also seen, though the distal portions and coarctation may not be optimally imaged to exclude coarctation. Many such patients present with cardiogenic shock and poor ventricular function. Echocardiography is valuable in assessing ventricular function.

Cardiac Catheterization

Echocardiography can provide all information needed to perform surgical procedures or cardiac transplantation. Occasionally, a Rashkind atrial septostomy is required to decompress the left atrium in the case of a restrictive PFO. This can be performed at the bedside (under echocardiographic guidance) or in the cardiac catheterization laboratory, depending on physician and institutional experience; however, the atrial septum in this lesion is usually thick and not amenable to septostomy. Dilation or stenting of the PFO can be performed in cases in which surgery cannot be performed in a timely fashion.

Management

Patients with HLHS typically present with acidosis and shock. The most important issue in management is recognition or suspicion of a critical underlying congenital heart abnormality. In this regard, prompt initiation of prostaglandin therapy is indicated. Careful observation with appropriate supportive treatment ought to be given with efforts to make a definitive diagnosis as soon as possible. Supportive treatment ought to be given along with treatment of any other suspected illnesses until the differential diagnosis is clarified. If the diagnosis is made, avoidance of maneuvers that decrease PVR such as endotracheal intubation and hyperventilation will usually lead to improved systemic cardiac output and correction of the underlying acidosis; however, patients are frequently treated with standard resuscitative measures (endotracheal intubation, correction of acidosis, fluid boluses, inotropic therapy) until the diagnosis is made. Therefore, management is one of prostaglandin therapy and discontinuing, weaning, or reversal of any therapies

that may be counterproductive to restoring systemic cardiac output. The sooner the suspicion of critical cardiac disease arises, the sooner the patient will be directed toward appropriate management.

Over time, as the ductus arteriosus is kept open, the pulmonary blood flow will increase significantly, particularly since prostaglandin causes pulmonary vasodilation. This will eventually lead to pulmonary overcirculation and pulmonary edema with systemic steal. Therefore, pulmonary blood flow should not be allowed to be excessive. This can be accomplished by a process of hypoventilation (reduced respiratory rate, measured increase of PCO_2 and decrease of PaO_2) to induce pulmonary vasoconstriction, which will prevent excessive pulmonary blood flow. This process not only minimizes pulmonary edema, but also allows more blood to the aorta via the PDA, thus increasing systemic cardiac output.

Surgical management includes the Norwood procedure or cardiac transplantation. The Norwood procedure includes an initial palliative procedure followed by the Glenn and then the Fontan procedure. Palliation includes using the pulmonary valve and proximal MPA as the neoaorta by ligating the distal main pulmonary artery and connecting the proximal main pulmonary artery to the aortic arch. The aortic arch is augmented (reconstructed) and any coarctation removed in the process. The PDA is ligated in this process as well. This will improve the systemic blood flow. The pulmonary arteries are then supplied with a 3.5–4 mm systemic to pulmonary arterial shunt (BT shunt). In addition, the atrial septum is removed surgically. The first stage of Norwood procedure is performed at 1–2 weeks of age and the second stage (Glenn) at about 6–9 months of age. The second stage of the Norwood procedure involves takedown of the systemic to pulmonary arterial shunt and connection of the SVC to right pulmonary artery (Glenn shunt). The third stage of Norwood, usually performed 1 year after the Glenn shunt, consists of connecting the IVC to the pulmonary arteries through a tunnel in the right atrium, thus separating the deoxygenated from the well-oxygenated blood. The stages of the Norwood procedure with appropriate figures are described in Chapter 49.

An alternative surgical solution to the Norwood procedure is cardiac transplantation. The newborn is maintained on prostaglandins until a suitable donor heart is made available. Neonatal heart transplantation is becoming difficult because of a lack of donor hearts suitable in size for these babies. Many institutions are now opting for the Norwood procedure as the primary method of treatment.

Many cardiologists still give parents the option of nonintervention and instead provide compassionate care without mechanical ventilation or use of prostaglandins, with the understanding that all such children will die once the ductus arteriosus closes. This dilemma is discussed in Chapter 58.

Controversies in the Management of Hypoplastic Left Heart Syndrome

Controversies continue to exist in the management of HLHS. Aside from the ethics of whether any intervention ought to be undertaken (which is becoming less frequent as results of intervention continue to improve), there is the question on which type of procedure to perform, and the timing of the procedures. The Fontan procedure was at one time being performed as the second stage, though studies showed that mortality was decreased with a staged approach. The type and size of systemic to pulmonary shunt used in the first stage continues to be problematic as it is initially difficult to control pulmonary (and systemic) blood flow with fluctuating PVR. A right ventricle to pulmonary artery conduit (shunt) has been proposed and is being currently assessed. Combined surgical/interventional catheterizations have been proposed and are being tried in an effort to minimize surgical risks. These include placement of an interatrial stent, stent and stenting the ductus arteriosus in the catheterization laboratory, and placement of bilateral pulmonary artery bands in a limited surgical procedure.

Suggested Readings

Allen HD, Gutgesell HP, Clark EB, Driscoll DJ: *Moss and Adams' Heart Disease in Infants, Children and Adolescents Including the Fetus and Young Adult*, 6th ed. Philadelphia, PA, Lippincott Williams & Wilkins, 2001.

Bove EL, Hennein HA: Hypoplastic left heart syndrome, Armonk, NY, Futura Publishing, 2002.

Garson A, Bricker JT, Fisher DJ, Neish SR: *The Science and Practice of Pediatric Cardiology*, 2nd ed. Baltimore, MD, Williams & Wilkins, 1998.

Malec E, Januszewska K, Kolcz J, Mroczek T: Right ventricle-to-pulmonary artery shunt versus modified Blalock-Taussig shunt in the Norwood procedure for hypoplastic left heart syndrome—influence on early and late haemodynamic status. *Eur J Cardiothorac Surg* 23(5):728–734, 2003.

Michel-Behnke I, Akintuerk H, Marquardt I, Mueller M, Thul J, Bauer J, Hagel KJ, Kreuder J, Vogt P, Schranz D: Stenting of the ductus arteriosus and banding of the pulmonary arteries: basis for various surgical strategies in newborns with multiple left heart obstructive lesions. *Heart* 89(6):645–650, 2003.

Rycik J, Wernovsky G: *Hypoplastic Left Heart Syndrome*. Boston, Kluwer Academic Publishers, 2002.

Shime N, Hashimoto S, Hiramatsu N, Oka T, Kageyama K, Tanaka Y: Hypoxic gas therapy using nitrogen in the preoperative management of neonates with hypoplastic left heart syndrome, *Pediatr Crit Care Med* 1(1):38–41, 2000.

Torres A Jr, DiLiberti J, Pearl RH, Wohrley J, Raff GW, Bysani GK, Bond LM, Geiss DM: Noncardiac surgery in children with hypoplastic left heart syndrome, *J Pediatr Surg* 37(10):1399–1403, 2002.

27

COARCTATION OF THE AORTA

David J. Waight

INTRODUCTION

Coarctation of the aorta is a constriction, stricture, or stenosis of a portion of the aorta or aortic arch. Coarctation of the aorta constitutes approximately 8% of congenital heart disease or approximately 1 in every 1200–1300 people.

ANATOMY AND EMBRYOLOGY

Coarctation of the aorta results from a thickening of the media of the aortic wall that forms a ridge on the inner surface of the aorta. It is felt that the narrowing is caused by tissue of the ductus arteriosus. The exact genetic and molecular abnormality of this defect is unknown; however, patients with Turner syndrome and an XO genotype have a high incidence of coarctation. Approximately 15–20% of Turner patients have coarctation of the aorta. During fetal life, a ductus arteriosus is almost always patent, and the area of coarctation may be minimal. Hypoplasia of the arch, if it occurs, may be more noticeable. After the newborn period, the ductus arteriosus closes, at which time blood flow

must traverse the area of narrowing and a pressure gradient develops.

The most common location of coarctation of the aorta is adjacent to the point of insertion of the ligamentum arteriosum or the remnant of the patent ductus arteriosus (PDA) (Figure 27-1). This area of coarctation just distal to the origin of the left subclavian artery is the most common location for coarctation of the aorta at any age. With severe coarctation of the aorta, there is often hypoplasia of the proximal descending aorta, which is often referred to as a long segment coarctation. There may also be narrowing of the transverse and isthmic portion of the aortic arch known as a hypoplastic aortic arch. This is different from the hypoplastic arch seen with aortic or mitral atresia. In this case, the ascending aorta is most hypoplastic with lesser degrees of hypoplasia of the transverse and isthmic aorta.

Distal to the narrowed segment, there is often an enlargement of the descending aorta referred to as a poststenotic dilatation. This is not as prominent in cases of a hypoplastic aorta unless there is a large ductus arteriosus supplying blood flow to the distal segment. The degree of stenosis can vary

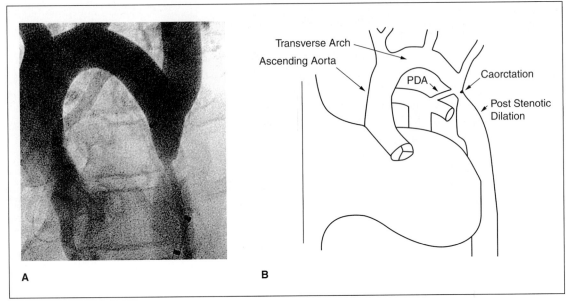

FIGURE 27-1

(**A**) Lateral projection of an aortic angiogram demonstrating a severe coarctation. (**B**) Diagram of arch anatomy and coarctation with a patent ductus arteriosus.

from a very mild degree of narrowing with a small pressure change across the aorta to severe obstruction or near interruption.

Coarctation of the aorta can also occur at other locations, including a rare incidence of abdominal coarctation.

ASSOCIATED ANATOMICAL DEFECTS

Coarctation of the aorta is often associated with a bicuspid aortic valve. A bicuspid aortic valve is the most common abnormality of the cardiovascular system and is associated with coarctation from 13–85% of the time. In contrast, only a small percentage of patients with a bicuspid aortic valve have coarctation of the aorta.

Coarctation can also be associated with other forms of left-sided obstruction, including mitral valve stenosis. Patients with several areas of obstruction in the left-sided circulation, including mitral stenosis, subaortic narrowing and coarctation, are often referred to as having Shone syndrome.

Coarctation can also be associated with more complex forms of congenital heart disease including

ventricular septal defect and cyanotic congenital heart disease including truncus arteriosus and transposition of the great arteries.

PATHOPHYSIOLOGY

Narrowing within the aorta leads to decreased pressure or hypotension, distal to the obstruction and may also cause hypertension proximal to the obstruction. The distal hypotension is associated with decreased blood flow to the abdominal organs and lower extremities, which may lead to ischemia of the organs and the muscles below the coarctation site. Hypertension proximal to the obstruction generally causes the head and neck vessels as well as the coronary arteries to be hypertensive. The left ventricle is subjected to this increased pressure (increased afterload), which may lead to significant left ventricular hypertrophy. With an acute increase in left ventricular afterload, the left ventricle may not be able to compensate and clinical heart failure may occur. If this occurs blood pressure may be decreased both proximal and distal to the area of obstruction since the ventricle cannot supply enough force to generate a pressure gradient. With uncorrected coarctation, this proximal hypertension may lead to early coronary and carotid artery disease, with an increased risk of myocardial infarction and stroke, respectively. Long-term LVH may also lead to myocardial dysfunction.

In the presence of complete, or near complete obstruction of the juxtaductal aorta, (usual site of coarctation) and the presence of a patent ductus arteriosus, blood can flow to the descending aorta if the pulmonary vascular resistance is elevated. This is the case in neonates. The blood flowing to the descending aorta is desaturated and lower extremity saturations will be decreased. A blood pressure difference may not be apparent as both the proximal and distal portions of the aorta may have good blood flow and relatively equal pressures.

People with significant obstruction across a coarctation may develop collateral vessels from the aorta above the obstruction to the aorta below the coarctation. These tortuous vessels provide a source of continuous flow from the high-pressure aorta to the lower pressure aorta and may produce a continuous murmur.

CLINICAL HISTORY

Coarctation of the aorta has two distinct presentations: (1) the neonatal period and (2) presentation in infancy, childhood, or adulthood. Neonates present with coarctation that is usually severe or critical. With later presentation, the coarctation is typically less severe and may have good flow to the descending aorta from collateral vessels.

When coarctation presents in the newborn period, it is often severe, and associated with a closing patent ductus arteriosus (Figure 27-1). Newborns with severe coarctation are often completely asymptomatic at birth and do not become symptomatic until they are 4–10 days of age. This delayed presentation is secondary to the presence of a patent ductus arteriosus, which allows flow to the descending aorta from the main pulmonary artery. Newborns have high pulmonary vascular resistance. The right ventricular, main pulmonary artery, and branch pulmonary artery pressures are elevated. This allows right-to-left shunting from the main pulmonary

artery across the patent ductus arteriosus to the descending aorta. This blood has a decreased oxygen content but provides adequate perfusion to the abdominal organs and lower extremities. After several days to a few weeks, the patent ductus arteriosus closes spontaneously, ending the right-to-left shunt and resulting in decreased perfusion to all areas below the coarctation site. Prior to ductal closure the only feature may be cyanosis of the lower extremities. Symptoms may be absent at this stage.

The primary presenting symptoms begin to occur with ductal closure or when there is associated left ventricular failure. These can include poor feeding with decreased volume of formula taken or abbreviated breast-feedings with diaphoresis during feeds. Newborns may also present with vomiting secondary to decreased bowel perfusion and intolerance of feedings. In newborns with critical coarctation, shock may occur.

In older infants, children, and adults, there are typically no symptoms, unless sequelae of coarctation occur (Table 27-1). These sequelae may include headaches (from hypertension), or left-sided heart failure from long-standing hypertension. Older children and adults may also present with claudication, which is leg pain with exercise, secondary to the inability of the body to increase the perfusion to the lower extremities during exercise owing to the fixed obstruction proximal to the descending aorta. Shock does not usually occur .

TABLE 27-1

FEATURES OF COARCTATION

Neonatal Presentation	Postneonatal Presentation
Shock	Symptoms of upper
Acidosis/distress	extremity hypertension
Poor perfusion	Headache
Lower extremity cyanosis	LV failure
Feeding difficulty	Symptoms of lower
Diaphoresis	extremity hypotension
	Calf pain
	Poor pulses
	Bruits/murmur because
	of collaterals

CLINICAL EXAMINATION

The physical signs observed on presentation may include diminished, absent, or delayed femoral and lower extremity pulses, or a prolonged capillary refill time of greater than 2 s in the lower extremities. Pulses in the right radial artery are normal, with pulses in the femoral, posterior tibial, or dorsalis pedis arteries poorly felt, delayed, or absent. This exam finding is confirmed with a differential blood pressure from the upper extremities to the lower extremities. Most commonly, this is obtained from the right arm and either lower extremity. An origin of the left subclavian in the area of the coarctation may lead to a lower blood pressure in the left arm than the right arm. In the rare case of an aberrant origin of the right subclavian artery from the descending aorta, a blood pressure differential will not be seen with coarctation.

In newborns with critical coarctation and a patent ductus arteriosus with right-to-left shunting, there may be differential oxygen saturations with the saturation in the upper extremities being normal and the saturation in the lower extremities being decreased. It is important to consider coarctation as a possible diagnosis in an infant presenting with significant signs of congestive heart failure in the first 2 weeks of life after being well for several days.

Infants, children, and adults do not generally present with signs of severe congestive heart failure or shock but do present with decreased femoral pulses, hypertension, or milder forms of congestive heart failure. A murmur may be noted corresponding to the location of the coarctation, heard best in the left infraclavicular area, the left axilla or, in the left posterior chest. This is a systolic murmur that may extend into diastole because of the continuous pressure difference between the upper and lower extremities. There may be an ejection click and ejection systolic murmur (from a mild gradient) at the right upper sternal border in patients with an associated bicuspid aortic valve. A murmur may also be heard from collateral vessels. The latter develop in the ascending aorta in response to distal hypoperfusion and connect to the descending aorta and provide a stable but diminished blood supply to the branches of the descending aorta. The murmur is often audible in the left axilla and possibly in the back. This is a continuous murmur from continuous flow of blood from the high pressure ascending aorta to the lower pressure descending aorta. Technically, it may be more appropriate to use the term bruit, rather than a murmur.

LABORATORY FINDINGS

Electrocardiogram or ECG

The ECG is most commonly normal in patients with coarctation. Increased left-sided voltages indicating left ventricular hypertrophy may be present in older children and adults with coarctation and longstanding hypertension. Right bundle branch block suggesting right ventricular hypertrophy is also noted in up to 50% of older children and adults.

Chest Radiograph

The plain film of the chest in patients with coarctation of the aorta generally demonstrates a normal heart size and normal pulmonary vascular markings, unless there is associated heart failure. An enlarged ascending aorta may produce a somewhat more prominent aortic bulge on the right side of the spine. In the area of the discrete coarctation, there may be an indentation visible with the proximal descending aorta seen on the left side of the spine. There may also be poststenotic dilatation of the aorta seen below the coarctation segment. This can appear as what is called a "three-sign" on the left para-mediastinal shadow in the anterior posterior chest radiograph. The phenomena of rib-notching visible on AP CXR is essentially pathognomonic of coarctation of the aorta. This notching is visible on the undersurface of the ribs because of dilation of the intercostal vessels that are serving as collateral supply from the ascending to the descending aorta. Rib-notching is commonly seen in older children and adults and is uncommon in children less than approximately 5 years of age.

Echocardiogram

The diagnosis of coarctation of the aorta can usually be confirmed with an echocardiogram after the diagnosis is established with clinical exam and blood pressure measurements. The prominent features noted on the echocardiogram include a two-dimensional view of the proximal descending aorta showing a narrowed aortic segment at the site of the coarctation, a tubular hypoplasia (in some newborns), and the poststenotic dilatation of the aorta. This is somewhat dependent on excellent imaging, which is usually possible in the neonate. In patients with difficult imaging, few or none of these features may be visible. This is more common in older or adult patients.

Doppler imaging of the aorta is the most diagnostic echocardiographic imaging for coarctation of the aorta. Doppler evaluation of the descending aorta shows an altered waveform with diastolic runoff that is diagnostic of coarctation of the aorta. With Doppler echocardiography, a high velocity signal may be noted in the area of the coarctation because of the pressure gradient across the narrowed area. Altered patterns of this jet may be seen as well, which further indicate a coarctation is present. The common finding is a double density with both low and higher velocity signals overlapping (a double envelope) and diastolic runoff.

Additional defects can also be noted by echocardiography including a bicuspid or stenotic aortic valve, subaortic stenosis, mitral stenosis, and left ventricular hypertrophy or dysfunction. Other defects, such as ventricular septal defects, or more complex forms of congenital heart disease may also be seen.

Magnetic Resonance Imaging

Magnetic resonance imaging, or MRI, is a useful tool in the evaluation of patients with coarctation owing to its ability to adequately image the entire aortic arch, including the abdominal aorta. The MRI is also used for follow-up of patients after surgical or catheter intervention when evaluating for recurrent coarctation.

Cardiac Catheterization

Cardiac catheterization remains a useful tool in the evaluation of patients with coarctation because of the excellent imaging available with aortic angiography. The precise gradient across the area of the coarctation is measured by evaluating the pressure above and below the area of the coarctation. Additional cardiac defects can also be imaged with angiography. The exact origin of the head and neck vessels and their relation to the coarctation is well defined by angiography. The coarctation segment and long segment coarctation are best viewed on the lateral plane angiogram.

TREATMENT

The treatment of patients with coarctation of the aorta include medical management, interventional cardiac catheterization, and surgery. The appropriate therapy for an individual patient varies with the time of presentation.

Newborns and small infants who present with severe coarctation are often initially managed with medical therapy. This therapy includes management of heart failure, acidosis, or shock. Intubation and mechanical ventilation may be required.

On initial presentation, newborns and infants in the first few weeks of life should also be treated with prostaglandin E1. Prostaglandin will pharmacologically keep a patent ductus arteriosus open and possibly allow a closed ductus arteriosus (prior to irreversible obliteration) to become patent again. The opening of the PDA serves two purposes for infants with coarctation. By allowing a patent passage from the main pulmonary artery to the descending aorta, it allows perfusion of the descending aorta from flow through the pulmonary artery. The ductus arteriosus is usually located directly adjacent to the site of the coarctation segment. When the PDA is open, it allows an increased diameter in the area of the coarctation. This will also allow improved antegrade flow from the ascending aorta through the narrowed portion of the aorta. The latter may occur even if the ductus arteriosus is not reopened. Thus, a trial of prostaglandin is almost always attempted in a neonate.

Definitive therapy of coarctation can be achieved with surgical repair, balloon dilatation, or a combination of balloon dilatation and stent implantation. Surgical management of coarctation of the aorta can be applied in any age group but is most commonly used in infants and small children as primary therapy.

Balloon dilatation of the coarctation segment is most commonly performed in children greater than 1 year of age. Therapy with balloon dilatation and stent implantation is generally reserved for older children and adults. In these patients the implantation of a stent that can be easily expanded to adult size is practical with a limited risk of damage to the femoral artery.

Surgical Management

The standard surgical approach for aortic coarctation is a left thoracotomy, which is usually muscle-sparing, meaning the lattissimus dorsi muscle is simply reflected and not divided. The isthmus of the aorta is approached by dividing the parietal pleura. Care is taken to preserve the vagus and recurrent laryngeal nerves as well as the phrenic nerve. The entire aortic arch and descending aorta are dissected circumferentially for prevention of tension on the anastomosis. Clamps are placed above and below the narrowed area. The stenotic portion is resected and both ends anastomosed together. In cases of aortic arch hypoplasia, a so-called extended end-end anastomosis is performed, which means that the incisions go up to the left carotid artery and beyond proximally, and down the posterior aspect of the descending aorta over several millimeters. Both openings are then much larger and are anastomosed in a similar fashion. This procedure enlarges the aortic arch to a significant degree and is mostly performed in infants. Complications include nerve injury, chylothorax, and residual or recurrent recoarctation. The overall results are excellent, with essentially no mortality and a <5% recoarctation rate in noninfants and <15% in infants. Surgery for recoarctation has virtually disappeared, since recoarctation is treated preferentially by balloon dilatation. Other surgical repairs such as the left subclavian flap (tying off the distal left subclavian artery and using the proximal portion as a patch to enlarge the coarctation area) and patch aortoplasty (prosthetic patch is used to enlarge the coarctation area) are used very infrequently.

Neonates presenting with large VSDs and aortic coarctation are sometimes better managed with a single-stage surgery via sternotomy. The VSD is closed using standard cardiopulmonary bypass techniques and the aortic arch repaired with an extended end-end anastomosis, sometimes adding a small proximal patch.

RECOARCTATION

There is a significant incidence of recurrent narrowing of the aorta (recoarctation) following both initial balloon angioplasty in smaller infants and surgical correction of coarctation. Recoarctation of the aorta presents in the same manner as primary coarctation but the therapy is generally confined to balloon dilatation of the recoarctation segment.

CONTROVERSIES

The management of patients with coarctation is controversial because of the three forms of therapy that may be used. Balloon dilatation can be done in any age group, although it has not been shown to be as successful in children under 6 months of age because of a high recurrence rate. The use of stent implantation in the coarctation segment combined with balloon angioplasty is a relatively new strategy in the treatment of coarctation of the aorta. Although stent implantation produces a minimal or no residual gradient, the need for a large sheath size limits its use to larger children and adults. Long-term follow-up of patients following stent implantation has not yet been studied because of the relatively recent use of this therapy. Early midterm results have been very encouraging.

Suggested Readings

Beekman RH: Coarctation of the Aorta, in: Emmanoulides GC, Riemenschneider TA, Allen HD, Gutgesell HP (eds.): *Moss and Adams Heart Disease in Infants, Children, and Adolescents*, 5th ed. Baltimore, MD, Williams & Wilkins, 1995.

Morris MJH, McNamara DG: Coarctation of the aorta and interrupted aortic arch, in: Garson A, Bricker JT, Fisher DJ, Neish SR (eds.): *The Science and Practice of Pediatric Cardiology*, 2nd ed. Baltimore, MD, Williams & Wilkins, 1998.

Quaegebeur JM, Jonas RA, Weinberg AD, Blackstone EH, Kirklin JW: Outcomes in seriously ill neonates with coarctation of the aorta. A multiinstitutional study. *J Thorac Cardiovasc Surg* 108:841–854, 1994.

28

TOTAL ANOMALOUS PULMONARY VENOUS CONNECTION

David G. Ruschhaupt

ANATOMY AND EMBRYOLOGY

Total anomalous pulmonary venous connection (TAPVC), also known as total anomalous pulmonary venous return (TAPVR) defines the condition where communication of the common pulmonary vein and the left atrium has been interrupted. This defect complex represents approximately 2–3% of all congenital heart defects. During normal embryologic development of the heart, the pulmonary veins from both lungs combine to form a common pulmonary vein, which then fuses into the left atrium to become its posterior wall (Figure 28-1). When this process fails to occur, alternative venous pathways develop. In TAPVC, all of the pulmonary and systemic venous blood return is to the right atrium. Patient survival requires that there be an atrial septal defect (fossa ovalis) or an unobstructed patent foramen ovale.

Embryologic interruption of the common pulmonary venous pathway to the left atrium results in supradiaphragmatic (70%), infradiaphragmatic (25%), and mixed (5%) alternative connections of the pulmonary veins to the right atrium. In virtually all cases, there is a common pulmonary venous sinus, which in turn connects to a systemic vein and then to the right atrium. The most common supradiaphragmatic connection is to the left vertical vein with the ultimate drainage site being the left superior vena cava (Figure 28-2) or to the coronary sinus. Other supradiaphragmatic drainage sites are to the right horn of the sinus venosus (right superior vena cava or the azygous vein) or the right atrium directly. Infradiaphragmatic sites of drainage have a long vertical common venous channel, which perforates the diaphragm and drains either to the portal vein or the ductus venosus (Figure 28-2). Less commonly observed drainage sites are the gastric vein, left or right hepatic veins, or directly to the inferior vena cava.

Stenosis of the pulmonary venous system is a common and serious associated lesion. Virtually all

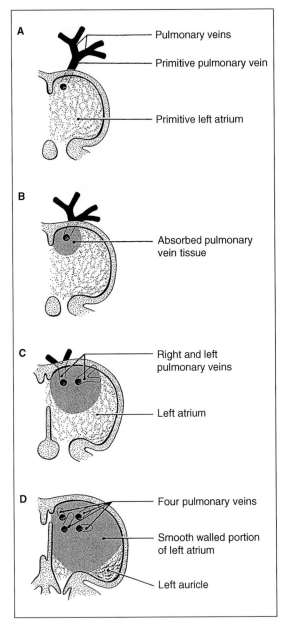

FIGURE 28-1

EMBRYOLOGY OF THE PULMONARY VEINS

Source: Moore KL. *The Developing Human. Clinically Oriented Embryology.* 4th ed. Philadelphia: WB Saunders, 1988.

of the infradiaphragmatic cases are obstructed. This is because the long, vertical common channel obstructs either at the level of the diaphragm or at its final venous insertion site. The supradiapragmatic connections also may have obstructions but this is less frequent. In general, when the connection is to the right atrium, obstruction is not found. Coronary sinus drainage has been found to be obstructed 20% of the time. The left superior vena cava may obstruct 40% of the time at the junction of the SVC and the innominate vein or in the uncommon situation where the vertical vein passes between the left pulmonary artery and the left main bronchus. Sixty-five percent of veins draining to the azygous vein are obstructed.

PATHOPHYSIOLOGY

Total anomalous venous connection is a cyanotic congenital heart defect. Since all of the systemic veins and pulmonary veins converge into the right atrium, there must be arterial desaturation. The severity of cyanosis, however, depends on the amount of pulmonary blood flow. The greater the pulmonary flow, the less the cyanosis. Adequate systemic cardiac output is dependent on sufficient right-to-left atrial shunting through the atrial septal defect. The left atrium is small. This is because the common pulmonary vein has not contributed to the anatomic volume of the left atrium. The left ventricle is significantly reduced in size because of the reduced volume of flow. In contrast, there is volume and pressure overload of the right ventricle and right atrium with enlargement of the tricuspid valve orifice (Figure 28-3).

When the pulmonary veins drain anomalously without obstruction, there usually is marked increase in pulmonary blood flow. This means that there will be a large increase in the volume of oxygenated pulmonary venous blood returning to the right atrium. The expected cyanosis, therefore, will tend to be concealed. Systemic arterial saturations will usually range between 87 and 95%. Pulmonary artery hypertension resulting from the increased pulmonary blood flow with pressures exceeding

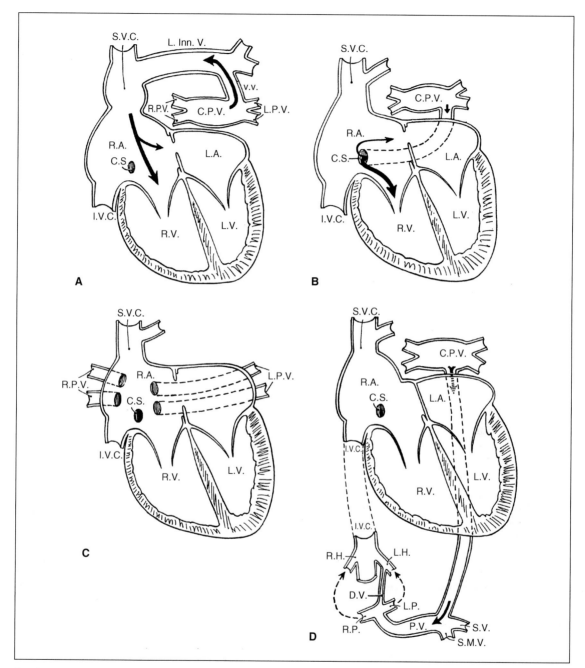

FIGURE 28-2

INSERTION OF PULMONARY VEINS IN TAPVC

Source: Moss' Heart Disease in Infants, Children, and Adults. 4th ed. Baltimore: Williams & Wilkins, 1989.

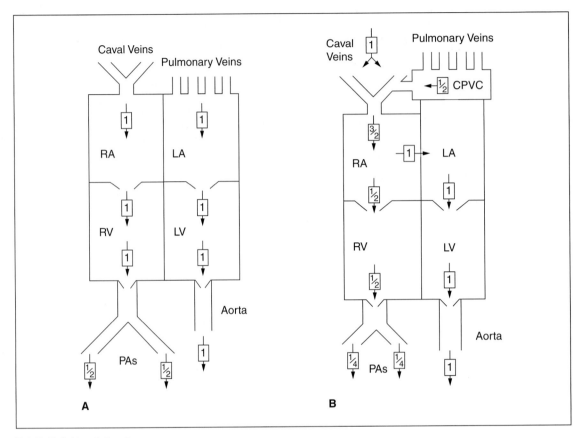

FIGURE 28-3

DIAGRAM OF A NORMAL HEART

Pathophysiology of TAPVC. (**A**) Normal heart with one relative cardiac output flowing to both the pulmonary and systemic circulations and in each cardiac chamber. (**B**) Diagram of TAPVC with elevated PVR. **A** demonstrates the changes seen with TAPVC and elevated PVR as seen in the neonate. As seen, the ratio of highly saturated pulmonary venous return (half relative cardiac output in this example) is less than the desaturated systemic venous return (one relative cardiac output). Thus, systemic oxygen saturations will be significantly decreased. The CPVC is the common pulmonary venous chamber. Note the need for an atrial communication (usually a PFO) to supply systemic output. (**C**) TAPVC with lower PVR. **C** demonstrates the changes that occur as PVR is lowered from the elevated levels in the neonate as shown in **B**. Note the increased pulmonary venous return (two relative cardiac outputs in this example) mixing with systemic venous return (one relative cardiac output) yielding a greater amount of saturated vs. desaturated blood mixed in the right atrium. In this example, there is twice the normal flow across the tricuspid and pulmonary valves, thus there is increased turbulence and pathologic murmurs of function tricuspid and pulmonary stenosis. (**D**) TAPVC with obstruction. **D** demonstrates the changes that occur with obstruction of blood flow between the common pulmonary venous chamber and the systemic venous system. Note the minimal amount of pulmonary venous return (one-eighth relative cardiac output) mixing with systemic venous return in the right atrium. Thus, there will be severe systemic oxygen desaturation. If the obstruction becomes complete, oxygenation will not occur at all.

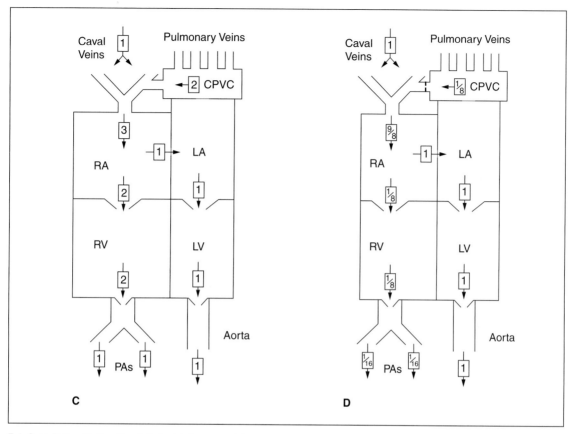

FIGURE 28-3 (continued)

50% of systemic levels, is a constant feature of this lesion.

Obstructed anomalous pulmonary veins produce a different physiologic picture. Severe pulmonary venous obstruction produces pulmonary edema and pulmonary arterial hypertension. Sometimes pulmonary arterial pressure will even exceed systemic pressure levels. Because of the venous obstruction, pulmonary arterial blood flow is significantly reduced. If the ductus arteriosus remains patent, there will be shunting of desaturated pulmonary arterial blood into the descending aorta. The combination of pulmonary edema, right-to-left ductal shunting, and reduced pulmonary artery blood flow produces severe cyanosis and acidosis.

Figure 28-3 demonstrates the underlying pathophysiology.

CLINICAL HISTORY

Because of the mild cyanosis and the unimpressive cardiac murmur, babies with unobstructed supradiaphragmatic type of anomalous pulmonary venous connection may initially escape detection; however, the large amount of pulmonary artery overcirculation and pulmonary edema reduce lung compliance. The resulting tachypnea, with respiratory rates often as high as 80 breaths per minute, poor feeding, sweating with feeds, and failure to thrive compel detection. Babies with the obstructed form of total anomalous pulmonary venous connection are quite ill with significant cyanosis and severe tachypnea and acidosis. Often these babies may be misdiagnosed with persistent fetal circulation or hyaline membrane disease because of cyanosis, acidosis, tachypnea, abnormal lungs by chest radiography and the absence of clearly pathologic cardiac murmurs.

CLINICAL EXAMINATION

The typical physical examination for a patient with unobstructed total anomalous pulmonary venous connection will show mild cyanosis. The arterial oxygen saturations may range from 85 to 95% depending on the volume of pulmonary blood flow. The precordium will be hyperdynamic, reflecting right ventricular volume enlargement and pulmonary arterial hypertension. The first heart sound will have an increased intensity, and is best appreciated at the 3rd and 4th left intercostal space. Likewise, there will be an increase in intensity of the second heart sound. Because of the increase in right ventricular volume load, there will usually be a prominent filling 3rd heart sound at the left lower sternal border accompanied by a diastolic rumble murmur indicating the increased flow volume across the tricuspid valve. The increased stroke volume of the right ventricle generates a grade 1–2 ejection systolic murmur at the pulmonary valve location. When the anomalous veins drain to the left superior vena cava, the turbulence of flow created at the

TABLE 28-1

CLINICAL PRESENTATION TAPVC

Supradiaphragmatic	
Cyanosis:	Mild; oxygen saturation between 88 and 94%
Respiration:	Tachypnea with rates up to 70–80 BPM[a]
Precordium:	Very hyperdynamic
Murmur:	Grade 1+ ejection systolic, LUSB S3; Grade 1+ diastolic rumble LLSB Possible left infraclavicular continuous murmur

[a]BPM: Breaths per minute.

TABLE 28-2

CLINICAL PRESENTATION TAPVC

Infradiaphragmatic	
Cyanosis:	Severe; oxygen saturation <60%
Respiration:	Tachypnea with retractions
Precordium:	Active
Murmur:	None

vertical vein's point of entry to the innominate vein may create a continuous "venous hum" murmur. This murmur may be confused with a patent ductus arteriosus (Table 28-1). Babies with the obstructed form of total anomalous venous connection are significantly cyanotic and tachypneic. The pulmonary venous obstruction causes increased pulmonary vascular resistance with pulmonary edema and pulmonary artery hypertension. Tachypnea results. The precordium is hyperdynamic. S1 and S2 are both increased. Cyanosis and acidosis are the dominant features of the clinical examination (Table 28-2).

LABORATORY FINDINGS

Electrocardiography: The ECG shows peaked p waves, reflecting right atrial enlargement. Severe right ventricular hypertrophy is also present, often with a qR configuration in lead V1.

Chest radiography: Cardiac enlargement and evidence for increased pulmonary arterial blood flow are present on the chest radiograph. Classically the chest radiograph of the older child with pulmonary venous drainage to the left superior vena cava would demonstrate a widened mediastinum, sometimes referred to as a "snowman" configuration of the heart. The "snowman" is created by the heart, a dilated vertical vein, a dilated innominant vein, and a dilated superior vena cava into which the latter drain. With pulmonary venous obstruction, the heart size may be normal; however, the lungs will show pulmonary edema that may resemble the findings of hyaline membrane disease.

TABLE 28-3

LABORATORY FINDINGS TAPVC

	Supradiaphragmatic	*Infradiaphragmatic*
Chest x-ray	Cardiomegally	Small heart
	Increased PBF	Pulmonary edema
	Widened mediastinum	
ECG	Right atrial enlargement	Right atrial enlargement
	RVH with qR in lead v1	RVH with qR in lead v1
Echo	Small LA and LV	Small LA and LV
	Large right ventricle	Large right ventricle
	Paradoxic septal motion	Right-to-left PDA shunt
	Right-to-left atrial shunt	Right-to-left atrial shunt
	Abnormal pulmonary vein	Abnormal pulmonary vein

Echocardiography: Cardiac ultrasound has created the possibility of making the diagnosis without cardiac catheterization. The right atrium and right ventricle are very dilated. The left atrium and left ventricle are small. Color flow Doppler echocardiography allows identification of the right-to-left shunting across the atria and, most importantly, the location and drainage site of the anomalous pulmonary venous channel. If there is tricuspid valve regurgitation, the pulmonary artery pressure may also be estimated. In the newborn with pulmonary venous obstruction and suprasystemic level pulmonary artery hypertension, color Doppler flow may also identify right-to-left shunting via the ductus arteriosus.

Cardiac catheterization and angiography: If catheterization is performed, the catheter may be placed directly into the common as well as the branch pulmonary veins to determine if there is obstruction within the channel. Oxygen saturation determinations will be highest at the site of the pulmonary venous channel's entry into the systemic veins. Once mixing of pulmonary and systemic venous blood has occurred, the oxygen saturation measurement will be similar, if not identical, in all of the cardiac chambers. Pulmonary arteriography and or selective pulmonary venous angiography will show the exact drainage pattern and show if there is mixed anomalous venous drainage.

The laboratory findings are summarized in Table 28-3.

TREATMENT

Once the diagnosis of total anomalous connection of the pulmonary veins is established, the treatment is surgical. In the case of obstructed pulmonary venous connection, immediate surgical intervention is required and will be life-saving. There may be a temptation to delay the surgery for the unobstructed infants since they are not critically ill; however, there is no technical advantage to this approach. The repair is usually performed under deep hypothermic circulatory arrest. The pulmonary venous confluence is identified and anastomosed to the back of the true left atrium. The vertical vein, whether infra or supradiaphragmatic, is most often ligated. Mortality for the obstructed form of TAPVC remains relatively high (20%). This is a function of the poor clinical condition prior to surgery, and may also be related to noncardiac or chromosomal anomalies. The unobstructed form of TAPVC has a lower mortality (<5%) because these patients are usually older and in better preoperative condition.

LONG-TERM OUTLOOK

The long-term outlook for repaired TAPVC is good. Complications include pulmonary venous restenosis. Atrial arrhythmias may be encountered but are not usually a long-term problem. In the absence of pulmonary venous stenosis, the long-term prognosis is good. SBE prophylaxis is required for life.

Suggested Readings

Allen HD, Gutgesell HP, Clark EB, Driscoll DJ: *Moss and Adams' Heart Disease in Infants, Children, and Adolescents Including the Fetus and Young Adult*, 6th ed. Philadelphia, PA, Lippincott Williams & Wilkins, 2001.

Garson A, Bricker JT, Fisher DJ, Neish SR: *The Science and Practice of Pediatric Cardiology*, 2nd ed. Baltimore, MD, Williams & Wilkins, 1998.

29

SINGLE VENTRICLE

Ernerio Alboliras

INTRODUCTION

Single ventricle is a heart that is missing the inflow or nontrabeculated portion of either ventricle. Most cases of tricuspid atresia and mitral atresia retain at least a remnant of this aspect of the right ventricle or left ventricle and are thus not considered single ventricle. Likewise, unbalanced complete common atrioventricular canal, where one ventricle is dominant and the other is hypoplastic, is not a single ventricle. All of the above conditions, however, may manifest with a similar pathophysiology. In a similar fashion, double outlet right ventricle may have a similar physiology of a single ventricle.

Single ventricle is rare, occurring in about 5 per 100,000 live births. Single ventricle can be classified based on the morphology of the ventricle:

1. Single left ventricle
2. Single right ventricle
3. Common ventricle

EMBRYOLOGY

The embryology of single ventricle is still unknown. Presumably, both ventricular septation and movement of the common atrioventricular orifice are disrupted.

ANATOMY

Both atria connect to the single ventricle via either a common atrioventricular valve (common inlet) or separate atrioventricular valves (double inlet).

Single left ventricle is the most common morphologic type. The main ventricular chamber has the characteristic numerous fine trabeculations of a left ventricle. A double inlet single left ventricle (often called double inlet left ventricle) is the most common inflow characteristic, but a common inlet could also occur. Rarely, a double inlet single left ventricle with two annuli fibrosi but with membranous atresia of either valve may be found. A single left ventricle commonly has an outlet chamber, a rudimentary outlet portion of the right ventricle, which is believed to have its embryonic origin from the bulbus cordis and not from the embryonic ventricle. This anteriorly located outlet chamber may be to the left (seen in l-looped heart) or right (seen in d-looped heart) of the ventricle. The ventricular chamber communicates with the outlet chamber through an outlet known as the bulboventricular foramen. The outlet chamber typically is aligned with the aorta, with the pulmonary artery arising from the main ventricular chamber. The great arteries may be l-malposed (aorta is anterior, to the left, and parallel to the main pulmonary artery), d-malposed (aorta is anterior, to the right, and parallel to the main pulmonary artery), or normally related (the so-called Holme's heart, wherein both arteries have a normal relationship, with the main pulmonary artery coursing obliquely from its anterior and rightward location to a leftward location). The most common arterial alignment is l-malposition, with the aorta arising anteriorly and leftward from the outlet chamber. Rarely, both great arteries may arise from the outlet chamber.

Single right ventricle is characterized by coarse trabeculae carnae. A common inlet single right ventricle is usual, although a double inlet single right ventricle may also be seen. There is no outlet chamber. There are rare instances reported of the presence of a slit-like compartment that is extremely small, presumed to be a left ventricle, posterior to the main ventricular chamber, with no atrioventricular valve or great arterial communication. The ventricle–great artery relationship is thus that of a double outlet right ventricle, unless there is atresia of one great artery. Various types of great artery malpositions can also occur—(e.g., d-malposition if the aorta is anterior and to the right of the main pulmonary artery, l-malposed if the aorta is anterior and to the left of the main pulmonary artery, or the aorta can be directly anterior or posterior to the main pulmonary artery).

Common ventricle is the rarest type of single ventricle, wherein components of both the right ventricle (coarse trabeculation) and left ventricle (fine trabeculation) are seen on each side of the single ventricle with no ventricular septum.

Other pathologic findings may be seen in single ventricle. The bulboventricular foramen of the outlet chamber in a single left ventricle may be obstructively small. This may result in various degrees of obstruction to the vessel arising from the outlet chamber such as aortic stenosis, atresia, arch interruption, or coarctation. It is a common observation that if the vessel arising from the main ventricular chamber is stenotic or atretic, the bulboventricular foramen is nonobstructive; however, if the aorta arises from the outlet chamber, pulmonary artery banding is known to lead to progressive obstruction of the bulboventricular foramen. Other anomalies that may be seen in single ventricle include (1) stenosis, regurgitation, cleft or dysplasia of the atrioventricular valve; (2) various systemic venous anomalies such as bilateral superior venae cavae; (3) patent ductus arteriosus; (4) secundum atrial septal defect; (5) double aortic arch; and (6) pulmonary stenosis or atresia. Additional rare findings that can be observed, especially in single right ventricle, are dextrocardia, asplenia, polysplenia, and multiple congenital anomalies.

PATHOPHYSIOLOGY

The lack of separation of the pulmonary circulation and systemic circulation causes mixing of oxygenated and unoxygenated blood, resulting in various degrees of cyanosis (Figure 29-1). The amount of effective pulmonary blood flow determines the amount of cyanosis. The presence of pulmonary stenosis or atresia, or elevated pulmonary resistance, may result in cyanosis that may be present early after birth. A single ventricle also acts as a common mixing chamber similar to a large ventricular septal defect. If there is no pulmonary stenosis, the normal reduction of pulmonary resistance after birth can result in gradually increasing pulmonary blood flow ultimately causing pulmonary overcirculation and later pulmonary vascular disease (Eisenmenger syndrome). In the presence of severe aortic outflow, obstruction there may be profoundly diminished systemic perfusion and shock.

CLINICAL FINDINGS

The near-routine use of obstetric ultrasonography with acquisition of the fetal cardiac four-chamber view has made antenatal diagnosis of single ventricle common. Postnatally, the majority of patients develop signs and symptoms in the first few days or weeks of life. Those that manifest early are usually

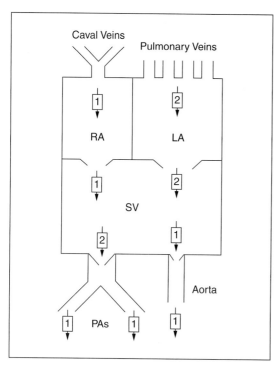

FIGURE 29-1

DIAGRAM SHOWING A SINGLE VENTRICLE

In this diagram, the aorta and pulmonary arteries arise from one ventricular chamber and there is no obstruction to pulmonary or systemic blood flow. There are two relative cardiac outputs flowing to the lungs compared to one cardiac output to the systemic circulation, which reflects the lower resistance in the pulmonary circulation. The saturation of the body is the same as the saturation of blood in the pulmonary circulation if adequate mixing occurs in the single ventricle. The saturation reflects the relative amounts of blood returning from the lungs via the pulmonary veins versus that returning from the body through the caval veins (superior and inferior vena cava). Thus, if there is obstruction to pulmonary blood flow (or elevated pulmonary vascular resistance), the net pulmonary arterial and venous flow will be less, and the saturations will be decreased. If there is aortic obstruction, pulmonary arterial and venous blood flow will be increased; if obstruction is severe, systemic cardiac output could be compromised.

patients with pulmonary stenosis who present with cyanosis, while those with aortic obstruction present with poor peripheral perfusion. In the absence of pulmonary stenosis, the presentation is later, with the appearance of signs and symptoms of pulmonary overcirculation. If there is aortic

obstruction as in coarctation or interruption, there may be a difference in blood pressure between the right arm and a lower extremity. The first heart sound is normal. The second heart sound is single. A systolic ejection murmur is present in those with outflow obstruction. A diastolic rumble of functional mitral stenosis may be seen if there is significant pulmonary blood flow, and thus increased flow across the atrioventricular valve.

DIAGNOSIS

The electrocardiogram is not usually helpful for diagnosis. It may demonstrate right, left, or combined ventricular hypertrophy. Deviation of the QRS axis and abnormalities in atrial depolarization or atrioventricular conduction may be seen. Chest radiography only provides assessment of cardiac size and position and the amount of pulmonary vascularity. The more decreased the pulmonary vascularity, the more cyanotic the patient, and the more increased the pulmonary vascularity the more likely the patient presents with tachypnea and other signs of pulmonary overcirculation.

Two-dimensional echocardiography is diagnostic for single ventricle. The information that is obtained from a high-quality echocardiographic study may be sufficient to send patients for palliative initial surgery without preoperative cardiac catheterization. Echocardiography identifies the morphologic type of single ventricle, ventricular function, atrioventricular valve anatomy and integrity, presence of bulboventricular foramen obstruction, presence of aortic arch obstruction, presence of pulmonary stenosis, presence of pulmonary artery distortion, the presence of systemic and pulmonary venous anomalies, and the caliber of the ductus arteriosus. Prior to the bidirectional Glenn or hemi-Fontan operation, echocardiography may identify pulmonary artery distortion, anomalies of systemic venous return (i.e., bilateral superior venae cavae), ventricular function and atrioventricular valve performance. Prior to the Fontan operation, echocardiography can be used to identify any pulmonary artery distortion, assess ventricular and atrioventricular valve function, and provide clues for the presence of pulmonary arteriovenous mal-formations. After the Fontan operation, echocardio-graphy can be used to assess cardiac function, the integrity of the systemic venous pathway, the fenes-tration (in cases in which a fenestrated Fontan oper-ation has been adopted), presence of pulmonary arterial distortion, thrombus formation, and the presence of pericardial or pleural effusions and ascites.

Cardiac catheterization is largely reserved for evaluating the systemic, pulmonary venous, and pul-monary artery architecture that may not be defined by echocardiography, characterizing pre- and post-Fontan hemodynamics, and for invasive electrophys-iologic studies and management of arrhythmias.

TREATMENT

Mothers with antenatally diagnosed fetal single ventricle are advised to deliver in a tertiary care institution with postnatal evaluation in an intensive care setting. Intravenous prostaglandin E_1 is indi-cated for cases with severe pulmonary stenosis or atresia and for severe aortic arch obstruction.

Surgical management is similar to tricuspid atresia or hypoplastic left heart syndrome. The eventual goal is a staged separation of the systemic venous from the pulmonary venous circulation with eventual creation of a cavopulmonary circulation or the modified Fontan operation. The management strategy of single ventricle physiology is complex and involves many decision points (Figure 29-2).

The modified Fontan operation cannot be safely accomplished in infancy because of the increased pulmonary vascular resistance, which takes several months to decline to acceptable levels. If pul-monary outflow obstruction exists, a systemic-to-pulmonary artery shunt may be needed. If aortic arch obstruction exists, the approach is reestab-lishing unobstructed aortic arch flow and limiting pulmonary blood flow. Banding of the pulmonary artery has been replaced by other methods be-cause patients frequently develop progressive bul-boventricular foramen obstruction. This bulbo-ventricular foramen obstruction is also seen in bidirectional Glenn and Fontan operations

because of conformational changes after reducing the volume load from the single ventricle. In order to avoid the possibility of a hemodynamically sig-nificant aortic obstruction, a Norwood-type recon-struction with proximal main pulmonary artery-to-aorta anastomosis is favored. A systemic-to-pul-monary artery shunt is then connected between the aorta and the pulmonary arterial confluence. Complete ligation of main pulmonary artery and placement of a systemic-to-pulmonary artery shunt can be another option in a single ventricle with no outlet chamber and with a large aortic outflow. The eventual creation of a cavopulmonary circulation is more safely accomplished in stages over 1–2 years because of the associated acute increase in ventric-ular wall thickness, acute decrease in ventricular chamber size, and acute impairment of myocardial performance because of acute volume unloading. An intermediate operation, the bidirectional Glenn shunt or the hemi-Fontan operation, results in less severe changes in ventricular wall thickness and chamber size, and is well tolerated. It can be safe-ly performed at around 6 months of age and is the preferred staging operation in most institutions.

The final stage is the creation of a cavopul-monary circulation, or the modified Fontan opera-tion. Atriopulmonary anastomosis has been replaced by placement of either a "lateral tunnel" or extracar-diac conduit between the inferior vena cava and the pulmonary confluence. This so-called final stage commonly takes the form of a fenestrated Fontan, a 4–5 mm hole between the systemic venous baffle and the pulmonary venous atrium or a 4–5 mm tube graft between the extracardiac conduit and the pul-monary venous atrium. The fenestrated Fontan oper-ation is associated with a decreased incidence of pericardial and pleural effusions, and a decreased incidence of protein-losing enteropathy.

OTHER DEFECTS WITH SINGLE VENTRICLE PATHOPHYSIOLOGY

Biventricular hearts may have presentations that are similar to the various types of single ventricle. These include unbalanced complete common atri-oventricular canal with hypoplasia of either right

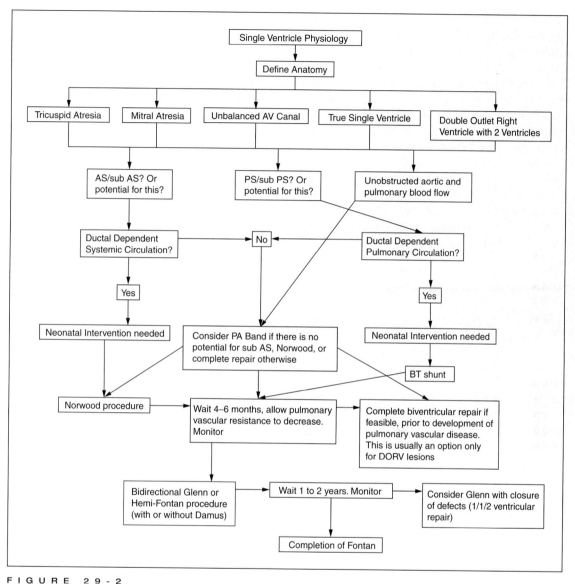

FIGURE 29-2

GENERAL MANAGEMENT STRATEGY FOR SINGLE VENTRICLE PHYSIOLOGY, THOUGH NOT EXHAUSTIVE

ventricle (left ventricular dominant) or left ventricle (right ventricular dominant). Left ventricular dominant complete atrioventricular canal is often associated with pulmonary artery stenosis/atresia or double outlet left ventricle. Right ventricular dominant complete atrioventricular canal may be associated with aortic stenosis/atresia or double outlet right ventricle. Management of both types of unbalanced atrioventricular canal is a pathway that leads to a single ventricular repair.

Double outlet right ventricle is a heart where both aorta and main pulmonary artery are aligned with the right ventricle. This occurs when both great arteries arise from two right ventricular coni, or if one great artery arises from a right ventricular conus and the other great artery has fibrous continuity with the tricuspid valve or the right ventricular aspect of a common atrioventricular valve. Tetralogy of Fallot with more than 50% override is not double outlet right ventricle because the aorta is in fibrous continuity with the mitral valve. Double outlet left ventricle is an extremely rare condition that occurs when both the aorta and the main pulmonary artery are aligned with the left ventricle. This occurs when one great artery arises from a left ventricular conus and the other great artery has fibrous continuity with the mitral valve or the left ventricular aspect of a common atrioventricular valve. Both double outlet right ventricle and double outlet left ventricle may be associated with numerous intracardiac or blood vessel anomalies. Most have a ventricular septal defect. If there are adequately sized right and left ventricles, there is the possibility that the great arteries can be aligned to their respective ventricle either through baffling, conduit placement or arterial switching, in which case a two-ventricle repair is possible. Otherwise, management is a pathway that leads to a single ventricle repair or the modified Fontan operation.

Suggested Readings

Allen HD, Gutgesell HP, Clark EB, Driscoll DJ: *Moss and Adams' Heart Disease in Infants, Children, and Adolescents Including the Fetus and Young Adult*, 6th ed. Philadelphia, PA, Lippincott Williams & Wilkins, 2001.

Garson A, Bricker JT, Fisher DJ, Neish SR: *The Science and Practice of Pediatric Cardiology*, 2nd ed. Baltimore, MD, Williams & Wilkins, 1998.

30

TRUNCUS ARTERIOSUS

David G. Ruschhaupt

ANATOMY AND EMBRYOLOGY

Truncus arteriosus communis is a rare cyanotic congenital heart lesion (approximately 2.8% of all congenital heart defects) that results from the failure of the spiral septum of the embryonic truncus to properly partition the pulmonary artery from the truncus arteriosus (common arterial trunk). Since the spiral septum makes an important contribution to the closure of the ventricular septum, a large ventricular septal defect (VSD) is also present in this lesion. The truncus arteriosus complex consists of a single large arterial vessel arising from the base of the heart and a large VSD. The arterial vessel supplies the coronary, systemic, and pulmonary arterial circulations. The truncal orifice is guarded by a single, large semilunar valve (truncal valve), which may straddle a VSD with a 60–100% displacement into the right ventricle. A right aortic arch may be present 20% of the time. If a patent ductus arteriosus is part of the complex, the ascending aorta and aortic arch is hypoplastic with coarctation or complete interruption of the aortic arch.

The Collet and Edwards classification of the pulmonary arteries has, for many, been a useful way to describe the variations in the truncus complex. The most common form, type I, has a short, single common pulmonary artery that arises from the left or posterior portion of the common truncal artery. It divides into the left and the right pulmonary arteries. Type II, often difficult to separate from type I, has two separate pulmonary arteries, which are very close to one another as they arise from the posterior portion of the truncus. Type III, the least common, has two distinctly separate pulmonary arteries arising from the lateral wall of the truncus. The origin of these vessels may be so close together as to make the type distinction very difficult. It is now generally agreed that type IV truncus is a form of pulmonary artery atresia and should not be included in the classification of truncus arteriosus.

While there may be a single coronary artery, most often there are two. The origin of the left is posterior, often very close to the orifice of the pulmonary artery. Occasionally, it arises from the pulmonary artery itself. The right coronary artery arises anteriorly. The coronary artery distribution is usually normal.

The truncal valve is always larger than the aortic valve would have been, as it is accommodating the combined cardiac output. Most commonly there are three leaflets but the valve may also be bicuspid or have four leaflets. The leaflets are abnormally thickened and very nodular.

Truncus arteriosus is a conotruncal abnormality and therefore is associated with the q22 chromosome deletion. The exact mechanism in which this abnormality translates into the phenotypic anatomic abnormalities described above remains unknown.

PATHOPHYSIOLOGY

Truncus arteriosus is an anomaly that allows for complete mixing of arterial and venous blood in the common arterial trunk and for pulmonary artery overcirculation. The truncal valve and artery are dilated because they accommodate the combined systemic and pulmonary artery blood volume. Figure 30-1

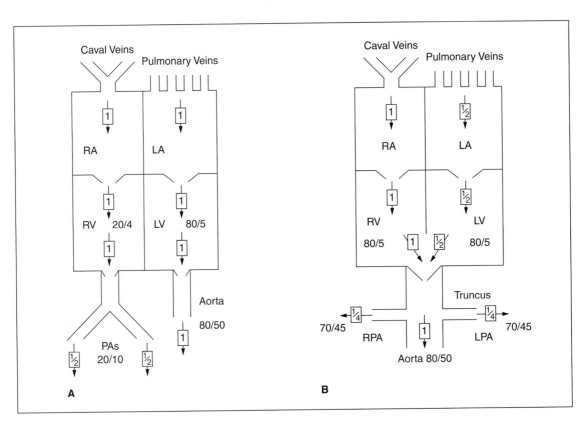

FIGURE   30-1

PATHOPHYSIOLOGY OF TRUNCUS ARTERIOSUS

A normal heart with pressures and labels is shown in part 1**A**. The pressures shown are hypothetic for this example. **B** shows a diagram of truncus arteriosus with elevated PVR. Note that there is minimal cardiac enlargement, and that the pressures in the right and left ventricles are equal. There is a 10 mmHg systolic gradient from the truncus into the branch PAs, reflecting mild narrowing, The diastolic pressures are slightly lower, reflecting slightly lower PVR vs. SVR. The net oxygen saturation in the aorta will be decreased as the ratio of pulmonary venous return (1/2 relative cardiac output in this example) vs. systemic venous return (1 relative cardiac output in this example) is decreased. As the PVR decreases, as shown in part **C**, the pulmonary venous return increases, as does the ratio of pulmonary venous return (2 relative cardiac outputs in this example) versus systemic venous return (1 relative cardiac output in this example). Thus, there is more saturated blood to mix with desaturated blood. In addition, the left heart is larger, and the diastolic pressure in the PAs has decreased (reflecting decreased PVR). Finally, the diastolic pressure in the aorta has also decreased, reflecting diastolic runoff into the PAs. Clinically this is seen by findings of an increased pulse pressure.

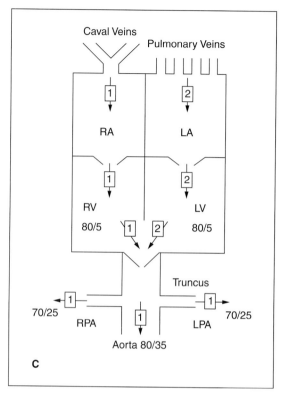

Truncus

C

FIGURE 30-1 (continued)

reduce cardiac output if the ventricles are unable to compensate for this. Incompetence of the valve will increase the volume overload of the heart (preload), further adding to the stress placed on the ventricle and the risk of heart failure. Interruption of the aortic arch, when present, superimposes the features of a ductal-dependent systemic circulation on the pathophysiology described above. The pathophysiology of the latter can be thought of as the pathophysiology of truncus arteriosus (as shown in Figure 30-1) and the pathophysiology of critical coarctation of the aorta (as described in the chapter on coarctation of the aorta).

CLINICAL HISTORY

The clinical expression of truncus arteriosus is governed by the volume of pulmonary artery blood flow and the presence or absence of truncal valve insufficiency. Truncus arteriosus is a cyanotic congenital defect; however, the increased pulmonary blood flow may cause the cyanosis to be overlooked. The newborn infant may initially maintain high pulmonary vascular resistance. Except for mild cyanosis, the usual clinical findings may not be obvious. If the defect has not been detected in the newborn nursery, signs of pulmonary overcirculation (congestive heart failure) and failure to thrive dominate the clinical picture as pulmonary vascular resistance decreases. As with all large ventricular and great vessel level shunting lesions, feeding and growing become the major clinical problems. Tachypnea, diaphoresis, and tachycardia are also observed secondary to pulmonary edema. Pneumonia, atelectasis, and sepsis may also occur, and may be multifactorial because of altered lung compliance, bronchial compression, and possibly immune deficiency as seen in DiGeorge syndrome.

Attempts at treating the heart failure and inducing weight gain fail. Unoperated, only 50% of patients with this defect survive the first month of life; 30% survive beyond 3 months and only 12% survive beyond the first birthday. Those patients who do survive infancy without surgery show gradual clinical "improvement" over the next several years. This is because there is increasing pulmonary

diagrams this flow pattern. The VSD is large, allowing for equalization of pressure in the right and left ventricle. The pressure loaded right ventricle, which ejects blood directly into the systemic circulation, is hypertrophied. The left ventricle and left atrium are volume loaded (enlarged) because of increased pulmonary artery blood flow. The amount of pulmonary blood flow is determined by the pulmonary vascular resistance, and any anatomic narrowing present in the pulmonary arteries. This pathophysiology is similar to a VSD. Over the first 3 months of life, the newborn elevation of pulmonary vascular resistance decreases with increasing pulmonary blood flow and systemic arterial oxygen saturation. These changes are shown in Figure 30-1.

Abnormalities of the truncal valve may alter the physiology. An obstruction of the valve will cause increased afterload to the ventricles, and may

vascular resistance with concomitant reduction in the pulmonary blood flow. Cyanosis and clubbing of the extremities become evident. Eisenmenger's physiology makes correction of the defect impossible at this point.

CLINICAL EXAMINATION

The clinical findings in truncus arteriosus are dependent on the volume of pulmonary blood flood flow and the presence or absence of truncal valve insufficiency. Pulse-oximetry will document mild systemic arterial desaturation. Tachypnea with intercostal retractions is evident. Significant volume load on the heart creates cardiac enlargement with a hyperdynamic precordium. The first heart sound is normal to increased in intensity. An ejection click follows the first sound and is appreciated best at the apex of the heart and at the third left intercostal space. This is a result of ejection of blood into the large common arterial trunk. The second heart sound is increased in intensity. Even though there is only a single semilunar valve, this second sound often sounds as if it were split. There is a third heart sound (filling sound) at the apex of the heart. A grade II-IV/VI harsh systolic murmur is created at the third left intercostal space by blood flow through the ventricular septal defect and across the truncal valve. The sound is mainly an ejection sound of flow across this area. It is not a result of the nonrestrictive VSD. In the presence of truncal valve stenosis, it will be much louder. Because of the significant increase in pulmonary blood flow, there will be increased diastolic blood flow across the mitral valve and a low frequency, rumbling diastolic murmur inside the cardiac apex. If there is truncal valve insufficiency, there will be a separate high frequency diastolic murmur at the third left intercostal space (Table 30-1).

LABORATORY FINDINGS

Electrocardiography

The ECG will show a sinus rhythm, most likely with right-axis deviation. Biventricular hypertrophy

TABLE 30-1

SUMMARY OF CLINICAL FINDINGS IN TRUNCUS ARTERIOSUS

History
Cyanosis
Failure to thrive
Poor feeding
Sweating
Physical Examination
Arterial desaturation
Tachypnea
Active precordium
Systolic murmur, grade II-IV, left sternal border (LSB)
S3, diastolic rumble, toward apex
High frequency diastolic murmur, 3rd left intercostal space (LICS) and apex

will be present. The T-wave configuration in lead V1 may be upright reflecting the right ventricular hypertrophy.

Chest Radiography

The chest plain film will demonstrate cardiac enlargement. In the lateral projection, left atrial enlargement will often be shown. The lung markings will reflect the increased pulmonary blood flow. The area of the main pulmonary artery will be shallow because the main pulmonary is not present in the usual location. A right aortic arch in the presence of increased pulmonary artery blood flow suggests truncus arteriosus and not tetralogy of Fallot, which will show decreased pulmonary blood flow with right aortic arch.

Echocardiography

The echocardiogram will establish the diagnosis. In the long axis view, the dilated truncal valve will be shown straddling a large ventricular septal defect. The pulmonary artery will not be demonstrated in the usual position. Careful imaging will identify the main pulmonary artery arising either from the lateral or posterior portion of the truncus arteriosus. With the use of pulse and color Doppler echocardiography, the presence of truncal valve obstruction and/or insufficiency can be identified.

Cardiac Catheterization and Angiography

Cardiac catheterization will demonstrate systemic arterial oxygen desaturation, usually 85% or higher. Systemic level pressure and an increase in oxygen saturation will be found in the right ventricle. Importantly, the catheter can be advanced into the main pulmonary artery from the truncus arteriosus. Any obstruction of blood flow to this vessel may be determined from pressure measurements or angiography (Table 30-2).

T A B L E   3 0 - 2

SUMMARY OF LABORATORY FINDINGS IN TRUNCUS ARTERIOSUS

Electrocardiogram
  Sinus rhythm
  Right-axis deviation
  Biventricular hypertrophy

Chest x-ray
  Cardiac enlargement
  Increased pulmonary blood flow
  Right aortic arch

Echocardiogram
  Dilated truncal root straddling ventricular septum
  Large VSD
  Pulmonary arteries arising from ascending aorta

Cardiac Catheterization
  Systemic arterial desaturation
  Systemic pressure in right ventricle
  Large VSD
  Straddling truncal valve
  Pulmonary arteries arising from ascending aorta
  Pulmonary artery hypertension

TREATMENT

The poor prognosis for this defect demands that surgery be performed early in the neonatal period. Banding of the pulmonary artery, once the main choice for palliation, is no longer attempted. Rather, the repair is primary with a Rastelli approach (internal LV to aortic baffle, and an RV to PA conduit) using cardiopulmonary bypass with moderate hypothermia. After complete dissection, the RV infundibulum is opened and the VSD closed with a patch, routing the left ventricle into the truncus. The pulmonary arteries are detached from the ascending aorta. The ascending aorta is reconstructed. A valved homograft is then placed to reconstruct the right ventricular outflow tract, connecting it distally to the branch PAs. Hypoplastic branch PAs or discontinuous branch PAs (truncus type II or III) are often a problem during the long-term follow-up. During the initial surgery, attempts are usually made to keep the branch PAs in continuity. This is achieved by harvesting aortic tissue along with the PAs and making a wide homograft to PA connection. Moderate truncal valve insufficiency can often be tolerated as the preoperative volume load will be gone, often reducing the insufficiency. Cases of severe truncal valve insufficiency are difficult to deal with. If truncal valve intervention is considered unavoidable, repair maneuvers include commissuroplasties and resection of accessory cusps with valve reconstruction. An interrupted aortic arch is no longer considered to be a significant risk factor. Repair of the arch is undertaken along with repair of the truncus. In experienced centers, survival after truncus surgery approaches 95%. Complications include pulmonary hypertensive crisis in older children (i.e., >3 months old), bleeding, infection, heart block, patch dehiscence, right ventricular outflow tract obstruction, and residual or recurrent aortic arch obstruction. The circulation is "corrected" but long-term care will focus on the need for homograft replacement, branch PA stenosis, and possible truncal (aortic) valve insufficiency. The timing of homograft replacement depends on the size of the original conduit as well as factors of calcification and intimal narrowing. The original homograft will often last 3–4 years, at which point it is "outgrown" because of body growth and the fact that the homograft has no growth potential. After successful surgery, growth and development are normal (unless there is an associated genetic abnormality) and the patient faces few if any restrictions in activity.

CONTROVERSIES IN MANAGEMENT

There are few controversies in the need for initial surgical intervention in this lesion. In the past, there were controversies on whether or not homograft tissue or synthetic material ought to be used for the initial RV to PA conduit. Now, the controversy arises on when to intervene in truncal valve insufficiency and when to replace the initial homograft as it becomes stenotic and regurgitant. This is less controversial in a symptomatic patient but becomes so in an asymptomatic patient.

LONG-TERM OUTLOOK

The long-term outlook for patients with this lesion is, in general, good. It is influenced by the status of the truncal valve, any associated ventricular dysfunction, and underlying genetic abnormalities.

Replacement of the RV to PA valve and homograft is required periodically because of body growth and deterioration (narrowing or regurgitation). The truncal valve usually requires replacement at some point in most patients. This is another risk factor and is similar to that of aortic valve replacement. The replacement valve may be a homograft versus a mechanical valve with the associated risks and benefits of each. Medications may be required if there is associated ventricular dysfunction or significant valve regurgitation. SBE prophylaxis is required for life. Restrictions in activity depend on the presence and degree of any residual defects or abnormalities (e.g., valve regurgitation, residual VSD, ventricular function, and so forth). In general, patients are expected to reach adulthood and lead productive lives.

Suggested Readings

Allen HD, Gutgesell HP, Clark EB, Driscoll DJ: *Moss and Adams' Heart Disease in Infants, Children and Adolescents Including the Fetus and Young Adult*, 6th ed. Philadelphia, PA, Lippincott Williams & Wilkins, 2001.

Garson A, Bricker JT, Fisher DJ, Neish SR: *The Science and Practice of Pediatric Cardiology*, 2nd ed. Baltimore, MD, Williams & Wilkins, 1998.

31

TRANSPOSITION OF THE GREAT ARTERIES (TGA)

Ra-id Abdulla

INTRODUCTION

Transposition of the great arteries (TGA) is a congenital heart disease in which the great vessels that emerge from the heart (aorta and main pulmonary artery) are switched such that the aorta emerges from the right ventricle and the main pulmonary artery emerges from the left ventricle. This lesion causes no hemodynamic complication while the fetus is in utero; however, soon after birth the child manifests with severe cyanosis owing to the fact that the aorta emerges from the right ventricle, which receives blood from the already oxygen-depleted systemic veins. Of note is that this description is of the entity known as "d-TGA" where the "d" denotes the location of the aorta. There are other types of transposition, one of which is known as "l-TGA," and usually refers to the condition where the ventricles are transposed or switched as well as the arteries, resulting in normal physiology and no cyanosis (physiologically corrected). Only d-TGA is discussed in this chapter.

INCIDENCE

Transposition of the great arteries occurs in 0.2–0.4/1000 live births. This is the second most common congenital heart disease encountered in early infancy. It is also the most common cause of transfer to the cardiac care unit in the neonatal and infancy period.

EMBRYOLOGY

There is no apparent genetic predisposition to this congenital heart disease. The incidence does not appear to be higher when there is a positive family history. It is uncommon in low birth weight and premature infants. It appears to have a higher incidence in rural areas and higher birth order as well as advanced maternal age. Mechanism of occurrence is not clear. It is typically not associated with other anomalies. Infants of diabetic mothers have a somewhat increased incidence when compared to the general population.

PATHOLOGY

The aorta is anterior and slightly to the right of the main pulmonary artery. The aortic valve is to the right of the pulmonary valve but still anterior to it. The right pulmonary artery receives more blood than the left. This is a result of its alignment secondary to abnormal main pulmonary artery position owing to transposition. The right pulmonary artery consequently becomes larger than the left. Most infants have a patent foramen ovale and a patent ductus arteriosus (PDA). Fifty percent of patients with TGA have ventricular septal defects and 50% have an intact ventricular septum. Pulmonary stenosis is the most commonly associated cardiac defect with transposition of the great vessels. Next are anomalies of the tricuspid valve, followed by coarctation of the aorta. These anomalies are more commonly associated in transposition of the great vessels with ventricular septal defect than with an intact ventricular septum.

Pulmonary stenosis in patients with transposition of the great arteries, particularly those with a ventricular septal defect (VSD), is typically a result of leftward bowing of the ventricular septum and close proximity of the mitral valve to the ventricular septum, leading to dynamic obstruction. Anatomic valvar pulmonic stenosis is rare. One-third of patients with d-TGA and VSD will have closure of the VSD in the first year of life. The VSD may be located anywhere in the septum.

Sixty percent of patients have a right coronary artery (RCA) emerging from a right sinus of valsalva. The left coronary artery (LCA) emerges from the left sinus and gives rise to the circumflex (CCX) and left anterior descending (LAD) coronary artery. In 10% of patients the RCA and CCX emerge from the right sinus with the LAD from the left sinus of valsalva. In these cases the CCX travels posterior to the pulmonary artery. In other cases, the CCX emerges from the right sinus and the RCA and LAD emerge from the left sinus of valsalva. In addition, the RCA may emerge from the right sinus and give rise to the LCA. The LCA in this case will give rise to the CCX and LAD branches.

PATHOPHYSIOLOGY

The pathophysiology of TGA is as described in Chapter 11. The diagrammatic representation is given in Figure 31-1. Parallel systemic and pulmonary circulations occur. The only way such children can survive after delivery is because of bidirectional shunting of blood at the atrial level via a

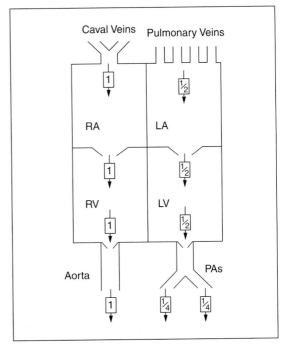

FIGURE 31-1

PATHOPHYSIOLOGIC DIAGRAM OF TGA WITH INTACT INTERATRIAL SEPTUM

Note that the aorta, which emerges form the right ventricle, receives deoxygenated blood from the systemic circulation (caval veins), thus causing severe cyanosis. There are two separate circuits of blood in transposition. The first returns deoxygenated blood from the body, then through the right atrium and ventricle and back to the body. The second circuit receives well-oxygenated blood from the lungs and sends it back to the lungs through the left atrium and ventricle. These two circuits are not completely isolated, otherwise that would be incompatible with life. A certain degree of blood mixing between the two circulations occurs at the ASD, PDA, and VSD (if present), resulting in a small or great increase in oxygen content of arterial blood, depending on the extent of defects between the left and right sides of the heart.

patent foramen ovale (PFO) or atrial septal defect (ASD). This bidirectional shunting will cause the blood in the two separate circuits to mix, allowing the deoxygenated blood destined to the body to be more oxygenated.

The drop in the pulmonary vascular resistance soon after birth will increase the pulmonary blood flow through the PDA (left-to-right or aortic-to-pulmonary shunting) and this will result in dilation of the left atrium and stretching of the patent foramen ovale with shunting of blood from the left atrium to the right atrium across the stretched patent

foramen ovale. This will allow mixing of blood and better oxygen saturation. A larger ASD, as seen after balloon atrial septostomy, will augment this atrial level mixing (Figure 31-2).

Patients with ventricular septal defects tend to have better mixing of the pulmonary and systemic circulations for a similar reason. Patients with a VSD may become more cyanotic as the VSD gets smaller. Patients with an intact ventricular septum tend to have dynamic left ventricular outflow tract (LVOT) obstruction usually reversible after arterial switch operation. Patients with an anatomic left ventricular outflow tract obstruction tend to have better left-to-right shunting across the VSD and less cyanosis.

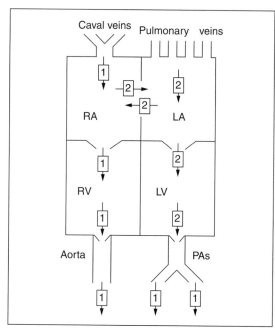

FIGURE 31-2

TGA AFTER BALLOON ATRIAL SEPTOSTOMY (OR WITH A LARGE ATRIAL SEPTAL DEFECT)

This theoretical diagram depicts a state with relatively low pulmonary vascular resistance. This is reflected by the fact that there is twice as much blood flow in the pulmonary circulation as in the systemic circulation. The increased pulmonary venous return causes an increased left atrial pressure which enhances atrial level mixing. Pulmonary blood flow can be further increased with a ductus arteriosus. The net saturation will reflect good mixing and the relative volume of pulmonary and systemic venous return (2 to 1 in this example).

CLINICAL FINDINGS

Babies are typically full term. Babies with d-TGA and intact ventricular septum, or a very small VSD, present early in the first day or two of life. Cyanosis not improving with oxygen therapy is the typical presenting clinical manifestation. Babies with TGA and ventricular septal defect may have less noticeable cyanosis, yet have tachypnea and respiratory distress in the first 2 weeks of life because of pulmonary overcirculation. Other than cyanosis, the physical examination may demonstrate a hyperdynamic precordium. On auscultation there is a single second heart sound. There may be a murmur across the pulmonary valve reflecting increased pulmonary blood flow (functional pulmonary stenosis). This is more apparent in patients with a VSD. The VSD itself may cause a murmur, though atypical for a VSD, as the blood flows from the RV to the LV. It is usually lower pitched and may be noted at the left mid to upper sternal border. In addition, left ventricular outflow tract obstruction may cause a systolic ejection murmur in the same general location.

LABORATORY FINDINGS

Electrocardiography

The typical ECG in TGA is within normal limits in the early neonatal period, with later development of right ventricular hypertrophy reflecting the systemic pressures in the RV.

Chest Radiography

The initial chest radiograph is typically within normal limits with the later finding, particularly in patients with a VSD, of cardiomegaly and increased pulmonary blood flow. At a later age the typical (egg-on-side) will be noted. This is because of biventricular dilatation and a narrow mediastinum owing to the positions of the great vessels. A right aortic arch is seen in 1% of patients with an intact ventricular septum and in 3% of patients with a VSD. A right aortic arch is more common (10%) in patients with d-TGA with pulmonary stenosis or pulmonary atresia.

Echocardiography

Echocardiography demonstrates the anatomy of the d-TGA. The particular features that may be assessed include:

1. Any VSD, its size and location.
2. The patent foramen ovale or ASD, and direction of shunting.
3. The presence of a patent ductus arteriosus.
4. The anatomy of the coronary arteries.
5. The aortic arch and its orientation.
6. The left ventricular outflow tract and the presence and nature (dynamic/anatomic) of any obstruction.
7. The presence of any pulmonary stenosis or pulmonary atresia.
8. The tricuspid valve, especially in association with an endocardial cushion defect.
9. The right ventricular size.

Echocardiography can also be used to guide atrial septostomy if the PFO is restrictive.

Cardiac Catheterization

Cardiac catheterization is indicated in patients in whom the coronary artery anatomy is not clear and when the LVOT obstruction is thought to be anatomic rather than dynamic. It may also be used

to perform a Rashkind atrial septostomy although this may be performed at the bedside using echocardiographic guidance.

TREATMENT

At birth, patients with TGA are very ill because of severe cyanosis, particularly in the absence of a VSD. Once the diagnosis is suspected, owing to severe cyanosis, and even before confirmation through an echocardiogram, prostaglandin intravenous infusion should be initiated to keep the ductus arteriosus patent. The PDA will help increase mixing of blood at the atrial level, thus improving oxygen saturation. Once the diagnosis is confirmed through echocardiography, the size of the atrial communication should be assessed. If small and restrictive, it is usually enlarged via a Rashkind balloon atrial septostomy performed at the bedside under echocardiographic guidance, or in the cardiac catheterization laboratory under fluoroscopic guidance. A large atrial communication facilitates more atrial mixing and improved oxygen saturation.

There is no role for medical treatment other than supportive care including prostaglandin to keep the ductus arteriosus patent and balloon atrial septostomy for a restrictive PFO. A d-TGA with intact ventricular septum is best repaired surgically with an arterial switch procedure, as the left ventricle is best suited to be the systemic ventricle. This is usually performed in infants less than 4 weeks of age (usually in the first 2 weeks of life) after the pulmonary vascular resistance has decreased (to avoid a pulmonary hypertensive crisis). A longer delay may cause the LV to become less hypertrophied (because of a drop in the pulmonary vascular resistance) and be less amenable to function as a systemic pump postoperatively. The latter is less important in the presence of significant left ventricular outflow tract obstruction or a large VSD, which maintains a pressure load on the LV; however, the latter will result in pulmonary overcirculation and require repair in the first month of life as well.

Patients with significant left ventricular outflow tract obstruction (anatomic) with a large VSD

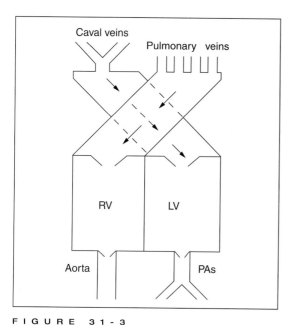

Caval veins

Pulmonary veins

RV   LV

Aorta   PAs

FIGURE 31-3

SCHEMATIC DIAGRAM OF A HEART WITH TGA AFTER THE SENNING (OR MUSTARD) PROCEDURE

performed using pericardium or prosthetic material. These patients are left with a right ventricle functioning as a systemic pump. They are at risk for right ventricular failure, as well as atrial dysrhythmias because of the extensive atrial suture lines. In some patients with right heart failure, conversion of the atrial switch to an arterial switch procedure is performed after preparing (conditioning) the left ventricle. Results of this are being investigated.

Main pulmonary artery banding is employed in patients with multiple VSDs or to prepare the left ventricle in older children for the arterial switch operation. Conversion of the atrial switch procedure to an arterial switch procedure will require that the MPA is first banded for a period of time until the left ventricle is able to tolerate the systemic pressure. In the past, palliative atrial switch procedures were performed in patients with d-TGA and a VSD and pulmonary vascular obstructive disease, in order to lessen the extent of cyanosis.

may be better candidates for a Rastelli procedure. This is a procedure in which the left ventricular outflow is baffled to the aorta through the VSD. The pulmonary valve is ligated (or left untouched if atretic), and a right ventricle to pulmonary artery conduit is placed. This is usually performed at 4–6 months of age as there is no risk of pulmonary overcirculation or LV "deconditioning" with this combination of defects.

The Mustard and Senning procedures were commonly performed 10 years ago (Figure 31-3). In both procedures, baffling the venous return is

Suggested Readings

Allen HD, Gutgesell HP, Clark EB, Driscoll DJ: *Moss and Adams' Heart Disease in Infants, Children and Adolescents Including the Fetus and Young Adult*, 6th ed. Philadelphia, PA, Lippincott Williams & Wilkins, 2001.

Garson A, Bricker JT, Fisher DJ, Neish SR: *The Science and Practice of Pediatric Cardiology*, 2nd ed. Baltimore, MD, Williams & Wilkins, 1998.

Losay J, Touchot A, Serraf A, Litvinova A, Lambert V, Piot JD, Lacour-Gayet F, Capderou A, Planche C: Late outcome after the arterial switch operation for transposition of the great arteries. *Circulation* 104:121–126, 2001.

32

PULMONARY ARTERIOVENOUS MALFORMATIONS (AVMS)

Hitendra T. Patel

INTRODUCTION

Pulmonary arteriovenous malformations (AVMs) are abnormal direct connections between the pulmonary arteries and pulmonary veins without entering the capillary network surrounding the alveoli. These connections may be single or multiple. The afferent pulmonary arteries and efferent pulmonary veins are typically dilated. The arteriovenous malformations may also be microscopic and multiple. The latter is usually associated with acquired defects. The natural history is for the lesions to increase in size and number over time. These lesions can occur in any part of the lung and may be localized or diffused.

ETIOLOGY

Pulmonary AVMs are acquired or congenital in origin (see Table 32-1). Congenital AVMs may be isolated or inherited as part of other vascular abnormality syndromes such as hereditary hemorrhagic telangectasia (HHT) or Rendu-Osler Weber disease. HHT is inherited as an autosomal dominant trait and is highly penetrant. The candidate gene has been mapped to chromosome 9q. It is a vascular dysplasia leading to telangectasia and arteriovenous malformations of the skin, mucosa, and viscera.

When pulmonary AVMs are acquired, they are usually seen in patients with liver disease (cirrhosis, biliary atresia), heterotaxia syndrome (usually polysplenia), or in those patients who have undergone certain types of cardiac surgery. The latter include a classical Glenn shunt, Kawashima procedure, or other systemic venous connection to the pulmonary artery in which hepatic blood does not drain to the pulmonary circulation. The common denominator in all the acquired causes of pulmonary AVMs appears to be the absence of an unidentified hepatic blood factor reaching the lung. It is believed that this hepatic factor is required in the lungs in order to prevent pulmonary AVMs from developing. In chronic liver disease, this factor does not appear

TABLE 32-1

ETIOLOGY OF PULMONARY AVM

Congenital:	Isolated
	Hereditary—hereditary hemorrhagic telangectasia (HHT)
Acquired:	Chronic liver disease
	Heterotaxia syndromes—usually polysplenia and associated with intrahepatic biliary cirrhosis
	Portal vein thrombosis
	Postcardiac surgery—classical Glenn shunt
	Kawashima procedure (bidirectional Glenn shunt in face of an interrupted IVC)
Trauma:	Lung contusion or penetrating lung injury

and AVMs have been shown to resolve with liver transplantation. In AVMs occurring following certain types of cardiac surgery, it is postulated that they occur because the hepatic venous blood flows directly to the systemic circulation bypassing the lungs. Some investigators suggest that the lack of pulsitile pulmonary flow is the etiologic factor. Resolution of pulmonary AVMs has been demonstrated in these patients once the hepatic venous flow is redirected to course through the pulmonary circulation.

PATHOPHYSIOLOGY

This is one of the anatomic causes of cyanosis or desaturation; however, it is an intrapulmonary right-to-left shunt rather than intracardiac. The magnitude of the shunt depends on the size and number of fistulae, as well as the relative resistances and pressures of the proximal arteries and distal venous system. Postural change in ventilation and perfusion (V/Q mismatch) may lead to increased shunting and hence cyanosis with an upright position (orthodeoxia).

This postural change in cyanosis depends in part on the location of the pulmonary AVM. Hypoxemia is increased with exercise, since exercise-induced changes in pulmonary vascular resistance (PVR) and systemic vascular resistance (SVR), and an overall increased pulmonary blood flow, will promote a right-to-left shunt.

CLINICAL HISTORY

Patients usually present with central cyanosis and exercise intolerance. On further questioning, there may be a history of orthodeoxia and platypnea (dyspnea induced by upright position and relieved by recumbency). Other presenting symptoms and signs may be neurologic from systemic emboli leading to stroke, cerebral abscess or the signs and symptoms of other arterial emboli. Another presentation may be recurrent hemoptysis, which may be massive and life threatening. The newborn period is a rare time of presentation, and if so, the AVMs are usually a result of large defects, which may result in marked cyanosis and metabolic acidosis. Asymptomatic patients may present for evaluation with a family history of HHT, or with manifestation of AVMs in other sites (nonpulmonary) causing frequent and massive epistaxis, stridor, abdominal pain, and/or bleeding. Asymptomatic patients may also be diagnosed with pulmonary AVMs during evaluation for a persistent density on a chest plain film.

PHYSICAL EXAMINATION

Cyanosis (especially orthostatic) and clubbing are usually the main clinical findings. The cyanosis may be minimal at rest, and therefore, oxygen saturations during exercise may be required to demonstrate the cyanosis or desaturation. The initial physical findings may be in other organ systems and include stridor, or the manifestation of systemic emboli. The cardiac exam is otherwise typically unremarkable. Rarely a continuous murmur may be appreciated directly over the area of a large lesion.

LABORATORY FINDINGS

Blood Testing

A complete blood count may demonstrate polycythemia if the cyanosis is severe and long-standing.

Electrocardiography

The ECG is either normal or may show left axis deviation (LAD) and left ventricular hypertrophy (LVH) in symptomatic newborns with large lesions.

Chest Radiography

The chest plain film will demonstrate large lesions as opacities. Small diffuse microscopic AVMs may be suspected by the finding of oligemic lung fields. The cardiac size (except in the symptomatic newborn) is typically normal.

CT Scan/MRI

Both of these modalities are excellent at visualizing the AVM except for the microscopic lesions.

Echocardiography

Contrast echocardiography (bubble study) may suggest the presence of an intrapulmonary AV shunt by the presence of contrast in the pulmonary veins and LA. The contrast is obtained by agitating normal saline with a small amount of air and blood, which creates microcavitations. This is then rapidly injected intravenously. The microcavitations, which appear as ECHO bright "bubbles," should be filtered in the pulmonary capillary bed. If a direct connection between the pulmonary arteries and veins exists, then the bubbles will be seen in the left atrium. Localization of this contrast to a particular pulmonary vein may help in localizing the site of the AVM.

Catheterization/Angiography

This will help define the anatomy and hemodynamics of an AVM. Blood oxygen sampling will usually demonstrate pulmonary venous desaturation. If there is a localized AVM, then isolated pulmonary vein desaturation may be seen. Usually, the intracardiac, pulmonary, and systemic pressures are normal, as is the cardiac output. Selective right and left lung angiography is typically performed in all patients. If isolated lesions are demonstrated, then selective injections into each lesion are usually performed to delineate the afferent arterial and efferent venous anatomy. Multiple or diffuse AVMs are characterized by the absence of the capillary blush phase of the pulmonary angiogram and early appearance of contrast in the PV.

TREATMENT

If there is a treatable underlying systemic disease (e.g., hepatic failure), then this disease is treated first (liver transplantation and so forth).

Transcatheter embolization is the treatment of choice and is used with isolated and well-defined AVMs. Many different methods are available, including coils, detachable balloons, or occluder devices. The aim is to occlude all lesions. Multiple attempts may be needed at different times, as the lesion anatomy changes over time or new lesions may appear.

If transcatheter therapy does not succeed, then surgical resection, lobectomy, or pneumonectomy of a large lesion become treatment options; however, surgical intervention is rarely required as long as the patient is not failing to thrive or severely hypoxic. Any intervention (catheter or surgical) does not prevent other pulmonary AVMs from developing. In extreme cases with total lung involvement, the only option is for lung transplantation.

SBE is indicated in all of these patients.

Treatment Controversies

It is still unclear when and how often to intervene in asymptomatic patients with diffuse microscopic AVMs because of an otherwise untreatable cause (HHT, isolated, or that associated with congenital heart disease). In patients with AVMs secondary to the creation of a direct systemic venous shunt to the pulmonary artery with no hepatic blood reaching the pulmonary circulation, it is unclear whether additional surgeries should be undertaken to redirect hepatic venous blood to the lungs. It has been demonstrated that inclusion of hepatic blood flow back into the pulmonary circulation does result in resolution of the AVMs. Long-term follow-up data, however, is not available. Whether this surgery should be undertaken prophylactically in at-risk patients prior to the development of pulmonary AVMs is a debated question.

Another topic of uncertainty is anticoagulation in patients with pulmonary AVMs. There is a significant risk of systemic embolization of thrombi; however, physicians vary in treatment from formal anticoagulation with warfarin, aspirin alone or in conjunction with another antiplatelet agent or no therapy.

Suggested Readings

Emmanoulides GC, Allen HD, Riemenschneider TA, Gutgesell HP (eds.): *Moss and Adams' Heart Disease in Infants, Children, and Adolescents: Including the Fetus and Young Adult*, 5th ed. Baltimore, MD, Williams & Wilkins, 1995, Chap. 57, pp. 799–804.

National Center for Biotechnology Information, http://www.ncbi.nlm.nih.gov/Omim/searchomim.html. Search word: Hereditary hemorrhagic telangectasia or HHT.

33

ACQUIRED HEART DISEASE

Peter Koenig

INTRODUCTION

Acquired heart disease is secondary to trauma, tumors, inflammatory diseases, or cardiomyopathies. Both cardiac tumors and cardiomyopathies may have genetic basis and can present in utero; however, they are not considered congenital as they manifest after completion of cardiac development. Acquired heart disease involves cardiac conduction tissue, myocardial and/or pericardial tissue. This chapter discusses the inflammatory and noninflammatory diseases of the heart. Cardiac tumors and trauma are discussed in Chapters 34 and 35.

Cardiomyopathies can be divided into physiologic groups as shown in Figure 33-1. The causes within each group of cardiomyopathy may be similar. Hypertrophic and restrictive cardiomyopathies tend to have different causes than dilated cardiomyopathies. The various etiologies of cardiomyopathies are shown in Figure 33-2.

PATHOPHYSIOLOGY OF CARDIOMYOPATHY

The pathophysiology of myocardial disease can be subdivided into dilated, restrictive, and hypertrophic muscle diseases or myopathies (Chapter 11). Myocardial disease may cause systolic and/or diastolic dysfunction. Typically one of these dysfunctions becomes more prominent.

Dilated cardiomyopathies typically have systolic dysfunction as the major component. Restrictive cardiomyopathy is typically a type of diastolic dysfunction. Hypertrophic cardiomyopathy is also typically a diastolic abnormality unless there is obstruction in which case, systolic function may be problematic. Clinically, the findings are related to the underlying pathophysiology and typically have components of "forward" and "backward" heart failure (Chapter 11).

INFLAMMATORY HEART DISEASE

Inflammatory diseases of the heart may manifest as myocarditis, endocarditis, pericarditis, or a coronary artery vasculitis. If all portions of the heart are inflamed, it is known as pancarditis. More frequent causes of inflammation are given in Tables 33-1 and 33-2.

*The author gratefully acknowledges John Marcinak for his contributions to the portions on infectious disease.

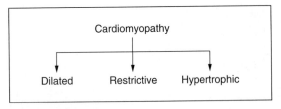

F I G U R E   3 3 - 1

TYPES OF CARDIOMYOPATHY, CLASSIFIED BY UNDERLYING PATHOPHYSIOLOGY

ENDOCARDITIS

Etiology

Endocarditis denotes endocardial inflammation and can be infectious or noninfectious. Causes of endocarditis are listed in Tables 33-1 and 33-2. Although the endocardium lines the entire heart, the term is usually used to denote valvar inflammation or valvulitis, which may result in valve dysfunction

or destruction. The extent of pathology is dependent on the type of inflammation and/or the organism involved. Infective endocarditis is usually bacterial and rarely viral. Bacterial endocarditis may be caused by a number of organisms, the most common organisms are alpha-hemolytic streptococci, followed by *Staphylococcus aureus*. Less common causes are beta-hemolytic streptococci, coagulase negative staphylococcus, and nonbacterial causes such as candida. Typically, strep viridans causes a less fulminant infection with subtle signs and symptoms such as fever, anorexia, and weight loss, as well as signs and symptoms of underlying cardiac pathology. Modification of a preexisting pathologic murmur may not be apparent. With a staphylococcal aureus cardiac infection, the signs and symptoms may be more severe with fever, sepsis, and signs and symptoms of significant cardiac pathology including failure from valve destruction (aortic, mitral, tricuspid, or pulmonary valve regurgitation).

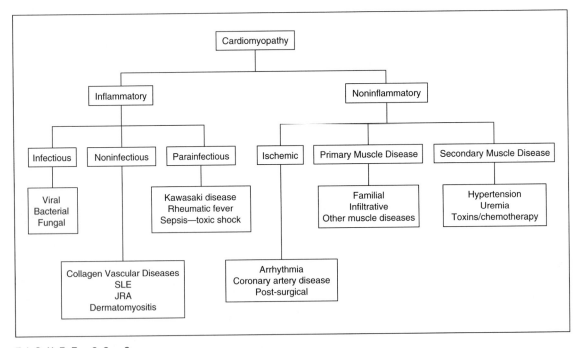

F I G U R E   3 3 - 2

TYPES OF CARDIOMYOPATHY, CLASSIFIED BY ETIOLOGY

TABLE 33-1

INFECTIOUS CAUSES OF ENDOCARDITIS, MYOCARDITIS, AND PERICARDITIS

Infected portion of the heart:			
	Endocarditis	Myocarditis	Pericarditis
Infectious Agent[a]			
Bacteria			
Actinomyces	Y		Y
Anaerobes	Y		Y
Bartonella	Y		
Brucella	Y	Y	Y
Clostridia		Y	
Corynebacterium (diphtheria)	Y	Y	
Enterobacteriaceae			
Klebsiella pneumoniae		Y	
Pseudomonas aeruginosa	Y		Y
Salmonella typhi		Y	Y
Erysipelothrix	Y		
Gram negative bacilli	Y		
Haemophilus influenzae type b			Y
Klebsiella		Y	
Legionella pneumophila	Y	Y	
Listeria moncytogenes	Y	Y	Y
Mycobacteria			
Mycobacterium avium complex			Y
Mycobacterium tuberculosis			Y
Mycoplasma pneumoniae		Y	Y
Neisseria meningitidis		Y	Y
Neisseria gonorrhoeae	Y		Y
Nocardia	Y	Y	
Staphylococcus			
S. aureus	Y[c]	Y	Y
S. epidermidis	Y		
Streptococcus			
Group A		Y	Y
Group B	Y		Y
Enterococcus	Y		
Pneumococcus	Y		Y
Viridans	Y[c]		
Chlamydia	Y	Y	
Chlamydia psittaci	Y	Y	
Chlamydia trachomatis	Y	Y	
Chlamydia pneumoniae	Y	Y	
Ehrlichia	Y	Y	
Fungi and Yeast			
Aspergillus spp.	Y	Y	Y
Blastomyces demafitidis	Y	Y	Y

(continued)

TABLE 33-1 (continued)

INFECTIOUS CAUSES OF ENDOCARDITIS, MYOCARDITIS, AND PERICARDITIS

Infected portion of the heart:	Endocarditis	Myocarditis	Pericarditis
Infectious Agent[a]			
Candida spp.	Y	Y	Y
Coccidiodes immitis	Y	Y	Y
Cryptococcus neoformans	Y	Y	Y
Histoplasma capsulatum	Y	Y	Y
Mucor	Y	Y	
Other Parasites			
Taenia solium (cysticercosis)		Y	
Echinococcus		Y	Y
Schistosoma spp.		Y	Y
Toxocara canis		Y	
Trichinella		Y	
Visceral larva migrans		Y	
Protozoal			
Entamoeba histolytica			Y
Leishmaniasis (kala-azar)		Y	
Malaria		Y	
Toxoplasma gondii		Y	Y
Trypanosoma cruzi		Y	
Rickettsia			
R. ricketsii, R. tsutsugamushi	Y	Y	Y
Spirochetes			
Borrelia burgdorferi (Lyme disease)		Y	
Borrelia recurrentis (relapsing fever)		Y	
Leptospira (leptospirosis)		Y	
Treponema pallidum (syphilis[d])		Y	Y
Viruses			
Adenoviruses			Y
Serotype 2		Y	
Serotype 5		Y[b]	
Arbovirus		Y	
Cytomegalovirus		Y	Y
Ebstein-Barr virus		Y	Y
Enteroviruses			
Coxsackie A		Y	Y
Coxsackie B[c]		Y[b]	Y
Echovirus		Y	Y
Poliovirus		Y	
Hepatitis A, B, C		Y	
Herpesvirus		Y	Y
Human immunodeficiency virus		Y	
Influenza A		Y	Y
Measles		Y	Y

TABLE 33-1 (continued)

INFECTIOUS CAUSES OF ENDOCARDITIS, MYOCARDITIS, AND PERICARDITIS

Infected portion of the heart:	Endocarditis	Myocarditis	Pericarditis
Infectious Agent[a]			
Mumps		Y	Y
Parvovirus		Y	
Rabies		Y	
Respiratory syncytial virus		Y	
Rubella		Y	Y
Rubeola		Y	
Smallpox/vaccinia		Y	Y
Varicella-Zoster		Y	Y

[a]Y= infectious agent has been shown to cause infection.
[b]Common cause of myocarditis.
[c]Common cause of endocarditis.
[d]Also causes aortitis.

Infectious endocarditis typically occurs with bacteremia (or fungemia) in individuals with an underlying cardiac pathology, particularly those with high velocity jet. A prior episode of endocarditis is an increased risk factor. Foreign bodies such as a prosthetic valve, material to close a defect, or a cardiac device are also risk factors, as are indwelling catheters, and intravenous injections via nonsterile techniques (e.g., intravenous drug abusers). Finally, if the organism is extremely virulent, endocarditis may occur without predisposing factors. The underlying cause for endocarditis in all these conditions appears to be the ability of a bacterium or fungus to attach to the endocardium and multiply. It appears that jet lesions will cause abnormalities in the endocardium, which will allow this to happen. Once the organism multiplies, inflammation will occur with further damage to the valve and endocardium. Noninfectious endocarditis can occur in anyone with an underlying inflammatory disease.

Pathophysiology

The pathology of infectious endocarditis usually involves a damaged or abnormal valve. Initially, a lesion is created via mechanical stress, usually through turbulence. The turbulence owing to the Venturi effect is the greatest in areas in which there is an elevated pressure gradient. Any condition (stenosis, regurgitation, or a high velocity left-to-right shunt) that causes turbulent flow may result in endothelial damage. In addition, endothelial injury may occur from direct damage (catheter), or high output states. The endothelial damage initiates platelet fibrin deposition. Growth of the platelet fibrin deposit leads to a nonbacterial thrombotic vegetation. Transient bacteremia, which occurs in normal individuals, can lead to bacterial entrapment within this meshwork. Colonization may then occur with organism multiplication and destruction of surrounding tissue. The infection may cause valve, muscle, or conduction system injury or destruction. Valve destruction will lead to regurgitation (Chapters 11 and 17). Myocardial involvement will lead to myocardial dysfunction (Chapter 11). Involvement of the conduction system may lead to rhythm abnormalities or heart block (Chapter 36). Abscess formation may also occur. If the abscess erodes into the pericardial space, tamponade may occur. In addition, the vegetation may fragment leading to embolic phenomena. These may cause strokes, embolic pneumonia, and renal or myocardial infarction. Embolization is more common in endocarditis caused by candida, haemophilis, and *S. aureus* infections. These septic emboli are the cause for bacteremia and fungemia. In general, viruses do not cause endocarditis or vegetations.

TABLE 33-2

NONINFECTIOUS CAUSES OF ENDOCARDITIS/MYOCARDITIS/PERICARDITIS

Inflamed portion of the heart:	Endocarditis	Myocarditis	Pericarditis
Causal Agent[a]			
Toxic			
Scorpion, spider bites, diphtheria		Y	
Drugs/Hypersensitivity			
Sulfonamides		Y	
Phenylbuzone		Y	
Neomercazole		Y	
Acetazolamide		Y	
Amphotericin B		Y	
Indomethacin		Y	
Tetracycline		Y	
Isoniazid		Y	
Methyldopa		Y	
Phenytoin		Y	
Penicillin		Y	
Chloramphenicol		Y	
Streptomycin			
Hydralazine			Y
procainamide			Y
Hypersenstivity/Autoimmune			
Rheumatoid arthritis	Y	Y	Y
Rheumatic fever	Y	Y	Y
Ulcerative colitis		Y	
Systemic lupus erythematosus	Y	Y	Y
Mixed connective tissue disease		Y	
Whipple's disease		Y	
Other			
Sarcoidosis		Y	Y
Kawasaki disease	Y	Y	Y
Other Inflammation			
Radiation		Y	Y
S/p myocardial infarction			Y
S/p myocardial trauma/surgery			Y

[a]Y= Agent has been shown to cause inflammation.

The underlying disease process of noninfectious myocarditis has been described for diseases such as rheumatic fever. In the latter, there is an inflammatory infiltrate and edema of the valve tissue as well as the chordae tendinae. Hyaline degeneration leads to verrucae formation at the leaflet edge preventing coaptation of the leaflets and thus, regurgitation. Later fibrosis and calcification of the valve occurs. The latter will result in decreased leaflet mobility and stenosis. In systemic lupus erythematosis, a lesion known as a Libman-Sacks lesion occurs, which is a verrucous, nonbacterial lesion of degenerating valve tissue with clumps of fibrin and platelet thrombi. This usually occurs on the ventricular side of the valve, as well as the chordae tendinae and papillary muscles. In addition, there may be an inflammatory infiltrate causing valve thickening with later fibrosis and calcification. The pathophysiology of noninfectious endocarditis is related to the amount of regurgitation and stenosis of the valves (Chapters 11 and 17).

Clinical Presentation

Clinical presentation of endocarditis consists of the signs and symptoms of an inflammatory process (fever), with associated cardiac involvement (signs and symptoms of forward and backward failure, and a pathologic murmur). Cardiac findings of endocarditis are related to the degree of underlying valve dysfunction (regurgitation), myocardial dysfunction, and conduction abnormalities, which are similar to the findings from other causes. These findings include a murmur and possible signs and symptoms of heart failure. Of note is the description of the murmur found in many textbooks as a "new or changing murmur." What is implied is a new *pathologic* murmur as an innocent murmur may be louder with associated fever and anemia and not be supportive evidence of endocarditis. The statement of a "changing" murmur implies that a previously noted pathologic murmur owing to structural heart disease will be "more pathologic" or "different" in character because of the infection of the valve or cardiac structure involved; however, the determination of a true change in a pathologic murmur may be difficult. The prior pathology is a risk factor itself, which should increase the index of suspicion of the possibility of endocarditis if suggested by other clinical and laboratory findings.

Clinical findings related to the inflammation and the infection itself includes fever. Other common findings are nonspecific symptoms such as myalgia,

arthralgia, headache, and malaise. Less common findings include petechiae, and other embolic phenomena (pneumonia, stroke, renal infarct), splenomegaly, neurologic findings, and the classically described findings (of infective endocarditis): Osler nodes (immunologic response with a palpable tender area in the pads of the fingers, toes, and sides of the fingers), Janeway lesions (nontender, hemorrhagic plaques occurring on the palms and soles owing to septic emboli of bacteria and WBC, with subsequent necrosis and subcutaneous hemorrhage), Roth spots (small pale retinal lesions with areas of hemorrhage near the optic disc) and splinter hemorrhages.

Laboratory Findings

Laboratory findings include a positive blood culture (if infectious), elevated acute phase reactants, anemia, hematuria, presence of rheumatoid factor, and leukocytosis. Of note is that the bacteremia with infective endocarditis is continuous and thus blood cultures need not only be obtained during fever. The volume of blood obtained for culture is more important than the number of times the blood is drawn. Echocardiography can be used to demonstrate endocardial vegetations as well as valve dysfunction (stenosis or regurgitation).

Diagnosis

The diagnosis of infective endocarditis may be difficult in some cases. Criteria, mainly for adults, have been made to aid in the diagnosis (Table 33-3). The diagnosis of noninfectious endocarditis is made after the finding of valve abnormalities in the presence of an inflammatory disease.

Treatment

Treatment of any bacterial process includes appropriate antibiotic therapy. In addition, supportive care of any underlying heart failure is similar to treating valve disease from other causes. Surgical repair or replacement of infected valves is needed if the valve destruction is severe, although it should be delayed as long as possible to allow adequate clearance of bacteria from the blood stream. Sometimes a delay is not possible and antibiotic

TABLE 33-3

DUKE CRITERIA FOR THE DIAGNOSIS OF INFECTIVE ENDOCARDITIS

Definite

1. Pathologic criteria
   a. Microorganisms: demonstrated by culture or histology in a vegetation, or in a vegetation that has embolized, or in an intracardiac abscess
   b. Pathologic lesions: vegetation or intracardiac abscess present, confirmed by histology showing active endocarditis
2. Clinical criteria
   a. Two major criteria or,
   b. One major and three minor criteria, or
   c. Five minor criteria

Possible

Findings consistent with infective endocarditis that fall short of definite, but not rejected

Rejected

1. Firm alternative diagnosis for manifestations of endocarditis, or
2. Resolution of manifestations of endocarditis with antibiotic therapy for 4 days or less, or
3. No pathologic evidence of infective endocarditis at surgery or autopsy, after antibiotic therapy for 4 days or less.

Criteria

Major Criteria

1. Positive blood culture for IE
   a. Typical microorganisms consistent with IE from two separate blood cultures, or
   b. Microorganisms consistent with IE from persistently positive blood cultures in:
      i. At least 2 positive blood cultures drawn >12 h apart
      ii. All of three or a majority of four or more separate blood cultures (with first and last sample drawn at least 1 hour apart)
2. Evidence of endocardial involvement
   a. Positive echocardiogram for IE
      i. Vegetation
      ii. Abcess
      iii. New partial dehiscence of prosthetic valve
   b. New valvar regurgitation (worsening or changing of preexisting murmur not sufficient)

Minor Criteria

1. Predisposition: predisposing heart condition or intravenous catheter/drug use
2. Fever: temperature greater or equal to 38.0°C
3. Vascular phenomena: major arterial emboli, septic pulmonary infarcts, mycotic aneurysm, intracranial hemorrhage, conjunctival hemorrhages, and Janeway lesions
4. Immunologic phenomena: glomerulonephritis, Osler's nodes, Roth spots, and rheumatoid factor
5. Microbiological evidence: positive blood culture but does not meet a major criterion as noted above or serologic evidence of active infection with organisms consistent with IE
6. Echocardiographic findings: consistent with IE but do not meet a major criterion as noted above

Source: Modified from Durack DT, Lukes AS, Bright DK: New criteria for diagnosis of infective endocarditis: utilization of specific echocardiographic findings. *Am J Med* 96:200–209, 1994.

therapy will need to be continued postoperatively. The duration of antibiotic therapy may be 4–6 weeks, though this is adjusted depending on the organism, and other clinical factors.

Treatment of noninfectious endocarditis is usually the same as treatment of the underlying inflammatory disease.

Prophylaxis

Prevention of infectious endocarditis, SBE prophylaxis, is discussed in Chapter 56.

MYOCARDITIS

Myocarditis is the inflammation of heart muscle. It has been described (Dallas criteria) as "an inflammatory infiltrate of the myocardium with necrosis and/or degeneration of adjacent myocytes not typical of the ischemic damage associated with coronary artery disease." Causes of myocarditis are given in Tables 33-3 and 33-4. Infectious myocarditis is usually viral in origin. Similar to bacterial endocarditis, viruses vary in their virulence and presentation. Most viral agents do not cause any significant myocardial injury and present with few if any signs and symptoms.

Pathophysiology

The pathophysiology is similar to a dilated cardiomyopathy with the addition of inflammation. The inflammation may be infectious or noninfectious. In the case of infectious myocarditis, the causative agent is usually viral although bacteria and fungi may also cause myocarditis. In both infectious and noninfectious myocarditis, there is an immune reaction (inflammation) in response to an infectious or noninfectious agent. The immunologic response includes the accumulation of mononuclear cells, including lymphocytes, plasma cells, and eosinophils. Edema as well as necrosis of the myocardium may be seen, the latter with severe infections. In some infections, neutrophils and macrophages will be seen as well. The immune response may cause further myocardial damage or may be protective. In addition, injured myocytes may release antigens causing a further immune response. The understanding of the exact mechanism of myocardial damage is still unclear.

TABLE 33-4

CLINICAL SIGNS AND SYMPTOMS TO DIAGNOSE KAWASAKI DISEASE

Diagnostic Criteria
1. Fever of at least 5 days duration plus
2. Presence of at least four of the following:
   - Extremity changes—initial erythema of palms and soles, later desquamation of tips of fingers/toes
   - Polymorphous rash
   - Bilateral nonpurulent conjunctivitis
   - Oral mucous membrane changes—red lips, "strawberry tongue," oral, and pharngeal erythema
   - Cervical lymphadenopathy
3. Exclusion of other disease with similar findings (measles, Stevens Johnson, scarlet fever)

Associated Findings
1. Cardiac—myocarditis, pericarditis, endocarditis
2. Neurologic—aseptic meningitis
3. GI—diarrhea, hydrops of the gallbladder, obstructive jaundice. Increase LFTs, low serum protein/albumin
4. GU—urethritis, sterile pyuria, proteinuria
5. Ophthalmolgical—uveitis
6. Hematologic—normochromic, normacytic anemia, thrombocytosis
7. Dermatologic—erythema and crusting at site of BCG innoculation
8. Other lab findings—negative ASO titer, increased acute phase reactants (CRP, ESR)

The amount of myocardial injury varies among the various causes. Coxsackie B viral myocarditis is known to cause fulminant myocarditis with myocyte necrosis and profound dysfunction.

With myocarditis, there may be an associated vasculitis. The latter may cause myocardial ischemia. This may lead to further changes in the myocardium such as cell injury and fibrosis. Cardiac enlargement with myocardial injury may cause dilation of the cardiac valves, leading to regurgitation. In addition, myocarditis may affect the conduction system and cause conduction abnormalities and/or arrhythmias.

Clinical Presentation

The clinical presentation of myocarditis will vary with the cause of inflammation and the resultant myocardial dysfunction. Viruses, bacteria, other infectious agents, and noninfectious causes of myocarditis vary in the amount of myocardial injury caused. Signs and symptoms of forward and backward failure will occur, correlating with the amount of muscle damage.

In addition to signs of muscle dysfunction, there will be signs and symptoms of inflammation (fever, increased serum markers of inflammation) as well as signs and symptoms of the specific inflammatory disease (e.g., measles will have the typical rash of measles, dermatomyositis will have the rash of dermatomyositis). The viral causes of myocarditis typically have a viral prodrome such as a rash or gastrointestinal symptoms (vomiting and diarrhea).

Finally, there may be signs and symptoms of conduction abnormalities such as bradycardia or syncope if there is complete heart block. Arrhythmias may occur as they can with any significant hemodynamic abnormality. Healing of the myocardial damage may include scar formation. Since scar tissue does not have the contraction and electrical conduction properties of the myocyte, overall heart dysfunction, conduction abnormalities, and arrhythmias may persist.

Diagnosis

Diagnosis of myocarditis is made in the presence of typical signs and symptoms. Laboratory studies may show findings of inflammation (increased acute phase reactants and erythrocyte sedimentation rate). The chest radiograph varies with the severity of disease, though it typically shows an enlarged, globular shaped heart with increased vascular markings consistent with pulmonary edema. An ECG may show ST segment and T-wave changes to suggest ischemia or a pattern suggestive of myocardial infarction. Echocardiography is diagnostic and can demonstrate the large, poorly functioning heart and the degree of dysfunction. Any associated valvar dysfunction may be seen as well.

Treatment

The treatment of myocarditis is first centered on supportive care. This may include diuretics to treat pulmonary edema and hepatic congestion because of backward heart failure, as well as inotropic support to improve myocardial contractility, and afterload reduction. Mechanical ventilation may be required as well as mechanical cardiac support such as a ventricular assist device or extracorporeal membrane oxygenation (ECMO). Refractory heart failure may require heart transplantation. Arrhythmias are treated via improving the hemodynamic derangement from the myocardial dysfunction as well as specific antiarrhythmic therapy.

In addition to supportive care, treatment of the underlying cause of the myocarditis is usually undertaken. In the case of a systemic inflammatory illness, this is treated in the usual fashion. Bacterial causes are treated with appropriate antibiotics. Treatment of viral myocarditis is made difficult by the lack of specific antiviral agents; however, it is felt that the inflammatory response may be the major cause of myocardial injury. Thus, treatment of the underlying inflammation is common practice. This may include intravenous gamma-globulin (IVIG) and steroids, though both are controversial. The use of IVIG is supported only with anecdotal evidence of efficacy.

Prognosis

Viral myocarditis has a wide range of outcomes. There may be little if any myocardial involvement with few if any sequelae. Conversely, there may be fulminant myocardial involvement resulting in cardiogenic shock, requiring intense cardiac support such as inotropic agents, mechanical ventilation, and cardiac assist devices (ECMO in small children and ventricular assist devices in older children). The latter has a high mortality; however, if supportive care can be maintained, myocardial recovery usually occurs. Recovery may be nearly complete (even with severe illness), partial, or poor. With partial recovery, continued pharmacologic therapy for heart failure and physical restrictions may be required. With poor recovery, the heart function remains poor, with the requirement of continued pharmacologic support and restrictions in activity. Heart transplantation will likely be required in these circumstances.

PERICARDITIS

Pericarditis is inflammation of the pericardium. It may be infectious or noninfectious with various etiologic factors (Tables 33-1 and 33-2). Of the infectious causes, both viral and bacterial are more common than fungal pericarditis. Viral pericarditis usually occurs with an associated viral myocarditis; however, the pericardial component is frequently more prominent than is the myocardial component. When there is a bacterial cause of pericarditis, there may also be a component of myocarditis. Again, the pericardial component is usually more prominent.

Of note is that there are causes of pericardial effusion, not necessarily inflammatory, thus no pericarditis; however, these are sometimes still referred to as pericarditis. These include pericardial effusions owing to direct trauma (central line erosion into the pericardial space), hypothyroidism and myxedema, and pericardial tumors (though these may have an inflammatory component). The physiology and presentation of these are similar to pericarditis, except for the lack of signs and symptoms of inflammation. Chronic pericardial effusions, termed chronic pericarditis, may not have the pathophysiology of acute tamponade (shock), but are similar in pathophysiology to the restrictive myocardial diseases.

Pathophysiology

The pathophysiology is one of restricted filling of the heart, therefore diastolic dysfunction. The ability of the heart to fill decreases as the pericardial pressure increases. The pressure is related to the amount of fluid and the rapidity of fluid accumulation. (Large volumes of fluid that accumulate slowly cause less of a pressure increase in the pericardial space.) Bacteria usually cause more rapid fluid accumulation, thus greater symptoms. If the pericardial pressure is severely elevated and causing shock, tamponade is said to be occurring.

Clinical Findings

Signs and symptoms are related to diastolic dysfunction. This includes signs and symptoms of backward failure with lesser degrees of forward failure. These include pallor, tachypnea, tachycardia, abdominal pain (owing to hepatic congestion), peripheral edema, muffled heart sounds, and a pericardial friction rub on auscultation. A rapid rise in pericardial pressure may not allow time for signs of venous congestion to occur, and forward failure (shock) may be the first symptom. Mild symptoms of pericardial inflammation may include sharp chest pain, which typically increases with lying supine and decreases with sitting. The reason for this appears to be the effect of position on stretching the pericardium.

In addition, there may be an exaggerated paradoxical pulse. The paradoxical pulse is generated by changes in intrathoracic pressure and its effects on diastolic filling of the heart. During inhalation, owing to an increase in the negative intrathoracic pressure, there is an increase in the systemic venous return to the right heart. As the right ventricle enlarges, it hinders left ventricular filling and output. Thus, there is a mild decrease in stroke volume and blood pressure in inspiration. From a practical standpoint, the paradoxical pulse is measured as follows: the blood pressure cuff is deflated and the pressure is noted when the first systolic sounds are noted. (These will vary between inspiration and expiration.) The blood pressure cuff is deflated until the systolic sounds are heard during both inhalation and exhalation. The difference between when one is able to auscultate every systolic sound during both inhalation and exhalation and when one is able to auscultate the systolic sound only during exhalation is the paradoxical pulse. The normal difference is less than 10 mmHg. With constriction from the pericardium (as from a pericardial effusion or constrictive pericardial disease), the space occupied by the LV and RV is relatively fixed. Therefore, any enlargement of one ventricle will cause an equal reduction of volume of the other ventricle. Thus, with a large pericardial effusion, inhalation causes RV enlargement, LV diminution, and a decreased stroke volume. This will be seen clinically with a decreased systolic blood pressure.

Finally, signs and symptoms of inflammation should be present. Fever is a common sign of inflammation, though it may be less pronounced in cases such as posttraumatic pericardial inflammation, and more marked in bacterial than viral pericarditis. Bacterial pericarditis usually presents with rapid hemodynamic compromise in the setting of fever and other systemic signs of a bacterial infection, whereas viral myocarditis has a more insidious onset.

Laboratory findings include an abnormal ECG. Conduction abnormalities do not typically occur as they may with endocarditis and myocarditis; however, there are typical ECG changes, such as the following:

1. Early, diffuse ST elevation, depressed PR segment
2. ST segment begins to return to normal, amplitude of T-wave diminished, PR segment depressed
3. ST segment normal, T-wave inversion
4. All changes resolve completely, though the T-wave abnormalities may persist

There is low overall voltage with large effusions. Arrhythmias may be seen, both ventricular and atrial, though these are more common with myocarditis.

The chest radiograph may be normal with a small effusion. With a larger effusion, the chest radiograph typically shows an enlarged pericardial shadow (water bottle shape of the cardiothymic silhouette), mediastinal widening, and a pleural effusion. Of note is the similar appearance with a dilated cardiomyopathy. Therefore, additional testing such as echocardiography may be required to differentiate the cardiac versus pericardial border.

Diagnosis

The diagnosis of pericarditis is made with the signs and symptoms described above and the finding of pericardial effusion by echocardiography. Supportive laboratory studies such as elevated acute phase reactants are noted. In the setting of a large pericardial effusion, pericardiocentesis can be diagnostic as well as therapeutic. Pericardial fluid should be sent for gram stain, culture, and cytology. Other evidence of tuberculosis (positive skin test) is helpful to diagnose tuberculous pericarditis in the absence of findings in the pericardial fluid.

Treatment

Treatment of a noninfectious pericarditis is usually the same as treatment of the underlying systemic inflammatory disease (e.g., rheumatic fever, systemic lupus erythematosus [SLE]). Treatment of viral pericarditis is usually one of observation and the use of nonsteroidal anti-inflammatory drugs. Viral pericarditis is usually self-limiting. Anti-inflammatory drugs usually cause rapid improvement in signs and symptoms. This rarely recurs, and if so, should suggest the possibility of an underlying noninfectious cause of inflammation.

Pericardiocentesis is required if there is evidence of tamponade and can be life-saving. Bacterial pericarditis requires placement of a large bore pericardial drain, and/or opening the pericardium (creation of a pericardial window) to allow the space to be irrigated, debrided, and to prevent tamponade.

VASCULITIS

Inflammation of the vessels of the heart, namely the coronary arteries, is typically seen only with Kawasaki disease. A small vessel vasculitis may be a part of viral myocarditis as well as other inflammatory conditions of the heart. Kawasaki associated coronary arteritis is discussed below.

SPECIFIC NONINFECTIOUS INFLAMMATORY HEART DISEASES

Noninfectious inflammation of the heart usually involves all portions of the heart (endocardium, myocardium, and pericardium). It is usually in response to systemic inflammatory disease such as collagen vascular disease (SLE, rheumatoid arthritis, and dermatomyositis, among others). It may also be a result of inflammatory diseases that are part of an infectious disease process such as rheumatic fever (poststreptococcal infection), Kawasaki disease (felt to be infectious though no single organism found thus far) Lyme disease, or septic shock. For lack of a better term, the latter may be referred to as parainfectious causes of inflammatory heart disease. Because of their unique presentation, Kawasaki disease and rheumatic fever are discussed below.

KAWASAKI DISEASE

Kawasaki disease, also known as mucocutaneous lymph node syndrome, is an illness manifest by fever, rash, edema of hands and feet, conjunctivitis, swollen lymph glands in the neck, and cracked red lips, as described in Table 33-4. It is a systemic inflammatory with the exact cause remaining unknown. In addition to other organ systems, it can affect the heart and cause coronary arteritis.

Etiology

Kawasaki disease usually occurs in children under 5 years of age, with an average age of 2 years. It is more common in those of Asian ethnicity but can occur in any racial or ethnic group. No known infectious agent has been isolated, but the seasonal pattern of occurrence suggests an infectious cause. It is rare, though possible, to have recurrence of this disease.

Pathophysiology

The pathophysiology of Kawasaki disease reflects the underlying endocarditis, myocarditis, and pericarditis. The physiology is similar to that of other inflammatory illnesses as described above.

Clinical Findings

The clinical course is triphasic with acute, subacute, and convalescent phases. The acute phase occurs on days 1–14 with an initial fever and upper respiratory or gastrointestinal symptoms. These are followed by a nonpurulent conjunctivitis, stomatitis and oral mucous membrane changes, induration or swelling and erythema of the hands and feet, a nonspecific rash, and cervical adenitis (usually unilateral and greater than 1.5 cm in diameter). The erythrocyte sedimentation rate is elevated early in the acute phase and remains elevated throughout the subacute phase and into the convalescent phase. Arthritis, desquamation of the tips of the fingers and toes, thrombocytosis, and cardiac changes begin at approximately 7–10 days during the subacute phase (2nd–4th week of the illness, days 10–32). The symptoms of the acute phase resolve during the subacute phase, and the signs and symptoms in the subacute phase resolve prior to or during the convalescent phase (days 32–42 and beyond). With current treatment, most symptoms disappear by the 4th–6th week of the illness.

Inflammatory cardiac disease can occur and usually begins in the subacute phase, and specifically causes coronary arteritis. Myocarditis, endocarditis, and pericarditis can occur. Coronary arteritis occurs in 15–20% of untreated patients. The endocarditis, myocarditis, and pericarditis are usually self-limited. The coronary arteritis can cause the development of coronary artery aneurysms. These range from small (a few mm) to large (6–8 mm). The large aneurysms are at risk of rupture acutely (a very rare occurrence) and thrombosis. Most small coronary artery aneurysms resolve completely. Large coronary artery aneurysms may appear to have resolved (normal appearing lumen via angiography), though do so via intimal proliferation. Thus, they are not normal and are risk factors for coronary artery stenosis and occlusion.

Signs and symptoms of cardiac involvement can include tachycardia and tachypnea owing to forward and backward heart failure from the associated myocarditis and endocarditis (valvulitis). In addition, there may be chest pain or angina if there is a significant coronary artery lesion.

Diagnosis

Diagnosis of Kawasaki disease is clinical (Table 33-4). Coronary artery aneurysms are a late manifestation and do not occur in a majority of patients; therefore, this finding is not part of the initial diagnostic criteria. The echocardiogram is not a diagnostic test unless aneurysms are found (which would be unusual in the absence of other symptoms). Thus, diagnosis of Kawasaki disease is an independent clinical diagnosis and the absence of coronary artery aneurysms on echocardiography does not exclude the diagnosis. The decision to treat is made regardless of the findings on echocardiography.

Treatment

Once the diagnosis is established or reasonably certain, current treatment consists of IVIG. Its efficacy has been demonstrated (reduction of the incidence of coronary artery aneurysms from 15 to 2%) if given within the first 10 days of the illness. There is evidence that use in the convalescent phase is also efficacious, though perhaps less than if given in the acute phase. The dose is 2 g/kg over 10–12 hours. In addition, high dose aspirin (80–100 mg/kg) is given initially every 6 hours until defervescence occurs for 2–3 days. After this, the aspirin dose is decreased to 3–5 mg/kg until all clinical and laboratory evidence of a continued inflammatory illness have subsided in the presence of a normal echocardiogram (no evidence of coronary artery abnormalities), usually 4–6 weeks. If the initial inflammation persists, repeated infusions of IVIG can be given. If the coronary arteries remain abnormal after resolution of inflammation, aspirin is continued indefinitely. Large coronary artery aneurysms may be treated with additional antithrombotic agents (e.g., warfarin, heparin).

Throughout treatment, supportive care is given for any underlying cardiac derangement. Pericardiocentesis is performed if signs of tamponade are present. Diuretic and inotropic agents are given for the treatment of heart failure, as are afterload reducing agents.

Controversies remain in the treatment of Kawasaki disease. The role of aspirin (recommended dose and length of treatment) remains to be redefined in the era of IVIG. Steroid therapy was used in the past, though the role of steroids is also unclear in this disease. Of note is the need to withhold certain immunizations following IVIG treatment. It is recommended that the following immunizations be withheld at least 11 months following IVIG therapy: MMR, varicella, or other live virus vaccines.

Initial Follow-Up

Medical follow-up of the patient with Kawasaki disease varies among institutions and may include general pediatricians, infectious disease specialists, and rheumatologists, as well as cardiologists. The initial diagnosis may be made by any of these individuals. The role of echocardiography in the assessment of cardiac sequelae has changed over time. Currently, a baseline echocardiogram is recommended at the time of diagnosis. A follow-up echocardiogram at 6 weeks of the illness is felt to be sufficient to exclude coronary artery involvement if the first was normal as well. Additional echocardiograms are indicated only if one of these prior studies are abnormal.

Long-Term Outlook

In patients who have had no cardiac involvement, specifically, no coronary artery abnormalities, the outlook is excellent. Most children recover completely and lead normal lives with no restrictions. Pediatric cardiology follow-up may be infrequent if at all. In patients who have had coronary artery abnormalities noted, continued follow-up and surveillance for coronary artery disease and myocardial ischemia is typically undertaken indefinitely. Follow-up tests such as echocardiograms, stress tests, and even cardiac catheterization may be required. Patients with giant coronary artery aneurysms require more frequent follow-up. Risks for the development of these aneurysms are: males less than 1 year, fever >16 days (or recurrence), WBC >30,000, ESR >101, ESR or CRP elevated >30 days, recurrence of elevated ESR or CRP, ECG abnormalities (Q waves in leads II, III, aVF), signs and symptoms of a myocardial infarction.

RHEUMATIC FEVER

Rheumatic fever is an inflammatory disease caused by a response to certain strains of beta-hemolytic streptococcus. These strains are not the same as those causing other diseases such as superficial skin infections, rather, they are caused by those strains causing streptococcal pharyngitis. The systemic inflammation of rheumatic fever can cause arthritis (typically the large joints such as the knees, ankles, wrists, and elbows), which is described as exquisitely painful (pain at rest or with little motion) and occurs with associated erythema and warmth. The arthritis is asymmetric and migratory (migrating polyarthritis). The central nervous system is involved and chorea (Sydenham's chorea) can occur. A rash may be seen and is described as red, macular, and nonpruritic, with a serpiginous border. It is seen over the trunk and limbs and may be fleeting. Subcutaneous nodules may be seen and are described as nontender nodules over the extensor surfaces of the joints (elbows, knuckles, knees, and ankles).

Cardiac involvement in rheumatic fever consists of endocarditis, myocarditis, and pericarditis. Myocarditis occurs, though less frequently than endocarditis. Pericarditis usually occurs in association with endocarditis or myocarditis. The aortic and mitral valves are the most commonly (noticeably) affected heart valves.

Observation of many cases of rheumatic fever has shown that those patients with initial severe joint involvement have minimal if any cardiac involvement and vice versa.

Pathophysiology

The exact mechanism in which the streptococcus causes rheumatic fever is not clear; however, the basic pathophysiology and histopathology are known. First there is an exudative degenerative inflammatory stage. This consists of edema of the ground substance with fragmentation of collagen fibers. An infiltrate consisting of T cells, macrophages, B cells, and mast cells is seen along with fibrinoid deposition. The transitory manifestations of this phase may last 2–3 weeks and respond to anti-inflammatory treatment. A second phase is seen which may persist for months to years. In this stage, the Ashoff nodule is seen. The latter, a hallmark of rheumatic fever, is a perivascular infiltrate of large cells with polymorphous nuclei and basophilic cytoplasm arranged in a rosette around an avascular center of fibrinoid. This stage probably does not respond to anti-inflammatory treatment.

The pathophysiology is the same as for other inflammatory illnesses of the heart and reflects the degree of valvar, myocardial, and pericardial dysfunction.

The Host

The role of genetic susceptibility is not clear; however, it is felt that this does exist, since the strains of streptococcus causing rheumatic fever do so in only a small percentage of people. Susceptibility is more likely caused by crowded conditions (close contact) as it occurs mainly in winter and spring.

Clinical Findings

The clinical findings of arthritis, a rash, subcutaneous nodules, and chorea are as described. Cardiac findings can include tachypnea, tachycardia, and frank shock if there is significant myocardial dysfunction or valvar regurgitation. A murmur of mitral or aortic regurgitation will be present if those are significant. The finding of a friction rub suggests pericarditis, though this is usually associated with findings of myocardial or valvar dysfunction.

Laboratory findings include a prolonged PR interval in the ECG as well as dysrhythmia if there is significant myocardial disease. The chest radiograph may show an enlarged heart, reflective of myocardial dysfunction and valvar regurgitation. Echocardiography can well demonstrate all of the cardiac features of this disease including cardiac function, valvar regurgitation, and pericardial effusion.

Diagnosis—History/Symptoms

The symptoms of rheumatic fever usually begin 1–6 weeks after a streptococcal pharyngitis. Diagnostic features and criteria are given in Table 33-5.

Treatment

Treatment of rheumatic fever has not changed significantly in the last few decades, except for the introduction of afterload reducing agents. Suppor-

TABLE 33-5

GUIDELINES FOR THE DIAGNOSIS OF RHEUMATIC
FEVER (MODIFIED JONES CRITERIA)*

1. Major criteria
Carditis
Migratory polyarthritis
Sydenham's chorea
Erythema marginatum
Subcutaneous nodules
2. Minor criteria
Clinical
Fever, arthralgia
Laboratory
Elevated acute phase reactants (ESR,
C-reactive protein—CRP)
Prolonged PR interval
3. Supporting evidence of prior strep infection
Elevated or rising ASO titers
Positive throat culture or rapid strep test

*Diagnosis is made with the presence of two major criteria, or one major and two minor criteria—in the presence of a preceding strep infection. The latter may not be seen with Sydenham's chorea due to the late appearance of the chorea.

tive care of any underlying cardiac hemodynamic derangements is given (diuretics, inotropic agents, and afterload reducing agents). Bedrest or a restriction of activity is prescribed during the acute phase (afterload reducing agents function as a pharmacological bedrest). The underlying inflammation is treated with aspirin and/or steroids. The latter may be continued from several weeks to several months, after which they are tapered with close monitoring for any exacerbation of inflammation. Eradication of streptococcal infection with antibiotic therapy is followed by prophylaxis against any recurrent streptococcal infection. This is usually performed with long-acting penicillin (intramuscular benzathine penicillin) given every 28 days. Oral prophylaxis has a much higher rate of recurrence of rheumatic fever. Whether or not to give prophylaxis, or what type to give in patients with arthritis and no history of carditis, is not clear.

Prophylaxis with an antibiotic other than penicillin is used for procedures with anticipated bacteremia if there is any valvar lesion (SBE prophylaxis).

Long-Term Outlook

Arthritis, chorea, rash, and skin findings of rheumatic fever are all self-limited and not known to cause long-term sequelae. Cardiac lesions tend to improve over time, though this is variable. Moderate or severe aortic or mitral valve regurgitation may progress or cause progression of other findings (cardiac enlargement and dysfunction, pulmonary edema, dysrhythmia). The long-term outlook is therefore dependent on the presence and severity of the underlying cardiac disease. Long-term afterload reduction, prophylaxis for recurrent rheumatic fever, and SBE prophylaxis are required. Exercise restriction may be needed with significant valvar or myocardial dysfunction, though this is an indication for intervention. The interventions and indications for them are the same as for other valve lesions with the exception of a Ross procedure for aortic regurgitation (using a patient's own pulmonary valve to replace the aortic valve). Although not usually clinically apparent (probably because of low pulmonary artery pressures), the pulmonary

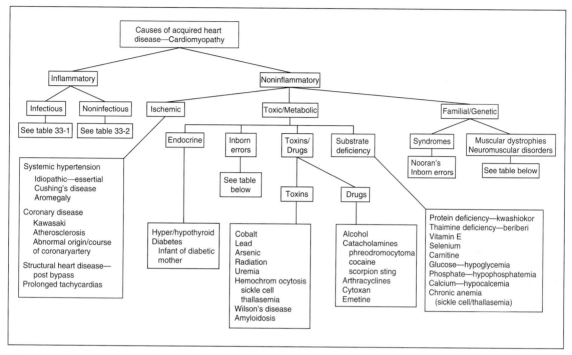

FIGURE 33-3

ACQUIRED HEART DISEASES/CARDIOMYOPATHIES BASED ON DISEASE CATEGORIES

valve is felt to be affected in most cases of rheumatic fever and fill to be unsuitable for this procedure. In the even longer term, valvar disease may progress from primarily regurgitation to stenosis. Management of this is similar to that of stenoses from other causes.

SPECIFIC CAUSES AND TREATMENT OF NONINFLAMMATORY HEART DISEASES/CARDIOMYOPATHIES

Noninflammatory heart diseases and cardiomyopathies are shown in Figures 33-3, 33-4, and 33-5.

Juvenile progressive (Duchenne)
Myotonic dystrophy (Steinert)
Limb-girdle (Erb)
Juvenile progressive spinal atrophy (Kugelberg-Welander)
Nemaline myopathy
Myotubular myopathy

        Hereditary dilated CMP—autosomal dominant/recessive, X-linked
        Friedeich's ataxia
        Emery Dreifuss dystrophy
        Fascioscapulohumeral dystrophy
        Beckers muscular dystrophy

FIGURE 33-4

MUSCULAR DYSTROPHIES/NEUROMUSCULAR DISORDERS

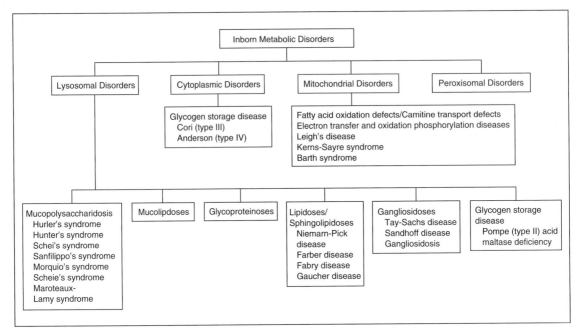

FIGURE 33-5

INBORN METABOLIC DISORDERS

The cardiac pathophysiology for all of these diagnoses is similar to that of other causes of cardiomyopathy (Chapter 11). The diseases listed in Figure 33-3 are associated with either a dilated, restrictive or hypertrophic cardiomyopathy.

Clinical Presentation and Diagnosis

The clinical findings of the diseases listed in Figure 33-3 may be related to the primary disease problem. Examples are seizures because of hypoglycemia in an infant of a diabetic mother, a history of drug or toxin use, renal failure or starvation. In these cases, the coexistence of the possibility of an underlying cardiac problem ought to be recognized. In other cases, the presenting clinical feature may be the signs and symptoms of cardiomyopathy (Chapters 11), findings of structural heart disease (usually valvar, especially with inborn errors of metabolism), or arrhythmia in the absence of inflammation. In all of these cases, a cardiac workup is indicated. Along with the findings on the history and physical examination, the ECG, and echocardiographic findings are usually sufficient to diagnose the cardiac pathology (cardiomyopathy and type, valve disease, conduction abnormalities). Sometimes tissue (heart, skeletal muscle or skin fibroblasts for metabolic testing) is required for the definitive diagnosis. Treatment is dependent on the underlying diagnosis, though supportive treatment for cardiac dysfunction is similar (diuretics for preload reduction, inotropic agents for poor contractility, and afterload reducing agents). Management may also include cardiac transplantation (Chapter 54) if the treatment of heart failure is unsuccessful, and the underlying disease process is resolved or nonprogressive. Treatment of isolated cardiac abnormalities (e.g., aortic valve repair or replacement for rheumatic fever, or coronary bypass grafting for Kawasaki disease) is also included in the cardiac management of theses diseases. Nevertheless, treatment of cardiac disease associated with another systemic disease requires optimal management of the primary disease process. Some diseases are irreversible and/or fatal. Other diseases are reversible with simple measures (thyroid hormone for hypothyroidism). Discussion of each individual disease is beyond the scope of this text; however, the general principles remain.

Suggested Readings

AHA scientific statement. Diagnostic guidelines for Kawasaki disease. *Circulation* 103:335, 2001.

Allen HD, Gutgesell HP, Clark EB, Driscoll DJ: *Moss and Adams' Heart Disease in Infants, Children, and Adolescents Including the Fetus and Young Adult*, 6th ed. Philadelphia, PA, Lippincott Williams & Wilkins, 2001.

Asai T, et al: Study of heart disease in Kawasaki disease ACTA. *Jpn J Pediatr* 9:1086, 1976.

Choudhary SK, Mathur A, Sharma R, Saxena A, Chopra P, Roy R, Kumar AS: Pulmonary autograft: should it be used in young patients with rheumatic disease? *J Thorac Cardiovasc Surg* 11(3):483–490, 1999.

Dajani AS, et al: Guidelines for long-term management of patients with Kawasaki disease. *Circulation* 89:916–922, 1994.

Dajani AS, et al: Guidelines for the diagnosis of rheumatic fever. Jones Criteria, updated 1992. *Circulation* 87:302–307, 1993.

Durack DT, Lukes AS, Bright DK: New criteria for diagnosis of infective endocarditis:utilization of specific echocardiographic findings. *Am J Med* 96:200–209, 1994.

Feigin RD, Cherry JD: *Textbook of Pediatric Infectious Diseases*, 3rd ed. Philadelphia, PA, WB Saunders, 1992.

Garson A, Bricker JT, Fisher DJ, Neish SR: *The Science and Practice of Pediatric Cardiology*, 2nd ed. Baltimore, MD, Williams & Wilkins, 1998.

Jenson HB, Baltimore RS: *Communicable Diseases in Children*. Appleton & Lange, 1995.

Long S, Pickering Prober: *Principles and Practice of Pediatric Infectious Diseases*, 2nd ed. New York, NY, Churchill Livingstone, 2003.

Mandell GL, Bennett JE, Dolin R. Mandell: *Douglas and Bennett's Principles and Practice of Infectious Diseases*, 5th ed. Philadelphia, PA, Churchill Livingstone, 2000.

Markowitz M, Gordis L: *Rheumatic Fever*, 2nd ed. Philadelphia, PA, WB Saunders, 1972.

Mauizio M, et al: Late intravenous gamma globulin treatment in infants and children with Kawasaki disease and coronary artery abnormalities. *Am J Cardiol* 68:796–797, 1991.

Melish ME: Clinical and epidemiologic aspects of Kawasaki disease. *Clin Cardiol* 14:II3–II10, 1991.

Scott JS, Ettedgui JA, Neches WH: Cost-effectiveness of echocardiography in children with Kawasaki disease. *Pediatrics* 104(5):e57, 1999.

Shingadia D, Shulman ST: New perspectives in the drug treatment of Kawasaki disease. *Paediatr Drugs* 1(4): 291–297, 1999.

34

CARDIAC TRAUMA

Peter Koenig

INTRODUCTION

It is rare to encounter cardiac trauma in pediatrics partly because of underdiagnosis. Cardiac trauma in children may be underdiagnosed from the lack of suspicion. This may be a result of the absence of external physical findings such as bruising since children have more compliant chests than do adults. Another reason for the lack of suspected cardiac trauma is the similarity in signs and symptoms with other diagnoses or sequelae of trauma (e.g., hypotension because of blood loss rather than cardiac dysfunction, or dysrhythmia because of electrolyte imbalances from resuscitation, and so forth). When present, cardiac trauma can be subdivided into nonpenetrating, or blunt, and penetrating cardiac trauma, with each of these subdivided into further categories.

BLUNT CARDIAC TRAUMA

Mechanisms of Blunt Cardiac Trauma

The mechanisms of blunt trauma include direct cardiac injury, indirect cardiac injury, bidirectional or compressive cardiac injury, concussive injury,

deceleration injury, blast injury, and combination injury. In direct injury, force is applied directly to the precordium in one direction, anterior to posterior. With indirect injury, there is a hydraulic ram effect with an abrupt increase in intravascular pressure, as seen with sudden compression of the abdomen. In bidirectional or compression injury, force is applied to the chest from two separate directions such as an automobile rolling over the chest, or being compressed or crushed in a hydraulic press. In each of these mechanisms of trauma, there is an elevated pressure or sustained force applied to the heart.

Concussion of the heart, "commotio cordis," is an acute cardiac dysfunction associated with sustained dysrhythmia because of a sudden impact or collision of the chest with an object such as a baseball or other object. The force is nonsustained. It should only be described in the absence of cardiac contusion. Resuscitation with this type of injury can be very difficult as it is probably electrical in nature, resulting from electrical alterations during a vulnerable period of the heart (R on T phenomenon). Electrical defibrillation may be required to successfully resuscitate these individuals.

Aortic tears can occur with acceleration or deceleration of the body. Since the heart is suspended in the chest as if on a pendulum (with the cardio-aortic junction as the fulcrum, and the aorta fixed in the chest at the brachiocephalic branches and the diaphragm), an acceleration or deceleration of the body can cause disruption or tearing of the aorta at the points of fixation.

Blast injury is a blunt injury to the chest and heart because of an explosion, and may involve both con-cussive or combination of traumatic mechanisms. Many other types of traumatic injuries may involve a combination of mechanisms discussed above.

TYPES OF CARDIAC INJURY WITH BLUNT TRAUMA

Although the mechanisms of blunt trauma may be varied, the injuries seen in the heart can be similar in each. The involved parts of the heart may be the pericardium, the myocardium, the valves, or the vessels in the vicinity of the heart. Diagnosis is based on suspicion (vague symptoms with a history to suggest the possibility of cardiac injury), exam-ination (usually nonspecific), and diagnostic tests (cardiac enzymes, electrocardiographic monitor-ing, and echocardiography).

Pericardial Injury

It is rare to have isolated pericardial injury to the heart with blunt trauma. Acute injuries to the peri-cardium can include lacerations or rupture of the pericardium. Bleeding into the pericardial space may be from the heart, or from other sources near the heart. Symptoms of pericardial injury may include sharp chest pain because of pericardial irri-tation, hypotension because of tamponade with associated signs of tachycardia, and an exaggerated paradoxic pulse (decrease in systolic pressure with inhalation). Echocardiography is usually diagnos-tic and will demonstrate fluid in the pericardial space. An isolated laceration of the pericardium without bleeding or other injuries may not be pos-sible to diagnose noninvasively.

In addition to acute pericardial injuries, a post-traumatic pericarditis may also occur 1–4 weeks after the traumatic event. The traumatic event may be forgotten at the time of presentation and may include things such as a football player being hit in the chest with the helmet of another football player. There is a resultant inflammation of the heart and may be associated with flu-like symptoms, though sharp chest pain is a common complaint. The chest pain is typically improved with sitting and worsens with lying. Signs may include tachycardia and an exaggerated pulsus paradoxus, or hypotension if tamponade is present. Physical examination may further reveal distant heart sounds, distended neck veins, and hepatomegaly. The chest pain should not be reproducible by pressing on the chest; however, there may be associated musculoskeletal trauma making the latter unreliable.

Myocardial Injury

Myocardial Contusion

Myocardial contusion is one type of traumatic car-diac injury and is seen in 25% of all serious thoracic trauma in adults. It is less frequently diagnosed and probably underdiagnosed in children because of a lack of suspicion and fewer physical findings, which may be a result of differences in the thoracic cage; however, the pathology is similar in children and adults and includes myocardial hemorrhage and hematoma, followed by myocardial fiber necrosis and later development of scar formation. Symptoms include precordial chest pain, which is anginal in nature, but not responsive to nitrates, as is angina arising from coronary artery disease. There may be symptoms of shortness of breath with exertion in the presence of decreased cardiac function, or pal-pitations if dysrhythmia occurs. Signs of shock may be present. The physical examination may be unre-vealing unless cardiac dysfunction is great enough to cause associated venous congestion, edema, hepatomegaly, pulmonary edema. An abnormal rhythm may be noted or an S3 or S4 with cardiac dysfunction. Laboratory findings can include an abnormal ECG showing tachycardia or dysrhyth-mias, ST changes, Q waves, conduction abnormali-ties (block), or prolongation of the QT interval. None of the latter are diagnostic for contusion. A plain film of the chest may show associated lesions such as rib, sternal or vertebral fractures, pneumo or hemothorax, or a pulmonary contusion, which may increase the suspicion of cardiac injury.

Serum studies including the cardiac enzymes CPK and more recently troponin T are sensitive markers of myocardial injury. LDH was used in the past for myocardial injury detection. It exceeds the normal range at 24–48 h, peaks at 3–6 days, and returns to normal at 8–14 days. The relatively cardiac specific isoform of CPK, CPK-MB is more sensitive and specific with a small amount being released early, though in general it exceeds normal within 4–8 h, peaks at 24 h and returns to normal in 3–4 days. There is overlap of CPK-MB with enzymes released from skeletal muscle and other organ systems. Troponins I and T are highly specific for cardiac muscle and rise above normal within 4–8 h similar to CPK-MB, however, these enzymes have a higher and later (1–2 days) peak with a sustained elevation for 7–10 days. The levels of cardiac troponin also correlate with prognosis.

Echocardiography is a sensitive test for global dysfunction, and wall motion abnormalities, which accompany myocardial contusion. It is also a sensitive test for aneurysms, septal defects, valvar injury, pericardial effusion, and thrombi. Nuclear scans are also sensitive tests for functional abnormalities, seen more frequently in the right than left ventricle; however, these are not predictive of morbidity or mortality. The history of myocardial contusions is usually that of complete recovery; however, late complications of muscle necrosis such as free wall or intraventricular septal rupture may occur. Muscle akinesis may occur leading to aneurysm formation.

Management consists of (1) supportive care: intropic, diuretic, and afterload reducing agents; (2) monitoring for dysrhythmia or the development of pericardial effusions are other late sequelae; (3) pain control; (4) rest with progressive increase in physical activity depending on the degree of injury; and (5) consideration of anticoagulation to prevent thrombus formation (balanced by the risk of extension of any hematoma).

Cardiac Rupture

Cardiac rupture is another type of myocardial injury that may be a result of an earlier myocardial

contusion, or an acute event from significantly elevated intracardiac pressures experienced with either direct impact or a hydraulic ram effect. It is more likely to occur if the impact takes place during diastole (when the ventricles are filled) and occurs in the right ventricle more than the left ventricle which occurs more than in the atria. In the acute setting, cardiac rupture is usually fatal. Rupture is less likely to be fatal as a result of a prior myocardial contusion in which case there may be chest pain and signs of impending cardiac tamponade.

Similar to rupture of the free wall of the myocardium, rupture of the interventricular septum may occur leading to a ventricular septal defect (VSD). The VSD may occur acutely owing to hydraulic changes and usually occurs in the apical septum. It may also occur a few weeks after the traumatic event as a late sequelae of a myocardial contusion. The ensuing signs and symptoms depend on the size of the VSD and may include signs and symptoms of pulmonary edema with a large left-to-right shunt. Treatment of a hemodynamically significant traumatic VSD is preferably delayed until the margins of the VSD are healed enough to allow stable closure.

Aneurysm Formation

Short of myocardial free wall rupture or VSD formation, an aneurysm of the ventricular free wall may occur. It may occur after a prior myocardial contusion, or because of injury of a coronary artery with secondary myocardial infarction and scar formation. The latter could potentially result in rupture as well. If a large portion of the cardiac muscle is dysfunctional, cardiac output may be impaired and signs and symptoms of congestive heart failure may occur. The injured myocardium may be a focus of rhythm abnormalities, thrombus formation, with signs and symptoms of these including embolic phenomenon.

Valve Injury

Isolated valve injury is rare in blunt myocardial trauma. If it occurs, it is felt to be due to abrupt increases in intracardiac pressure against a closed valve from direct impact or indirect hydraulic ram effect. The aortic valve is the most frequently injured valve owing to the higher pressures of the left ventricle and aorta as well as the location in the heart (at the fulcrum of the pendulum). The valve injury is usually a laceration amenable to repair. In the case of cusp avulsion, valve replacement may be required. Valve injury may also be a result of perivalvar edema or hematoma. The second most common valves injured are the mitral and tricuspid valves with mechanisms of injury similar to the aortic valve leading to valvar or chordal damage. In addition, there may be papillary muscle damage because of contusion or ischemia leading to valvar dysfunction unlike the aortic valve. The latter may improve with time. Symptoms of valve injury depend on the valve involved and severity of the valve injury, which are similar to signs and symptoms of valvar regurgitation discussed in the valve disease section of this book.

Vessel Injury

Large arterial or venous injury may occur owing to deceleration forces described above. This may result in vessel laceration, with bleeding into the pericardial space (and subsequent tamponade), pleural or other large spaces (and subsequent exsanguination). Venous injury, such as that in the inferior vena cava, has a high mortality because of the thin vessel walls. Arterial injury may have lower mortality because of adventia that may remain intact, preventing bleeding and leading to aneurysm formation. This false aneurysm formed may lead to dissection of the intimal flap. This process may be asymptomatic or may be associated with dyspnea (airway compression), back pain, dysphagia (esophageal compression), hoarseness (recurrent laryngeal nerve injury), asymmetric pulses, or aortic regurgitation.

Injury to small arteries or veins is rarely seen with blunt cardiac trauma. Coronary artery injury, if it occurs, may lead to myocardial ischemia and signs and symptoms and laboratory studies similar to a myocardial contusion. Angiography may be necessary to demonstrate that the myocardial injury occurred because of a coronary artery injury. Laceration of a coronary artery can lead to cardiac

tamponade. Thrombosis of a coronary artery may be a result of primary coronary artery injury, or embolism from a mural thrombus.

PENETRATING CARDIAC TRAUMA

The causes of penetrating trauma to the heart are numerous. It is less common in children than adults, and most often because of violence; however, it may also occur during cardiac interventions (e.g., catheterization, indwelling catheter placement, cardiac resuscitation). The severity of the injuries depends on the type of penetration (gunshot, knife, catheter) and the location of the injury. The precordial wound is the most common; however, the heart may be lacerated from other locations as well, including posterior puncture via the esophagus.

Diagnosis of a penetrating cardiac injury relies on a combination of history and physical findings. Neither is conclusive as a precordial penetration may have missed the heart. The right ventricle, followed by the left ventricle and right atrium are the most frequently involved cardiac chambers from external penetrating trauma. The left atrium is most frequently involved with transesophageal penetration. Pericardial injury is almost always present. Depending on the size of the pericardial defect, signs and symptoms of tamponade (small defect) or exsanguination (large defect) may be present. The coronary arteries may also be injured with signs and symptoms of tamponade or exsanguination and/or myocardial ischemia/infarction. The right coronary artery is relatively more protected within the thorax than the left coronary artery. Laceration of the left anterior descending coronary artery can be a complication of pericardiocentesis. Coronary artery lacerations may lead to coronary-cameral fistulae if the communication with a cardiac chamber persists. This may be a complication of endomyocardial biopsy and is not infrequently seen in heart transplant patients. Valve injuries are rare, but can occur owing to direct injury to the valve, or its supporting structures. Myocardial injury from penetrating trauma includes pseudoaneurysm formation (defect of the myocardium covered by an outer layer of fibrous tissue) and septal defects.

Posttraumatic infections can occur, as can post-pericardiotomy syndromes. The latter is an inflammatory response to pericardial injury. It is also seen after cardiac surgery and myocardial infarction (both of the latter may disrupt the pericardium).

Management of penetrating injury includes stabilization (including pericardiocentesis or emergent surgical treatment for bleeding) followed by surgical repair. Small injuries in a hemodynamically stable patient may be followed with surgical intervention postponed. The latter may be the case with needle injuries or catheters.

OVERVIEW OF TRAUMA

1. Obtain a medical history to include details on the mechanism of injury and decide whether or not there is reason to increase the level of suspicion.
2. Look for subtle abnormalities in the vital signs such as tachycardia, exaggerated paradoxic pulse, or extremity pulse/BP differential to raise the level of suspicion.
3. Complete physical examination with a focus on the thoracic skeletal, pulmonary, and cardiac systems. Look for outward signs of trauma in the chest. Examine four extremity pulses and look for rate, volume, differential, and paradoxic change with breathing. Perform careful auscultation looking for muffled heart sounds, and pathologic murmurs. Assess for liver enlargement, peripheral edema, and peripheral versus central perfusion.
4. Order additional tests based on the suspicions raised from the history and physical examination. Consider a chest radiograph, an electrocardiogram, serum cardiac enzymes, and echocardiography. Strong consideration for consultation by a pediatric cardiologist in the presence of raised suspicion prior to additional lab testing. The latter may eliminate unnecessary tests and false positives and negatives on the tests ordered.
5. Management will depend on the data collected from the history, physical examination, and laboratory testing. Frequently, observation for cardiac trauma will require cardiac monitoring such as telemetry and frequent vital signs found in an intensive care setting. Management may include surgical repair of valve damage or drainage of blood from the pericardial space. Traumatic ventricular septal defects may be repaired in the operating room or the catheterization laboratory, the timing of which is dictated by the clinical status. Delay in repair may allow tissue healing and improved suture stability. Blunt trauma may be managed conservatively.

Suggested Readings

Allen HD, Gutgesell HP, Clark EB, Driscoll DJ: *Moss and Adams' Heart Disease in Infants, Children and Adolescents Including the Fetus and Young Adult*, 6th ed. Philadelphia, PA, Lippincott Williams & Wilkins, 2001.

Bromberg BI, Mazziotti MV, Canter CE, Spray TL, Strauss AW, Foglia RP: Recognition and management of nonpenetrating cardiac trauma in children. *J Pediatr* 128(4):536–541, 1996.

Garson A, Bricker JT, Fisher DJ, Neish SR: *The Science and Practice of Pediatric Cardiology*, 2nd ed. Baltimore, MD, Williams & Wilkins, 1998.

Tiao GM, Griffith PM, Szmuszkovicz JR, Mahour GH: Cardiac and great vessel injuries in children after blunt trauma: an institutional review. *J Pediatr Surg* 35(11):1656–1660, 2000.

35

TUMORS AND CARCINOMAS INVOLVING THE HEART

Joel T. Hardin

INTRODUCTION

Cardiac neoplasms are rare during infancy and childhood, diagnosed at a prevalence of less than 0.03% in a large autopsy series conducted in the era prior to widespread availability of echocardiography.[1] A recent retrospective review shows an increased prevalence of this diagnosis, from 0.06% in the early 1980s to 0.3% in the early 1990s.[2] These data more likely reflect increased recognition in asymptomatic patients with cardiac tumors (including a growing number of fetal diagnoses) rather than incidence. The recognition is also enhanced through more routine and focused investigations for cardiac tumors on populations known to be at risk (e.g., patients with tuberous sclerosis).

Over 90% of primary cardiac tumors are histologically benign, although the clinical importance may not be. Affected patients can present with serious cardiac arrhythmia, heart failure, ductal-dependent univentricular heart physiology, stroke, and pericardial effusion. The most common

pediatric cardiac tumor (rhabdomyoma), on the other hand, has a favorable natural history including spontaneous regression in a majority of cases. This chapter will review the most common cardiac neoplasms presenting during infancy and childhood (Table 35-1), the spectrum of clinical presentation (Table 35-2), and various treatment strategies for selected cardiac tumors.

THE CLINICAL PRESENTATION OF CARDIAC TUMORS

The clinical presentation of cardiac tumors is increasingly an incidental discovery during echocardiography of an asymptomatic child (or fetus) performed for other indications. In the fetus, cardiac tumors are easily recognized and rarely impair the fetal circulation. Echocardiography in the infant or older child has a similar diagnostic reliability; however, echocardiography often cannot sufficiently discriminate among different tumor

TABLE 35-1

CARDIAC TUMORS MOST LIKELY TO PRESENT
DURING INFANCY OR CHILDHOOD

Benign	Malignant
Rhabdomyoma	Rhabdomyosarcoma
Fibroma	Angiosarcoma
Myxoma	Extranodal non-Hodgkin's lymphoma
Angioma	Intracardiac extension of infradiaphragmatic tumors
Purkinje cell tumor	(e.g., Wilms tumor, malignant hepatic tumors)
Teratoma	

TABLE 35-2

VARIABLE CLINICAL PRESENTATION
OF CARDIAC TUMORS

Asymptomatic
Arrhythmia
Syncope
Pathologic murmur
Cyanosis
Incidental discovery on fetal or transthoracic
  echocardiography
Obstruction to ventricular inflow or outflow
Univentricular heart disease physiology
  (e.g., simulating HLHS)
Cardiogenic shock
Congestive heart failure
Pericardial effusion
Superior vena cava obstruction syndrome
Abnormal ECG (e.g., left atrial enlargement)
Extra heart sounds (e.g., atrial myxma's plop)
Cardiomegaly on chest radiography
Sudden death
Stroke
Peripheral embolic event
Underlying disorder at risk for a cardiac
  tumor (e.g., tuberous sclerosis)

subtypes, and there are limits on imaging resolution, especially in the anterior mediastinum for transthoracic studies. High resolution computed tomography or MRI can further enhance diagnostic sensitivity, while also providing correlation of MRI tumor characteristics to histologic tissue type.[3] Although historically important for cardiac tumor diagnosis, cardiac catheterization and angiocardiography have generally been replaced with these more sensitive noninvasive imaging techniques.

In a neonate presenting with cardiogenic shock, especially in an infant with apparent univentricular heart disease physiology, cardiac tumor should be included in the differential diagnosis. The pathophysiology in these cases can include a tumor obstructing the ventricular inflow or outflow, and many such patients will have functionally ductal-dependent systemic circulation.

Fetuses, infants, and children of all ages can present with cardiac arrhythmia as the sole manifestation of a cardiac tumor. Virtually every type of cardiac arrhythmia can be observed, including heart block (from tumor infiltration into conduction system elements), atrial and ventricular premature depolarizations, reentrant supraventricular tachycardia, ventricular tachycardia, and ventricular fibrillation. In some cases, a ventricular arrhythmia may be a result of tumor embolization to the coronary circulation. There are case reports of such patients being resuscitated with extracorporeal support (ECMO).[4]

Thromboembolic complications of cardiac tumors represent another mode of clinical presentation, more often seen in patients with cardiac myxoma. Pulmonary embolism, stroke, and peripheral embolism have all been reported. In the evaluation of a pediatric patient presenting with pulmonary embolism or stroke, the possibility of cardiac tumor should be included in the larger evaluation of potential cardioembolic etiologies. Embolism to the coronary circulation can present as sudden death.

Pericardial effusion can represent a clue to possible cardiac tumor. This is much more common in patients with primary cardiac lymphoma. It is therefore important to include cytology when planning diagnostic studies of pericardial fluid. Some of the more common pediatric solid tumors such as Wilms tumor can invade the inferior vena cava and extend into the right atrium. Obstruction of the IVC may present as ascites or hepatomegaly. Lastly, many cardiac tumors can occlude flow through the superior vena cava, thus presenting a rare cause of the superior vena cava (SVC) syndrome (truncal, facial and upper extremity plethora/edema; sometimes raising cerebral venous impedance sufficiently to cause hydrocephalus).

Except in the cases of incidental discovery during echocardiography for other purposes, symptomatic presentations such as the scenarios outlined above should prompt cardiology consultation, chest radiography, electrocardiography, echocardiography, and in selected cases, computed tomography or cardiac magnetic resonance imaging (MRI) evaluation. Anterior mediastinal masses or potentially malignant pericardial effusion should jointly be evaluated by cardiology and hematology-oncology consultants.

SELECTED PEDIATRIC CARDIAC TUMORS

Rhabdomyoma

Rhabdomyoma is the most common cardiac tumor in the pediatric age group. Roughly half of affected patients have tuberous sclerosis; slightly less than half have isolated cardiac rhabdomyoma; and only rarely is rhabdomyoma associated with other types of congenital heart disease. If a cardiac tumor is identified during fetal echocardiography, the prevalence of tuberous sclerosis increases to approximately 70%.[5]

Rhabdomyomas are composed of large round cells with clear cytoplasm, often with eosinophilic strands stretching from the nucleus to the cell membrane. The cells are therefore often referred to as "spider cells." There is controversy regarding the embryonic origin of cardiac rhabdomyomas, which are felt by many to be hamartomas. Rhabdomyomas

do not infiltrate adjacent myocardium, but they lack true encapsulation. They frequently protrude into intracavitary cardiac positions, affect all cardiac chambers, and frequently exist as multiple discrete tumors. The left ventricle is the most frequently involved site. These tumors can range in size from less than 1 mm to as large as 10 cm in diameter. In general, larger rhabdomyomas occur as sporadic lesions in patients who do not have tuberous sclerosis.

Approximately 50% of rhabdomyomas spontaneously decrease in size and may eventually disappear, perhaps involving a mechanism of selective tumor cell apoptosis.[6] Regression rates are higher among infants or young children, and in those with smaller tumors, although time to regression is variable. As rhabdomyomas regress, there is usually no associated dystrophic calcification. This is a useful distinction relative to the next most common type of pediatric cardiac tumor, the fibroma, which frequently becomes calcified, and typically does not spontaneously regress.

The majority of patients with cardiac rhabdomyoma also have tuberous sclerosis. Tuberous sclerosis is a syndrome comprised of distinctive clinical findings including cardiac rhabdomyoma, intracranial hamartomas, cutaneous angiofibromas, linear epidermal nevi, and renal angiomyolipomas. Loci linked to tuberous sclerosis have been mapped to chromosomes 9 and 16.[7] Unfortunately, even though cardiac rhabdomyomas in tuberous sclerosis can spontaneously regress, the same is not true for associated intracranial hamartomas. Various seizure types including infantile spasms can occur in these patients, and corticotrophin used to treat infantile spasms can stimulate growth of cardiac rhabdomyomas.[8]

Asymptomatic patients with rhabdomyoma do not require treatment. Cardiac arrhythmias controlled with antiarrhythmic medications can be expectantly managed, with the knowledge that many of these tumors will regress such that treatment can be discontinued. In a neonate presenting with univentricular heart disease physiology, initial treatment is directed at maintaining ductal patency and is similar to the preoperative management of a patient with hypoplastic left heart syndrome.

Surgical intervention is rarely required to alleviate critically obstructed ventricular inflow or outflow, or manage an intractable cardiac arrhythmia. Aggressive surgical tumor resection that may involve surrounding muscle may produce more severe cardiac dysfunction than was originally attributed to the tumor.

Fibroma

Fibromas occur less commonly than rhabdomyomas, and are less likely to coexist with other disorders. Histologically, these tumors consist of fibroblasts and collagen, and there is often extensive infiltration and interdigitation of tumor fibers with adjacent myocardium. Within these tumors, there may be cystic degeneration and ectopic calcification, differentiating them from the more common rhabdomyoma. They can grow to sizes as large as 5 cm. Unlike rhabdomyoma, fibromas do not regress, and can even demonstrate continued slow growth into previously unaffected portions of the heart.

A common location for cardiac fibroma is within the ventricular septum. The septum may enlarge to such proportions so as to mimic the clinical presentation of hypertrophic cardiomyopathy. Echocardiographic distinction between these two conditions can also be difficult; therefore one should consider additional imaging techniques such as cardiac MRI in these situations.

Asymptomatic patients with fibromas can be expectantly managed, with the caveat that the parent should understand the potential for ongoing tumor growth and future symptomatic presentation. Symptomatic patients with cardiac fibroma are usually referred for surgical resection. These tumors are more difficult to resect, and as with the surgical strategy in cardiac rhabdomyoma, subtotal resection is often a better goal. Cardiac transplantation has occasionally been required in infants and children with life-threatening symptoms of cardiac fibroma.

Myxoma

Cardiac myxomas are the most common cardiac tumors in adults, and rarely present during infancy or childhood. More females than males are affected. These tumors grow as intracavitary masses, usually affixed to structures within the left atrium. They rarely grow from surfaces elsewhere in the heart. Myxomatous cells form small nests around nutrient blood vessels within the tumor. The surrounding stroma may calcify or undergo fibrosis. The tumor surface can either be smooth or irregular, and surface elements are prone to embolization.

In childhood, presence of a cardiac myxoma may imply an underlying myxoma-endocrine neoplasia syndrome (often referred to as the Carney complex). This familial disorder has been linked to a major locus on chromosome 17.[9] Affected patients have spotty skin pigmentation, cardiac myxomas, dysfunction of multiple endocrine systems, and a tendency to develop schwannomas. Therefore, if a diagnosis of childhood myxoma is established, first-degree relatives of the index case should also be subjected to screening cardiology evaluation.

Clinical presentation of a cardiac myxoma usually involves one of three primary pathways: congestive heart failure, palpitations, or neurologic symptoms. A neonate with cardiac myxoma may present with cyanosis. The classic auscultatory "plop" of myxoma occurs infrequently, in as few as 15% of cases. Given the propensity for embolic complications with cardiac myxoma, symptomatic patients are usually referred for surgical resection. Unlike rhabdomyoma and fibroma, the surgical objective with myxoma is complete resection, as inadequate resection risks tumor recurrence. Recurrent myxomas also occur more frequently in patients with the Carney complex.

Purkinje Cell Tumor

This rare cardiac tumor has only been described in young infants presenting with cardiac arrhythmia. Histologic characteristics of these lesions include clusters of eosinophilic and highly vacuolated myocardial cells with a foamy appearance. Purkinje cell tumors are smaller than other cardiac tumor subtypes, usually less than 5 mm in diameter. These tumors are usually subendocardial and can be dispersed throughout the myocardium.

Clinical presentation with Purkinje cell tumor is often with a life-threatening ventricular arrhythmia. Given that some of these tumors are quite small and beyond the resolution of transthoracic echocardiography, many experts recommend cardiac MRI evaluation in the patient with otherwise unexplained ventricular arrhythmia. Surgical resection or cryoablation of Purkinje cell tumors has been reported, but is often complicated by the dispersed nature of multiple nests of tumor cells throughout the myocardium.

Primary Cardiac Lymphoma

Primary cardiac lymphoma represents the most common malignant cardiac tumor. This is an extranodal malignant lymphoma that can exist as any lymphocyte cell type (e.g., Burkitt's lymphoma, B-cell lymphoma). Clinical presentation includes congestive heart failure, cardiac arrhythmias, pericardial effusion, or SVC obstruction syndrome. This diagnosis is often established relatively late, and after advanced myocardial infiltration has occurred. Immunocompromised patients are at greatest risk. Cardiac lymphoma is usually managed with systemic chemotherapy rather than surgery.

SUMMARY

Pediatricians and family physicians may never encounter an infant or child with a cardiac tumor, as these are very rare diagnoses. An increasing number of fetuses (most with tuberous sclerosis) have cardiac tumors diagnosed by fetal echocardiography, usually performed for other indications. Symptomatic presentation in the neonate can simulate ductal-dependent univentricular heart disease, or may present with cardiac arrhythmias. Older children with cardiac tumors can present with pericardial effusion, cardiac arrhythmia, cardioembolic stroke, or sudden death.

Diagnosis is usually predicated on noninvasive imaging techniques such as echocardiography, computed tomography, and cardiac MRI. The most common cardiac tumor in childhood is rhabdomyoma, frequently associated with tuberous sclerosis, and possessing a favorable natural history of spontaneous resolution in the majority of cases. Fibromas, myxomas, Purkinje cell tumors, and primary cardiac lymphoma are more likely to present with symptoms. Surgical resection is usually reserved for patients with symptoms referable to a cardiac tumor, or in situations where the likelihood of future symptoms is high.

References

1 Nadas AS, Ellison RC: Cardiac tumors in infancy. *Am J Cardiol* 21:363–366, 1968.
2 Freedom RM, Lee KJ, MacDonald C, Taylor G: Selected aspects of cardiac tumors in infancy and childhood. *Pediatr Cardiol* 21:299–316, 2000.
3 Kiaffas MG, Powell AJ, Geva T: Magnetic resonance imaging evaluation of cardiac tumor characteristics in infants and children. *Am J Cardiol* 89(10):1229–1233, 2002.
4 McElhinney DB, Carpentieri DF, Bridges ND, Clark BJ, Gaynor JW, Spray TL: Sarcoma of the mitral valve causing coronary arterial occlusion in children. *Cardiol Young* 11(5):539–542, 2001.
5 Tworetzky W, McElhinney DB, Margossian R, Moon-Grady AJ, Sallee D, Goldmuntz E, van der Velde ME, Silverman NH, Allan LD: Association between cardiac tumors and tuberous sclerosis in the fetus and neonate. *Am J Cardiol* 92(4):487–489, 2003.
6 Wu SS, Collins MH, de Chadarevian JP: Study of the regression process in cardiac rhabdomyomas. *Pediatr Dev Pathol* 5(1):29–36, 2002.
7 van Slegtenhorst M, de Hoogt R, Hermans C, et al: Identification of the tuberous sclerosis gene TSC1 on chromosome 9. *Science* 277:805–808, 1997.
8 Arcinegas EG, Hakimi M, Farooki ZQ, Truccone NJ, Green EW: Primary cardiac tumors in children. *J Thorac Cardiovasc Surg* 79:582–591, 1980.
9 Stratakis CA, Kirschner LS, Carney JA: Carney complex: diagnosis and management of the complex of spotty skin pigmentation, myxomas, endocrine overactivity, and schwannomas. *Am J Med Genet* 80:183–185, 1998.

C H A P T E R

36

CARDIAC ARRHYTHMIAS

Frank Zimmerman

INTRODUCTION

This chapter is meant to serve as a practical review of the mechanisms, clinical features, natural history, and management of cardiac arrhythmias in children. While the mechanisms of arrhythmias in children are the same as in adults, the natural history and age distribution are unique for the pediatric population. This affects management decisions and choice of therapy, particularly with concern to the timing of interventions such as electrophysiology studies, implantable devices, or catheter ablation. Furthermore, the association of arrhythmias and congenital heart disease in children necessitates a thorough cardiac evaluation for structural abnormalities along with investigation of the specific electrical disturbance.

BRADYCARDIA AND HEART BLOCK

Definition

Bradycardia is a slow heart rhythm with a rate below the lower limits of normal for age. Younger patients have higher normal average heart rates that decrease to adult values by the late teenage years.

Guidelines for bradycardia based on 24-h ambulatory monitoring are as follows:

1. Newborn, less than 60 bpm while asleep and less than 80 bpm while awake
2. One year, less than 60 bpm while asleep and less 80 bpm while awake
3. 2–6 years, less than 60 bpm
4. 7–11 years, less than 45 bpm
5. Adolescents, less than 40 bpm
6. Well-trained athlete, less than 30 bpm

SINUS BRADYCARDIA

Sinus bradycardia is characterized by a normal sinus appearing P wave on 12-lead ECG with a heart rate below normal for age. The term sinus node dysfunction has a broader definition encompassing any disorder of the sinus node. This includes sinus bradycardia, severe sinus pauses, the tachycardia/bradycardia syndrome, sinus node reentry tachycardia and sinoatrial exit block. The incidence of sinus bradycardia in children is unknown mainly because most young patients with bradycardia are asymptomatic. In a 24-h ambulatory study of asymptomatic individuals less than

25 years of age, approximately 25–35% demonstrated heart rates below the lower limits of normal for age.

Etiology of Sinus Bradycardia

Familial

Familial bradycardia is a rare disorder which has been described to occur in young patients. An autosomal dominant pattern of inheritance has been reported in one family.

Congenital Heart Disease

Sinus bradycardia and sinus node dysfunction have been associated with atrial septal defects before and after surgery, the Mustard or Senning operation and following the Fontan operation. The cause of bradycardia includes surgery near the sinus node, chronic hemodynamic effects to the atrium or congenital sinus node abnormalities associated with the underlying structural heart disease.

Acquired or Familial Myocardial Disorders

Sinus bradycardia is associated with myocardial disorders such as cardiomyopathy, inflammatory myocardial diseases such as myocarditis or following ischemia or infarction.

Medications

Various medications, especially antiarrhythmic agents, may cause sinus bradycardia.

Hypervagotonia

Vagal stimulation can result in sinus bradycardia under the following circumstances:

1. Placement of nasogastric or endotracheal tubes or during suctioning in intubated patients
2. GE reflux (also may be associated with apnea)
3. Well-trained athletes
4. Carotid sinus hypersensitivity (usually seen in older patients)
5. REM sleep
6. Breath-holding spells
7. Increased intracranial pressure
8. Obstructive sleep apnea

Miscellaneous

1. Long QT syndrome (mechanism is unknown, but maybe secondary to autonomic nervous system dysfunction)
2. SIDS
3. Tumors
4. Obstructive jaundice
5. Anorexia
6. Apnea, bradycardia of prematurity (also occasionally seen in full-term infants)

Clinical Features of Sinus Bradycardia

Most young patients with sinus bradycardia are asymptomatic or have mild symptoms of fatigue or exercise intolerance. Symptoms of significant fatigue, exercise intolerance, dizziness, or syncope may be associated with more severe forms of bradycardia. The diagnosis of sinus bradycardia is usually made with a 12-lead ECG or 24-h ambulatory monitoring. Exercise stress testing may be used to determine heart-rate response with activity and has been used to differentiate sinus node dysfunction from increased vagal tone seen in athletes, the former having an abnormally low heart-rate response to exercise while the latter able to achieve normal peak heart rates. Invasive electrophysiology testing is rarely a primary indication to assess for sinus node dysfunction with sinus bradycardia; however, it may be performed in conjunction with routine electrophysiology studies for other indications.

Management

Therapy for sinus bradycardia is usually based on the presence or absence of symptoms. In asymptomatic young patients without structural heart disease, there is no accepted lower heart-rate limit that. would warrant intervention; however, severe sinus bradycardia in children with congenital heart disease is often treated, even if asymptomatic, as this may be associated with further development of congestive heart failure or hemodynamic compromise. Acute treatment of symptomatic sinus bradycardia includes medical therapy with atropine or isoproterenol or with transcutaneous or transvenous temporary pacing. Chronic medical therapy for symptomatic sinus bradycardia is usually not effective because of variable response over time and unacceptable side effects of the medications. Pacemaker implantation is recommended if chronic therapy for symptomatic sinus bradycardia is indicated.

HEART BLOCK

Heart block refers to the disturbance of the normal conduction between the atria and the ventricles. Heart block is categorized into first-degree AV block, second-degree AV block (type 1 and type 2), and third-degree or complete AV block.

First-Degree AV Block

First-degree AV block occurs when the PR interval is greater than the upper limits of normal for age. While this is not a cause of bradycardia, because there is intact AV conduction, it may be associated with sinus node dysfunction or AV node disease. First-degree AV block can be seen in up to 6% of normal neonates. Conditions associated with first-degree AV block include rheumatic fever, Chagas' disease, rubella, mumps, hypothermia, cardiomyopathy, metabolic abnormalities, and hypervagotonia. Treatment is usually not indicated for asymptomatic first-degree AV block but routine monitoring may be recommended if there is any evidence of coexisting sinus or AV node dysfunction. Pacemaker implantation is rarely indicated for individuals with pacemaker syndrome because of extreme PR interval prolongation.

Second-Degree AV Block

Second-degree AV block is divided into two types. Mobitz type 1 block (Wenckebach) occurs when there is progressive lengthening of the PR interval followed by a nonconducted P wave. Mobitz type 2 block occurs when lengthening of the PR intervals does not precede the nonconducted P wave. Type 1 second-degree AV block is often seen in normal individuals at times of high parasympathetic tone such as during sleep or in well-trained athletes. As the location of block occurs at the level of the AV node and varies with parasympathetic tone, it is usually not associated with significant conduction system disease.

Type 2 second-degree AV block is less commonly seen but is thought to indicate more significant conduction system disease. It is associated with various forms of congenital heart disease or can occur following cardiac surgery. It has a less predictable course with variable progression to complete heart block.

Intervention for type 1 second-degree AV block is usually not indicated unless there is evidence for more significant conduction system disease. Type 2 second-degree AV block warrants close observation and some have recommended elective pacemaker implantation when diagnosed, especially when this occurs following the cardiac surgery.

Complete Heart Block

Third-degree or complete heart block is characterized by the absence of communication of electrical activity from the atria with the ventricles. The etiology of complete heart block is as follows:

1. Congenital AV block
   a. This is most commonly associated with neonatal lupus syndrome in children born to mothers who have antibodies to RO-SSA and LA-SSB antibodies.
   b. Abnormal development of the AV node because of complete interruption of the AV conduction system.
   c. Various forms of congenital heart disease including L-transposition of the great arteries and heterotaxy syndromes.
2. Acquired AV block
   a. Myocarditis
   b. Acute rheumatic fever
   c. Lyme disease or infection
   d. Myocardial infarction
   e. Surgical or catheter induced
   f. Trauma
   g. Cardiomyopathy

Many young infants and children with complete heart block may be asymptomatic. The presence and severity of symptoms are usually related to the rate of the escape rhythm and also to the heart-rate response to exercise. When symptoms occur, they include fatigue, exercise intolerance, heart failure, or syncope. Patients with complete heart block and associated congenital heart disease are at higher risk for heart failure or sudden cardiac death, with one report showing increased mortality of up to 29% in untreated patients.

Acute therapy for complete heart block associated with symptoms includes the use of medications such as isoproterenol and atropine as well as the use of transcutaneous or transvenous temporary pacing. Chronic medical therapy for complete heart block is not acceptable because of variable response to medications over time and therefore implantable pacemakers are the mainstay of chronic therapy.

SUPRAVENTRICULAR TACHYCARDIA

Mechanisms

A thorough understanding of the mechanisms of tachycardia allows for more targeted therapy for specific arrhythmias as well as for the development of new antiarrhythmic agents. Despite great advances in the understanding of the mechanisms and basic principles for specific arrhythmias, much remains unknown and many exceptions to rules occur. The mechanisms of tachycardia are as follows:

Abnormal Automaticity

Enhanced abnormal automaticity or inappropriate firing of a cluster of cells outside of the sinus node may occur either in single beats or in runs of tachycardia. The abnormal cluster of cells may exist in the atrium, AV junction, or ventricle. They display electrophysiologic properties similar to the pacemaker cells seen in the sinus node area. The features of automaticity include a warm-up and cool-down phenomenon at the onset and termination of the tachycardia, variation in the tachycardia rate both during a single episode and between separate episodes, the inability to terminate the tachycardia with cardioversion or pacing, and finally the response to antiarrhythmic medications.

Reentry

Reentry tachycardias are a result of a continuous circuit of electrical activity as opposed to abnormal firing from a single focus. The circuit may be contained in the atrium, the AV node or ventricle or may use both atrial and ventricular tissue. Regional differences in the conduction properties and refractory properties of the tissue are needed in order to propagate this form of tachycardia. Reentry circuits may revolve around fixed areas of obstruction such as surgical scars or around areas of function block. Clinical features of reentry tachycardia include the ability to terminate tachycardia with critically timed paced atrial or ventricular beats or with direct current (DC) cardioversion. There is an abrupt onset and offset of tachycardia with minimal heart-rate variation during a single episode.

Triggered Automaticity

Tachycardias with features of both abnormal automaticity and reentry are categorized as triggered automaticity. The cause of triggered automaticity is the occurrence of oscillations in cell membrane potentials during repolarization that lead to the reactivation of tissue and result in a self-propagating tachycardia. Clinical features of trigged automaticity include a warm-up and cool-down phenomenon and variation in tachycardia rate during a single episode similar to that seen with abnormal automaticity; however, this tachycardia may be terminated with critically timed paced beats or with DC cardioversion as seen with reentry tachycardias.

PREMATURE BEATS

Atrial Premature Beats

Definition

Premature atrial beats are early beats from an atrial focus outside of the sinus node usually because of abnormal automaticity. The ECG features include a P wave before each QRS complex with morphology different from that seen during sinus rhythm.

Clinical Features

Atrial premature beats are a common and usually benign finding noted as an irregular heart rhythm on examination. They are often asymptomatic; however, in a small group of patients, they may cause significant symptoms of palpitations, anxiety or dizziness. Atrial premature beats may occur in the setting of metabolic abnormalities, hyperthyroidism, or in association with atrial tumors. Rarely, atrial premature beats are associated with supraventricular tachycardias (SVT).

Management

Initial management is to document the arrhythmia and confirm the diagnosis of atrial premature beats. This can be done with event recorder, 24-h ambulatory monitoring or 12-lead ECG. If there are no other abnormal findings on the examination and no symptoms of sustained tachycardia, then the patient may be followed conservatively on no medications. Occasionally, antiarrhythmic medications are used to suppress the atrial premature beats in patients who have significant symptoms. Associated metabolic abnormalities or hyperthyroidism should be treated as indicated.

Ventricular Premature Beats

Definition

Ventricular premature beats are early beats arising from a focus in the ventricle usually because of abnormal automaticity or triggered automaticity. The ECG features include an early wide QRS complex beat, which is not associated with a preceding P wave. There may or may not be a retrograde P wave associated with the premature ventricular beat. A compensatory pause following the premature beat does not reliably help to distinguish ventricular premature beats from atrial premature beats with aberration.

Clinical Features

Ventricular premature beats occur in approximately 1–2% of the normal population. They occur rarely in infants while increasing to an incidence of 50–60% in adolescents and adults. In the past, ventricular

premature beats have been classified based on the frequency, morphology, and association with ventricular couplets or triplets; however, this classification is not used clinically to predict future cardiac events such as ventricular tachycardia (VT). Ventricular premature beats are more worrisome than atrial premature beats because they may be associated with diseases of ventricular myocardium. This is especially true if there are multiple QRS morphologies of ventricular premature beats. Most patients are asymptomatic but some may have significant symptoms of palpitations, chest pain, or anxiety.

Management

Similar to atrial premature beats, the initial goals of management are to document and confirm the diagnosis of ventricular premature beats. The quantification of the occurrence of ventricular premature beats as well as assessment for any occult arrhythmias can be achieved with 24-h ambulatory monitoring. There is divergence of opinion about evaluation for asymptomatic patients with ventricular premature beats and no structural heart disease. Exercise stress testing has been advocated for evaluation of these patients with the thought that resolution of the premature ventricular beats with exercise usually signifies a benign prognosis; however, there are many exceptions to this finding and thus exercise testing is not a sensitive enough tool to assess risk in this population. Because of the association of ventricular ectopy and structural heart disease evaluation with echocardiogram or even cardiac magnetic resonance imaging (MRI) may be indicated. Treatment with antiarrhythmic medications can be used for symptomatic patients or for those who are felt to have a high frequency of premature beats placing them at risk for the development of a tachycardia-induced cardiomyopathy. RF catheter ablation is usually reserved for those resistant to medications.

Sinus Tachycardia

Definition

Sinus tachycardia is an accelerated rhythm arising from the sinus node area. The sinus node is normally sensitive to catecholamines and vagal inputs and therefore, sinus tachycardia is usually in response to external influence to the sinus node. The ECG features include a narrow complex QRS tachycardia with a one-to-one relationship between the atria and ventricles and P wave morphology identical to that seen during normal sinus rhythm.

Clinical Features

Sinus tachycardia may result in symptoms of palpitations or dizziness. Other associated symptoms are related to the cause of sinus tachycardia. A syndrome of inappropriate sinus tachycardia is characterized by the absence of structural heart disease or other identifiable causes for sinus tachycardia. The syndrome occurs most often in adolescents or young adults and may be associated with debilitating symptoms of dizziness or palpitations. The etiology of this syndrome is unknown.

Management

The management of sinus tachycardia is directed at the underlying etiology. The syndrome of inappropriate tachycardia can be treated with antiarrhythmic medications or with RF catheter ablation of the sinus node.

Ectopic Atrial Tachycardia

Definition

Ectopic atrial tachycardia is a result of impulses arising from a single focus in the atrium outside of the sinus node. The ECG typically shows a narrow complex QRS tachycardia with an abnormal P wave morphology different than that seen during sinus rhythm preceding each QRS complex. There may be one-to-one AV conduction or AV dissociation with persistence of tachycardia. The PR interval may be longer than that seen during normal sinus rhythm.

Clinical Features

Ectopic atrial tachycardia accounts for about 5–10% of supraventricular tachycardia seen in children. When this is diagnosed in early infancy, as significant proportion of patients have complete resolution of tachycardia within the first year of life.

Symptoms associated with ectopic atrial tachycardia are related to the rates of a tachycardia, which may range from 120 to 300 beats per minute. It is an important cause of tachycardia-induced cardiomyopathy because it may occur undetected until patients present with the symptoms of congestive heart failure. Ectopic atrial tachycardias may be associated with congenital heart disease as well as metabolic abnormalities or hyperthyroidism.

Management

Initial management includes assessment for associated structural cardiac anomalies as well as assessment of cardiac function. Ambulatory monitoring is often used to assess the frequency and duration of tachycardia and to help assess efficacy of medical or interventional therapy. Ectopic atrial tachycardia is often refractory to medical therapy; however, an acceptable goal of therapy may be to simply reduce the rate of tachycardia to avoid the development of tachycardia-induced cardiomyopathy. Initial medical therapy includes the use of beta-blockers, digoxin, or calcium channel blockers, followed by class 1C or class 3 antiarrhythmic agents if tachycardia persists. RF catheter ablation procedure is an effective means for definitive therapy for ectopic atrial tachycardia. DC cardioversion and adenosine are usually are not effective measures for acute treatment of ectopic atrial tachycardia.

Multifocal Atrial Tachycardia

Definition

The premature firing of multiple foci in the atrium causes multifocal atrial tachycardia. The ECG demonstrates frequent ectopic atrial premature beats with multiple P wave morphologies different from that seen during sinus rhythm.

Clinical Features

Multifocal atrial tachycardia is rare in pediatrics and has been associated with pulmonary disease or following surgery for congenital heart disease. It is also seen as an idiopathic form in infants.

Management

Management of multifocal atrial tachycardia is similar to that of ectopic atrial tachycardia and again is difficult to control with medication. DC cardioversion and adenosine are not helpful for this arrhythmia and because of the multiple sources of the ectopic rhythm, RF catheter ablation is usually not indicated.

Junctional Ectopic Tachycardia

Definition

Junctional ectopic tachycardia (JET) is an automatic or triggered tachycardia arising from the AV node or AV junction resulting in a narrow QRS complex tachycardia with variable heart rates. The ECG features demonstrate a narrow complex QRS with variable VA relationship and no demonstrable P waves.

Clinical Features

JET is most commonly seen in the postoperative period following surgery for congenital heart disease and is hypothesized to occur secondary to stretching or trauma near the AV junction. It may also be related to poor hemodynamics or the use of inotropes in the postoperative period. There is a familial disorder of JET that is also associated with the later development of complete heart block.

Management

The management of postoperative JET has evolved with time and currently involves cooling the patient and avoidance of fever. Inotropes are decreased as much as possible. If the rates are less than 180 beats per minute, AV synchrony is reestablished by overdrive atrial pacing. If these maneuvers are not effective, then intravenous procainamide or amiodarone can be used. In the congenital disorder, antiarrhythmic medications are used to control heart rates to avoid the development of tachycardia-induced cardiomyopathy; however, careful attention should be paid as to the late development of complete heart block.

Atrial Flutter

Definition

Atrial flutter is a single reentry loop contained within the atrium. The typical form of atrial flutter revolves around the tricuspid valve ring and is dependent on an area of slowed conduction between the IVC and coronary sinus os, also known as the tricuspid valve isthmus area. On viewing the tricuspid valve ring from below, this circuit revolves in a counterclockwise fashion in the typical form of atrial flutter and revolves in a clockwise fashion in the atypical form of atrial flutter. The 12-lead ECG during typical atrial flutter demonstrates a "saw tooth" pattern in the baseline because of inverted P waves best seen in the inferior leads II, III, aVF. Atrial rates range from 250 to 500 bpm with variable AV conduction. The atypical form of atrial flutter results in upright P waves in the inferior leads. The ECG pattern of atrial flutter in newborns or in those with structural heart disease is variable. It is not unusual to see distinct P waves rather than the "saw tooth" pattern in these situations.

Clinical Features

Atrial flutter is most commonly seen in children in the newborn period and accounts for approximately 5–10% of SVT at this age. Atrial flutter in the setting of a structurally normal heart is usually self-limited and resolves by 1 year of age. Because of variable AV conduction, ventricular rates during tachycardia are approximately 240–260 bpm. Atrial flutter occurring after the newborn period is almost always associated with congenital heart disease. It is most commonly seen following the Fontan or Mustard procedures but can also be seen before or after surgery for atrial septal defects or tetralogy of Fallot. In the setting of congenital heart disease, atrial flutter is associated with higher mortality rates if not controlled with medications or intervention such as radio frequency (RF) catheter ablation. Atrial flutter persisting greater than 48 h is associated with increased risk of stroke although the risk is not as high as that seen in the patients with atrial fibrillation. Symptoms of palpitations or mild congestive heart failure are commonly associated with atrial flutter but because of the variable AV conduction and relatively slower ventricular rates, it is unusual to see syncope or cardiac arrest.

Management

Acute management of atrial flutter is dependent on the duration of the episode of tachycardia. If the episode is greater than 48 h, anticoagulation is required before cardioversion. Acute termination of tachycardia can be achieved with transesophageal pacing, which is effective in 75% of patients with atrial flutter. DC cardioversion with initial energy of 0.5–1 J/kg is effective in nearly 100% of cases but this requires the use of anesthesia. Medical therapy is directed at rate control with the use AV nodal blocking agents such as beta-blockers or calcium channel blockers or acute conversion with ibutilide, amiodarone or class I antiarrhythmic agents. Chronic therapy for atrial flutter consists of AV nodal blocking agents as first line therapy or in combination with class IA or IC or class III antiarrhythmic agents to prevent recurrences of tachycardia. RF catheter ablation is used for definitive treatment and is most successful for atrial flutter circuits that are dependent on the tricuspid valve isthmus. RF catheter ablation in patients with structural heart disease and atypical forms of atrial flutter (known as intraatrial reentry tachycardia) is associated with an approximately 80% acute success rate but is limited by a 50% risk for recurrence of tachycardia. Surgical options include the modified Maze procedure, which can be performed either as an isolated surgery or in conjunction with other cardiac surgeries. Results have shown good success rates with lower risks of recurrences as compared with RF catheter ablation. Some patients with atrial flutter who require antibradycardia pacemakers may be candidates for antitachycardia pacing devices. These are able to detect atrial flutter and attempt overdrive pace termination of the flutter automatically.

Atrial Fibrillation

Definition

Atrial fibrillation is a chaotic atrial tachycardia owing to multiple wavelets of electrical activity involving both the right and left atrium. In some cases, the tachycardia is initiated by ectopic atrial foci originating from the pulmonary veins. The 12-lead ECG demonstrates disorganized, low amplitude, irregular baseline activity consisting of coarse or fine fibrillation waves. At times, the electrical activity may organize and appear to be similar to atrial flutter but this is transient and the electrical activity eventually disorganizes into atrial fibrillation. Ventricular response is variable but irregular opposed to the regular rates seen with atrial flutter.

Clinical Features

Atrial fibrillation is an uncommon arrhythmia in children accounting for less than 1% of SVT in young patients but increases to an incidence of up to 10% after 60 years of age. It is associated with congenital and structural heart disease, hyperthyroidism, drugs or medications, hypertrophic cardiomyopathy, mitral valve disease, and hemochromatosis. There is a higher incidence of atrial fibrillation in patients with accessory atrioventricular connections (seen in the Wolff-Parkinson-White (WPW) syndrome) and there is a familial form of atrial fibrillation triggered during times of increased vagal tone. Atrial fibrillation occurring in the absence of structural heart disease is known as lone atrial fibrillation and appears to have a somewhat benign course with minimal risk for tachycardia-induced cardiomyopathy or stroke.

Management

Important considerations for the management of atrial fibrillation include the risk of stroke, which occurs in patients who have atrial fibrillation lasting longer than 48 hours and thus anticoagulation is required prior to cardioversion. Acute management options include: (1) rate control (with beta-blockers, digoxin, or calcium channel blockers), (2) chemical cardioversion (with class IA, IC or class III antiarrhythmic agents), or (3) DC cardioversion. DC cardioversion with energy of 1-2 J/kg is effective in most patients and may be repeated after administration of antiarrhythmic medications in resistant cases. Chronic management decisions are dependent on the frequency of symptoms and presence of structural hearts disease. Rate control with AV nodal blocking agents or prevention of recurrent episodes with class IA, IC, or class III antiarrhythmic agents are used for chronic management of atrial fibrillation. The catheter ablation procedure may be performed in selected patients with no structural heart disease and lone atrial fibrillation. The cause of tachycardia in this population is thought to be a result of ectopic foci arising from the pulmonary vein ostia. Surgical options include the modified Maze procedure, which can be performed as isolated surgery or in conjunction with other cardiac surgery.

Sinus Node Reentry Tachycardia

Definition

Sinus node reentry tachycardia is a rare form of atrial tachycardia in children. The reentry circuit is localized to the sinus node area. The 12-lead ECG demonstrates typical features of reentry tachycardia with abrupt onset and offset and P waves with the same morphology as seen during sinus rhythm. The PR interval may be slightly longer during tachycardia than what it is seen during sinus rhythm.

Clinical Features

Sinus node reentry tachycardia accounts for less than 1% of tachycardia seen in children and may be associated with symptoms of palpitations, low energy, or dizziness. Heart rates are variable and affected by catecholamines or vagal tone.

Management

Acute management for sinus node reentry tachycardia includes vagal maneuvers, which can potentially terminate the tachycardia, or DC cardioversion. Chronic therapy with antiarrhythmic medications includes the use of beta-blockers, calcium channel blockers, digoxin, or class I or class III antiarrhythmic agents. RF catheter ablation procedure can be performed targeting the circuit near the sinus node.

AV Node Reentry Tachycardia

Definition

AV node reentry tachycardia is a result of reentry within the AV node or peri-AV nodal tissue. The reentry circuit consists of both fast and slow conducting AV node pathways. Some atypical forms of AV node reentry tachycardia are because of AV node pathways with intermediate conduction properties. The typical form of AV node reentry tachycardia occurs with conduction proceeding from the atrium to the ventricle down the slowly conducting pathway and proceeding back to the atrium over the fast conducting AV node pathway. The atypical form of AV node reentry tachycardia occurs in less than 10% of cases and results from conduction from the atrium to the ventricle over the fast conducting AV node pathway and back up to the atrium over the slow or intermediate AV node pathway. The ECG during typical AV node reentry tachycardia demonstrates a narrow complex SVT with rates of 200–300 bpm and a VA interval of less than 70 ms. The P wave is usually not visible as it is buried in the QRS complex. The ECG pattern during atypical AV node reentry tachycardia is that of a long RP tachycardia with retrograde P waves in the inferior leads.

Clinical Features

AV node reentry tachycardia is rarely seen in children less than 2 years of age, but accounts for 30% of SVT at 6–10 years of age and greater than 50% of SVT in adults. Interestingly, dual AV node physiology can be seen in up to 30–40% of children without tachycardia; however, factors leading to the later development of AV node reentry tachycardia have not been described.

Management

Acute management for AV node reentry tachycardia includes the use of vagal maneuvers such as ice or water to the face in infants. Intravenous adenosine is highly effective for conversion of this tachycardia. The use of longer acting AV nodal blocking agents such as calcium channel blockers or beta-blockers is indicated if tachycardia recurs after adenosine. Of note, intravenous calcium channel blockers are not recommended in children less than 1 year of age because of the increased risk of hypotension. DC cardioversion or transesophageal pacing is rarely needed for acute management of AV node reentering tachycardias because of the effectiveness of adenosine. Chronic therapy includes the use of AV nodal blocking agents such as digoxin, beta-blockers, or calcium channel blockers or class IA, IB or class III agents for resistant cases. RF catheter ablation targeting the slow AV node pathway is an effective definitive therapy for AV node reentry tachycardia.

AV Reentry Tachycardia

Definition

AV reentry tachycardia is a result of a reentry circuit using both atrial and ventricular tissue. The AV node is often involved with one limb of the circuit and an accessory AV connection is involved with the other limb. Accessory AV connections are described as muscle fibers or strands, possibly embryologic remnants, that allow for electrical activity to essentially short circuit the normal AV node and His-Purkinje conduction system. Accessory AV connections have been described based on anatomic location:

1. *Kent fiber.* This is a short AV connection between the atrium and ventricle crossing the fibrous AV annulus on the right or left side of the heart. It results in ventricular preexcitation and is the cause of WPW syndrome.
2. *Mahaim fiber.* These are long, insulated fibers connecting the atria to the right bundle branch. They have electrophysiologic properties similar to the AV node. Early descriptions of Mahaim fibers suggested connections between the AV node and the right bundle branch or directly from the AV node to the right ventricle.
3. *James fibers.* These short accessory connections course from the atrium to the bundle of His resulting in a short PR interval without ventricular preexcitation and are the cause of the Lown-Ganong-Levine (LGL) syndrome.

The presence of accessory AV connections results in a number of syndromes and tachycardias as described below:

Preexcitation: Ventricular preexcitation is defined as a short PR interval with a slurred, widened QRS complex because of the presence of an accessory AV connection. The initial portion of the slurred QRS complex is known as the delta wave. The preexcitation pattern on the 12-lead ECG during normal sinus rhythm helps to identify the anatomic location the accessory AV connection.

Orthodromic reciprocating tachycardia (ORT): ORT is the most common form of tachycardia seen in patients with accessory AV connections. The reentry circuit consists of conduction from the atrium to the ventricle over the AV node and back to the atrium via the accessory AV connection. The ECG shows a narrow QRS complex tachycardia with a VA interval greater than 70 ms. Tachycardia rates range from 200 to 320 bpm.

Antidromic reciprocating tachycardia (ART): ART accounts for less than 10% of AV reentry tachycardias. The tachycardia circuit is opposite of that seen with ORT with conduction from the atrium to the ventricle over the accessory connection in an antegrade fashion. This results in a wide complex QRS tachycardia with a QRS pattern consistent with the ventricular preexcitation pattern seen on the ECG during normal sinus rhythm. It is the only type of tachycardia seen with Mahaim fibers.

Permanent form of junctional reciprocating tachycardia (PJRT): PJRT is an uncommon form of AV reentry tachycardia because of a slowly conducting accessory AV connection usually located in the posterior septal area. Because of the slow conduction properties of this accessory connection, the tachycardia is often incessant and the rates are variable between 150 and 280 bpm. The ECG demonstrates a narrow complex tachycardia with a long RP interval.

Clinical Features

The relative incidence of AV reentry tachycardia varies with age. It accounts for approximately 90% of tachycardias in infancy but decrease to less than 50% in adults. The incidence of WPW syndrome occurrence is 0.15–0.3% and increases to an incidence of 1% in patients with congenital heart disease. Approximately 20% of patients with Ebstein anomaly have accessory AV connections. Although typically associated with ventricular preexcitation, 60–70% of patients with accessory AV connections have no preexcitation on the baseline ECG and are termed concealed accessory connections. Among those patients with AV reentry tachycardia, 20% have associated structural heart disease. As mentioned, orthodromic reciprocating tachycardia accounts for approximately 90% of AV reentry tachycardia. There is a bimodal distribution of the occurrence of tachycardia with 40% of episodes occurring in the first 2 months of life and 40–70% occurring at approximately 5–10 years of age. In patients with accessory AV connections and WPW syndrome, there is an increased risk of atrial fibrillation with incidence of approximately 5% in infants. Rapid conduction over the accessory AV connection during atrial fibrillation is the cause of sudden cardiac death in this population with an incidence of approximately 1.5/1000 patient years. Risk factors for sudden cardiac death in patients with WPW syndrome include rapid antegrade conduction of the accessory AV connection (defined as the shortest preexcited RR interval of less than 220–250 ms during atrial fibrillation), the presence of multiple accessory AV connections, and male gender.

Management

Acute management of AV reentry tachycardia includes vagal maneuvers or intravenous adenosine. AV nodal blocking agents such as beta-blockers, digoxin, or calcium channel blockers, DC cardioversion or transesophageal pacing can be used if tachycardia recurs; however, it is important to note that the use of digoxin or verapamil is contraindicated in patients with ventricular preexcitation on the baseline ECG owing to the risk of accelerated antegrade conduction over the accessory AV connection increasing the risk of sudden cardiac death. Chronic therapy includes the use of AV nodal blocking agents, class IA, IC or III antiarrhythmic agents. RF catheter ablation is an effective definitive therapy for AV reentry tachycardia. PJRT is particularly difficult to treat

with chronic medications and often times requires the use multiple antiarrhythmic medications.

The management of asymptomatic patients noted to have a ventricular preexcitation on the baseline EKG continues to be debated. Determination of the antegrade conduction properties of the accessory AV connection with intracardiac or esophageal pacing studies has been suggested to assess the risk for sudden cardiac death.

Ventricular Tachycardia

Definition

Ventricular tachycardia is defined as an abnormal accelerated rhythm arising from below the bundle of His. The mechanisms of VT include reentry (the most common), abnormal automaticity or triggered automaticity. While VT in children can occur in the setting of a normal heart, it is important to investigate for structural heart disease. VT occurring in association with structural heart disease carries a more serious prognosis because of the susceptibility to hemodynamic compromise and possible degeneration to ventricular fibrillation.

The ECG features of VT include a wide complex QRS greater than the upper limits than normal for age at accelerated rates usually >120 bpm. The P wave may occur at the end of the QRS complex in a retrograde fashion or may be completely dissociated from the tachycardia. The appearance of the QRS morphology varies based on the etiology of tachycardia but is often classified as monomorphic (uniform QRS morphology) or polymorphic (multiple QRS morphologies). A specific type of polymorphic VT that has a sinusoidal pattern of QRS variation is known as "torsade de pointes."

Clinical Features

The incidence of VT in children is not well described. Data from ambulatory monitoring in children suggest that the incidence of ventricular ectopy (including VPBs) is approximately 0.5% in infants increasing to 18–50% in adolescents. This is in comparison to a study of young athletes demonstrating a 10% incidence of VT on ambulatory monitoring. The differential diagnosis of a wide complex tachycardia includes SVT with aberrancy, antidromic reciprocating tachycardia, or atrial tachycardia with a bystander accessory connection. Specific conditions associated with VT are as follows:

Idiopathic ventricular tachycardia: Idiopathic VT occurs in healthy infants, children and adults with no identifiable heart disease. Long-term studies suggest a benign prognosis with spontaneous resolution in some patients. Two specific forms of idiopathic VT have been described. Right ventricular outflow tract tachycardia is a result of triggered automaticity of a group of muscle cells characterized by catecholamine and adenosine sensitivity. The QRS morphology is that of LBBB with an inferior axis. Left ventricular tachycardia has been described arising from His-Purkinje system in the inferior LV septum. It is characterized by sensitivity to verapamil and programmed stimulation. The QRS morphology is that of RBBB with a superior axis. Symptoms of idiopathic VT are dependent on the rate of tachycardia, which is variable, and are often absent in many patients.

Accelerated idioventricular rhythm: This arrhythmia occurs most often in infants and is characterized as an accelerated ventricular rhythm slightly greater than the baseline sinus rate. The mechanism is poorly understood but it is not associated with structural heart disease and has a benign prognosis.

Arrhythmogenic right ventricular dysplasia: ARVD is characterized by RV dilatation associated with myocardial thinning and fatty replacement of the myocardium. The abnormal ventricular myocardium gives rise to VT with a LBBB morphology as well as specific ECG findings. The RV abnormalities are difficult to detect by echocardiography and thus cardiac catheterization or MRI is used to confirm the diagnosis. There is a familial pattern of inheritance in some patients and an increased risk of sudden death because of arrhythmia or cardiac dysfunction.

Cardiac tumors: Tumors involving the ventricular myocardium often serve as a substrate for VT. Common tumors include rhabdomyomas associated with tuberous sclerosis. Hamartomas have been reported to be associated with rapid, hemodynamically significant VT in infants. The VT is usually monomorphic but can vary based on the location of the tumor. Therapy includes surgical resection or cryoablation of the arrhythmia focus.

Catecholamine-related polymorphic VT: This tachycardia occurs with emotion or stress and often results in syncope. It is characterized by an irregular polymorphic VT that can degenerate to ventricular fibrillation. A disorder of cardiac ion channels may account for this disorder in some patients. Therapy consists of beta-blockers to prevent recurrent episodes or an ICD in refractory cases.

VT associated with cardiomyopathy or myocarditis: Nonsustained VT is often associated with hypertrophic or dilated cardiomyopathy. The incidence ranges from 30–60% and the presence of VT increases the risk for sudden death in these populations. The mechanism of tachycardia and ECG features are variable. VT may occur in the acute phase of myocarditis or late after recovery because of residual abnormalities of the myocardium. VT is also associated with cardiomyopathy because of coronary artery abnormalities, metabolic abnormalities, drugs, or medications.

VT associated with congenital heart disease: VT mainly because of reentry or triggered automaticity can occur before or after surgery for congenital heart disease. This is most often associated with tetralogy of Fallot or aortic stenosis. The substrate of tachycardia includes ventricular hypertrophy and scarring from hemodynamic factors as well as surgical scars following ventriculotomy or myomectomy.

Torsade de pointes and the long QT syndrome: A specific type of polymorphic VT with a sinusoidal pattern of QRS complexes "twisting" around the baseline is known as torsade de pointes. This specific VT is thought to be a result of triggered automaticity and is seen in the setting of prolonged repolarization. Prolonged repolarization is manifest as a prolonged QT interval on the ECG (corrected QT interval greater than upper limits of normal for age). Causes of prolonged QT interval include acquired or inherited disorders. The inherited disorders are known as the long QT syndrome and were first described in 1957 in family members with the ECG findings and recurrent syncope or sudden death owing to episodes of torsade de pointes. The long QT syndrome can occur in families with autosomal recessive inheritance (Jervell and Lange-Nielsen syndrome) or with autosomal dominant inheritance (Romano-Ward syndrome). The repolarization abnormality is because of defects in sodium or potassium ion channels in the heart. To date, six genes that encode sodium and potassium channels and one gene that encodes a cytoskeletal gene (ankyrin B) that may affect sodium transport have been associated with the long QT syndrome. Over 150 different mutations in the seven known genes accounts for approximately 50% of those patients identified with the long QT syndrome. The clinical diagnosis of long QT syndrome is based on the prolonged corrected QT interval on ECG; however, it is estimated that approximately 20% of gene carriers will have a normal ECG. Therefore, a family history of long QT syndrome or a history of recurrent unexplained syncope, near-sudden death, or torsade de pointes should alert the physician to the possible diagnosis of long QT syndrome. Triggers for cardiac events include exercise (especially swimming or diving), emotion or stress and in some, symptoms occur at rest. The risk of sudden death or recurrent syncope can be significantly reduced with beta-blocker therapy. Occasionally, surgical sympathectomy or implantable pacemaker or defibrillators are used for those with recurrent symptoms despite beta-blocker therapy.

Management of VT

Management of VT begins with documentation of the arrhythmia ideally with 12-lead ECG to confirm the diagnosis. Acute therapy for symptomatic VT includes DC cardioversion for monomorphic VT or defibrillation for polymorphic VT or ventricular fibrillation. Intravenous lidocaine or amiodarone may be used in more stable situations. Acute therapy for torsade de pointes includes magnesium, isoproterenol, overdrive pacing, or defibrillation.

Chronic management depends on the age of the patient, occurrence of symptoms, presence of structural heart disease, and natural history of the specific type of VT. In patients with asymptomatic, idiopathic VT and no structural heart disease, observation and careful follow-up may be appropriate. Antiarrhythmic therapy is effective for control of symptoms because of certain forms of VT but may not alter the risk for sudden death in high-risk situations. Implantable defibrillator therapy for refractory patients or those thought to be at high risk is gaining increasing use in the pediatric population.

Suggested Readings

Deal BJ: Supraventricular tachycardia mechanisms and natural history. in: Deal BJ, Wolff GS, Gelband H (eds): *Current concepts in diagnosis and management of arrhythmias in infants and children.* Armonk, NY, Futura Publishing Company, 1998, pp. 117–144.

Garson A Jr: Arrhythmias. in: *The Electrocardiogram in Infants and Children: A Systematic Approach,* Philadelphia, PA, Lea & Febiger, 1983, pp. 195–375.

Michaelson M, Engle MA: Congenital complete heart block: an international study of the natural history.

in: Brest AN, Engle MA (eds): *Cardiovascular Clinics*, Philadelphia, PA, FA Davis, 1972, pp. 85–101.

Moss AJ: Long QT syndrome. *JAMA* 289:2041–2044, 2003.

Pinsky WW, Gillette PC, Garson A Jr, McNamara DG: Diagnosis, management, and long-term results of patients with congenital complete atrioventricular block, *Pediatrics* 69(6):728–733, 1982.

Richards JM, Alexander JR, Shinebourne EA, de Swiet M, Wilson AJ, Southall DP: Sequential 22-hour profiles of breathing patterns and heart rate in 110 full-term infants during their first 6 months of life, *Pediatrics* 74(5):763–767, 1984.

Schwartz PJ: Idiopathic long QT syndrome: progress and questions, *Am Heart J* 109(2):399–411, 1985.

Southall DP, Johnston F, Shinebourne EA, Johnston PG: 24-hour electrocardiographic study of heart rate and rhythm patterns in population of healthy children, *Br Heart J* 45(3):281–291, 1981.

Walsh EP, Saul JP: Cardiac arrhythmias. in: Fyler DC (ed): *Nadas' Pediatric Cardiology*, Philadelphia, PA, Hanley & Belfus, 1992, pp. 377–434.

37

THE RESTING ELECTROCARDIOGRAM AND AMBULATORY ECG MONITORING

Frank Zimmerman

INTRODUCTION

Einthoven first introduced a 3-lead electrocardiogram (ECG) as a noninvasive means to record electrical activity of the heart. This has now evolved into the 12- or 15-lead pediatric ECG commonly used today. Although other modalities are available for anatomy and diagnoses, the ECG remains a quick, noninvasive method for evaluation of arrhythmias, conduction abnormalities, and to an extent, anatomic or myocardial abnormalities. This chapter presents an overview of pediatric electrocardiography, and discusses features specific to pediatrics and patients with congenital heart disease.

ECG BASICS

The ECG is a graphic representation of the summation of all the voltage potentials of the heart for a given point of view at a given time. As a wavefront of electrical activity moves through the heart, an electrocardiographic signal is produced. A depolarizing wavefront moving toward an electrode creates a positive deflection above the baseline (P wave, R wave). A repolarizing wavefront toward the electrode creates a negative deflection (Pa wave, often hidden in the QRS complex). In the ventricle, repolarization occurs in the opposite direction of depolarization, resulting in a positive deflection (T wave) in the same direction as the QRS complex

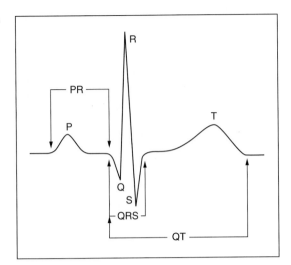

FIGURE 37-1

STANDARD ECG INTERVALS

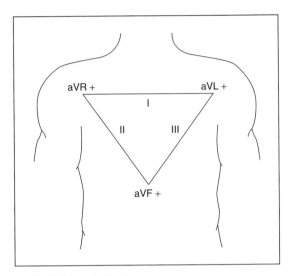

FIGURE 37-2

STANDARD FRONTAL PLANE (LIMB) LEADS

Orientation of frontal plane leads I, II, III and augmented leads aVR, aVL, aVF.

(Figure 37-1). When depolarizing wavefronts move in opposite directions, the smaller wavefront is subtracted from the larger wavefront and the result is a smaller "net" positive deflection in the electrode facing the larger wavefront.

ECG LEADS AND RECORDING

The standard 12-ECG leads are divided into two main groups: limb leads (I, II, III, aVR, aVL, aVF), and precordial leads (V1–V6) (Figures 37-2 and 37-3). Additional leads V7, V3R, and V4R are often used in pediatric patients. The "augmented" leads (aVR, aVL, aVF) record from a single point in reference to a central terminal. The limb and augmented leads form a frontal plane axis around the heart by which to describe the direction of movement of electrical wavefronts (Figure 37-4). The ECG is recorded at standard speed of 25 mm/s and a gain of 10 mm/mv (Figure 37-5). The speed can be increased to 50 mm/s and the gain increased to help visualize waveforms and deflections.

ECG INTERPRETATION

The normal values for the ECG vary depending on the age of the patient and are shown in Table 37-1.

These values are derived from healthy children and presented as the range ±2 standard deviations. A systematic method for the interpretation of pediatric ECGs is given below.

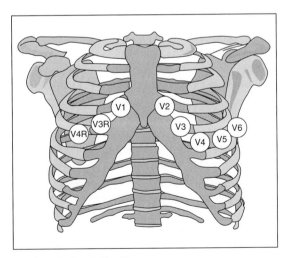

FIGURE 37-3

STANDARD HORIZONTAL PLANE (PRECORDIAL) LEADS

Location of the precordial leads V1–V6 and V3R, V4R.

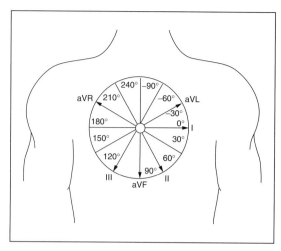

FIGURE 37-4

FRONTAL PLANE AXIS

The frontal plane axis is oriented as shown using limb leads I, II, III and augmented leads aVR, aVL, aVF.

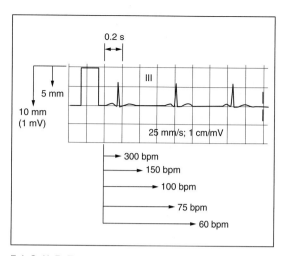

FIGURE 37-5

STANDARD ECG RECORDING SPEED AND GAIN

Rate

The ventricular rate can be measured on the ECG by adding the number of small boxes between two consecutive QRS complexes and dividing that number into 15,000 (Figure 37-5). This will give the heart rate in beats per minute. Another method is to count the number of complexes in a 6-sec period using the 3-sec markers on the 12-lead ECG. Another method is to count the large boxes in between the QRS complexes and divide that number into 300. This gives the heart rate again in beats per minute. Finally, one can calculate the cycle length in milliseconds (each small box on the ECG is 40 ms and a large box is 200 ms when recorded at 25 mm/s) and divide that number into 60,000 converting it to heart

TABLE 37-1

NORMAL ECG VALUES

Age	HR (bpm)	QRS Axis (degrees)	PR Interval (seconds)	QRS Interval (seconds)	R in V1 (mm)	S in V1 (mm)	R in V6 (mm)	S in V6 (mm)
1st week	90–160	60–180	0.08–0.15	0.03–0.08	5–26	0–23	0–12	0–10
1–3wks	100–180	45–160	0.08–0.15	0.03–0.08	3–21	0–16	2–16	0–10
1–2 mo	120–180	30–135	0.08–0.15	0.03–0.08	3–18	0–15	5–21	0–10
3–5 mo	105–185	0–135	0.08–0.15	0.03–0.08	3–20	0–15	6–22	0–10
6–11 mo	110–170	0–135	0.07–0.16	0.03–0.08	2–20	0.5–20	6–23	0–7
1–2 yr	90–165	0–110	0.08–0.16	0.03–0.08	2–18	0.5–21	6–23	0–7
3–4 yr	70–140	0–110	0.09–0.17	0.04–0.08	1–18	0.5–21	4–24	0–5
5–7 yr	65–140	0–110	0.09–0.17	0.04–0.08	0.5–14	0.5–24	4–26	0–4
8–11 yr	60–130	–15–110	0.09–0.17	0.04–0.09	0–14	0.5–25	4–25	0–4
12–15 yr	65–130	–15–110	0.09–0.18	0.04–0.09	0–14	0.5–21	4–25	0–4
>16 yr	50–120	–15–110	0.12–0.20	0.05–0.10	0–14	0.5–23	4–21	0–4

rate in beats per minute. The normal heart rate varies by age and can be seen in Table 37-1.

Rhythm

Determination of the heart rhythm is assessed by first locating the P waves and observing the following points:

1. The relationship between the P waves and the QRS complexes
2. The P-wave axis
3. The P-wave morphology

Normal sinus rhythm is characterized by a 1:1 relationship between the P wave and QRS complex. The P-wave axis during sinus rhythm is usually between 0 and 90° (see below) and the P-wave morphology is relatively constant. A common and benign finding in children is that of sinus arrhythmia, which is defined as beat-to-beat variation in the heart rate with no significant change in the P-wave morphology. This is because of variations in sympathetic and parasympathetic input to the heart and is especially pronounced with breathing.

Axis

Determination of the frontal plane electrical axis is performed individually for the P wave, the QRS complex, and the T wave. The axis defines the predominant direction of the summation of electrical wavefronts. Determination of the axis in the frontal plane can be performed as follows:

1. In lead I, measure the area of deflection above the baseline and subtract the amount below the baseline. If the net result is positive, then the axis is between +90 and −90°.
2. In lead aVF, perform the same calculation. If the sum is positive, then the axis lies between 0 and 180°. Using these two leads, one can then superimpose the results and determine the quadrant within which the axis lies (Figure 37-4).

Another method is to identify a lead that has equal forces both above the baseline and below the baseline, which would indicate that the axis vector is perpendicular to that lead.

The normal axis for normal sinus P waves lies between 0 and 90°, which would indicate movement from the high lateral right atrium toward the low medial crux (center) of the heart. The QRS axis varies with age and is dependent on the relationship of right and left ventricles (normal vs. ventricular inversion) as well as the relative muscle mass of each ventricle. In the newborn period, there is relative right ventricular mass dominance with respect to the left ventricle and thus the QRS axis is directed rightward. With time, the right ventricular mass decreases relative to that of the left ventricle and thus the axis moves into the 0 to 90° range. The T-wave axis is usually in the same direction or within 90° of the QRS axis. There is specific T-wave axis changes in lead V1 seen in infants. At birth, the T wave in lead V1 is usually upright but then becomes inverted within 3–7 days. The T wave remains inverted in lead V1 until adolescence and then it becomes upright.

THE P WAVE

The P wave represents atrial depolarization and is dependent on the origin of depolarization (sinus vs. ectopic focus), conduction through the atrium (prolonged conduction results in wider P wave), and atrial size (see hypertrophy below). The P-wave axis helps determine the source of atrial depolarization. An axis between 0 and 90° suggests a sinus origin of the P wave. An axis between −90 and 0° denotes a low right atrial rhythm, which may be seen in normal conditions, especially while at rest. An axis between 90 and 120° would indicate a left atrial rhythm or an ectopic atrial rhythm. The P wave should not be taller than 0.3 mV or wider than 0.12 seconds in duration.

THE PR INTERVAL

The PR interval is measured from the beginning of the P wave to the onset of the QRS deflection. It is the measure of conduction from the high right atrium through the AV node and into the ventricle. The normal PR intervals for age are shown in Table 37-1.

A prolonged PR interval can be a result of increased vagal tone, medications, hyperthyroidism, or diseases that slow conduction through the atrium, AV node or His-Purkinje system. A short PR interval may be seen with ventricular preexcitation in Wolff-Parkinson-White (WPW) syndrome or enhanced AV node conduction because of increased sympathetic tone, which is commonly seen in younger patients.

THE QRS COMPLEX

The QRS complex begins when the wavefront of depolarization reaches the ventricles. The first downward deflection is designated the Q wave and the first upward deflection designated as the R wave. A negative deflection following a Q wave or R wave is the S wave. The QRS duration represents the time to depolarize the ventricles. A prolonged QRS duration is seen with intraventricular conduction delay or with bundle-branch block. The amplitude of the QRS complex reflects the relative forces directed toward a specific lead and reflects the relative sizes of the right and left ventricles. As mentioned, the relative mass of the right ventricle is larger than that of the left ventricle at birth and thus the amplitude of the R wave is larger in the right-sided precordial leads (V1 through V3) early in life; however, as the relative size of the ventricles changes with growth, the R-wave amplitudes shift from the initial right-sided dominance to a left-sided dominance. Q waves are normally seen in the lateral leads (I and aVL), inferior leads (II, III, and aVF) and the precordial leads V5 and V6. This represents the depolarization of the ventricular septum directed from the left to the right ventricle. Q waves that are both deeper and wider than normal may be seen with ventricular hypertrophy or myocardial infarction.

THE ST SEGMENT

The ST segment begins at the end of the QRS complex until the onset of the T wave. During this phase, ventricular muscle cells are isoelectric (between depolarization and repolarization).

Therefore, the ST segment should not deviate more than 1 mm from the baseline and has a typical upsloping appearance as it transitions to the T wave. The J point is the junction between the end of the QRS segment and the beginning of the ST segment and may normally deviate downward to 1 mm from the baseline.

ST segment deviation can be caused by myocardial ischemia or injury, inflammation, hypertrophy, and secondary to medication such as digoxin. Early repolarization is a term describing ST segment elevation of up to 2–4 mm seen usually in the midprecordial leads (V2 through V5) and the inferior leads (II, III, and aVF). Early repolarization is seen in healthy adolescents and is distinguished from other pathologic causes of ST elevation by the presence of normal upsloping ST segments and normal or large amplitude T waves.

THE T WAVE

The T wave corresponds to repolarization of the ventricles. Since the ventricle repolarizes in an opposite direction to depolarization, the T wave and QRS deflections are usually in a similar direction. Normal T-wave variation seen in lead V1 during infancy through adolescence has been previously described. Abnormal T-wave changes can be seen with ischemia, cardiomyopathy, ventricular hypertrophy, mitral valve prolapse, electrolyte abnormalities, or medications.

THE QT INTERVAL

The QT interval is measured from the onset of the Q wave to the end of the T wave. The normal QT interval varies with heart rate: it is longer at slower heart rates and shorter at faster heart rates. Therefore, a standard correction of the QT interval is required to account for changes with heart rate. The Bazett formula is commonly used to "correct" the QT interval based on the heart rate: QT interval divided by square root of RR interval. The "corrected" QT interval (QTc) should be less than 450 ms in infants and 440 ms in children and adults. Prolongation of the QTc interval can be seen in inherited forms of potassium or sodium channel defects known as the long QT syndrome or secondary to medications, electrolyte abnormalities, cardiomyopathy, or CNS disease.

THE U WAVE

The U wave when present is a low amplitude deflection seen following the T wave. It is seen with hypokalemia, antiarrhythmic drugs, or in long QT syndrome. The U wave is usually not incorporated into the QT interval unless it is greater than half the height of the T wave, then a QTU interval can be calculated.

THE ABNORMAL ECG

Enlargement and Hypertrophy

Right atrial enlargement is defined by a peaked P wave higher than 3 mm and is usually seen best in the inferior leads or anterior precordial leads. This is historically known as P pulmonale, which occurs in cor pulmonale because of pulmonary hypertension and right ventricular hypertrophy (RVH) (Figure 37-6A).

Left atrial enlargement is identified by a prolonged P wave duration of greater than 100 ms. Also, a broad or notched P wave in lead II or a deep, slurred terminal portion of a biphasic P wave in lead V1 can be seen with left atrial enlargement. Historically, this is termed P-mitrale because of the association of left atrial hypertrophy with mitral stenosis. A combination of both a tall and broad P wave is indicative of biatrial enlargement (Figure 37-6B).

Right ventricular hypertrophy by ECG in children is complicated by the age-related changes in the relative mass of the right and left ventricles. A list of the proposed criterion for right ventricular hypertrophy is as follows:

1. *R wave greater than the 98th percentile in lead V1.* This finding is a result of the fact that increase in right ventricular mass results in

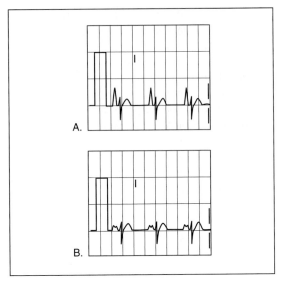

FIGURE 37-6

RIGHT AND LEFT ATRIAL ENLARGEMENT

Lead I of the standard 12-lead ECG is shown. Panel A demonstrates tall, peaked P waves consistent with right atrial hypertrophy (p-pulmonale). Panel B demonstrates broad, notched P waves consistent with left atrial hypertrophy (p-mitrale).

more electrical force directed toward the right-sided lead V1, and is a specific finding for right ventricular hypertrophy outside of the newborn period. In older patients, the height of the R wave in millimeters × 5 has been used to estimate the right ventricular systolic pressure in mmHg; however, the use of echocardiography is more accurate than the ECG to determine this value.

2. *S wave in lead V5 or V6 greater than the 98th percentile.* This finding is also a useful measurement indicating increased right ventricular pressure in older patients. It is seen in patients with RVH owing to chronic lung disease or pulmonary hypertension and is often associated with right atrial enlargement.

3. *Abnormal T-wave direction in lead V1.* As previously mentioned, the normal T-wave changes in lead V1 seen with age have been described. An upright T wave in lead V1 after 5–7 days of

age is indicative of right ventricular hypertrophy secondary to elevated right ventricular pressure. This finding may be seen with mild degrees of right ventricular hypertrophy before the R-wave amplitude in V1 becomes increased. The T wave becomes upright normally as early as 6–8 years of age.

4. *Right axis deviation.* Isolated right axis deviation can be seen in conjunction with other criterion for right ventricular hypertrophy, but should not be used alone as a specific feature of this finding.

5. *Increased RS ratio in V1 or decreased RS ratio in V6.* The normal values for these ratios vary with age and are less sensitive for the diagnosis of right ventricular hypertrophy.

6. *QR pattern in V1.* This pattern suggests severe right ventricular hypertrophy because of elevated right ventricular pressure; however, it may be seen in 10% of normal newborns and children. It can also be seen in patients with ventricular inversion because of depolarization of the ventricular septum from the anatomic left ventricle to the anatomic right ventricle.

7. *The rSR′ pattern in V1.* An rSR′ pattern in V1 may be associated with right ventricular volume overload such as seen in patients with atrial septal defects (Figure 37-7A); however, this pattern may be seen in the normal population but usually does not extend beyond V1 in normal children. Therefore, right ventricular hypertrophy should only be diagnosed when the R′ wave is greater than the 98th percentile for age. An rSR′ pattern associated with a prolonged QRS duration for age is suggestive of right ventricular conduction delay or right bundle branch block (see below).

Left ventricular hypertrophy is more difficult to predict than right ventricular hypertrophy from the electrocardiogram. This is especially true in healthy adolescent children where large R wave amplitudes are commonly seen the mid-precordial and lateral-precordial leads. The specificity for ECG diagnosis for LVH increases if multiple criteria can be identified.

1. *R wave greater than the 98th percentile for age in lead V6.* This "voltage criterion" used alone

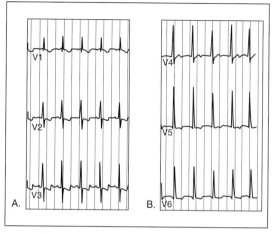

FIGURE 37-7

RIGHT AND LEFT VENTRICULAR HYPERTROPHY

Right ventricular hypertrophy is shown in a 15-year-old male with a large atrial septal defect (panel A). There is an rSR′ pattern in lead V1 with an R′ voltage greater than the upper limits of normal. Left ventricular hypertrophy is shown in an infant with dilated cardiomyopathy (panel B). The R wave in lead V6 is greater than the upper limits of normal for age and there are associated ST segment and T-wave abnormalities.

for left ventricular hypertrophy is not specific as many healthy adolescents may have R-wave amplitude exceeding the 98th percentile in the lateral precordial leads.

2. *S wave greater than the 98th percentile in lead V1.* This finding in conjunction with a large R wave in V6 adds to the specificity of diagnosing left ventricular volume overload.

3. *Increased RS ratio in V6 or decreased RS ratio in V1.* As is true with RVH, this criterion alone is a poor predictor of ventricular hypertrophy but may be used in conjunction with other criterion to improve specificity.

4. *Abnormally deep Q wave in leads V5 and V6.* While small Q waves are normally seen in leads V5 and V6, deep Q waves greater than 5 mm in amplitude are suggestive of left ventricular diastolic overload or left ventricular septal hypertrophy. The sensitivity of this finding is

increased if associated with peaked T waves in these leads.

5. *Lateral T-wave inversion.* T-wave inversion in leads V5 and V6 in combination with R-wave amplitude greater than the 98th percentile is suggestive of left ventricular hypertrophy with strain (Figure 37-7B). It is seen in conditions of increased left ventricular pressure such as aortic stenosis or coarctation of the aorta. Inverted T waves not associated with other features of left ventricular hypertrophy are suggestive of myocardial ischemia.

6. *Left axis deviation.* Left axis deviation is rarely associated with left ventricular hypertrophy; however, in the neonate, left axis deviation may indicate other congenital anomalies such as AV canal defect or left anterior hemiblock.

Biventricular hypertrophy occurs when both criterion for RVH and LVH exists together or if the R wave and S wave amplitudes in the mid-precordial leads are greater than the 98th percentile for age. This former condition is known as Katz-Wachtel criterion.

Intraventricular Conduction Abnormalities

Right bundle-branch block (RBBB) occurs when the QRS duration is greater than the upper limits of normal for age and the QRS morphology is suggestive of right bundle-branch block. In right bundle-branch block, the septal and left ventricular conduction are normal, thus the initial QRS complex appears normal. There is late activation of the right ventricle and the terminal portion of the QRS complex is oriented toward the right precordial leads. This results in the typical rSR′ pattern in leads V1, V2, and aVR (Figure 37-8A). The terminal portion of the QRS complex in the opposing left leads (V5, V6, lead I) shows a deep slurred S wave. Right axis deviation may occasionally be associated with RBBB. The ability to diagnose ventricular hypertrophy in the presence of bundle-branch block is difficult, if not completely inaccurate. Furthermore, evaluation of ST or T wave segments is also inaccurate.

Incomplete right bundle-branch block (IRBBB or RVCD) refers to the finding of a QRS pattern as

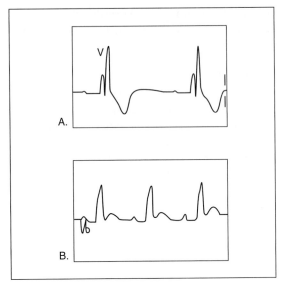

FIGURE   37-8

RIGHT AND LEFT BUNDLE-BRANCH BLOCK

Right bundle-branch block is shown as a prolonged QRS complex and an rSR′ pattern in lead V1 (panel A). Left bundle-branch block is shown as a prolonged QRS complex and broad R waves in lead V6.

seen with RBBB (rSR′) in the right precordial leads; however, the QRS duration may be normal or slightly prolonged for age. This may be seen in conditions of right ventricular volume overload such as with atrial septal defects.

Left bundle-branch block (LBBB) occurs when the QRS duration prolonged for age but the morphology reflects terminal forces oriented toward the left precordial leads. This results in large R waves leads V5 and V6 with deep, slurred S waves in lead V1 (Figure 37-8B). The ST and T wave segments and ventricular hypertrophy are difficult to interpret in the presence of LBBB.

The left bundle branch is known to quickly divide into a left anterior fascicle and a left posterior fascicle once it crosses to the left side of the ventricular septum. Isolated conduction block in either of these fascicles can result in the shift in the QRS axis. Left axis deviation occurs if the left anterior fascicle is interrupted (*left anterior hemiblock*). This may occur as an isolated finding or in combination with RBBB (*bifascicular block*). Left axis deviation seen in certain congenital heart lesions such as AV canal defects or tricuspid atresia are not typically because of left anterior hemiblock but rather because of displacement of the conduction system. *Left posterior hemiblock* is less commonly seen and occurs when the posterior fascicle of the left ventricle is interrupted resulting in a rightward shift of the QRS axis.

Nonspecific intraventricular block occurs if the QRS duration is greater than the upper limits of normal for age but the QRS morphology is not specific for RBBB or LBBB. This may be seen with myocardial infarction, myocarditis, electrolyte abnormalities or it may be because of medications.

Abnormal Depolarization/Repolarization

Preexcitation

Preexcitation results from anomalous activation of the ventricle that occurs earlier than expected from a sinus beat if it traveled through the AV node and His-Purkinje system. This is manifest on the ECG as widening and slurring of the QRS complex. The most common etiology of ventricular preexcitation is because of an accessory connection of muscle fibers between the atrium and ventricle. This is known as WPW syndrome when associated with Subraventricular tachycardias (SVT). Conduction over this accessory connection is usually more rapid than conduction over the AV node and thus the ventricular muscle at the insertion site of the muscle fibers is activated before the normal wavefront of activation via the His-Purkinje system. This produces a short PR interval and a "delta wave" or slurring of the initial deflection of the QRS complex (Figure 37-9). The pattern of ventricular preexcitation with WPW syndrome varies, depending on the location of the accessory pathway, and algorithms are available to estimate the location along the mitral or tricuspid valve rings or within the posterior coronary sinus. A less common form of preexcitation occurs when the accessory connection runs from the atrium to the distal right bundle and is known as a Mahaim fiber. This type of accessory connection is unique in that it has conduction properties similar to the AV node

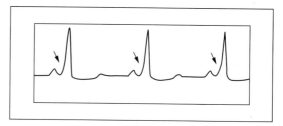

FIGURE 37-9

VENTRICULAR PREEXCITATION

Ventricular preexcitation manifest as a "delta wave" (arrows) is shown during sinus rhythm.

(possibly is a fetal remnant) and is associated with antidromic reciprocating tachycardia (wide-complex SVT that travels from the atrium to the ventricle over the accessory pathway). Another type of "preexcitation" that has been described manifests as a short PR interval on ECG with a normal QRS complex. This is known as Lown-Ganong-Levine syndrome and is thought to be a result of an accessory connection between the atrium and the His bundle. It is possible that this ECG finding is simply because of enhanced AV node conduction as is seen in many infants and young children and not to the presence of an accessory connection. Assessment of ventricular hypertrophy or repolarization abnormalities is not accurate in the presence of ventricular preexcitation.

Repolarization

Q waves are normally present in the inferior leads II, III, and aVF and the left precordial leads V5 and V6. The appearance of new onset, wide and deep Q waves is suggestive of myocardial infarction or ventricular hypertrophy. Causes of myocardial infarction in children include Kawasaki's disease, cardiomyopathy, hypoxic events, myocarditis, or drugs such as cocaine. A specific cause of myocardial infarction seen in infants is a result of anomalous coronary artery to the pulmonary artery (ALCAPA). In this entity, abnormal Q waves may be seen in leads I, aVL, and V4–V6 because of ischemia/infarction of the anterolateral left ventricle.

The ST segment is normally isoelectric with a typical upstroke pattern as it merges with the T wave.

Abnormal elevation greater than 1 mm above or below the baseline may be seen with various diseases that are distinguished by the location and number of ECG leads involved, the upstroke pattern of the ST segment, and the sequence of changes seen over time.

1. *Myocardial ischemia/infarction.* The typical sequence of events begins with the ischemia phase manifest as tall, peaked T waves and mild ST changes recorded in the leads facing the affected myocardium. This is followed by the injury phase manifest as ST segment elevation in the case of epicardial injury or ST depression with endocardial injury. T-wave inversion occurs during the ST segment change with myocardial injury. This distinguishes injury from changes seen during pericarditis in which the T-wave changes occur after the ST segment has returned to the baseline. The final phase is myocardial ischemia signified by the return of the ST segment to the baseline, decrease in the R wave voltage and the appearance of Q waves.

2. *Pericarditis.* Pericardial inflammation results in diffuse, generalized ST segment elevation with maintenance of the T wave amplitude and direction. This is followed by return of the ST segment to the baseline and then followed by T wave inversions. The T wave changes may last for weeks before resolving.

3. *Myocarditis.* Myocardial inflammation results in variable ECG changes included ST segment flattening, elevation or depression, T-wave inversions, and reduced QRS voltages.

4. *LVH.* Left ventricular hypertrophy owing to pressure overload may result in a "strain" pattern consisting of ST segment flattening or depression, T-wave inversion in leads II, III, aVF, V5, and V6, and voltage criterion for LVH.

5. *Hypertrophic cardiomyopathy.* ST segment and T-wave changes with hypertrophic cardiomyopathy may be seen prior to echocardiographic changes and are similar to that seen with LVH with strain.

6. *Digoxin.* A specific pattern of ST segment depression can be seen with digoxin therapy at therapeutic levels.

The T wave normally follows the same direction as the QRS complex and is upright in leads I, II, III, aVF, V5, and V6. T-wave inversion can occur with ischemia/infarction, myocarditis, pericarditis, cardiomyopathy mitral valve prolapse or LVH with strain. Peaked T waves can occur with hyperkalemia, ischemia, LVH, or head injury. Flattened T waves can occur with hypokalemia (also associated with the presence of U waves) or hypothyroidism.

The QT interval varies normally with heart rate and, therefore, should be "corrected" using the Bazett formula as previously mentioned. A prolonged corrected QT interval can occur with the congenital long QT syndrome, or with acquired causes such as hypokalemia, hypocalcemia, head injury, hypomagnesemia, select medications, or antiarrhythmic drug therapy (Figure 37-10). A shortened corrected QT interval can be caused by hypercalcemia.

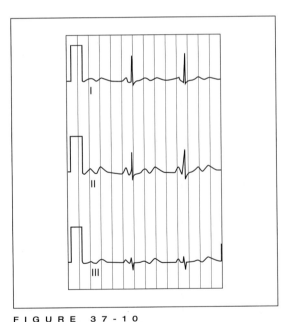

FIGURE   37-10

PROLONGED QTU INTERVAL

An abnormally prolonged QTU interval on standard ECG leads I, II, and III is shown in a patient with congenital long QT syndrome. The abnormal U wave is included in the corrected QTU interval because it is greater than one-half of the height of the T wave.

CLINICAL UTILITY

Although specific indications for performing a 12-lead ECG vary, it is commonly used in the assessment of patients who present with symptoms such as palpitations, heart murmur, syncope, and cyanosis or in patients with family history of cardiac abnormalities. Evidence for the use of the ECG suggests that there is some utility in the evaluation of murmurs, which is affected by many false positives and negatives (Chapter 2). The use of the ECG for the palpitations, syncope or other suspicion of an arrhythmia or conduction abnormality is clear; however, it ought to be realized that the ECG is a very brief sample of the rhythm, but can uncover underlying conduction abnormalities, which may be associated with an arrhythmia (e.g., long QT syndrome or WPW). In a similar fashion, the ECG is useful as a baseline prior to cardiac surgery as the surgery may cause conduction abnormalities. The use of the ECG for a screening tool (e.g., athletes) is not cost effective, though this changes with a strong family history of cardiomyopathy, where the ECG may offer a relatively sensitive first screening method; however, it also should be noted that this is limited because of the variable expression of cardiomyopathy. Thus, other tests or follow-up screening/consultation may be necessary. Finally, the use of the ECG for the evaluation of cyanosis is secondary, as other testing and evaluations are more diagnostic.

AMBULATORY MONITORING

Holter Recording

The Holter monitor is a continuous ECG tape recording able to store two to three ECG channels for 24–48 h. The device is a small tape recorder or digital recorder attached to leads worn by the patient for the prescribed time. The data are downloaded to a computer where they are analyzed, reviewed, and a final report is generated. Variables reported with a Holter monitor include heart rate trends, atrial or ventricular ectopy or arrhythmias, bradycardia or sinus pauses, ST segment trends, heart rate variability, and selected ECG waveforms.

The patient keeps a diary and is instructed to record the time of any symptoms while wearing the Holter monitor. Approximately 20–50% of older patients have symptoms during a Holter monitor, with 2–15% because of arrhythmia.

The most efficacious use of Holter monitoring is in situations where symptoms occur frequently (several times per week). If the history elicits that symptoms occur infrequently, then event recorder monitoring may be more appropriate (see below). Holter monitoring is also used to assess for any acute changes following an intervention (surgery or catheterization), the frequency of ventricular ectopy detected on ECG or exam, and as surveillance for occult arrhythmias in high-risk patients (e.g., following surgery for tetralogy of Fallot).

Event Recorder Monitoring

Event recorders are small devices capable of recording a single ECG lead for several minutes. The device may be attached to leads that are worn continually by the patient or can be worn as a wristwatch. Other devices have built-in electrodes that are placed directly in contact with the skin when recording the ECG. Patient activation is required for these devices to record the rhythm; however, newer devices are attached to leads with programmable auto activation parameters. The recorded ECG data are transmitted over the phone by the patient, processed by a computer and sent to the physician.

Event recorders are ideal for evaluation of infrequent symptoms of palpitations or near-syncope. Their use is limited in younger children and those with syncope since most require patient activation. A newer, implantable loop recorder is now available for situations with infrequent symptoms that are difficult to document with current devices. The implantable loop recorder is a small device that is surgically placed in a subcutaneous pocket in the chest similar to a pacemaker. There are no leads directly placed in the heart but are built-in electrodes that record a single ECG lead. These devices have both a patient-activated feature as well as programmable auto-activated parameters. Current battery life is approximately 1 year at which time the device is removed.

Suggested Readings

Dubin D: *Rapid Interpretation of EKGs*, 3rd ed. Tampa, FL, Cover Publishing, 1982.

Fisch C: Electrocardiography, in: Braunwald E (ed): *Heart Disease. A Textbook of Cardiovascular Medicine*, 5th ed. Philadelphia, PA, WB Saunders, 1997;108–153.

Marriot HJL: *Practical Electrocardiography*, Baltimore, MD, Williams & Wilkins, 1988.

Park MK, Gunteroth WG: *How to Read Pediatric ECGs*. Chicago, IL, Year Book, 1987.

Walsh EP: Electrocardiography and introduction to electrophysiologic techniques, in: Fyler DC (ed): *Nadas' Pediatric Cardiology*, Philadelphia, PA, Hanley & Belfus, 1980, pp. 117–158.

38

TILT TABLE TESTING

Frank Zimmerman

INTRODUCTION

Tilt table testing is a means of evaluating recurrent unexplained syncope in otherwise healthy persons. It is the only clinical laboratory diagnostic tool available for vasovagal or neurocardiogenic syncope. Tilt table testing was developed over 50 years ago to assess the body's heart rate and blood pressure response to changes in position. It was noted during such studies that occasionally people would have what is known as a vasovagal reaction and faint during upright tilt table testing.

MECHANISM

The most popular mechanism proposed to account for neurocardiogenic syncope during tilt table testing can be seen in Figure 38-1. In brief, passive upright tilt prevents effective pumping of blood via skeletal muscle contraction resulting in decreased venous return to the heart and decreased left ventricular filling. This elicits an increased sympathetic output that results in increased left ventricular contractility and activation of vagal C-fibers located within the left ventricle. The C-fibers normally send afferent signals to the brain; however, this

signal becomes overamplified in some patients and the brain responds by decreasing the heart rate and decreasing the blood pressure resulting in a syncopal episode. Other theories about the mechanism of neurocardiogenic syncope include changes in epinephrine or renin, decreases in cerebral blood flow, or changes in serotonin, norepinephrine or other neurotransmitters.

DESCRIPTION OF TEST

The head-up tilt table test is relatively easy to perform and very safe. The patient is usually asked not to eat or drink immediately prior to the procedure. The procedure usually takes place in a quiet room. The patient is asked to lie supine on a special table, which can automatically move the patient from a supine position to a standing position. Continuous ECG recordings are obtained and blood pressure monitoring is performed. This is usually achieved by noninvasive blood pressure cuff monitoring but can also be obtained by arterial line. Once the patient is lying comfortably on the table, an IV is usually inserted. Some protocols recommend that no IV be placed as this may increase the false positive rate of the study. The patient is then secured to

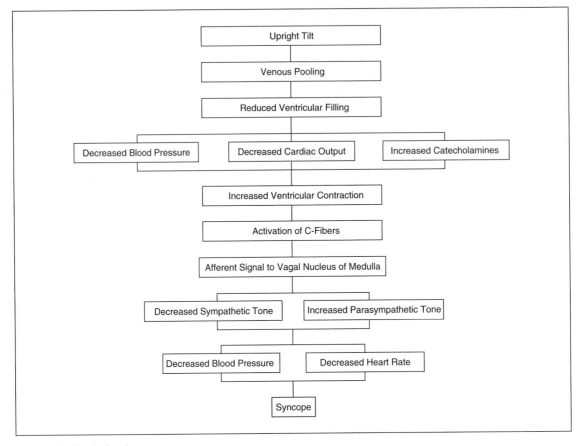

FIGURE 38-1

MECHANISM OF NEUROCARDIOGENIC SYNCOPE DURING HEAD-UP TILT TABLE TESTING

the table with seat belts around the legs and chest. The table is then raised to an angle of approximately 60°–80°. The patient is asked to stand motionless for a period of 20 min to 1 h based on the institutional protocol. If there are no symptoms or syncope, then the table is brought back to the supine position and the test may be repeated after challenging the patient with medication. The most common challenge is with an isoproterenol infusion, which is used to increase sympathetic output and has been shown to increase the sensitivity of the test. Other protocols have included challenge with sublingual nitroglycerine or IV adenosine.

RESPONSE TO THE STUDY

The head-up tilt table test is performed in attempt to reproduce the clinical symptoms of patients with neurocardiogenic syncope. Acute development of hypotension is known as a vasodepressor reaction while acute bradycardia or sinus pause is known as a cardioinhibitory reaction. In most circumstances, both of these reactions occur together, resulting in syncope (Figure 38-2); however, in some select cases, one response may be more predominant than the other and this may effect management. For instance, in patients with predominately cardioinhibitory responses, pacing may be a therapeutic

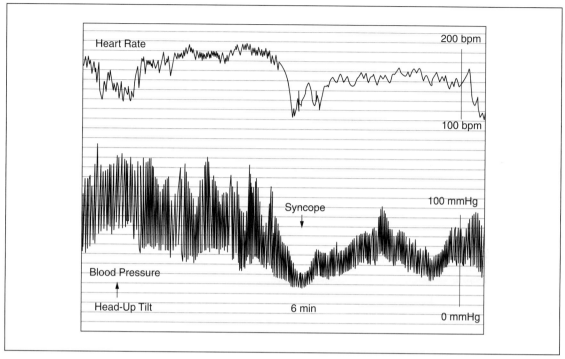

FIGURE 38-2

MIXED VASODEPRESSOR AND CARDIOINHIBITORY RESPONSE TO HEAD-UP TILT

Continuous monitoring of the heart rate and blood pressure tracings shown during head-up tilt. At 6 min into the test, there is a drop in heart rate from 180 to 100 bpm (cardioinhibitory response) associated with a drop in blood pressure from 110/50 to 40/25 mmHg (vasodepressor response) resulting in syncope. Both heart rate and blood pressure increase when the patient is brought to the supine position at the end of the study.

option if medications fail to alleviate symptoms. Once the patient is brought back to the supine position and normal venous blood flow returns to the heart, the abnormal vasovagal reaction ends and the blood pressure and heart rate return to normal. Some unusual exaggerated responses to head-up tilt table testing include episodes of asystole lasting up to 30 s, which again resolve when the patient is brought to the supine position and seizures because of central hypoperfusion.

INDICATIONS

The indications for tilt table testing are shown in Table 38-1. These indications were formulated for adults and reported in the ACC expert consensus document in 1996. Tilt table testing is usually considered warranted for the evaluation of recurrent syncope or a single episode accompanied by physical injury or accident occurring in high-risk settings, such as a commercial pilot or a competitive athlete, when the cause is not conclusively known to be vasovagal in origin. Other situations include evaluation of recurrent exercise-induced syncope when previous evaluation has been normal. In general, patients with single or infrequent syncopal episodes in which the clinical features clearly support the diagnosis of vasovagal syncope usually do not require tilt table testing.

TABLE 38-1

RECOMMENDED INDICATIONS FOR TILT TABLE TESTING

Tilt Table Testing Warranted

1. Recurrent syncope in a high-risk patient and
   a. No evidence of structural heart disease

      or

   b. Structural heart disease present but not thought to contribute to syncope
2. Evaluation in patients with known cause of syncope (e.g., heart block) but if susceptible to neurocardiogenic syncope would change treatment plans
3. Evaluation of exercise-induced syncope

Tilt Table Testing Possibly Warranted

1. Differentiation of neurocardiogenic syncope from seizures
2. Evaluation of elderly patients with frequent falls
3. Assessment of recurrent dizziness or presyncope
4. Evaluation of unexplained syncope in the setting of dysautonomias or peripheral neuropathies
5. Evaluation of efficacy of medical therapy for neurocardiogenic syncope

Tilt Table Testing Not Warranted

1. Single syncopal episode with features consistent with neurocardiogenic syncope not in high-risk setting
2. Syncope owing to a specific cause in which additional diagnosis of neurocardiogenic syncope would not alter treatment plan

SENSITIVITY AND SPECIFICITY OF THE TEST

Although tilt table testing is the only method available at this time for evaluation of neurocardiogenic syncope, its utility is limited because of several factors. The sensitivity of the test (i.e., chance that a patient with true neurocardiogenic syncope will have a positive head-up tilt table test) is approximately 43–57% in children and approximately 32–85% in adults. The sensitivity can be improved up to 77% in children with the use of isoproterenol; however, the addition of isoproterenol or other medications decreases the specificity of the test. Without pharmacologic challenge, the specificity is approximately 83–100% in children; however, this decreases to 35–100% with infusion of isoproterenol. Another limitation of tilt table testing is that the reproducibility of findings is variable. Reproducibility of test results in pediatric patients ranges from 65–85%. This means that patients who

have a positive tilt table test one day may have a completely different response on another day, even with no changes in their medical management.

CONCLUSION

In summary, tilt table testing is one of the only methods available for clinical evaluation of neurocardiogenic syncope. The utility of tilt table testing is limited because of the fact that there is a high incidence of false negative tests in the baseline state and an increased incidence of false positive tests when isoproterenol infusion is used.

Suggested Readings

Benditt DG, Ferguson DW, Grubb BP, Kapoor WN, Kugler J, Lerman BB, Maloney JD, Raviele A, Ross B, Sutton R, Wolk MJ, Wood DL: Tilt table testing for assessing syncope. *J Am Coll Cardiol* 28(1):263–275, 1996.

Calkins H, Zipes DP: Hypotension and syncope, in: Braunwald E, Zipes DP, Libbey P (eds): *Braunwald: Heart Disease: A Textbook of Cardiovascular Medicine*, 6th ed. Philadelphia, PA, WB Saunders, 2001, pp. 932–939.

Krongrad E: Syncope and sudden death, in: Emmanouilides GC, Riemenschneider TA, Allen HD, Gutgesell HP (eds): *Moss and Adams Heart Disease in Infants, Children and Adolescents*, 5th ed. Philadelphia, PA, Williams & Wilkins, 1995, pp. 1604–1619.

Stewart JM: Orthostatic intolerance in pediatric. *J Pediatr* 140:404–411, 2002.

Tanel RE, Walsh EP: Syncope in the pediatric patient. *Cardio Clin* 15(2):277–294, 1997.

C H A P T E R

39

STRESS TESTING

Frank Zimmerman

INTRODUCTION

Exercise stress testing in children is less commonly performed than in adults. It is primarily used to determine exercise tolerance or evaluate symptoms related to exercise rather than to evaluate for ischemic heart disease. While exercise stress tests are generally safe, they require a certain degree of cooperation and motivation thus posing many technical limitations in children. Performance on exercise stress testing is dependent on cardiac function and reserve, pulmonary function and reserve, metabolic function of the body, and overall coordination and motivation.

EQUIPMENT AND PROTOCOL

The goal for any stress testing protocol is to have the patient motivated to be active and exercise with a gradual increase in the workload until maximum exertion or symptoms occur. In most cases, maximum exertion should be achieved after 8–12 min of exercise, otherwise young patients become bored or disinterested. The two main types of exercise testing include the treadmill test (walking or running on a treadmill) or the cycle ergometer test (riding a stationary bicycle). There are a number of protocols for each modality and there are benefits and limitations for each. For instance, the commonly used Bruce protocol for the treadmill test requires fast walking or running at the later stages of exercise that may be difficult for younger children to perform. Thus, modified pediatric protocols can be used that increase workload by increasing the grade of the treadmill rather than increasing the speed. In general, cycle ergometers require more coordination to perform correctly and maximum exertion is difficult to achieve unless the patients are pretrained on the bicycle; however, it may be easier for children if they already know how to use a bicycle. The advantages of cycle ergometers include greater ease in obtaining physiologic data and that the patient is not required to be ambulatory.

If patients are unable to exercise, stress testing can be performed by the infusion of medications such as dobutamine. While this serves to artificially increase cardiac output and myocardial oxygen consumption, it does not result in the normal metabolic response to exercise. Thus, exercise tolerance cannot be measured and clinical symptoms related to exercise might not be reproduced. In patients with ischemic heart disease or suspected coronary artery anomalies, more detailed information can be obtained with imaging of the heart either by a nuclear scan or echocardiogram.

A technician, nurse, or physician with specific expertise in the field often supervises the exercise test. Standard testing includes continuous 12-lead ECG monitoring, intermittent blood pressure recordings by cuff and oxygen saturation recordings. If detailed information regarding metabolic function is desired, expired gas analysis can be performed during the test. This is accomplished by having the patient breathe into a mouthpiece connected to an analyzer that can perform breath-by-breath gas analysis. Because additional cooperation and coordination are required, it is difficult to obtain this data in children younger than 6–8 years of age.

RESPONSE TO EXERCISE

The overall response and tolerance to exercise is based on many factors. Muscles involved with exercise require adequate oxygen delivery to meet increased metabolic demands. If metabolic demands exceed oxygen delivery, aerobic metabolism can no longer continue and anaerobic metabolism ensues. This results in lactic acid production and limits the duration of exercise. Increased oxygen delivery is dependent on the lungs ability to increase oxygen uptake and the hearts ability to increase cardiac output. The normal cardiac response to exercise is seen in Figure 39-1. Although not all of these factors can be measured directly (e.g., cardiac output, lactic acid production), the following parameters can be obtained during the exercise test:

Endurance

This is measured as the total amount of time exercised or the amount of work that was performed. It is compared to standardized normative values based on the patient's age, sex, and the type of test performed. It is important that the patient has

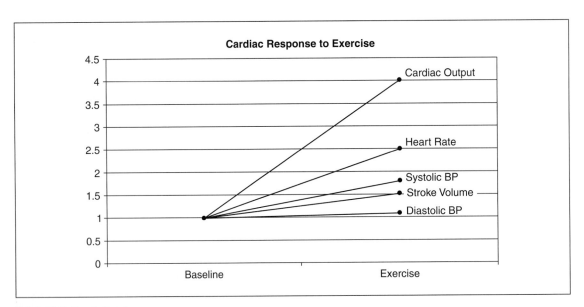

FIGURE 39-1

CARDIAC RESPONSE TO EXERCISE

The four-fold increase normally seen in cardiac output is related to the product of heart rate and stroke volume. Systolic blood pressure increases while there is minimal change in diastolic blood pressure owing to decreased systemic vascular resistance with exercise.

TABLE 39-1

CAUSES OF REDUCED EXERCISE ENDURANCE

1. Poor fitness
2. Poor effort
3. Cardiac disorder
4. Pulmonary disorder
5. Metabolic disorder

performed a maximum effort during the stress test in order to assess endurance. For instance, a patient with a poor effort who stops exercising after only a few minutes should not be labeled as being physically unfit. Causes of reduced exercise endurance or tolerance are listed in Table 39-1. Comparison of performance on serial exercise tests over time is often used to assess the patient's overall status or to assess the effects of a training program.

Heart Rate

The peak heart rate achieved during exercise is compared to standardized normative values for age and the type of test performed. Heart rate response to exercise in various conditions is shown in Figure 39-2. A maximal effort must have been put forth during the exercise study in order to assess peak exercise heart rates. A low peak heart rate response to exercise owing to sinus node dysfunction can be seen following surgery for congenital heart disease or may be a result of medications such as beta-blockers. Other etiologies of low peak heart rates include chronic heart block or the development of heart block with exercise (rate-related). Because cardiac output is dependent on the product of heart rate and stroke volume, a reduced heart rate response has profound effects on exercise endurance in conditions which stroke volume is limited. This is seen in younger patients and those with various forms of congenital or acquired heart disease.

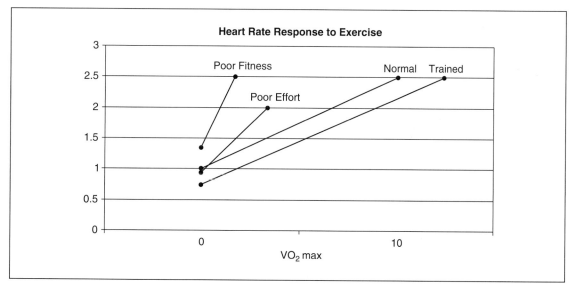

FIGURE 39-2

HEART RATE RESPONSE TO EXERCISE

The normal 10-fold increase in peak oxygen consumption (VO_2 max) is associated with a 2.5–3-fold increase in heart rate. The low peak heart achieved with poor effort can also be seen in patients with chronotropic incompetence.

Blood Pressure

The normal response of blood pressure during exercise is seen in Figure 39-1. Increases in systolic blood pressure are because of the proportionally greater increase in cardiac output compared to the decrease in systemic vascular resistance; however, because of the drop in systemic vascular resistance, diastolic blood pressure does not increase significantly during exercise. Inadequate rise in blood pressure may indicate poor cardiac function, ischemia, or left ventricular outflow tract obstruction. A significant increase in blood pressure during exercise can be seen in patients with familial hypertension or in those with coarctation of the aorta.

Oxygen Saturation

Oxygen saturation during exercise should remain unchanged. Decreases in oxygen saturation may be seen in patients with cyanotic heart disease if the amount of right-to-left shunting increases during exercise. Also, patients with pulmonary disease may demonstrate decreased oxygen saturation with exercise.

ECG

Continuous recording of the 12-lead ECG during exercise can be used to detect myocardial ischemia or infarction. Although this is a rare finding in children, it may be associated with congenital coronary artery anomalies, Kawasaki disease, cardiomyopathy or left ventricular outflow obstruction or aortic insufficiency. The ECG can be assessed for abnormal prolongation of the corrected QT interval at peak exercise. Some suggest that this is specific for diagnosing the long QT syndrome in patients with normal resting ECGs; however, the predictive value of this finding is unknown. Assessment of arrhythmias with exercise testing is commonly used. Ventricular ectopy (premature ventricular contractions [PVCs], nonsustained ventricular tachycardia) at baseline is often classified by the response to stress testing. Although there are important exceptions, resolution of ventricular ectopy during exercise is considered benign while persistence or worsening of the arrhythmia is more ominous and may indicate underlying cardiac disease.

Oxygen Consumption and Anaerobic Threshold

Exercise endurance and fitness is often measured in terms of peak oxygen consumption. This is the maximal amount of oxygen consumed during exercise and is reported as a percentage of the predicted normal value based on age and sex. The causes of low peak oxygen consumption are shown in Table 39-1. Serial measurements of oxygen consumption can be followed to determine optimal timing for heart transplantation in patients with cardiac dysfunction. Anaerobic threshold is defined as the point at which oxygen supply cannot meet the demands of the exercising muscles. The by-product of anaerobic metabolism is lactic acid leading to muscle fatigue and carbon dioxide resulting in a rise in the respiratory rate. The point at which anaerobic threshold is reached as a percentage of the predicted peak oxygen consumption is used as a measure of fitness that is not dependent on maximal effort during the stress test. Oxygen consumption, anaerobic threshold, and many other metabolic variables are measured with breath-by-breath analysis during the stress test.

INDICATIONS

The ACC/AHA guidelines regarding the indications for exercise stress testing in children are listed in Table 39-2. Class I indications are conditions for which there is evidence and/or general agreement that stress testing is useful and effective. Class IIa indications are conditions for which the weight of evidence/opinion is in favor of the usefulness/efficacy. Class IIb indications are conditions where usefulness/efficacy is less well established by evidence/opinion. The measurement of exercise capacity in children with congenital heart disease is often performed in order to guide therapy with medical treatment or intervention with surgery. Exercise stress testing is also useful for the evaluation of the

TABLE 39-2

INDICATIONS FOR EXERCISE STRESS TESTING IN CHILDREN

Class I

1. Evaluation of exercise capacity in children with congenital heart disease, those who have had surgery for congenital heart disease and those with acquired myocardial or valvular disease
2. Evaluation of the child with anginal chest pain
3. Assessment of the response of an artificial pacing system to exertion
4. Evaluation of exercise related symptoms in young athletes

Class IIa

1. Evaluation of the response to medical, surgical, or RF ablation therapy for children with a tachyarrhythmia induced during stress testing before therapy
2. As an adjunct to the assessment of congenital or acquired valvular lesions such as aortic stenosis
3. Evaluation for exercise-induced arrhythmias

Class IIb

1. Evaluation of children with a family history of sudden death with exercise
2. Follow-up of Kawasaki disease or systemic lupus erythematosus
3. Assessment of children with congenital complete heart block
4. Assessment of heart rate response in children treated with beta-blocker therapy
5. Measurement of the response of shortening or prolongation of the corrected QT interval
6. Evaluation of blood pressure response after repair of coarctation of the aorta
7. Assessment of the degree of desaturation with exercise in patients with cyanotic heart disease

rare patient who presents with typical anginal chest pain, described as burning or squeezing, or atypical chest pain that is consistently associated with exercise. It is usually not necessary to perform formal exercise testing in patients with complaints of chest pain not associated with exercise or activity. Other symptoms related to exercise such as dizziness or syncope are often evaluated with exercise stress testing.

CONTROVERSIES IN EXERCISE TESTING

There is currently debate regarding the indications for exercise stress testing in patients that have had Kawasaki disease. While most would follow patients that have persistent coronary artery lesions with stress tests, the prognostic value of stress testing in asymptomatic patients with resolved coronary lesions is unknown. Another use of the stress test is in the assessment of patients who present with isolated premature ventricular contractions. Resolution of the PVCs with exercise is thought to be a benign finding; however, there are some pathologic conditions associated with arrhythmias that may not be reproduced during stress testing. Therefore, because of lack of sensitivity, formal stress testing is usually not necessary for the evaluation of PVCs in the absence of structural heart disease or symptoms with activity. Stress testing has also been used to evaluate patients with either mild unrepaired or repaired coarctation of the aorta. Recent evidence has shown that blood pressure response to exercise in this group does not identify those with significant gradients across the coarctation.

Suggested Readings

Driscol DJ: Exercise testing, in: Emmanouilides GC, Riemenschneider TA, Allen HD, Gutgesell HP (eds): *Moss and Adams Heart Disease in Infants, Children and Adolescents*, 5th ed. Philadelphia, PA, Williams & Wilkins, 1995, pp. 293–309.

Gibbons RJ, Balady GJ, Beasley JW, Bricker JT, et al: ACC/AHA guidelines for exercise testing: A report of the American college of cardiology/American heart association task force on practice guidelines (committee on exercise testing), *J Am Coll Cardiol* 30(1):260–315, 1997.

Swan L, Goyal S, Hsia C, Hechter S, Webb G, Gatzoulis MA: Exercise systolic blood pressures are of questionable value in the assessment of the adult with a previous coarctation repair, *Heart* 89:189–192, 2003.

40

CHEST RADIOGRAPHY

S. Bruce Greenberg

GENERAL PRINCIPLES

Conventional chest radiography remains the most common imaging tool in medicine. Although, echocardiography has become the keystone of congenital heart disease imaging, the chest radiograph still provides a global view of the chest and of the pulmonary vascularity. Noncardiac causes of patient symptoms may also be suggested by chest radiography. Finally, the chest radiograph may suggest congenital heart disease in children presenting with apparently noncardiac symptoms such as wheezing.

A systematic approach to the chest radiograph in the child with suspected congenital heart disease is summarized in Table 40-1. A checklist provides an approach that ensures that no important information on the chest radiograph is overlooked. In analyzing the chest radiograph it is best to read the study in a consistent manner. It makes no difference if you prefer to look at the corners first and work your way to the center of the image or begin in the center and work your way to the corners; however, once an approach is determined it is best to read the images following the same pattern. The patient demographics and clinical history are part of the chest radiography examination. This includes information such as the age and gender. Certain forms of congenital

heart disease are more likely to present at different ages and the frequency may be different in boys and girls. In addition, different clinical presentations will occur. Thus, an indication for the chest radiograph other than performing it as a "screening" test is essential. A newborn with congestive heart failure may have a hypoplastic left heart, but this anomaly would not be considered likely in a 3-year-old. The chest radiograph showing increased pulmonary arterial vascularity suggests an admixture lesion rather than a left-to-right shunt in the child presenting with cyanosis. *A normal chest radiograph does not exclude congenital heart disease.*

THE CARDIAC SILHOUETTE

The cardiac silhouette is evaluated for size, shape, and position. Traditionally it is taught that the right heart border is formed by the right atrium and that the left heart border by a combination of the left atrium superiorly and left ventricle inferiorly on frontal radiographs. On lateral radiographs, the anterior heart border is formed by the right ventricle and the posterior border by a combination of the left atrium superiorly and the left ventricle inferiorly; however, the thymus may be border forming

TABLE 40-1

CHECKLIST APPROACH TO READING THE CHEST RADIOGRAPH FOR CONGENITAL HEART DISEASE

Checklist Item	Findings
Demographics	Age, sex, clinical history
Heart	Size and position
Main pulmonary artery	Location and size
Peripheral pulmonary arterial vascularity	Symmetry and volume
Pulmonary venous vascularity	Volume and sharpness
Aorta arch	Location and number
Abdominal situs	Solitus, inversus, or ambiguous
Bones	Spine, rib, and sternum anomalies

on frontal radiographs. Cardiac size must be evaluated on both frontal and lateral chest radiographs in infants and small children. The thymus can make the mediastinum appear wide in normal infants and small children giving the false impression of cardiomegaly on frontal radiographs. The lack of mass effect by the thymus and a characteristic wavy border helps identify the presence of a robust thymus, but obscures the true cardiac size. The thymus is predominantly located in the anterior mediastinum filling in the retrosternal space. The anterior position of the thymus makes identification of heart size easier on lateral radiographs in infants and small children. The inferior vena cava can be identified on the lateral radiograph as it enters the right atrium. Minimal protrusion of the heart posterior to the inferior vena cava is seen in the lateral radiographs. Since the retrosternal space is normally filled in by thymus on the lateral radiograph, the right ventricle size cannot be evaluated on chest radiographs in infants and young children. As the retrosternal space becomes more air filled in older children and adults, the right ventricle becomes visible on the lateral chest radiograph as the anterior border of the heart. Once the size of the thymus decreases relative to other mediastinal

structures so that it is no longer border forming on the frontal chest radiograph, the right lateral border will be the right atrium and the left heart border the left atrium and left ventricle.

The cardiac silhouette can be normal, large, or small. Congenital heart disease is not associated with a small heart size, but can be normal or large. Cardiac chambers and vessels that carry shunted blood will enlarge. Chambers that pump blood against increased pressure will hypertrophy. The chest radiograph portrays only the silhouette of the heart. As a result, an enlarged cardiac silhouette on both frontal and lateral chest radiographs will identify cardiac enlargement. Ventricle hypertrophy results in thickening of the muscle at the expense of the lumen. Hence, the heart silhouette will remain normal in size; however, the configuration of the heart will be altered. Right ventricle hypertrophy causes the cardiac apex to appear elevated. Left ventricle hypertrophy is characterized by rounding of the cardiac apex.

A normal heart may appear enlarged when in an abnormal thorax. The heart appears enlarged in a child with asphyxiating thoracic dystrophy because of the small chest volume associated with short ribs. More commonly, the heart size will appear to be enlarged if there is poor inspiration at the time of the chest radiograph. Hyperinflated lungs may give the appearance of a normal sized heart in a child with cardiomegaly. Any cardiac congenital anomaly that sustains intrauterine life and permits a live birth is not associated with cardiomegaly except for severe obstructions, arteriovenous malformations, and cardiomyopathies at the time of birth. Cardiomegaly associated with congenital heart disease is usually caused by left-to-right shunts and admixture lesions. The overcirculation of the lungs and cardiomegaly are not present in the newborn because of the increased intrauterine pulmonary resistance. As pulmonary resistance to flow decreases, the shunts become more manifest and cardiac size increases.

The cardiac silhouette can be located predominantly in the left hemithorax with the apex pointed to the left (levocardia), right hemithorax with the apex pointed to the right (dextrocardia), or in the middle (mesocardia). Most children with levocardia do not have congenital heart disease. Although congenital heart disease is common with dextrocardia, the association of heart position with congenital heart disease is complex. Dextrocardia can be associated with noncardiac abnormalities such as Kartagener's syndrome or congenital absence of the right lung.

Situs solitus includes levocardia, a left aortic arch, trilobed right lung, bilobed left lung, stomach, and spleen on the left side of the abdomen and liver and inferior vena cava on the right side. Situs solitus is associated with an incidence of congenital heart disease of about 1%. Situs inversus totalis, the complete reversal of situs solitus is associated with only a slightly increased incidence of congenital heart disease. Other combinations of organ position have a high incidence of associated congenital heart disease. Children with levocardia but situs inversus have a 99% chance of congenital heart disease.

THE PULMONARY ARTERY AND VASCULARITY

The main pulmonary artery is visible as a shadow superior and to the left of the cardiac silhouette. In infants and children the main pulmonary artery is not border forming, but can be visualized as a circular density through the thymus on frontal radiographs. The main pulmonary artery is evaluated for position and size. The main pulmonary artery can be in an abnormal position in some forms of congenital heart disease such as transposition or truncus arteriosus or elevated in left-to-right shunts such as ventricular septal defects in young children. Pulmonary artery enlargement is identified in children on chest radiographs with left-to-right shunts, some admixture lesions, and abnormalities of the pulmonary valve. A small or inapparent pulmonary artery is characteristic of right-to-left shunts and some admixture anomalies.

The peripheral pulmonary arteries are identified by an arborizing pattern of densities radiating from the main pulmonary artery. The pulmonary arterial vascularity is the most difficult of the chest radiograph to evaluate even for experienced cardiac radiologists. The descending right pulmonary artery is about the same size as the right bronchus and

peripheral pulmonary arteries are similar in size to their associated bronchi. Few pulmonary artery branches should be visible in the outer third of the lungs. In newborns, the pulmonary vascularity is normally less than that identified in older children and adults. The peripheral pulmonary arterial vascularity is normal, increased, or decreased. The peripheral pulmonary arterial vascularity must be interpreted along with heart size and the main pulmonary artery. A left-to-right shunt would be expected to result in cardiomegaly along with a large main pulmonary artery and increased peripheral pulmonary vascularity; however, pulmonary valve stenosis typically is associated with a normal sized heart and normal peripheral pulmonary vascularity but an enlarged main pulmonary artery segment.

Pulmonary veins are evaluated as being normal or increased. The pulmonary veins follow a more horizontal course than the pulmonary arteries. Pulmonary hypertension results in redistribution with an increase in the upper lobe pulmonary veins seen in older children and adults. Peribronchial cuffing and a fuzzy appearance to the pulmonary veins characterize pulmonary edema. Severe pulmonary edema makes evaluation of both the peripheral pulmonary arteries and veins difficult.

THE AORTA

The aortic arch is evaluated primarily for position and also for size. The aortic arch is easily identified in adults as a density adjacent to the spine on frontal radiographs that displaces the adjacent trachea to the opposite side. The aortic arch is more tightly coiled in infants and small children and may not be border forming and the trachea is frequently in the midline or difficult to identify. The spine pedicles will be denser on the side of the aortic arch making proper identification of the position possible in any properly exposed, straight radiograph of the chest. The aortic arch is normally on the left side. A right-sided aortic arch suggests a vascular ring or congenital heart disease. Virtually all right aortic arches with mirror image branching are associated with congenital heart disease. A higher incidence of congenital heart disease than normal is present for children with a right aortic arch and an aberrant left subclavian artery. Tetalogy of Fallot is associated with a 25% chance of having a right aortic arch. Ninety percent of children with a right aortic arch and congenital heart disease have tetralogy of Fallot because tetralogy of Fallot is such a common form of congenital heart disease. Truncus arteriosus is associated with a right aortic arch in 37% of cases, but is a less common form of congenital heart disease than tetralogy of Fallot.

THE SKELETON

Congenital heart disease is frequently associated with other anomalies. Down syndrome is associated with a double manubrial center and 11 rib pairs. A shield chest may be found in children with Turner syndrome. Spine anomalies can be detected in children with VATER association (a syndrome of vertebral defects, and atresia, radial dysplasia, renal dysplasia, and congenital heart defects) or Marfan syndrome. All of these syndromes and countless others are associated with congenital heart disease. While it is important to identify all the abnormalities on the chest radiograph, the associated syndromes are usually first identified by nonradiologic means.

SPECIFIC CATEGORIES OF CONGENITAL HEART DISEASE

Left-to-Right Shunts

Left-to-right shunts is the largest group of anomalies causing congenital heart disease presenting in childhood. A shunt ratio of 2:1 is generally considered the minimal size to enable detection of it on conventional radiographs. All significant left-to-right shunts present with cardiomegaly, a large main pulmonary artery and increased pulmonary arterial vascularity. Ventricular septal defects constitute the majority of left-to-right shunts and will have left heart enlargement on chest radiography since the left atrium and left ventricle carry shunted blood. The right ventricle does not significantly enlarge since most of the blood shunted across the ventricular septal defect does so during ventricular

systole when both ventricles are decreasing in volume. Patent ductus arteriosus also has left atrial and ventricular enlargement, but will also have enlargement of the ascending aorta and aortic knob since these structures also carry shunted blood. Unlike ventricular septal defect, the chest radiograph in patent ductus arteriosus may show asymmetric blood flow with increased flow to the right lung secondary to a jet effect of flow through the ductus. A complete atrioventricular septal defect will also have left-sided cardiac enlargement with increased pulmonary blood flow. A prominent right atrium with a characteristic shelf may be present.

Atrial septal defects frequently have normal chest radiographs. When abnormal, pure right side cardiac enlargement is present since the right atrium and right ventricle carry the shunted blood. Unlike ventricular septal defects, blood flows continuously across the atrial septal defect during atrial diastole. As a result, the left atrium and left ventricle do not carry the shunted blood and will be of normal size. Partial atrioventricular septal defects have the same physiology as secundum atrial septal defects, but may have the characteristic right atrial appearance described above for complete atrioventricular septal defects. Patients with partial anomalous pulmonary venous return usually have normal chest radiographs, but may have a similar appearance as an atrial septal defect.

Admixture Lesions

Children with admixture lesions have cardiomegaly and increased pulmonary arterial vascularity, but are cyanotic unlike those with left-to-right shunts. The main pulmonary artery is large and easy to visualize in left-to-right shunts. The main pulmonary artery is frequently abnormal in position or may be entirely absent in children with admixture lesions. D-transposition of the great arteries is the most common admixture lesion, but because of the position of the pulmonary artery dorsal to the ascending aorta, it is not visible on chest radiographs. The branch pulmonary arteries can be identified since they are enlarged, but when traced back to the mediastinum, they are seen to converge medial to the expected location of the main pulmonary artery. Some forms of truncus arteriosus do not have a main pulmonary artery, rather origins of the branch pulmonary arteries directly from the truncus or patent ductus arteriosus. A child with cyanosis, cardiomegaly, prominent arterial pulmonary vascularity, and a difficult-to-identify main pulmonary artery most likely has D-transposition of the great arteries or truncus arteriosus.

Total anomalous venous return without obstruction of the pulmonary veins will present with an enlarged main pulmonary artery segment as well as cardiomegaly and increased pulmonary arterial vascularity. Supracardiac anomalous venous return may have a characteristic "snowman" or "figure of 8" configuration on chest radiographs caused by a large vertical vein on the left side of the chest and enlargement of the superior vena cava on the right side of the chest. Double outlet right ventricle and single ventricle do not have a characteristic appearance, but will be in the differential diagnosis in a child presenting with cyanosis, cardiomegaly, and increased pulmonary arterial vascularity on chest radiography.

Right-to-Left Shunts

Children with right-to-left shunts will be cyanotic and have decreased pulmonary arterial vascularity on chest radiographs. Tetralogy of Fallot is the most common lesion with a right-to-left shunt. Pulmonary outflow obstruction results in right ventricle hypertrophy and can cause elevation of the cardiac apex on chest radiographs giving the classic boot shaped heart. Most children with tetralogy of Fallot do not have boot shaped hearts. The heart is normal in size and the main pulmonary artery is diminished, frequently resulting in a concave appearance of the mediastinum in the expected location of the main pulmonary artery. Pulmonary atresia with a ventricular septal defect and tricuspid atresia may have the same appearance as tetralogy of Fallot on radiographs.

Children with right-to-left shunts and cardiomegaly are less common. These children will have severe obstruction causing atrial enlargement. Pulmonary atresia with an intact ventricular septum and tricuspid valve regurgitation and Ebstein anomaly, are the two most common abnormalities

in this small category. Children with pulmonary atresia and an intact ventricular septum will present early in infancy, but children with Ebstein anomaly can present at any time since the tricuspid valve abnormality and amount of regurgitation may vary from mild to severe.

Cardiomegaly with Pulmonary Congestion

Cardiomegaly with pulmonary congestion may be caused by three categories of disease: obstruction of the heart at or distal to the mitral valve, cardiomyopathies, and high output states. Mitral atresia (hypoplastic left heart syndrome), mitral stenosis, critical aortic stenosis, coarctation of the aorta, and interruption of the aorta all cause obstruction of the heart distal to the mitral valve. In the latter lesions, the chamber proximal to the obstruction will be dilated unless decompressed via a septal defect, which may be seen on the chest plain radiograph. In addition, the right ventricle may be dilated because of increased pulmonary artery pressure and volume loading (e.g., hypoplastic left heart syndrome). In addition, the obstruction causes pulmonary venous hypertension resulting in pulmonary edema.

Coarctation of the aorta has two entirely different radiographic presentations. In infants, coarctation presents with signs of obstruction shortly after the ductus arteriosus closes. The heart will be enlarged and pulmonary congestion present on radiographs. Older children presenting with coarctation do not have cardiomegaly but may have a rounded appearance of the left heart border consistent with left ventricle hypertrophy. Rib notching associated with collateral blood flow does not appear until 5 years of age. The prominent aortic knob and poststenotic dilatation of the descending aorta are responsible for the "3 sign" on chest radiographs present in half of the children with coarctation of the aorta. A reliable sign of coarctation is the presence of a prominent descending aorta with a difficult to visualize proximal descending aorta on a frontal chest radiograph. The thymus should be identified in children suspected of interruption of the aorta because of the association with DiGeorge syndrome.

Cardiomyopathies resulting in pump failure, regardless of etiology, will result in global cardiomegaly and pulmonary edema. The cardiac silhouette may have a globular appearance. The radiographic picture is nonspecific but common causes of congenital cardiomyopathy include viral infection, anomalous origin of the left coronary artery, glycogen storage disease such as Pompei's disease, and endocardial fibroelastosis. Syndromes (e.g., Noonan's syndrome) and metabolic disease (e.g., infant of a diabetic mother) can also be associated with cardiomyopathies. Finally, cardiomyopathies can be acquired in children (e.g., Kawasaki's disease).

High output states are associated with cardiomegaly and pulmonary edema. In infants and small children vascular malformations such as vein of Galen malformation, liver hemangiomas, and peripheral arterial venous malformations can all result in heart failure. Children with vein of Galen malformations may have prominent jugular veins identified on chest radiographs. Anemias such as sickle cell disease can also lead to congestive heart failure.

The age of presentation can offer clues as to the most likely cause of congestive heart failure.

TABLE 40-2

COMMON LEFT-TO-RIGHT SHUNTS (CARDIOMEGALY AND INCREASED PULMONARY VASCULARITY)

Anomaly	Key Findings
Ventricular septal defect	Large left atrium and left ventricle, small aortic arch
Patent ductus arteriosus	Large left atrium, left ventricle, and aortic arch; rarely has associated pulmonary asymmetry with more vascularity to the right lung
Atrial septal defect	Large right atrium and right ventricle
Atrioventricular septal defects	Any chamber may be enlarged, right atrium is frequently prominent with a shelf

TABLE 40-3

COMMON RIGHT-TO-LEFT SHUNTS (DECREASED PULMONARY VASCULARITY)

Anomaly	Key Findings
Tetralogy of Fallot	Right ventricle hypertrophy causing elevation of cardiac apex, small or inapparent pulmonary artery segment, 25% have right aortic arch
Tricuspid atresia	Normal sized heart unless a large bulboventricular foramen is present
Pulmonary atresia with a ventricular septal defect	Same appearance as tetralogy of Fallot
Ebstein anomaly	Large heart from right atrium enlargement
Pulmonary atresia with intact ventricular septum	Large heart from right atrium enlargement

Congestive heart failure presenting in the first hours of life is most likely caused by volume overload or arrhythmia. Hypoplastic left heart syndrome is the most common cause of heart failure in the first week of life. Coarctation of the aorta is the most common cause of congestive heart failure in the second and third weeks of life. After the first month of life, heart failure is most commonly caused by overcirculation associated with left-to-right shunts.

Normal Sized Heart with Pulmonary Congestion

Both congenital heart disease and noncardiac disease can result in a pattern of pulmonary edema with a normal sized heart. Obstructive anomalies proximal to the mitral valve impede venous flow to the left atrium and result in pulmonary edema. Total anomalous pulmonary venous return with obstruction, pulmonary vein atresia or stenosis, and cortriatriatum can all present with a normal sized heart

TABLE 40-4

COMMON ADMIXTURE LESIONS (CARDIOMEGALY AND INCREASED VASCULARITY)

Anomaly	Key Findings
D-transposition of the great arteries	Mild cardiomegaly and increased vascularity with absent pulmonary artery segment
Truncus arteriosus	Cardiomegaly with a superiorly located pulmonary artery segment (Van Praagh type 1 or 4) or absent main pulmonary artery segment (Van Praagh type 2 or 3)
Total anomalous pulmonary venous return	Unobstructed: large main pulmonary artery and prominent vertical vein and superior vena-cava Obstructed: normal sized heart with pulmonary congestion

and pulmonary edema. Although any type of anomalous pulmonary venous return can be obstructed, the infracardiac type of anomalous pulmonary venous return is the most common. Multiple noncardiac causes of noncardiogenic pulmonary edema may have a similar appearance including transient tachypnea of the newborn and lymphangiectasia.

Rings, Slings, and the Anomalous Brachiocephalic Artery

Children with abnormal vascular impressions on the trachea and esophagus present with wheezing or feeding problems. The aortic arch and trachea positions are identified on the frontal chest radiograph. The presence of a right aortic arch without other stigmata of congenital heart disease suggests the presence of a double aortic arch or right aortic arch with an aberrant left subclavian artery. The trachea is midline within the ring rather than shifted away from the dominant arch. In children with a double aortic arch, the right arch is usually larger and more superior. An incomplete ring may be present in children with an aberrant left subclavian artery.

TABLE 40-5

EXPECTED RADIOGRAPHIC FINDINGS WITH CHD*

Cyanosis?	Heart Size	Location of Aortic Arch	Pulmonary Vascular Markings	Lesion(s) to Consider
No	LVE, LVE	Usually left	Increased	VSD, PDA
No	RVE, RAE	Usually left	Increased	ASD
Yes	RVE, RAE	Usually left	Increased	TAPVR
Yes	Normal size	Mainly left, right 25%	Decreased	TOF
Yes	LVE	Mainly left, right 37%	Increased	Truncus arteriosus

*Given the clinical finding in column 1 and the radiographic findings in columns 2–4, the most likely cardiac lesions to consider are shown in column 5.

CHD = congenital heart defect
LVE = left ventricular enlargement
RVE = right ventricular enlargement
RAE = right atrial enlargement
VSD = ventricular septal defect
PDA = patent ductus arteriosus
ASD = atrial septal defect
TAPVR = total anomalous pulmonary venous return
TOF = tetralogy of Fallot

TABLE 40-6
CLASSIC FINDINGS OF CHD ON THE CHEST PLAIN FILM

Finding	Cause	Explanation
Egg on a string	TGA	Direct rather than side by side position of great arteries causing superior mediastinal narrowing
Snowman	TAPVR—supracardiac	Dilated vertical vein and superior vena cava creating a rounded, enlarged superior mediastinum
Boot shaped heart	TOF	Absence of MPA segment and elevation of cardiac apex

CHD   = congenital heart defect
TGA   = transposition of the great arteries
TAPVR = total anomalous pulmonary venous return
TOF   = tetralogy of Fallot

The pulmonary sling or anomalous left pulmonary artery makes an impression on the right side of the trachea just above the carina. A separate impression on the trachea by the aortic arch will be identified more superiorly. On the lateral radiograph, a round density at the level of the carina between the trachea and esophagus is identified which corresponds to the aberrant left pulmonary artery. Malacia of the trachea and right bronchus may result in right lung atelectasis or hyperinflation from air trapping. In young children, the brachiocephalic artery originates to the left of the midline and makes an impression on the anterior edge of the trachea as it courses to the right. During development the aortic arch lengthens and the brachiocephalic artery origin eventually rotates to the right of the trachea. The impression of the trachea is seen on lateral radiographs and can cause wheezing if severe.

SUMMARY

The interpretation of the plain film of the chest by the radiologist is very similar to the history and physical examination by a clinician. There is a history (demographics, reason for the test/visit), followed by a directed radiological examination as outlined in Table 40-1. From these, a differential diagnosis is rendered, which is influenced by the history given. Tables 40-2 through 40-4 outline differential diagnoses for common left-to-right shunt lesions, right-to-left shunt lesions, and admixture lesions. It should be noted that all septal defects or shunts are a form of admixture, with the direction of the shunt and degree of desaturation dependent on loading conditions. In converse, findings on the plain film may lead to certain diagnoses as outlined in Table 40-5. Classic radiographic findings are listed in Table 40-6. These "classic" findings are frequently not necessarily "common" findings.

Suggested Readings

Cleveland RH: A radiologic update on medical diseases of the newborn chest. *Pediatr Radiol* 25:631–637, 1995.

Crowley JJ, Oh KS, Newman B, Ledesma-Medina J: Telltale signs of congenital heart disease. *Radiol Clin North Am* 31:573–582, 1993.

Fayad LM, Boxt LM: Chest film diagnosis of congenital heart disease. *Semin Roentgenol* 34:228–248, 1999.

Harris MA, Valmorida JN: Neonates with congenital heart disease: an overview. *Neonatal Netw* 19:37–41, 2000.

Harris MA, Valmorida JN: Neonates with congenital heart disease, part II: congenital cardiac defects with increased pulmonary blood flow. *Neonatal Netw* 15:61–65, 1996.

Markowitz RI, Fellows KE: The effects of congenital heart disease on the lungs. *Semin Roentgenol* 33:126–135, 1998.

Strife JL, Sze RW: Radiographic evaluation of the neonate with congenital heart disease. *Radiol Clin North Am* 37:1093–1107, 1999.

41

NUCLEAR IMAGING

S. Bruce Greenberg

INTRODUCTION

All cardiovascular nuclear medicine studies rely on the intravenous injection of a radiopharmaceutical. Photons or gamma rays are released during radionuclide decay while in the cardiovascular blood pool or myocardium. A detector external to the patient records the photon energy allowing for the creation of images. Except for positron emission tomography (PET), the detector is a gamma scintillation camera that consists of a lead grid, iodine crystals, photomultiplier tubes, pulse height analyzer, cathode ray tube, and control console. Different types of lead grids allow for increased spatial resolution (small grid holes) or temporal resolution (large grid holes). Single photon emission tomography (SPECT) is performed by rotating the gamma camera detector around a central axis. The acquired data can then be displayed in a tomographic format similar to computed tomography or magnetic resonance imaging. Typically, SPECT will be performed in multiple orthogonal planes. Technetium-99m and thallium-201 are the two most commonly used radionuclides for cardiac imaging.

Data analysis allows for determination of cardiac function, myocardial viability, and shunt size calculation in children with either congenital heart disease or acquired heart disease. The acquired images do not have the resolution of echocardiography, computed tomography or magnetic resonance imaging but the computer acquisition allows for quantitative analysis not possible by echocardiography.

BLOOD-POOL STUDIES

First-pass or gated blood-pool scintigraphy can perform radionuclide angiography for evaluation of cardiac function. Both techniques have low radiation exposure and require no geometric assumptions. The first-pass technique requires tracking a radiopharmaceutical bolus in the vascular system. A tight bolus of a technetium-99m radiopharmaceutical is injected into a peripheral vein. The vein is then flushed with saline. Pertechnetate is the most commonly used agent, but any technetium radiopharmaceutical except macroaggregated albumin (MAA) can be used. MAA embolizes in lung capillaries is used for lung scans. The technetium bolus is tracked as it passes through the systemic venous system, right heart, pulmonary circulation, left heart, and aorta by a gamma camera. Overlapping structures are temporally resolved by rapid data acquisition. A multicrystal camera with a high-sensitivity, low-resolution collimator is ideal for data collection.

The right and left ventricles are identified and the lumen of each ventricle outlined by a region of interest. The maximum activity within the region corresponds to end-diastole and the minimum activity to end-systole. The ejection fraction for each ventricle is then determined by the formula: ejection fraction = [(counts in diastole – counts in systole)/counts in diastole] × 100. The technique is good for both ventricles.

The first-pass technique can also be used to quantify left-to-right shunts. A normal time-activity curve in the lungs will show a rapid rise and fall in activity before a second rise following recirculation. In left-to-right shunts, rapid recirculation associated with the shunt will result in a shoulder of activity following the initial peak when decreasing activity is expected. The size of the shoulder is compared to the expected shape of the time-activity curve by gamma variate analysis to quantify the shunt size.

The short data acquisition time associated with first-pass technique is an advantage for patients who cannot remain still for the more prolonged periods required to perform multigated blood-pool imaging or magnetic resonance imaging. The technique also does not require gating and can be performed on patients with irregular heartbeats.

The technique requires a good bolus for temporal resolution of different anatomic structures. First-pass technique requires good vascular access and is compromised by a poor bolus or inadequate cardiac function. Wall motion can only be identified in one view.

Gated blood-pool scintigraphy requires a radionuclide to remain in the blood-pool. Blood treated with stannous pyrophosphate binds technetium-99m pertechnetate to red blood cell membranes and hemoglobin. The tagged red blood cells remain in circulation and gated images of the heart are obtained in multiple projections. A large number of counts are collected allowing for better resolution than the first-pass technique.

Wall motion abnormalities, such as dyskinesia and akinesia, are evaluated using cine-loops in multiple projections. Ejection fractions are determined by outlining the ventricle lumens as regions of interest and applying the formula for ejection fraction noted above. Unlike the first-pass technique that uses temporal resolution to separate different heart chambers, all of the cardiac chambers have continuous activity during the examination. Acquiring data in a left anterior oblique projection separates the ventricles. Incomplete separation of the left atrium and left ventricle will result in a slight underestimation of left ventricle ejection fraction. The right ventricle is poorly separated from the right atrium using gated blood-pool imaging. Time-activity curves can be generated either by first-pass or gated blood-pool scintigraphy, allowing for evaluation of diastolic filling and systolic ejection abnormalities.

Blood-pool studies are useful for detecting and quantifying abnormal cardiac function associated with congenital heart disease such as primary cardiomyopathies or congenital heart disease. An increased use has been to identify early cardiomyopathy associated with the use of chemotherapy in the treatment of cancer. Cardiac aneurysms are detected by abnormal wall motion.

MYOCARDIAL STUDIES

Thallium is a potassium analog that crosses cell membranes by active transport. Thallium-201 is extracted rapidly by myocardium and then undergoes redistribution as washout and continued extraction occurs. Thallium-201 chloride is injected following exercise. Typically, exercise is performed on a bicycle or treadmill and should represent near maximal stress. Stress images of the heart are obtained as soon as possible following the thallium injection since redistribution will begin almost immediately. Imaging should be performed using SPECT in three orthogonal planes. Three or four hours later, a booster dose of thallium-201 chloride is injected and rest images are performed. The two sets of images are displayed in rows so that direct comparison of stress and rest images can be performed. The left ventricle walls should have homogeneous thickness and uptake except for normal thinning of the apex, inferior surface of the heart, and membranous portion of the ventricular septum. The distribution pattern for stress and rest images is the same.

Abnormalities should be identified on at least two views. A reversible defect is an area of decreased activity on stress imaging that is normal on rest imaging. Ischemic myocardium is characterized by reversible defects. A fixed defect will have decreased activity on both rest and stress images. Fixed defects are characteristic of scar following infarction but can also be seen in hibernating myocardium. Hibernating myocardium is chronically ischemic but viable tissue that is poorly perfused and has poor contraction. Hibernating myocardium can be distinguished from scar on 24-h delayed images. The poorly functioning but viable myocardium will exhibit uptake on delayed imaging.

Technetium-99m sestamibi with its improved imaging characteristics and reduced radiation dose has largely replaced thallium-201 for myocardial imaging. Sestamibi binds to the mitochondrial cytoplasm of the myocardium, but is also taken up by other organs, most notably the liver. Activity in the liver can interfere with image interpretation, but will clear following a fatty meal.

The lack of myocardial redistribution requires separate injections for rest and stress imaging. Rest and stress imaging can be performed on two different days, but a 1-day protocol can also be performed. For the 1-day protocol, rest imaging is performed with a smaller dose. Rest imaging is performed 1 h after an intravenous injection. Exercise is performed following rest imaging and a second, larger dose is administered. A fatty meal following the second injection will remove activity from the liver that might interfere with imaging. The stress images are obtained at least 1 h following the second injection. Technetium sestamibi images are interpreted in the same manner as thallium studies, but no 24-h delay images are performed to detect hibernating myocardium since sestamibi does not redistribute.

Myocardial studies are performed in children to identify infarctions associated with congenital heart abnormalities such as anomalous origin of the left coronary artery or acquired infarctions associated with Kawasaki's disease. Postoperative myocardial abnormalities can also be detected.

LUNG PERFUSION

Lung perfusion scanning is used to determine relative flow to the lungs. MAA is tagged to technetium-99m prior to intravenous administration in a peripheral vein. The radiopharmaceutical flows centrally to the heart and embolizes in the capillary system of the lungs. The emboli do not obstruct enough capillaries to cause clinical symptoms of pulmonary emboli. A gamma camera is then used to image the lungs in multiple views. Technetium-99m MAA that bypasses the lungs through a right-to-left shunt will embolize in the brain, kidneys, and other visceral organs. Postoperative anatomy can also limit the usefulness of lung perfusion scans. A child with bilateral Glenn procedures will require separate right and left upper extremity injections to view both lungs. Fontan procedures can also cause apparent asymmetric distribution of the radiopharmaceutical in the lungs since returning venous flow is not adequately mixed before distribution to the lungs. Systemic to pulmonary shunts such as Blalock-Taussig or central shunts will appear as defects in the perfusion scan since this blood flow will contain none of the technetium-99m MAA particles from a venous injection.

Perfusion scanning is useful in children with congenital heart disease to identify branch pulmonary artery occlusion or determine the significance of branch pulmonary artery stenosis. An occluded branch pulmonary artery will show flow only to the contralateral lung. Branch pulmonary artery stenosis is commonly detected by echocardiography, magnetic resonance imaging, or angiography. The relative flow to each lung determined by the lung perfusion scan quantifies the significance of the stenosis. The study can be repeated to determine the degree of improvement following surgery, angioplasty, or stent placement.

POSITRON EMISSION TOMOGRAPHY

Positron emission tomography scanning is different than thallium and technetium sestamibi scanning discussed above and has had limited availability to the present. PET uses specialized radionuclides that produce positrons that are annihilated by electrons. Two 511-keV photons are produced that travel in opposite directions. A specialized detector isolates the location of the annihilation by coincident detection of the photons. The very short radiopharmaceutical half-lives require an on-site cyclotron. PET radiopharmaceuticals include perfusion and metabolism agents.

Suggested Readings

Greenberg SB, Sandhu SK: Ventricular function, *Radiol Clin North Am* 37: 341–359, 1999.

Gelfand MJ, Hannon DW: Nuclear studies of the heart and great vessels, in: Miller JH, Gelfand MJ (eds): *Pediatric Nuclear Imaging.* Philadelphia, PA, WB Saunders, 1994, pp. 83–101, Chap. 5.

Mettler FA, Guiberteau MJ: *Cardiovascular System, Essentials of Nuclear Medicine Imaging*, 4th ed. Philadelphia, PA, WB Saunders, 1998, pp. 129–190, Chap. 8.

Treves ST, Hurvitz G, Kurux A, Strauss HW: Heart, in: Treves ST (ed): *Pediatric Nuclear Medicine.* New York, NY, Springer-Verlag, 1985, pp. 245–287, Chap. 16.

Treves ST, Newberger J, Hurwitz R: Radionuclide angiocardiography in children, *J Am Coll Cardiol* 5:120S–127S, 1985.

42

MAGNETIC RESONANCE IMAGING

S. Bruce Greenberg

Magnetic resonance studies provide both morphologic and functional evaluation of congenital heart disease. The physics of magnetic resonance imaging is beyond the scope of this chapter, but the reader is referred to one of several good reviews of the subject. The core of the magnetic resonance scanner is a powerful, static magnetic field that partially polarizes or magnetizes the child within it. The magnetic field is always on unlike x-ray or ultrasound equipment. A combination of radio frequency pulses and small magnetic fields are used to disturb the large static magnetic field. Following these disturbances, body tissues begin to recover magnetization. Coils record the recovery as electronic signals that can be converted to images. The amount of signal detected is dependent on the intrinsic properties of the tissue and regional heterogeneity. Images with excellent contrast resolution are created because of different tissue recovery rates following the disturbance in the static magnetic field.

Special problems concerning cardiovascular imaging include cardiorespiratory motion and blood flow. The heart moves continuously unlike the brain, spine, or musculoskeletal system. The chest also has periodic movement with respiration. Conventional imaging sequences have unacceptable motion artifacts that are overcome primarily by cardiac gating. Gating allows for images to be built up over multiple heartbeats by collecting signal only during the same period of the cardiac cycle. Multiple images can be built at different phases of the cardiac cycle either in the same location to create a cine loop or at different locations to increase coverage. Respiratory motion can be approached in three different ways. First, it can be ignored. In long sequences, the respiratory motion is averaged out to minimize its importance. In some sequences, respiratory gating can be added to cardiac gating which has the disadvantage of lengthening scan time since data will not be collected during respiration. Finally, shorter sequences can be performed during breath holding. The latter strategy is becoming the dominant approach for adult cardiac magnetic resonance imaging examinations, but cannot be employed in sedated children or children with limited cognitive skills.

Blood flow creates unique problems and opportunities for magnetic resonance imaging. Other tissues in the chest are static, but blood flows through a slice during the time that the scan is performed. Blood that leaves the imaging slice after the radio pulse and before coils record signal will not contribute data to the final image. The blood volume will appear black in contrast to the surrounding vessel wall and other mediastinal structures. This is the basis of "black-blood" imaging techniques. Blood has intrinsic signal and if a sequence is selected that samples the blood for signal prior to its leaving the selected slice, the blood will be white. This is the basis of "white-blood" techniques.

CARDIOVASCULAR MAGNETIC RESONANCE TECHNIQUES

Magnetic resonance imaging can be divided into "black-blood" and "white-blood" techniques. In "black-blood" imaging, blood flow is seen as a black image, and static tissue appears white in the final image. Cardiac gated black-blood images are "spin echo" sequences that form the backbone of magnetic resonance anatomic imaging. Flowing blood leaves the imaged slice during the spin echo sequence so that no signal remains in vessels or cardiac chamber lumens. Spin echo sequences include a refocusing pulse that removes some artifacts associated with local field heterogeneity. Nonflowing blood as occurs in diastole or sluggish flow that can occur in veins will have a signal that can occasionally be confused for thrombus or tumor. Flowing blood receiving a radio pulse in one slice might contribute signal to a vessel lumen in an adjacent slice if that blood bolus moves into another slice as signal is recorded in the second slice. The use of additional pulse sequences in the double inversion recovery fast spin echo sequence produces a black-blood image regardless of the blood velocity by nulling signal from blood outside of the slice being imaged; however, this technique requires breath holding.

In "white-blood" imaging, blood flow is shown in white, and static tissue appears black in the motion sequence. This is similar to contrast angiography. White-blood images are produced by

gradient echo sequences that are fast enough to record signal in blood within a slice. Gradient echo sequences lack the refocusing pulse present in spin echo imaging that corrects for local field heterogeneity. These images will be more susceptible to artifacts caused by metal clips or wires in the chest. The images are not as sharp as spin echo images, but are acquired much faster. The rapid acquisition of images allows for multiple images within the cardiac cycle to be generated. A cine loop can be produced for both qualitative and quantitative analysis of cardiac and vascular motion. Functional measurements of ventricular volumes and the calculation of stroke volume, ejection fraction, and cardiac index use white-blood images. Both breath-hold and nonbreath-hold techniques are available. The breath-hold techniques yield sharper, whiter images of the blood. A specialized form of gradient imaging is sensitive to velocity and flow direction. This sequence is used to map blood velocity and flow patterns and can be used to calculate stroke volume, cardiac index, and regurgitant fraction.

Gadolinium enhanced magnetic resonance angiography requires a peripheral venous contrast injection. The available gadolinium chelates are much less toxic than radiographic contrast. X-ray contrast creates an image by impeding the passage of x-rays through a vessel or chamber filled with the contrast. Gadolinium is a paramagnetic element that affects the surrounding blood to increase the signal from the blood rather than directly creating a signal. The imaging sequence is very rapid capturing images of the selected arteries or veins during the circulation of the contrast agent through the vessels. The sequence must be well timed so that contrast is near its peak at the time of imaging. Various bolus-tracking systems allow for triggering the scan to begin when the bolus reaches a predetermined location. The same contrast bolus can be used to temporally resolve different vessels. A predominantly pulmonary artery acquisition can be followed by an aorta phase on the same contrast bolus. The source images are reconstructed into three-dimensional or multiplanar views. The technique requires breath holding but can be performed with respiration in sedated infants and small children without breath holding because of the small excursions of the chest with respiration. Respiration can be interrupted briefly in intubated patients during the examination.

The imaging results are approximately equal to conventional angiography, but some important advantages of gadolinium enhanced magnetic resonance angiography are important. Unlike conventional angiography, no invasive arterial catheterization or nephrotoxic contrast is used. The high dose of ionizing radiation associated with cine angiography is avoided. The gadolinium enhanced magnetic resonance angiography source images can be reconstructed in any imaging plane eliminating the need for multiple contrast injections and radiation exposures. Disadvantages include the need for breath holding in older children and artifacts caused by metal clips and coils in the chest.

PREPARATION FOR CARDIOVASCULAR MAGNETIC RESONANCE EXAMINATION

The cardiovascular magnetic resonance imaging examination requires preparation prior to scanning. Preparation can be subdivided into three categories: indications and clinical queries, contraindications, and sedation/patient cooperation issues. The indications for cardiovascular magnetic resonance imaging continue to grow but should be identified as they apply to each child. Five general indications for cardiovascular magnetic resonance imaging examinations in children are listed in Table 42-1. Children with congenital heart disease frequently will have more than one of the listed indications. For example, a child with suspected arrythmogenic right ventricular dysplasia requires both an anatomic study to evaluate the right ventricle wall for thinning or fat infiltration and a functional study to detect abnormal regional cardiac wall motion. A preoperative examination of the child with D-transposition of the great arteries should include anatomic images of anomalies and associated shunts, but requires quantitative measurement of the left ventricle mass for surgical planning.

A hierarchy of queries should be established during the scheduling of the magnetic resonance imaging examination. The selection of sequences

and the order in which they are performed is dependent on answering the most important questions first. For example, a prior history of tetralogy of Fallot is not sufficient. Is the study being scheduled because of inadequate visualization of the peripheral pulmonary arteries by echocardiography? Is a search for collateral vessels important? Is quantification of the right ventricle function or pulmonary regurgitation more important? The study should be tailored to answer the most important questions first since patient cooperation or sedation time is limited. Additional areas of investigation may be important but not intuitive from the primary diagnosis. A patient for follow-up of a coarctation may also need the aortic valve and proximal ascending aorta evaluated if an associated bicuspid aortic valve is present. Clear communication between referring clinician and cardiac radiologist during the scheduling process is essential.

Echocardiography is the primary imaging and functional analysis tool for congenital heart disease in children. Portability, universal availability, and high quality imaging of intracardiac anatomy with Doppler qualitative and quantitative function make echocardiography the backbone of cardiac imaging. Echocardiography has a limited field of view with bone and air creating blind spots. Intrathoracic fibrosis following surgery degrades ultrasound images. The right side of the heart is best visualized in infants and young children since the thymus can provide an extended window. The right ventricle and peripheral pulmonary arteries may not be well identified in older children and adults with congenital heart disease. Although cardiovascular magnetic resonance imaging can identify and measure virtually any lesion identified by echocardiography, this is unnecessary. The magnetic resonance imaging examination is used to complement echocardiography by adding important information that remains opaque to echocardiography. Occasionally, magnetic resonance imaging can help clarify confusing complex intracardiac lesions such as a criss-cross heart. In addition to the right ventricle and peripheral pulmonary arteries, magnetic resonance imaging is clearly superior to echocardiography for evaluation of cardiac tumors and the pulmonary veins. Primary coarctation is

TABLE 42-1

INDICATIONS FOR CARDIOVASCULAR MAGNETIC RESONANCE IMAGING

General Indication	Common Examples
Primary congenital heart disease: anatomy not adequately visualized by echocardiography	1. Right side of the heart 2. Branch pulmonary arteries and pulmonary veins 3. Coarctation of the aorta 4. Vascular rings and anomalous left pulmonary artery (pulmonary sling) 5. Complex intracardiac anatomy 6. Identification and quantification of collaterals 7. Cardiac tumors 8. Aneurysms (e.g., Marfan's syndrome)
Primary congenital heart disease: anatomy not adequately visualized by angiography	1. Lack of vascular access 2. Overlapping structures 3. Arteries distal to an atresia 4. Complex anatomy such as anomalous right pulmonary artery (cannot visualize the anomalous right pulmonary artery and main pulmonary artery simultaneously)
Postoperative imaging	1. Follow-up shunt for patency or stenosis 2. Follow-up palliative procedures (e.g., Fontan procedure, Norwood procedure) 3. Follow-up complete repairs
Postoperative vascular function (flow or velocity mapping examinations)	1. Recoarctation 2. Pulmonary artery and branch pulmonary artery stenosis 3. Shunts (e.g., Central, Blalock-Tausig, Glenn) 4. Fontan's procedure
Cardiac function	1. Qualitative evaluation of cardiac wall motion 2. Quantitative measurement of right and left ventricle volumes to determine ejection fractions, stroke volumes, cardiac index, shunts, and regurgitant fractions 3. Measure left ventricle mass

adequately evaluated by echocardiography alone in most children, but magnetic resonance imaging can be performed to better evaluate the size of the coarctation and to quantify collateral blood flow. Vascular rings, anomalous origin of the left pulmonary artery and the anomalous brachiocephalic artery are best evaluated by magnetic resonance imaging since both the vascular anomalies and the airway compression are identified. Children with aneurysms such as

Marfan disease are initially followed by repeat echocardiograms. In time, the child size and body habitus limit the field of view and magnetic resonance angiography should be used.

Cine angiography uses by far the highest dose of ionizing radiation for any medical diagnostic test. Recent studies have shown that even the lower radiation doses from computed tomography are associated with a small increased risk of cancer over the lifetimes of children. The risk is greatest in infants and small children. Cine angiography remains important to clinical care of children with congenital heart disease, but should be limited to gathering information not available by noninvasive technology. Echocardiography and magnetic resonance imaging can adequately visualize relevant anatomy in most children. Catheterization is most important for collecting physiologic data (i.e., pressure measurements) and interventional procedures. Peripheral access may be "used up" by repeated catheterizations making later interventional procedures problematic. Intracardiac anatomy is best evaluated by echocardiography with supplemental evaluation by magnetic resonance imaging. Magnetic resonance imaging of the great arteries and pulmonary veins is comparable to angiography for most patients. Small peripheral vessels and some collateral arteries are better identified by angiography. Overlapping structures, arteries distal to an obstruction and complex anatomy may be better identified by magnetic resonance imaging.

Both cardiac-specific and noncardiac contraindications for cardiovascular magnetic resonance imaging exist. A child must be clinically stable to undergo a magnetic resonance imaging study. Ferrous cerebral aneurysm clips and metal fragments in the eye are contraindications for magnetic resonance imaging. Cardiac-specific contraindications include an erratic heartbeat that precludes cardiac gating, the presence of an active pacemaker, pacemaker wires, an implanted automated defibrillator or the presence of certain older era prosthetic valves. Nitroglycerin and nicoderm patches can cause skin burns if present on patients in the scanner. Baclofen pumps and nerve stimulators are not contraindications but will need to be reset following the examination.

Patient cooperation is a prerequisite for magnetic resonance imaging. Older children and adults with congenital heart disease frequently require no sedation and can perform breath holding adequately to complete the examinations. Some patients who suffer from claustrophobia can be managed with a mild oral sedative such as diazepam. Infants and young children usually require deeper sedation or general anesthesia. Oral, rectal, and intravenous sedation can all be used effectively for sedation. The ideal level of sedation for magnetic resonance imaging in infants and small children is for the child to be asleep, while retaining all autonomic reflexes. This approaches deep sedation and requires a high level of monitoring, frequently by a pediatric anesthesiologist or experienced pediatric radiologist. Continuous monitoring with pulse-oximetry and a cardiac monitor by a dedicated observer from the time of administration of sedation to arousal is required. Sedation can be safely performed in children with cyanotic heart disease. In children, the sedation risk is predominantly from respiratory failure than cardiac disease. Nonbreath-holding techniques are used in sedated children and those unable to coordinate breath holding with imaging. Breath-holding techniques can sometimes be applied to sedated children with small respiratory excursions.

INTERPRETATION OF CARDIOVASCULAR MAGNETIC RESONANCE IMAGING

A systematic approach to reading cardiovascular magnetic resonance imaging is mandatory. A typical study can include hundreds of individual images, additional postprocessed three-dimensional images, and displays of functional data. A tailored examination might not include all of the following elements, but the approach is the same for interpreting all cardiovascular magnetic resonance imaging examinations. Quality control is first and foremost. The images must be evaluated to insure that an adequate examination has been performed. All of the relevant anatomy must be included and the image quality must be adequate for interpretation. Functional elements of the study require that proper gating is present and no aliasing occurs.

An anatomic checklist should be performed to ensure that no structures are inadvertently ignored. Systemic and pulmonary veins should be traced to the atria. The number of veins, size, and concordance are noted. The atria are identified and evaluated for situs, size, atrioventricular concordance, and septal defects. The ventricles are evaluated for situs, size and wall thickness, ventriculo-arterial concordance, and septal defects. The great arteries are examined for conal defects, size, and position. The trachea and bronchi are examined along with the great arteries to evaluate for situs and compression associated with vascular abnormalities. The aortic arch and major branches are identified and studied for arch position, branching pattern, and size. The main pulmonary artery and branch pulmonary arteries are examined for branching pattern and size. Finally, anatomic images should be examined for associated noncardiovascular disease that may incidentally be noted on the images.

Functional imaging should include viewing cine loops of the heart and great vessels to evaluate cardiac wall motion and identify turbulent flow in the heart or great vessels. Turbulent flow will appear as black within the white-blood images and is associated with stenosis and regurgitation. Qualitative evaluation of cine loops allows for segmental wall motion abnormality detection. There are no blind areas as may occur with echocardiography, limited projections as occurs in angiography, or poor spatial resolution as in nuclear cardiology. Muscle tagging further refines the technique, which increases the conspicuity of smaller abnormalities.

Magnetic resonance imaging is the gold standard for quantifying cardiac function. Quantification of ventricular volumes does not require any geometric assumptions. Both the right and left ventricle volumes are measured from the same images. End-diastolic and end-systolic images from the short axis of the heart cine loops are identified and the ventricle lumens and left ventricle muscle outlined. The slice volumes are summated to determine the end-diastolic and end-systolic volumes. The stroke volume and ejection fractions can be calculated for each ventricle. The cardiac index and left ventricle mass index are calculated to normalize for child size. Shunts or regurgitant fractions can also be calculated by comparing differences in the ventricle stroke volumes.

Flow analysis allows measurement of velocity and flow across a cross-section. This can be used to measure flow across a cardiac valve or within an artery or vein. The measurement of velocity is useful for determining the significance of stenosis. The modified Bernolli equation is applied to the measured velocity acquired from flow analysis just as it is used in echocardiography. Flow patterns can be used to quantify stroke volume and measure cardiac index. Unlike the technique of measuring ventricular volumes noted above, ventricular volumes and ejection fractions are not obtained; however, the measurements are not compromised by atrioventricular valve regurgitation. Flow analysis can also be used to quantify shunts.

THE CLINICAL UTILITY

Cardiovascular magnetic resonance imaging is both a compliment to the older, more established modalities echocardiography and angiography and an independent modality that provides unique information. The former use has been discussed above. Postoperative imaging is especially difficult for echocardiography because of poor windows associated with fibrosis. The large field of view allows for better visualization of systemic-pulmonary shunts such as Blalock-Tausig and central shunts and veno-pulmonary shunts such as Glenn's shunts and Fontan's procedures. The anatomic imaging is complemented by flow analysis with significant stenosis causing increased velocities. Recoarctation of the aorta is easily detected by magnetic resonance imaging and elevated velocities with associated collateral flow can be quantified by flow analysis. Pulmonary artery abnormalities in children with a history of shunts are common and best identified by magnetic resonance imaging. This is especially true for children following complete repair of tetralogy of Fallot.

Qualitative evaluation of cine cardiac cine loops can detect regional wall motion defects that occur in arrhythmogenic right ventricular dysplasia or cardiac infarction. Paradoxic septal motion in patients with pulmonary hypertension and right ventricle hypertrophy is also identified. Ventricular function is quantified in patients with cardiomyopathy. Pulmonary regurgitation following repair of tetralogy of Fallot is common which leads to eventual ventricular dysfunction. Right ventricular enlargement, ventricular function, and pulmonary regurgitant fraction are all quantified and help determine the timing for further surgical repair of the right ventricle outflow tract. Other causes of right or left ventricular dysfunction are less common but approached in the same manner. In children without regurgitant valves, shunts can be calculated by comparing the ventricular volumes.

The left ventricle muscle mass is an important indicator for success in performing an arterial switch procedure in children with D-transposition of the great arteries. The left ventricle mass index is calculated from measurements of the left ventricle.

Suggested Readings

Beerbaum P, Korperich H, Barth P, et al: Noninvasive quantification of left-to-right shunt in pediatric patients: phase-contrast cine magnetic resonance imaging compared with invasive oximetry. *Circulation* 103:2476–2482, 2001.

Chung T: Assessment of cardiovascular anatomy in patients with congenital heart disease by magnetic resonance imaging. *Pediatr Cardiol* 21:18–26, 2000.

de Roos A and Roest AA. Evaluation of congenital heart disease by magnetic resonance imaging. *Eur Radiol* 10:2–6, 2000.

Didier D, Ratib O, Beghetti M, et al: Morphologic and functional evaluation of congenital heart disease by magnetic resonance imaging. *J Magn Reson Imaging* 10:639–655, 1999.

Fogel MA: Assessment of cardiac function by magnetic resonance imaging. *Pediatr Cardiol* 21:59–69, 2000.

Geva T, Greil GF, Marshall AC, et al: Gadolinium-enhanced 3-dimensional magnetic resonance angiography of pulmonary blood supply in patients with complex pulmonary stenosis of atresia: comparison with x-ray angiography. *Circulation* 106:473–478, 2002.

Greenberg SB, Sandhu SK: Ventricular function. *Radiol Clin North Am* 37:341–359, 1999.

Greenberg SB: Assessment of cardiac function. Magnetic resonance and computed tomography. *J Thorac Imaging* 15:243–251, 2000.

Heibling WA, de Roos A: Clinical applications of cardiac magnetic resonance imaging after repair of tetralogy of Fallot. *Pediatr Cardiol* 21:70–79, 2000.

Mulkern RV, Chung T: From signal to image: magnetic resonance imaging physics for cardiac magnetic resonance imaging. *Pediatr Cardiol* 21:5–17, 2000.

Nienaber CA, Rehders TC, Fratz S: Detection and assessment of congenital heart disease with magnetic resonance techniques. *J Cardiovasc Magn Reson* 1:169–184, 1999.

Powell AJ, Geva T: Blood flow measurement by magnetic resonance imaging in congenital heart disease. *Pediatr Cardiol* 21:47–58, 2000.

Rebergen SA, de Roos A: Congenital heart disease. Evaluation of anatomy and function my MRI. *Herz* 25:365–383, 2000.

Roest AA, Helbing WA, van der Wall EE, de Roos A: Postoperative evaluation of congenital heart disease by magnetic resonance imaging. *J Magn Reson Imaging* 10:656–666, 1999.

Tonkin IL: Imaging of pediatric congenital heart disease. *J Thorac Imaging* 15:274–279, 2000.

43

ECHOCARDIOGRAPHY

Peter Koenig

Echocardiography has revolutionized cardiology, especially pediatric cardiology with its ability to noninvasively diagnose a multitude of congenital and acquired cardiac abnormalities in the pediatric age group.

PRINCIPLE OF CARDIAC ULTRASOUND

Echocardiography or ultrasound of the heart is based on basic physical principles of sound. Two major principles result in echolocation and assessment of direction and velocity of blood flow. Echolocation is based on the fact that the speed of sound is approximately constant in living tissue. Since tissue is mainly composed of water, the speed of sound in tissue (regardless of type: fat, muscle, connective tissue) is close to the speed of sound in water. The mathematical equation Velocity = distance/time becomes constant = distance/time, or distance = constant × time, or time = distance × 1/constant.

Thus, time and distance are related to one another by a constant. If either variable is known, the other can be solved through this mathematical equation. In practice, an ultrasound machine sends a pulse of sound out, and measures the time for the sound to return after reflection off a surface or interface. Once time is measured, distance can be calculated. This is done by dividing the total time in half (to account for sound travelling twice the distance, to and from the reflector) and multiplying by a constant.

In a manner similar to sonar in submarines, an object is then located at a certain distance from the sound transmitter (the probe in the case of ultrasound). The reflected object can then be graphically displayed in a fashion which represents distance (or time) to reflect from the origin (or time 0). Multiple reflections after one sound impulse can be displayed on the same line. If amplitudes of the reflected sound are displayed, this is known as A-mode or amplitude mode (Figure 43-1A). If dots of different size and brightness are displayed, this is known as B-mode or brightness mode (Figure 43-1B). If multiple sound pulses are sent and received, motion of the reflectors towards and away from the sound source can be recorded on a strip chart recorder showing multiple B-mode displays in a continuous fashion. This is known as M-mode or motion mode (Figure 43-1C). An M-mode

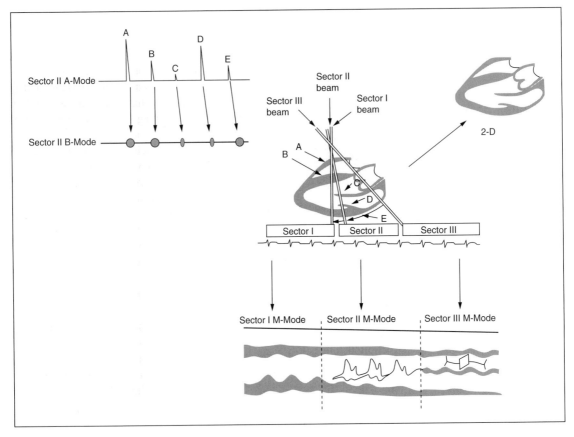

Parts **A–D** show corresponding ultrasound images using different modalities. In **A**, the A-mode corresponding to walls labeled **a** through **e** are shown. The corresponding B-mode pictures of these same walls are shown in **B**. In these cases, the x axis corresponds to distance (from the origin of the ultrasound) and the y axis corresponds to amplitude or brightness of returning sound. Part **C** shows an M-mode diagram for three sectors (B-mode over the time as shown with the corresponding ECG). In this case, the x axis corresponds to time, and the y axis corresponds to distance or depth from the origin of the ultrasound beam. In this example, the image changes as the ultrasound beam passes through varying portions of the heart as shown in A. A 2D image is shown in **D**, which corresponds to simultaneous B-mode imaging and scanning in a motion from sectors III to I as shown. In this case, the x and y axes represent distance in 2-d space.

recording can be made by varying the angle in which the sound penetrates the body. When this is performed from the chest while with an angle toward the heart, varying M-mode recordings can be made showing different parts of the heart (Figure 43-1C). If multiple pulses of sound are sent into the chest, while rapidly changing the angle of sound penetration (scanning), the result is the same as moving the ultrasound probe manually while

obtaining an M-mode picture, except that the image will be two-dimensional as it captures multiple M-mode planes in an instant. The net result is a 2D picture known as a 2D echocardiogram (Figure 43-1D). If multiple 2D echocardiographic images are obtained in succession, motion of the heart can be recorded. This is known as real-time 2D imaging or motion 2D imaging. If the sound pulse can be sent into the chest (M-mode), rapidly angled or "swept" back and forth (2D imaging) and either rotated, "swept" in another plane, or combined with other simultaneous 2D images, a 3D reconstruction of the heart can be made. If this is performed rapidly enough to allow multiple 3D images to be obtained in succession, a real-time 3D image or "4D" image can be obtained. Thus, simple reflection of sound can demonstrate a linear, 2D or 3D image in either a single frame, or over time to show motion. The method in which this principle is applied to show a picture of the heart will be discussed in sections to follow.

In addition to simply showing the distance of a reflector (echolocation), information can be obtained from analyzing the change in the transmitted and reflected sound. It is known that the sound reflected off a moving object will change in frequency depending on the direction and speed of the moving object. Similar to train whistles, ambulance sirens, and other moving objects, the relationship of sound to velocity was discovered by Christian Doppler in 1843.

The mathematical relationship is as follows:

$$f_d = [2(f_o)(V)(\cos \theta)]/c$$

or, with rearrangement,

$$V = (cf_d)/(2 f_o)(\cos \theta).$$

where c (the velocity of sound in human tissue) and f_o (the transmitted frequency) are constants and f_d (the observed frequency shift) can be measured. V is the velocity of the moving sound reflector (blood), and theta is the intercept angle between the transmitted sound and the moving reflector (blood).

Using this relationship, the ultrasound machine analyzes changes in the frequency of the transmitted and reflected sound and automatically applies the Doppler equation to calculate the velocity of the moving reflector. The angle of incidence is important. An object moving perpendicular to the direction of sound will have a calculated velocity of zero. The Doppler shift over time can automatically be displayed as velocity versus time as shown in Figure 43-2. Alternatively, the Doppler shift can be converted into a velocity scale, which is then converted to a color corresponding to the velocity of blood flow. This color Doppler map is usually displayed directly over the 2D image. By convention, red denotes flow towards the probe, and a blue color

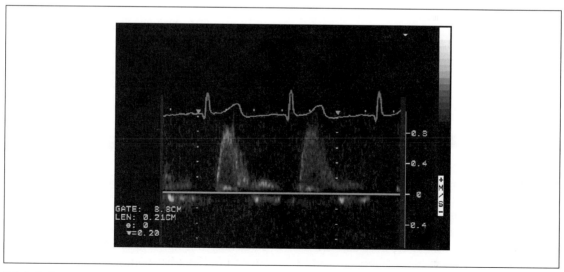

FIGURE 43-2

This figure demonstrates a pulse Doppler recording. The x axis represents time (with the tracing shown varying with paper speed), and the y axis represents velocity of blood flow in meters per second.

is assigned to flow away from the probe. Varying shades of red and blue correspond to the respective velocities.

Using the Doppler principle to determine the velocity of blood flow also allows for the calculation of pressure gradients using the Bernoulli equation. This applies the principle of conservation of mass. The total amount (volume) of blood flow prior to an area of narrowing must be equal to the amount (volume) of blood flowing through the area. If the diameter is narrowed, the only manner in which there can be conservation of mass is if the flow velocity increases. The complete equation takes into account items such as viscosity, but can be simplified, for practical purposes, to become:

$$\text{Pressure gradient} = 4\left(V_f^2 - V_i^2\right)$$

where V_f is the final velocity and V_i is the initial velocity. If the velocities are in m/s, the pressure gradient will be in mmHg using this equation. If the initial velocity is low in comparison to the final velocity, then it can also be dropped from the equation for further simplification to:

$$\text{Pressure gradient} = 4V_f^2$$

Thus, if the velocity of blood can be determined prior to a stenotic valve, and again distal to the stenotic valve, the gradient across the valve can be calculated. Using Doppler echocardiography and the principle of echolocation, blood flow velocity in a particular area (sample volume) can be measured allowing the above equation to be used.

HOW TO PERFORM

An echocardiogram is performed using the above principles, with an appropriate ultrasound machine for the object (patient) being assessed. The machines used in pediatrics are similar to those used for adults, but some of the transducers used as well as machine settings have to be adjusted for the size of the patient. Using a number of standard imaging planes, and "rules" of imaging (so not to confuse right and left, superior and inferior, and so forth), images are produced in order to directly reflect the anatomy. In pediatrics, the standard

imaging views are obtained and displayed in an anatomic fashion to allow easier interpretation. A segmental method of imaging is also used in pediatrics to help understand the relation of different chambers and vessels to one another as these are more frequently abnormal than in the typical adult patient. Because the machine settings and methods of imaging are so different from adults, it is best that the pediatric echocardiogram is performed by a technician trained to perform stuies in the pediatric age group (infants, children, and adolescents). In adults with congenital heart disease, many technical aspects (machine settings and transducers used) of the echocardiogram are similar to those without congenital heart disease, but the segmental techniques of assessing the anatomy are similar to those used in infants and children. Thus, echocardiography of complex congenital heart disease in adults may also best be performed by a technician trained in pediatric cardiac ultrasonography.

The net result of imaging in a programmed, segmental fashion is the acquisition of multiple 2D images with which the interpreter can construct a mental 3D image of the heart. In addition to the 2D images, color Doppler information is obtained which may disclose defects not seen with 2D imaging such as a patent ductus arteriosus (PDA), atrial septal defect (ASD), ventricular septal defect (VSD).

In addition to anatomic information, 2D imaging with Doppler interrogation can also provide a large amount of functional or indirect hemodynamic information. Chamber size and thickness can be compared to normals to assess for hypertrophy or dilation. Anatomic derangements can therefore be quantified by their affects on the heart. Gradients across valves, and pressure differences between chambers can also be indirectly measured using the Bernoulli equation. Heart function can be assessed by measuring shortening or ejection fraction. The latter is difference between the end-diastolic volume and end-systolic volume (also known as stroke volume) divided by the end-diastolic volume. Shortening fraction is conceptually the same as ejection fraction; however, it is the fractional difference of the diameters rather than volumes. The ejection fraction is related to preload, afterload, and contractility, each of which can be inferred if the other parameters are known. Further quantitative

TABLE 43-1

INDICATIONS FOR NEONATAL ECHOCARDIOGRAPHY

Indication	*Indication Class*
1. Cyanosis, respiratory distress, congestive heart failure, or abnormal arterial pulses	I
2. Chromosomal abnormality or major extracardiac abnormality associated with a high incidence of coexisting cardiac abnormality	I
3. Lack of expected improvement in cardiopulmonary status in a premature infant with a clinical diagnosis of pulmonary disease	I
4. Systemic maternal disease associated with neonatal comorbidity	I
5. Loud or abnormal murmur or other abnormal cardiac finding in an infant	I
6. Presence of a syndrome associated with cardiovascular disease and dominant inheritance or multiple affected family members	I
7. Presence of a syndrome associated with heart disease, with or without abnormal cardiac findings, for which an urgent management decision is needed	I
8. Cardiomegaly on chest radiograph	I
9. Dextrocardia, abnormal pulmonary, or visceral situs by clinical, electrocardiographic, or radiographic examination	I
10. Arrhythmias or other abnormalities on standard ECG suggesting structural heart disease or peripartum myocardial injury	I
11. Clinical suspicion of residual or recurrent abnormality, poor ventricular function, pulmonary artery hypertension, thrombus, sepsis, or pericardial effusion after cardiovascular surgical therapy for congenital heart disease	I
12. Nonimmunologic fetal hydrops	I
13. Follow-up assessment of a neonate with patent ductus arteriosus who has undergone medical or surgical intervention	I
14. Short, soft murmur at the lower left sternal border in the neonate	IIa
15. Failure to thrive in the absence of definite abnormal clinical findings	IIa
16. Presence of a syndrome associated with a high incidence of congenital heart disease for which there are no abnormal cardiac findings and no urgency of management decisions	IIIb
17. History of nonsustained fetal ectopy in the absence of postpartum arrhythmias	III

Source: Melvin D et al., *ACC/AHA Guidelines*, 1997.

TABLE 43-2

INDICATIONS FOR ECHOCARDIOGRAPHY IN THE INFANT, CHILD, AND ADOLESCENT

Indication	Indication Class
1. Atypical or pathological murmur or other abnormal cardiac finding in an infant or older child	I
2. Cardiomegaly on chest radiograph	I
3. Dextrocardia, abnormal pulmonary or visceral situs on clinical, electrocardiographic, or radiographic examination	I
4. Patients with a known cardiac defect to assess timing of medical or surgical therapy	I
5. Immediate preoperative evaluation for cardiac surgery of a patient with a known cardiac defect to guide cardiac surgical management and inform the patient and family of risks of surgery	I
6. Patient with known cardiac lesion and change in physical finding	I
7. Postoperative congenital or acquired heart disease with clinical suspicion of residual or recurrent abnormality, poor ventricular function, pulmonary artery hypertension, thrombus, sepsis, or pericardial effusion	I
8. Presence of a syndrome associated with cardiovascular disease and dominant inheritance or multiple affected family members	I
9. Patients with a family history of genetically transmitted myocardial disease, with or without abnormal cardiac finding	I
10. Phenotypic findings of Marfan's syndrome or Ehlers-Danlos syndrome	I
11. Baseline and follow-up examinations of patients with neuromuscular disorders having known myocardial involvement	I
12. Presence of a syndrome associated with a high incidence of congenital heart disease when there are no abnormal cardiac findings	I
13. Exercise-induced precordial chest pain or syncope	I
14. "Atypical," "nonvasodepressor" syncope without other cause	
15. Failure to thrive in the absence of definite abnormal clinical findings	IIb
16. In a child or adolescent, an asymptomatic heart murmur identified by an experienced observer as functional or an insignificant cardiovascular abnormality	III
17. In an otherwise asymptomatic child or adolescent, chest pain identified by an experienced observer as musculoskeletal in origin	III

Source: Melvin D et al., *ACC/AHA Guidelines*, 1997.

measurements can be made using echocardiography, but are beyond the scope of this textbook.

INTERPRETATION OF ECHOCARDIOGRAMS

Final interpretation of the echocardiogram is based on the anatomic findings and quantitation above. Comparison to known anatomy and normal measurements is needed for this final interpretation. Because of the vastly different types of anatomic abnormalities encountered in pediatrics, as well as the wide range of normal because of the wide size and age range in pediatrics, interpretation is best performed by individuals trained in pediatric cardiology.

INDICATIONS FOR ECHOCARDIOGRAPHY IN PEDIATRIC PATIENTS WITH ARRHYTHMIAS/CONDUCTION DISTURBANCES

Indication	Indication Class
1. Arrhythmia in the presence of an abnormal cardiac finding	I
2. Arrhythmia in a patient with a family history of a genetically transmitted cardiac lesion associated with arrhythmia, such as tuberous sclerosis or hypertrophic cardiomyopathy	I
3. Complete atrioventricular block or advanced second-degree atrioventricular block	I
4. Complete or high-degree secondary atrioventricular block	I
5. Arrhythmia requiring treatment	I
6. Ventricular arrhythmia in a patient referred for evaluation for competitive sports	IIa
7. Evidence of preexcitation on ECG	IIa
8. Preexitation on ECG in the absence of abnormal cardiac findings	IIb
9. Recurring arrhythmia not requiring treatment in the presence of normal findings on examination	IIb
10. Sinus arrhythmia or isolated extrasystoles in a child with otherwise normal cardiac findings and no family history of a genetically transmitted abnormality associated with arrhythmia	III

Source: Melvin D et al., *ACC/AHA Guidelines,* 1997.

THE CLINICAL UTILITY OF ECHOCARDIOGRAPHY

Echocardiography has revolutionized the diagnosis and management of congenital heart disease. Prior to echocardiography, anatomic diagnosis was inferred by the history, physical examination, and simple tests such as an ECG and plain film of the chest. The correlation of these with the true diagnosis was not optimal. Cardiac catheterization was performed for more accurate diagnosis, though lacks in its ability to demonstrate important anatomic features (e.g., chordal attachments in an AV canal defect) and is invasive. In the current era, most intracardiac abnormalities are diagnosed noninvasively via echocardiography and patients frequently undergo cardiac surgery or other interventions without further diagnostic studies. Echocardiography, however, is limited in its ability to image the coronary arteries, pulmonary arteries, and the aorta distal to the arch. Hemodynamic measurements may also not be accurately measured (e.g., pulmonary vascular resistance). Therefore, echocardiography remains complementary to other diagnostic studies available to cardiologists. In addition, certain conditions (obesity, hyperaeration of the lungs as seen with lung diseases, postoperative scarring, and so forth) may inhibit good echocardiographic imaging and require modifications such as the transesophageal approach to visualize certain structures.

Specific indications and uses of echocardiography are outlined throughout this book. In general, it is indicated anytime a noninvasive measure of cardiac size, thickness and overall function are needed, there is suspicion of an acquired or congenital anatomic abnormality, or follow-up such an abnormality, or if there is a desire to obtain hemodynamic information as described above. The American Heart Association and American College

TABLE 43-4

INDICATIONS FOR ECHOCARDIOGRAPHY IN PEDIATRIC ACQUIRED CARDIOVASCULAR DISEASE

Indication	Indication Class
1. Baseline studies and reevaluation as clinically indicated on all pediatric patients with suspected or documented Kawasaki's disease, myoperi-carditis, HIV, or rheumatic fever	I
2. Postcardiac or cardiopulmonary transplant to monitor for signs of acute or chronic rejection, thrombus, and cardiac growth	I
3. Baseline and reevaluation examinations of patients receiving cardiotoxic therapeutic agents	I
4. Patients with clinical evidence of myocardial disease	I
5. Patients with severe renal disease and an abnormal cardiac finding	I
6. Donors undergoing evaluation for cardiac transplantation	I
7. An acutely ill child with suspected bacterial sepsis or rickettsial disease	IIa
8. Follow-up examinations after acute rheumatic fever in patients with normal cardiac findings	IIb
9. A single late follow-up study after acute pericarditis with no evidence of recurrence or chronic pericardial disease	IIb
10. Long-term follow-up studies in patients with Kawasaki's disease who have no coronary abnormalities during the acute phase of the disease process	III

Source: Melvin D et al., *ACC/AHA Guidelines,* 1997.

of Cardiology published guidelines for the indications of echocardiography. Class I indications are for those conditions for which there is evidence and/or general agreement that a given procedure or treatment is useful and effective. Class II indications are for those conditions for which there is conflicting evidence and/or a divergence of opinion about the usefulness/efficacy of a procedure or treatment. These are subdivided into IIa, where the weight of evidence or opinion is in favor of usefulness and or efficacy, and IIb, where the usefulness/efficacy is less well established by evidence or opinion. Class III indications are for those conditions for which there is evidence and/or general agreement that the procedure or treatment is not useful or effective and in some cases may be harmful.

The above indications for the use of echocardiography are guidelines, as efficacy of a diagnostic test is more difficult to rate in terms of value than a therapeutic procedure; however, these guidelines provide just that. They take into account the technical aspects of the study, and the impact on patient management. Using these guidelines, the usefulness of echocardiography in the evaluation of common pediatric complaints is shown in Tables 43-1–43-8. These guidelines are taken directly from the AHA/ACC statement.

TABLE 43-5

INDICATIONS FOR ECHOCARDIOGRAPHY IN PEDIATRIC CARDIOPULMONARY DISEASE

Indication	Indication Class
1. Any patient with clinical findings of pulmonary artery hypertension	I
2. Baseline study of patients with cystic fibrosis and no findings of cor pulmonale	IIa

Source: Melvin D et al., *ACC/AHA Guidelines,* 1997.

TABLE 43-6

INDICATIONS FOR ECHOCARDIOGRAPHY IN PEDIATRIC THROMBOEMBOLIC DISEASE STATES

Indication	Indication Class
1. Thromboembolic event in an infant, child, or adolescent	I
2. Finding or family history of tuberous sclerosis	I
3. Appearance of sepsis, cyanosis, or right-heart failure in a patient with a long-standing indwelling catheter	I
4. Systemic embolization or acute-onset hypertension in a patient with right-to-left-shunting and an indwelling catheter	I
5. Superior vena caval syndrome in the presence of central venous catheter	I
6. Patient with indwelling catheter and fever but without evidence of pulmonary or systemic embolization	IIb
7. Routine surveillance of asymptomatic patients with indwelling catheter	III

Source: Melvin D et al., ACC/AHA Guidelines, 1997.

TABLE 43-7

INDICATIONS FOR TRANSESOPHAGEAL ECHOCARDIOGRAPHY IN PEDIATRIC PATIENTS

Indication	Indication Class
1. Any patient with congenital or acquired heart disease needing echocardiography when significant diagnostic information cannot be obtained by TTE	I
2. Monitoring and guidance during cardiothoracic procedures when there is a risk for residual shunting, valvular insufficiency, obstruction, or myocardial dysfunction	I
3. Guidance of catheter/device placement during interventional catheterization/radiofrequency ablation in patients with congenital heart disease	I
4. Study of patients with intra-atrial baffle in whom the potential for thrombus is of concern because of elevated central venous pressures, atrial chamber dilation, increasing cyanosis, or the appearance of arrhythmia	I
5. Patients with long-term placement of intravascular devices in whom thrombus or vegetation is suspected	I
6. Patients with a prosthetic valve in whom thrombus or vegetation is suspected	I
7. Any patient with suspected endocarditis and inadequate transthoracic acoustic window	I
8. Performing TEE in a patient who has not previously had careful study by TTE	III
9. Patients with structural esophageal abnormality	III

Source: Melvin D et al., ACC/AHA Guidelines, 1997.

TABLE 43-8

INDICATIONS FOR FETAL ECHOCARDIOGRAPHY

Indication	Indication Class
1. Abnormal-appearing heart on general fetal ultrasound examination	I
2. Fetal tachycardia, bradycardia, or persistent irregular rhythm on clinical or screening ultrasound examination	I
3. Maternal/family risk factors for cardiovascular disease, such as a parent sibling, or first-degree relative with congenital heart disease	I
4. Maternal diabetes	I
5. Maternal systemic lupus erythematosus	I
6. Teratogen exposure during a vulnerable period	I
7. Other fetal system abnormalities (including chromosomal)	I
8. Performance of transplacental therapy or presence of a history of significant but intermittent arrhythmia Reevaluation examinations are required in these conditions	I
9. Fetal distress or dysfunction of unclear etiology	IIa
10. Previous history of multiple fetal losses	IIb
11. Multiple gestation	IIb
12. Low-risk pregnancies with normal anatomic findings on ultrasound examination	III
13. Occasional premature contractions without sustained tachycardia or signs of dysfunction or distress	III
14. Presence of a noncardiovascular system abnormality when evaluation of the cardiovascular system will not alter either management decisions or fetal outcome	III

Source: Melvin D et al., ACC/AHA Guidelines, 1997.

Suggested Readings

Feigenbaum H: *Echocardiography*, Philadelphia, PA, Lea & Febiger, 1994.

Melvin D, Cheitlin MD, Alpert IS, Armstrong WF, et al; ACC/AHA Guidelines for the Clinical Application of Echocardiography: A Report of the American College of Cardiology/American Heart Association Task Force on Practice Guidelines (Committee on Clinical Application of Echocardiography) Developed in Collaboration With the American Society of Echocardiography, *Circulation* 95:1686–1744, 1997.

Meyer RA: *Pediatric Echocardiography*, Philadelphia, PA, Lea & Febiger, 1977.

Snider AR, Serwer GA: *Echocardiography in Pediatric Heart Disease*, Chicago, IL, Year Book, 1997.

Silverman NH: *Pediatric Echocardiography*, Baltimore, MD, Williams & Wilkins, 1993.

44

CARDIAC CATHETERIZATION

Ziyad M. Hijazi and Hitendra T. Patel

INTRODUCTION

Cardiac catheterization is the term used to describe the technique of transcutaneous insertion of a catheter into the venous or arterial system and advancement into the heart. This is followed by further catheter advancement and/or manipulation to obtain cardiac, pulmonary and systemic hemodynamic and angiographic data. Although the primary care physician or health care provider may never enter a catheterization laboratory, it is felt that knowledge of what is involved in the procedure will help the health care provider counsel patients and be a more knowledgeable participant in the health care system. Details of the equipment used and the manner in which the procedure is performed is outlined, as well as the hemodynamic calculations, indications, and risks of the procedure.

The pediatric cardiac catheterization laboratory is a relatively large investment by the hospital in both human resources, and capital expenditure. Basic requirements (personnel and equipment) of the pediatric cardiac catheterization laboratory are listed in Tables 44-1 and 44-2. It is useful for the

primary care provider to have some knowledge of this to better understand the reason for the costs to his/her patient.

PERFORMANCE OF PEDIATRIC CARDIAC CATHETERIZATION

Indications

It is important to understand the need for the cardiac catheterization. A full discussion regarding the cardiac diagnosis and the information to be obtained from the catheterization should occur with the primary cardiologist, noninvasive and invasive cardiologist and cardiothoracic surgeon. This will ensure optimal information is obtained and, if appropriate, potential interventional strategies discussed and implemented. In general, the indications are diagnostic, therapeutic, or both. The diagnostic indications are to provide anatomic or hemodynamic information that is unable to be obtained, or unreliable with noninvasive studies. The therapeutic indications are to palliate or cure an underlying cardiac abnormality.

TABLE 44-1

**PERSONNEL INVOLVED IN
PEDIATRIC CARDIAC CATHETERIZATION**

1. Pediatric cardiologist—interventional
2. Pediatric cardiologist—echocardiographer
3. Pediatric cardiothoracic surgeon
4. Pediatric cardiac anesthesiologist
5. Cardiovascular technologist
6. Echocardiography technologist
7. Nurse for patient monitoring and conscious sedation
8. Radiation physicist

Precatheterization

Once the decision for catheterization is made, a number of preprocedural details need to be defined. The generalities may be similar with minor differences from institution to institution. After the date, time, and place (or where to arrive) of the procedure is confirmed with the family, there are usually instructions as to when to stop eating and drinking and which medications should be given and which held. In rare circumstances (unlike years prior), the patient may be admitted the day prior to the procedure.

TABLE 44-2

**EQUIPMENT NEEDED IN
PEDIATRIC CARDIAC CATHETERIZATION**

1. Large procedure room
2. Biplane x ray machine for fluoroscopy and cine or digital angiography
3. Coagulation time analyzer
4. Oxygen saturation and blood gas analyzer
5. Metabolic cart to measure oxygen consumption
6. Electronic data storage
7. Inventory (and storage room) of catheters, and so forth, to accommodate complex and varied cardiac anatomy and range of patient sizes

It is important for the primary care physician to know the above details as there may be intervening illnesses or important details, which may need to be communicated to the cardiologist. Some of these illnesses (e.g., suspicion of respiratory syncytial virus [RSV] bronchiolitis) may require the procedure to be postponed and is best done prior to the day of the procedure.

The day of the procedure, a preprocedure history and physical examination is performed by the cardiologist. A final discussion with patient and family is usually held immediately prior to the procedure. This is the best opportunity for the cardiologist performing the procedure (invasive or interventional cardiologist) to meet the family and discuss the diagnosis and the need for cardiac catheterization and potential intervention. It is the role of the cardiologist to explain what cardiac catheterization entails and discuss any possible interventions. This is also the time for a full and open discussion outlining the risks and benefits prior to obtaining consent. It should allow for the patient and parents to ask questions. The latter has become more important over the last 5 years with the availability of investigational devices in many centers. The patient and the family should be oriented to the catheterization laboratory and the medical team who will be performing the procedure.

The Catheterization Procedure

Premedication and whether the procedure will be performed using conscious sedation or general anesthesia will vary amongst institutions. The premedication drug combination should have anxiolytic, sedative, and amnesic properties.

After premedication, parents are usually allowed to accompany the patient until asleep. Appropriate vascular access is obtained and the patient is positioned, restrained, draped, and kept warm. Skin preparation routine for any sterile procedure is performed. Blood for type and screen, and other laboratory studies are sent. If an intervention is planned then crossed matched blood should be available. This can be done as soon as access is achieved at the start of the case.

Throughout the procedure, continuous monitoring of heart rate, rhythm (ECG strip), respiratory rate, blood pressure, chest movement, oxygen saturation, and temperature (usually a rectal probe) is performed. During long procedures, with hemodynamic instability or with renal disease, a Foley's catheter may be placed to monitor urine output. Blood glucose is measured at regular intervals, which is especially important in small infants. A defibrillator unit as well as emergency resuscitation equipment and medications should always be available.

The site of intravenous access depends on the anatomy and presence of occluded vessels secondary to previous indwelling catheters or cardiac catheterization. Possible venous sites include the umbilical, femoral, subclavian, internal jugular, or brachial vein. In addition, with multiple venous occlusions, direct transhepatic puncture into the inferior vena cava is possible. Arterial sites include the umbilical, femoral, brachial, or carotid arteries. A vascular cut-down used to be a standard access procedure decades ago; however, the Seldinger technique has made this practice virtually unnecessary. A surgical cut-down may still be required if percutaneous access is not obtained or in small infants where large sheaths are required for the planned intervention. The best example is a carotid cut-down for balloon dilation of critical aortic stenosis. This allows for vessel repair and preservation. As material technology improves, most interventional procedures, even in low weight infants is possible using the percutaneous transcatheter approach without the need for a surgical cut-down for intravascular access.

Most diagnostic catheter studies can be performed using 3 or 4 French sheaths in the newborn and up to 6–7 French in adults. Larger sheaths and catheters are needed for interventional treatment. As technology improves, therapeutic catheters and the required sheath sizes continue to decrease making some interventions feasible even in premature infants, with probable fetal interventions in the future as well.

After vascular access is obtained, complete hemodynamic data are obtained. A routine method is usually applied to all cardiac catheterizations to reduce the possibility of omissions. Complete data are obtained regardless of other available noninvasive data that may be false.

Oxygen saturation and pressure data are compared to normal. From this data the pulmonary, effective pulmonary and systemic blood flow is calculated using the Fick equation. Using these relative blood flows, the left-to-right and right-to-left shunts can be calculated. In the absence of shunts, cardiac output can also be measured using thermodilution catheters. Using the pulmonary and systemic flow data with the pressure data the pulmonary vascular resistance (PVR) and systemic vascular resistance (SVR) can be calculated. If medical intervention is given to alter resistance (usually PVR), then the hemodynamic data are repeated for each intervention and the subsequent changes in flow and resistance are calculated.

DIAGRAMS OF NORMAL VALUES

Typical normal hemodynamic values are given in Figure 44-1. Oxygen saturations are given in percent. Mean (*m*) pressures are given in mmHg. Systolic over end-diastolic (in the ventricles) or

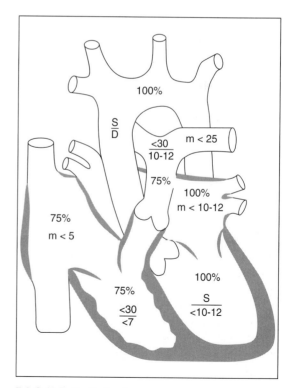

FIGURE 44-1

NORMAL PRESSURES AND O₂ SATURATIONS IN THE DIFFERENT CARDIAC CHAMBERS diastolic (in the arteries) and ranges of these are given in mmHg. Of note is that the systolic pressure in the left ventricle (S) is nearly equal to the systolic pressure in the aorta (S), with a range of 50 in neonates to 120 in adolescents similar to blood pressure ranges given in Chapter 10. The diastolic pressure (D) in the aorta is approximately 50% of the systolic pressure. A lower diastolic pressure may be seen with diastolic runoff or vasodilation. These values are also given in Chapter 10. The typical end-diastolic pressure in the left ventricle is 5–8 mmHg.

Hemodynamic Calculations

Fick equation: Oxygen consumption (either measured or derived from a table based on age, sex, and heart rate) = flow rate × oxygen extraction.

Oxygen consumption, VO_2 mL/min = blood flow (Q) L/min × oxygen extraction or $Q = VO_2/$ oxygen extraction.

Oxygen Content of Blood

This is dependent on the amount of oxygen bound to hemoglobin plus the amount of oxygen dissolved in the blood.

Maximum O_2 carrying capacity of Hb = 1.36 × Hb g/L = mL of O_2/L. If a patient has a Hb of 10 g/dL then the O_2 capacity of the blood is 1.36 × [10 g/dL × 10] = 136 mL/L. This is at 100% saturation. Thus, if a blood sample with a Hb of 10 g/dL has a saturation of 70% then the amount of oxygen it is carrying is 136 × 0.7 = 95.2 mL/L.

Dissolved O_2(mL/L) = 0.03/partial pressure of O_2 (mmHg). Therefore, if the measured PO_2 of a blood sample is 100 mmHg then the dissolved oxygen would be 0.03 × 100 = 3 mL/L.

Pulmonary Blood Flow

Pulmonary blood flow (Q_p) is the oxygen consumption divided by the oxygen extraction in the lungs. Oxygen extraction in the lungs is equal to the oxygen gain in the blood. Thus, $Q_p = VO_2/$ Pulmonary venous blood oxygen content − pulmonary arterial blood oxygen content.

Systemic blood flow (Q_s) is the oxygen consumption divided by the oxygen extraction in the

blood. Thus, $Q_s = VO_2/$systemic arterial blood oxygen content − systemic venous oxygen content.

Pulmonary venous (PV) O_2 content = [O_2 sat of PV blood/100 × O_2 capacity] + [dissolved O_2 = PO_2 × 0.03].

Pulmonary arterial (PA) O_2 content = [O_2 sat of PA blood/100 × O_2 capacity] + [dissolved O_2 = PO_2 × 0.03].

Systemic arterial O_2 content, aortic or arterial (Ao) [O_2 sat of Ao blood/100 × O_2 capacity] + [dissolved O_2 = PO_2 × 0.03].

Systemic venous blood content (mixed venous, MV) [O_2 sat of MV blood/100 × O_2 capacity] + [dissolved O_2 = PO_2 × 0.03].

Note that normally the dissolved oxygen quantity is small and is ignored during calculation; however, when studies are performed in 100% oxygen the dissolved oxygen becomes significant and should be used during the calculations.

The mixed venous blood sample is a theoretical sample that exists when all systemic venous return of the body has mixed. It is representative of the desaturated blood prior to coursing through the lungs and oxygenation. When no intracardiac shunts exist, the pulmonary artery blood is a good representation of mixed venous blood. If there are intracardiac shunts, then by convention the superior vena cava blood sample is used as a representation of the mixed venous sample.

Another concept to understand in the calculation of possible shunts is the concept of effective pulmonary blood flow (Q_{ep}). This is the amount of desaturated blood that is actually oxygenated as the pulmonary blood courses through the lungs. This concept is important when an intracardiac right-to-left and left-to-right shunts coexist. Normally, Q_p equals Q_{ep}, which equals Q_s. If there is a left-to-right shunt, the pulmonary blood flow may actually be a combination of systemic venous return plus the amount of the shunt flow. Thus, Q_p equals the Q_{ep} plus the shunt flow. Effective pulmonary blood flow is calculated using the SVC saturation as pulmonary artery or mixed venous saturation. Note if there is anomalous PV return to the SVC then a high SVC sample should be obtained. Q_{ep} is always calculated using a mixed venous sample that is from a site prior to any shunt.

Shunts

Pure L to R = $Q_p - Q_s$ (or Q_{ep})
Pure R to L = $Q_s - Q_p$ (or Q_{ep})

If there are bidirectional shunts in the same patient, i.e., R to L and L to R, then it is important to use Q_{ep} since the shunting alters the PA and arterial saturation.

L to R = $Q_p - Q_{ep}$
R to L = $Q_s - Q_{ep}$

Resistance

Ohms law states that the pressure difference between two points is directly related to the flow rate and resistance. In electrical flow: volts (potential difference) = current (flow rate of electrons) × resistance.

In the human circulation two resistance beds exist, the pulmonary and systemic. As long as no stenoses exist and the right and left pulmonary artery pressures are the same, then the mean PA pressure (mPAP) – mean LA pressure (mLAP) represents the pressure drop across the pulmonary vascular bed. Hence PVR or R_p = mPAP – mLAP/Q_p.

These calculations are usually indexed to body surface area in the pediatric population. If stenoses exist and the mean right and left PA pressures are different, resistance can still be calculated if the total pulmonary blood flow and the distribution of flow to the right and left lungs is known. This flow is in parallel and therefore, $1/R$ (pulmonary) = $1/R$ (right lung) + $1/R$ (left lung).

R (right lung) = mRPA pressure – mLAP/PBF × (% flow to right/100)
R (left lung) = mLPA pressure – mLAP/PBF × (% flow to left/100)

Angiography

Contrast agents (usually low ionic agents, visipaque or omnipaque) are injected through the catheter positioned at the area of interest. The amount and speed of injection of contrast is dependent on the size of patient, catheter type and size, the site of injection, the heart rate and blood flow rate. As contrast is injected it mixes with the blood and flows with it. This enables real-time visualization of cardiac function and measurement of filled structures. Real-time acquisition (digital or cine), of the image is obtained. Angiography is used to assess ventricular size and function, atrioventricular and semilunar valve size and function, visualize sites of intra and extracardiac shunts, and to visualize pulmonary and systemic vasculature. Biplane angiography (x ray imaging in two planes at one time) is essential in pediatrics to minimize the contrast load and it allows for angled views to better profile cardiac and extracardiac lesions. Angiography is essential for most interventional procedures to facilitate accurate sizing of structures and proper positioning of balloons, coils, devices, and stents.

Postcatheterization Care

Postcatheterization care is dependent on the type of procedure performed. For most diagnostic catheterizations, patient recovery with strict observation of cardio-respiratory status and hemostasis for 4–6 h is adequate. For complex and long procedures, inpatient observation with telemetry may be indicated. Discharge instructions usually include puncture site care, activity restrictions, and a problem list of what to expect and what side effects to watch for. The site of the catheter may have an occlusive dressing which may be left in place for a number of days. If the dressing becomes dirty or wet, the area can be cleaned with soap and water and a clean dressing can be applied. (If the site becomes erythematous, or develops purulent drainage, the cardiologist needs to be notified.) Showering or sponge bathing is usually allowed at which time the site of the catheter insertion site can be cleaned with soap and water; however, sitting in bath water and swimming is usually prohibited for at least 3 days after the procedure, or until the site is completely healed. This is done to prevent infection. Bruising at the site is normal, and may look larger in the first few days after the catheterization. If the bruised area appears to increase or swelling occurs (possible hematoma), the cardiologist should be notified. Soreness in the leg on the side of catheterization and limping are normal for the first few days. This discomfort can be treated with over-the-counter pain relievers such as acetaminophen. The leg should be checked twice daily by the family to look for swelling, pallor, coolness, or loss of sensation or movement in the leg on the side of the vascular access. Any of these findings should prompt notification of the cardiologist. Fever is another concern. It is normal to have low-grade fever the night of the procedure; however, if the temperature is more than 101.5°F, the cardiologist or primary health care provider should be notified. In terms of activity, resumption of normal activities can occur the day after the procedure with the possible following exceptions: bike riding, swimming, or strenuous exercise. These may be prohibited for a number of days following the procedure along with avoidance of squatting or sitting crossed-legged. Return to school (or work) usually occurs 2 days after the procedure. Prior medications, unless told otherwise, are usually resumed immediately after the catheterization.

Conclusions

After the procedure, the information learned, the outcome of intervention and the future plan is discussed fully with the family and patient (if old enough to understand). Some of the information may be preliminary and plans tentative, with final conclusions following analysis and discussion with the cardiology team. Most institutions have a formal cardiac catheterization conference to review procedures, data, and discuss management. This information should also be provided promptly to the primary care physician.

Complications

The morbidity and mortality associated with cardiac catheterization is dependent on the overall condition of the patient. The pulmonary function, nutritional state, and renal function of the patient all impact on the complication rate. Morbidity in the modern laboratory is about 2–4% with mortality less than 1%.

1. Complication of access site
   Minor: Bruising, hematoma, or loss of arterial pulse, which may require heparin or thrombolysis using streptokinase or tissue plasminogen activator.
   Major: Arterio-venous fistula, or limb compromise (ischemia) requiring surgical embolectomy.
2. *Embolic phenomena.* Air or thrombus may enter the circulation through catheters or the sheaths. Meticulous techniques minimize such a complication. If air is seen in the heart, administration of 100% oxygen to the patient until the air is absorbed is usually sufficient.
3. *Arrhythmias.* Arrhythmias are frequent, though usually transient. They include premature atrial and ventricular beats (both common) as well as atrial tachycardia, AV reentry tachycardia and atrial flutter (less common). Rarely, life-threatening arrhythmias may occur requiring cardioversion or overdrive pacing.
4. *Cardiac perforation.* This can occur during any catheterization, though there is a higher risk with larger, stiffer catheters and wires, intracardiac interventions, and endomyocardial biopsy. Extreme caution is usually exercised during catheter and wire manipulation, especially in the neonatal heart.
5. Intramyocardial injection of contrast may lead also to myocardial injury as well as rhythm disturbances.
6. Infection is rare from the procedure owing to meticulous sterile technique.
7. Allergic reactions can occur owing to the contrast agent or latex. This is relatively rare in occurrence.
8. Excessive blood loss is uncommon in an older infant, though occurs in a small fraction of neonates, especially after an intervention.
9. Complications related to specific interventions are described in the chapter dealing with interventional cardiac catheterization.

Suggested Readings

Allen HD, Gutgesell HP, Clark EB, Driscoll DJ: *Moss and Adams' Heart Disease in Infants, Children and Adolescents Including the Fetus and Young Adult*, 6th ed. Philadelphia, PA, Lippincott Williams & Wilkins, 2001.

Keane JF, Lock JE: Hemodynamic evaluation of congenital heart disease, in: James E Lock, John F Keane, Stanton B Perry (eds): *Diagnostic and Interventional Catheterization in Congenital Heart Disease*, 2nd ed. Kluwer Academic Publishers, 2000, pp. 37–72.

Lock JE: Evaluation and management prior to catheterization, in: James E Lock, John F Keane, Stanton B Perry (eds): *Diagnostic and Interventional Catheterization in Congenital Heart Disease*, 2nd ed. Dordrecht, Holland, Kluwer Academic Publishers, 2000, pp. 1–12.

Waldman JD, Young TS, Pappelbaum SJ, et al: Pediatric cardiac catheterization with same day discharge. *Am J Cardiol* 50:800–803, 1982.

45

THE ELECTROPHYSIOLOGIC STUDY

Frank Zimmerman

INTRODUCTION

Electrophysiologic (EP) studies were initially used to record intracardiac electrical activity and later used in conjunction with surgical treatment for arrhythmias. Currently, EP studies are performed to evaluate supraventricular and ventricular arrhythmias, often in anticipation of RF catheter ablation procedures, or to evaluate cardiac conduction disturbances. An evolving role of EP testing in pediatric patients is its use as a tool for predicting future cardiac arrhythmias, especially in the setting of congenital heart disease. While EP testing is now considered an essential component of the evaluation for many cardiovascular disorders, it is often reserved for use after other preliminary tests such as ECGs or ambulatory monitoring have been performed.

INDICATIONS

Bradycardia/Heart Block

Bradyarrhythmias suspected as the etiology for syncope or near-syncope are often evaluated using serial ECG or ambulatory monitoring. EP testing is reserved for select cases in which there is a strong suspicion for a rhythm disorder, but preliminary testing is normal. There is only a weak correlation between findings at EP testing, and EP testing is no better than noninvasive testing in predicting the development of heart block in patients with conduction abnormalities on resting ECG.

Tachycardia

The most common reason for performing EP studies in children is for the evaluation of tachycardias. Supraventricular tachycardias are the predominate arrhythmia in children. EP testing is performed to assess the mechanism of tachycardia and is usually combined with RF catheter ablation procedures. It is rarely performed to assess the adequacy of medical therapy for supraventricular tachycardia. Ventricular arrhythmias are less common in children but are more likely to be associated with underlying cardiac abnormalities. EP testing is used to determine the mechanism of tachycardia with or without RF ablation or as a predictive tool to assess the risk for future cardiac arrhythmias (see below).

WPW Syndrome

The Wolff-Parkinson-White (WPW) syndrome consists of ventricular preexcitation on the resting ECG associated with episodes of supraventricular tachycardia. While prospective studies in children are not available, it is estimated that the risk for sudden death in this population is approximately 1 per 1000 patient years. The mechanism is rapid antegrade conduction from atrium to ventricle over the accessory connection during atrial fibrillation. Adult studies have shown that EP testing can be used as a tool to assess risk for sudden death in this population. Those with rapid antegrade conduction properties of the accessory connection (preexcited RR interval less than 250 ms during atrial fibrillation or effective refractory period of the accessory connection less than 250 ms) are thought to be at higher risk for sudden death. The role of EP testing in asymptomatic children with WPW syndrome continues to be debated.

Documented Ventricular Tachycardia/Cardiac Arrest

Electrophysiologic testing is usually performed in patients with documented ventricular tachycardia or cardiac arrest to help guide management, assess medical therapy, or in anticipation of RF ablation. It remains common practice to perform such testing even if ICD placement is anticipated.

Congenital Heart Disease/Cardiomyopathy

Electrophysiologic testing is shown to be moderately useful for risk assessment in select patients with congenital heart disease such as tetralogy of Fallot; however, the predictive value is not specific enough to warrant testing in all patients. Decisions for EP testing in this population are made on an individual basis. EP testing is not a specific or predictive tool for risk assessment in patients with idiopathic dilated cardiomyopathy or hypertrophic cardiomyopathy.

PROCEDURE

Patient evaluation prior to the EP procedure begins with a thorough history and physical examination. Documentation of the arrhythmia is sought with ECG or ambulatory monitoring if possible and is important in order to correlate findings of the EP study with the patient's clinical symptoms. Antiarrhythmic medications are usually stopped for five half-lives prior to the procedure so as to not reduce the sensitivity of the test. The EP procedure is similar to a catheterization procedure and may be performed either with conscious sedation or with general anesthesia, depending on the patient's age and the patient's hemodynamic status. While the patient's comfort must be optimized, it is possible that deep anesthesia may decrease the likelihood of inducing a clinically relevant arrhythmia. This is especially true for automatic atrial or ventricular arrhythmias or AV node reentry tachycardia. Infusion of isoproterenol may help overcome the effects of anesthesia but can increase the chance of inducing arrhythmias that are not clinically relevant. The EP study is performed in a catheterization laboratory with specialized personnel and with equipment for intracardiac recording and pacing. The EP catheters used range in size from 2 to 8 French and are placed in the femoral vein or via the internal jugular vein or subclavian vein. An arterial line may also be placed for monitoring purposes. The capability for defibrillation and administration of cardiac medications must be available during the study.

BASELINE INTRACARDIAC MEASUREMENTS

Electrophysiologic catheters are placed in standard positions of the heart depending on the type of study being performed. The standard positions include the right atrium, the AV junction (AV node and His bundle), and the ventricle. A coronary sinus catheter may be placed to obtain recordings from the left side of the heart (mitral valve annulus). Normal values for intracardiac measurements in children are shown in Table 45-1. Intracardiac intervals studied during the procedure include the following:

NORMAL VALUES FOR INTRACARDIAC MEASUREMENTS IN CHILDREN

Corrected SNRT	<275 ms
AH interval	40–100 ms
HV interval	25–50 ms
RV conduction	15–35 ms
Atrial ERP	150–200 ms
AV node ERP	200–350 ms
Ventricular ERP	200–300 ms

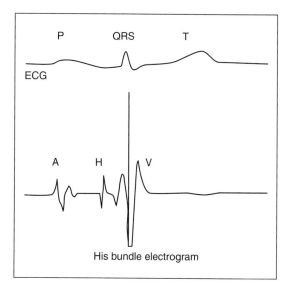

His bundle electrogram

FIGURE 45-1

SURFACE ECG AND INTRACARDIAC

His bundle electrogram. This intracardiac recording is obtained from an EP catheter placed at the AV junction in close proximity to the AV node. A, atrial electrogram; H, His bundle electrogram; V, ventricular electrogram

Intraatrial Conduction

Atrial conduction from high right atrium to low right atrium can be prolonged (slowed) following surgery for congenital heart disease surgery because of scarring or suture lines in the right atrium. Conduction delay or dispersion of conduction in the right atrium can result in the development of atrial arrhythmias.

AV Node Conduction

One of the earliest uses of intracardiac recordings was to study conduction of the AV node (Figure 45-1). This consists of conduction through the AV node proper (AH interval) and through the His-Purkinje system to the ventricles (HV interval). Drugs or medications, increased vagal tone, or diseases of the AV node can affect AV node conduction and prolong the AH interval. A short AH interval may represent the presence of an accessory atriofascicular connection seen in patients with Lown-Ganong-Levine syndrome, or can be seen in normal young patients with high adrenergic tone.

A significantly prolonged HV interval denoting conduction delay in His-Purkinje system is considered an ominous sign for heart block. It can be seen with disease of the His-Purkinje system or postoperatively because of damage of the conduction system. Prolonged HV intervals are also seen in patients with congenitally corrected transposition (l-transposition) of the great arteries in which the conduction system between the AV node and the right and left bundle branch is known to be susceptible to conduction delay or heart block. A short HV interval is indicative of an accessory atrioventricular connection such as that seen in WPW syndrome.

RV Conduction

Right ventricular (RV) conduction is measured from the onset of the surface QRS complex to the local ventricular electrogram at the RV apex. Prolonged RV conduction or right bundle-branch block is commonly seen following ventricular surgery for congenital heart disease. Right bundle-branch block following congenital heart disease surgery is usually considered benign; however, recent evidence suggests that RV conduction delay can be associated with RV enlargement and poor RV mechanics. Significant QRS prolongation owing to RV conduction delay has been suggested as a risk factor for ventricular arrhythmias following surgery for tetralogy of Fallot.

FUNCTIONAL INTRACARDIAC STUDIES

Once baseline recordings are obtained, functional studies are performed using various pacing maneuvers. The normal values for functional studies in children are shown in Table 45-1.

Sinus Node Function

Sinus node function may best be assessed by non-invasive studies such as ECGs or ambulatory monitoring as mentioned; however, assessment during intracardiac EP testing can be performed by several methods. The most common is the sinus node recovery time. This is performed by first pacing the atrium at a fixed rate (above the resting sinus rate heart rate) for 30–60 s. Pacing is then stopped and the time to the next sinus beat to occur is known as the sinus node recovery time. It is usually "corrected" by subtracting the baseline heart rate from the sinus node recovery time. Prolongation of sinus node recovery time suggests sinus node disease that can occur as a result of drugs or medications, or with conditions of increased fibrosis around the sinus node area (as seen following certain surgeries for congenital heart disease).

AV Node Function

AV node function is assessed by the response to paced premature atrial beats. The AV node effective refractory time is defined as the longest atrial premature beat that fails to conduct through the AV node. The refractory time is prolonged with diseases of AV node conduction (either congenital or acquired). This can also occur as a result of drugs such as digoxin, beta-blockers, or calcium-channel blockers or with high vagal tone. An abrupt prolongation or jump in the conduction time through the AV node with progressive premature atrial beats is evidence for the presence of dual AV node pathways. This phenomenon occurs when conduction is blocked in the fast AV node pathway but continues through the slow AV node pathway. Dual AV node pathways are the substrate for AV node reentry tachycardia but have been reported to occur in up to 30% of normal children

during EP testing. Rapid pacing at fixed rates may also be performed to assess the fastest rate at which 1:1 AV conduction occurs.

Effective Refractory Periods

Atrial, ventricular, and His-Purkinje effective refractory times can also be assessed using premature paced atrial beats. Prolonged effective refractory times can occur with diseases of the atrium, ventricle, and His-Purkinje system. Increased vagal tone may affect atrial or ventricular refractoriness but does not affect the His-Purkinje system. Assessment of the effective refractory period of an accessory pathway is used to assess risk for sudden death in patients with WPW syndrome. Adult studies have shown that risk factors include an accessory pathway effective refractory period of less than or equal to 250 ms (Figure 45-2).

EVALUATION OF SUPRAVENTRICULAR TACHYCARDIA (SVT)

Once conduction intervals and functional studies are obtained, atrial extra-stimulus testing is performed to assess for inducibility of arrhythmias. This is performed with the placement of premature atrial beats or with rapid atrial pacing. If pacing in the baseline state fails to induce the arrhythmia, the protocol may be repeated during infusion of isoproterenol. Important features of induced tachycardias include the method of induction and termination, atrial and ventricular relationships during SVT, and the pattern of atrial activation. This information is used to determine the mechanism of tachycardia (reentry, triggered, or automatic) and to target the source of the arrhythmia for RF ablation.

EVALUATION OF VENTRICULAR TACHYCARDIA (VT)

Intracardiac EP testing may be performed to assess patients with documented or suspected

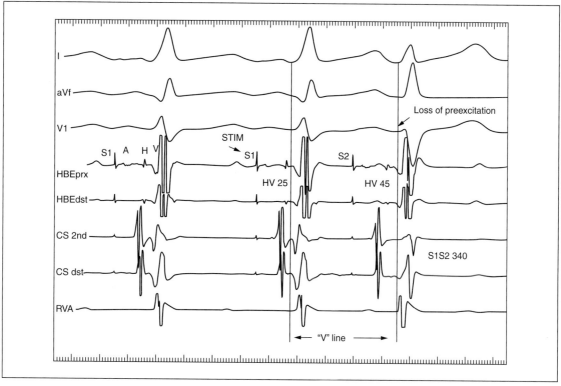

FIGURE 45-2

ACCESSORY PATHWAY EFFECTIVE REFRACTORY PERIOD

This intracardiac recording consists of three surface ECG leads (I, aVF, V1), two His bundle recordings (HBEprx, HBEdst), two coronary sinus recordings (CS 2nd, CS dst) and one right ventricular recording (RVA). The first two beats seen are atrial paced (S1, Stim) beats with ventricular preexcitation. The third beat is a premature atrial paced beat (cycle length 340 ms) and results in loss of preexcitation because of conduction block in the accessory pathway (effective refractory period). The HV interval is short during preexcited beats (25 ms) and becomes normal (45 ms) with loss of preexcitation.

ventricular tachycardia. The mechanism of wide complex tachycardias can be evaluated using the methods described for evaluation of SVT. An important use of EP testing is to assess for inducibility of VT in select patients to stratify risk for future cardiac arrhythmias. Pacing is usually performed in the RV apex as well as in the RV outflow tract and ventricular premature beats are usually limited from one to three beats in order to prevent induction of nonspecific ventricular arrhythmias. EP testing can also be performed to assess the efficacy of antiarrhythmic medical therapy.

RISKS

The safety of EP studies has improved by limiting the aggressiveness of pacing protocols to avoid induction of nonspecific atrial or ventricular arrhythmias. The incidence of cardiac perforation, thrombosis, or development of inadvertent heart block owing to catheter manipulation is less than 1%.

TRANSESOPHAGEAL PACING STUDIES

Atrial pacing studies can also be performed using a transesophageal approach. Atrial recordings from the esophagus were first described in adults and were used to assess supraventricular arrhythmias. Advantages of the esophageal recording and pacing study (TEP) over intracardiac EP studies include less invasive nature of the procedure and avoidance of risk for bleeding or thrombosis (Figure 45-3).

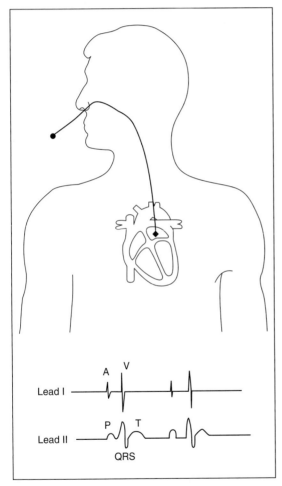

FIGURE   45-3

ESOPHAGEAL LEAD PLACEMENT AND RECORDING

Picture depicts placement of esophageal pacing lead via the nares to a depth at the level of the left atrium. Lead I depicts the electrogram recorded from the esophageal lead and lead II depicts the corresponding surface ECG.

Indications

The indications for TEP are similar to those for intracardiac EP testing. They include evaluation of SVT, risk assessment in patients with WPW syndrome and evaluation of sinus and AV node function. TEP is also used to help guide long-term medical management children with a history of SVT in infancy. TEP can be used as a therapeutic tool for atrial overdrive pacing to terminate reentrant SVTs. It is shown to be 98% effective for conversion of AV reentry tachycardias and 73% effective for conversion of atrial flutter.

Procedure

The procedure consists of either a conscious sedation or general anesthesia followed by placement of a 3–5 French esophageal pacing catheter via the nares to the midesophagus. In this position, the catheter is in close proximity to the left atrium and thus atrial electrograms are readily obtained. Pacing is usually performed at higher outputs than those used with intracardiac pacing. The protocol for pacing is similar to that described for intracardiac EP studies but is limited only to atrial pacing. This is usually performed in a baseline state and also can be repeated after infusion of isoproterenol. The results of functional studies obtained with TEP show good correlation with the results from intracardiac EP testing.

Risks

The TEP is a safe and well-tolerated procedure with minimal risks. There have been no reported instances of esophageal damage although minimal irritation would be difficult to document. Induction of nonspecific atrial arrhythmias (atrial fibrillation) is rare and usually self-limited. Nonetheless, appropriate precautions should be taken in the event of any emergencies.

Limitations

The limitations to the TEP include the need for adequate sedation to account for the discomfort caused by esophageal pacing; however, many children can tolerate TEP studies with minimal sedation. Inability to capture the atrium with esophageal pacing is also an issue for some patients, especially following cardiac surgery. Finally, the diagnostic capabilities of the TEP are limited in that a His recording obtained during intracardiac EP testing is not available with esophageal recordings.

SUMMARY

While EP studies play an important role for the evaluation of children with heart disease, long-term randomized controlled trials assessing the efficacy of electrophysiology studies in predicting future arrhythmic events are lacking. The predictive value of EP studies in postoperative patients with congenital heart disease continues to be debated. Furthermore, the use of EP studies in asymptomatic patients with WPW remains unclear.

Suggested Readings

Benson DW Jr, Dunnigan A, Benditt DG, et al: Transesophageal cardiac pacing: history, application, technique. *Clin Prog Pacing Electrophysiol* 1984; 2:360–372.

Pass RH, Walsh EP: Intracardiac electrophysiology testing in pediatric patients, in: Walsh EP, Saul JP, Triedman JK (eds): *Cardiac Arrhythmias in Children and Young Adults with Congenital Heart Disease.* Philadelphia, PA, Lippincott, Williams & Wilkins, 2001, pp. 57–94.

Walsh EP, Keane JF: Electrophysiologic studies and related procedures in congenital heart disease, in: Lock JE, Keane JF, Fellows KE (eds): *Diagnostic and Interventional Catheterization in Congenital Heart Disease.* Boston, MA, Kluwer Academic, 1987, pp. 161–181.

C H A P T E R

46

INTERVENTIONAL CARDIAC CATHETERIZATION

Ziyad M. Hijazi and Hitendra T. Patel

INTRODUCTION

The last 10 years have seen tremendous advancement in the field of interventional cardiology and this is likely to continue. This chapter describes the tools used in interventional catheterization, the procedures performed, and results. Some of the technical details are listed for interest purposes only as this detail most likely will not be useful to the primary care provider.

TOOLS USED IN INTERVENTIONAL CATHETERIZATION

Tools used in interventional catheterization consist of balloons for septostomy, valvuloplasty, and angioplasty, stents to maintain patency of stenotic vessels or conduits, occlusion devices for closure of atrial septal defects (ASD), ventricular septal defects (VSDs), and patent ductus arteriosi, and coils for occlusion of vessels.

Balloons are used to open vessels or create openings in walls (septae). This is sometimes referred to as dilation; however, the balloons actually create tears in either a septum (atrial septum during a balloon atrial septostomy) or in semilunar or AV valves (during valvuloplasty). In the case of arterial narrowing, balloons are used to create an intimal tear (during balloon angioplasty).

Coils are made of stainless steel or platinum. They have a thrombogenic polyester fibrous strand coating (a "fuzzy" portion, which provides a good nidus for clot formation). They are available in different core wire thicknesses for different vessel sizes. Furthermore, they are preformed to conform to a certain diameter coil after they are deployed or released from the sheath. The diameter and the length of the coil will determine the number of loops formed.

Stents are used to keep blood vessels patent. Stent implantation is frequently used for native or recurrent coarctation of the aorta in older children and adults. Furthermore, stents are used to keep pulmonary arteries patent since balloon angioplasty for pulmonary arteries is frequently not successful. The main drawback of stent implantation in smaller vessels is the development of neointimal proliferation (tissue growth inside the stent), which may require repeat angioplasty. Newer stent designs (drug eluting stents) may help solve this problem in the pediatric age group.

Closure devices are used to close secundum type atrial septal defects, ventricular septal defects, and patent ductus arteriosi. There are number of products available for each type of defect. The pros and cons of each device are beyond the scope of this book, though this information can be obtained. Overall, risks of any closure device include embolization (migration of the device from its location), thrombus formation on the surface, obstruction of blood flow, and entrapment of chordae or leaflets. Devices are available in different sizes. The ease of implantation, fracture of the device, and other changes over time remain areas of research.

PROCEDURES PERFORMED IN THE CATHETERIZATION LABORATORY

Atrial Septostomy

Atrial septostomy is the oldest interventional procedure (1966) and is performed to: (1) improve atrial level mixing in transposition of the great arteries (2) enable R-L shunt in patients with a restrictive atrial septal communication in tricuspid atresia (rare) or end-stage pulmonary hypertension with intact atrial septum, and (3) permit L-R shunting in newborns with hypoplastic left heart syndrome with an intact or very restrictive atrial septal communication. Initially, this procedure was performed surgically; however, with the advent of balloon or blade septostomy, the procedure is performed in the cardiac catheterization laboratory. Balloon septostomy is effective in the first month of life. After this the septum becomes too thick to tear with a balloon. In these cases a blade catheter is used to cut the septum after which the hole is dilated with a balloon. The procedure can be performed at the bedside or in the cardiac catheterization suite. It can be done via the umbilical vein in neonates, or the femoral vein and usually requires a 6 or 7 French sheath.

Complications include cardiac perforation, and tearing or avulsion of the inferior vena cava (IVC) in addition to the usual complications of cardiac catheterization.

Balloon Valvuloplasty of the Pulmonary Valve

Balloon pulmonary valvuloplasty is performed to relieve stenosis (obstruction) of a unicommisural or bicuspid pulmonary valve with a pressure gradient of 40 or 35 mmHg with right ventricular hypertrophy (RVH) on the ECG or echocardiogram. Balloon valvuloplasty is usually not effective in patients with dysplastic valves such as those seen in Noonan's syndrome. The type of access required depends on the size of the balloons required, although this procedure can be performed in newborn infants using a 4–6 French sheath. The balloon used is usually 120% of the pulmonary valve annulus. The balloon is passed through the valve such that it sits halfway between the valve annulus. The balloon is inflated until narrowing from the annulus (the waist) disappears. This may be repeated a number of times. Complications are rare and include rupture of the tricuspid valve apparatus, perforation of the pulmonary artery or right ventricular outflow tract, or balloon rupture and embolization.

Pulmonary Atresia with Intact Ventricular Septum

In patients with a well-developed main pulmonary artery and a pulmonary valve plate that is well developed and membranous rather than muscular, the atretic pulmonary valve can be perforated and the annulus dilated in the cardiac catheterization laboratory. After obtaining access to the femoral vein, the pulmonary valve is perforated using a fine, stiff wire or catheters able to generate radiofrequency energy at their tip. Following perforation, balloon dilation is performed similar to pulmonary valve stenosis as described above. Complications are similar to those described for balloon pulmonary valvuloplasty.

Peripheral Pulmonary Artery Stenosis

One of the indications for intervention in patients with severe pulmonary artery stenosis is RV hypertension, with the RV systolic pressure equal to or greater than 60–70% of the systemic systolic pressure. In the case of isolated right or left pulmonary artery stenosis, the decision to intervene is also based on the relative distribution of blood flow via a nuclear perfusion scan as well as the presence of any associated cardiac defects. Normal lung perfusion is 55–60% flow to right lung and 40–45% to the left lung. Intervention is considered if the flow to the left lung is less than 30%, and that to the right lung is less than 40%. Access is achieved from the femoral, internal jugular, or subclavian vein. Balloons able to tolerate very high pressures (high pressure balloons) are required. For very severe stenotic lesions with thick arterial walls, cutting balloons (balloons with blades on the outside) have been used to create the initial intimal tear. Balloon angioplasty for peripheral pulmonary artery stenosis has a 50–60% success rate. Therefore, for lesions where balloon dilation is ineffective, stent placement is considered. Since stents do not grow with the patient, the stent used should be able to be dilated sequentially to adult pulmonary artery dimensions to avoid relative stenosis because of body growth. Complications of this procedure include reperfusion lung injury, pulmonary artery rupture or aneurysm formation, stent migration, and balloon rupture and embolization. Complications of stent placement include the lack of stent growth with body growth, and neointimal proliferation (growth of tissue within the stent causing narrowing).

Balloon Valvuloplasty of the Aortic Valve

The indication for catheter intervention with valvar aortic stenosis is similar to that of surgical intervention. In centers with a large volume of interventions, balloon valvuloplasty is the preferred treatment for aortic stenosis. The indications to perform the valvuloplasty include a mean echocardiographic gradient greater than 30 mmHg or catheterization derived peak to peak catheter gradient across the aortic vale greater than 50 mmHg. Left ventricular hypertrophy (increased wall thickness) as measured by echocardiography should be present, and confirms the presence of a significant obstruction. The measurement of the degree of stenosis and the lack of correlation with echocardiographic and catheterization gradient are areas of continued controversy, as is the exact timing of intervention which may vary by age. Valvuloplasty is not very effective with dysplastic valves, or with a small aortic valve annulus.

Access for the procedure is via the umbilical artery or vein (transseptal) or femoral artery. Carotid artery cut-down and femoral artery access allow a retrograde technique to be used rather than the anterograde technique via the umbilical or femoral venous approach. The advantage of the carotid approach is the direct, straight course of the catheter into the left ventricle, unlike the tortuous route required with the other approaches, especially the venous approach. A 3–4 French sheath is required in neonates and infants. In older patients 4–8 French sheaths are required depending on the size and type of balloon chosen. Low-pressure balloons are used to reduce the risk of valve injury. Long balloons are chosen for stability during inflation since LV contraction will push the balloon into the aorta. Some operators have advocated the use of adenosine to produce reversible cardiac standstill at the time of inflation or right ventricle pacing to decrease the cardiac output during balloon inflation. A balloon diameter that is 80–100% of the valve annulus is usually used. This conservative approach is used to minimize the resultant aortic regurgitation with effective gradient reduction.

Complications of balloon aortic valvuloplasty include vessel trauma with a loss of the distal arterial pulse, balloon rupture, and embolization. Aortic regurgitation is another risk of this procedure and is difficult to avoid completely. At least trivial regurgitation is a known and expected complication. Nevertheless, owing to the risk of creating significant aortic regurgitation, plans for this possibility ought to be made prior to the intervention, and the patient ought to be a candidate for aortic valve repair, replacement or a Ross procedure.

Ventricular arrhythmias including ventricular tachycardia and fibrillation are known rhythm complications and are usually transient with no therapy required. Complete heart block is also a potential complication of this procedure.

Angioplasty of Recurrent or Native Coarctation

Aortic angioplasty is the treatment of choice for residual or postoperative gradients in the aorta of >20 mmHg, with hypertension proximal to the coarctation or left ventricular hypertrophy. Balloon dilation of native coarctation is somewhat controversial; however, most centers will advocate balloon dilation in patients older than 1 year with a discrete coarctation and a well-developed aortic isthmus. Balloon dilation of native coarctation in infancy remains controversial, although there is increasing evidence of its effectiveness in patients with discrete coarctation and a well-developed isthmus.

Access for the procedure is via the femoral artery. Balloons with a low burst pressure are used for native coarctation in order to reduce the risk of aortic rupture. Balloons with a high burst pressure may be required for residual postoperative coarctation, which has less of a risk of rupture because of scar formation. A balloon is selected with a diameter of two to three times the minimum diameter of the coarctation but not exceeding the diameter of the aortic isthmus or descending aorta at the level of the diaphragm. In adolescents and adults with a fully developed aorta, most interventionists advocate stent placement and dilation as the initial procedure to further reduce the risk of aortic rupture and recurrence of the coarctation.

Complications of aortic angioplasty include vessel trauma leading to the loss (usually transient) of the distal arterial pulse. Aortic rupture is very rare with the guidelines outlined above. Aortic aneurysm formation secondary to weakening of the aortic wall at the site of balloon angioplasty occurs in <5% of cases. Initial reports of aortic angioplasty cited an aneurysm incidence of 15–50%; however, with more conservative balloon sizes and improved techniques, this has significantly decreased to around 5%.

Closure of Patent Ductus Arteriosus (PDA)

There are number of methods used to close a patent ductus arteriosus in the cardiac catheterization laboratory. These include coil embolization, device closure, and the use of Gianturco Grifka Vascular Occlusion Device.

Coil Embolization of Small/Moderate PDA

Requirements for coil embolization of a PDA include the presence of a patent ductus arteriosus with a maximum diameter of 4 mm as well as a well-developed ampulla. Most PDAs have a conical shape with the narrowest portion at the pulmonary artery end. PDAs with a short or no length continue to be difficult to close with the available technology. Access for the procedure is via a femoral artery or vein with the need for a 4–5 French sheath. A coil which is two to three times the minimum diameter of the PDA is used. The PDA can be closed anterogradely from the pulmonary artery or retrogradely from the aorta. Small PDAs are easier to cross from a retrograde fashion. Ideally, one-half to one loop is opened in the pulmonary artery and the remaining 2–3 loops are positioned in the ductal ampulla. The length of the coil selected is based on the coil diameter and its ability to form at least 3–4 loops. The goal of the procedure is complete closure, which may require multiple coils, especially if the PDA >2–2.5 mm.

Complications of coil embolization of a PDA include coil embolization (migration). Until recently only free release coils were available in the United States. In order to decrease the risk of coil embolization and improve precise placement, a snare, bioptome, or other method to secure the coil on deployment has been proposed. Detachable coils are now available, which render this technique much easier to perform.

After closure, SBE prophylaxis is required for 6 months.

Coil or Device Closure of Moderate to Large PDA (>4 mm)

As with the smaller PDAs, complete closure of the vessel remains the goal of intervention. If coils are used for embolization, multiple, thicker coils will be required. Simultaneous delivery of multiple coils has been proposed to stabilize the coil. Bioptome technique or detachable coils should be used as described above; however, it is felt that closure using an occluder device may be more optimal. The Amplatzer duct occluder received approval from the U.S. Food and Drug Administration to close PDAs of various sizes. The use of the Amplatzer Duct Occluder eliminates the need for multiple coils, improves the rate of complete closure, and is easier to deliver. The Gianturco Grifka Vascular Occlusion Device is another approved device to close PDAs; however, this device is used to close certain types (shapes) of PDAs.

As with smaller PDAs, coil or device embolization remains a risk of the procedure. Other risks include left pulmonary artery stenosis, narrowing or coarctation of the aorta, and hemolysis if a residual shunt remains. The latter is a result of the shearing effect of small shunts with a large pressure gradient.

After closure, SBE prophylaxis is required for 6 months.

Device Closure of Secundum Atrial Septal Defects (ASD)

Multiple occluder devices have been and still are being tested for the closure of secundum ASDs. (Sinus venosus and primum ASDs are not yet amenable to device closure). At this time, the only Food and Drug Administration approved device to close a secundum ASD is the Amplatzer Septal Occluder device. It is an occluder device made out of Nitinol (a nickel and titanium alloy), with left and right disks and a central connecting waist. The size of the connecting waist (which corresponds to a size slightly larger than the size of the defect to be occluded) ranges from 4 to 40 mm. The diameter of the left disc and right discs are larger than the connecting waist (with the left being slightly larger than the right as the pressure in the left atrium is higher than the right). Secundum ASDs with diameters of approximately 32–34 mm can be closed provided the atrial size can accommodate the device. Access for the procedure is through the femoral vein with a

6–12 French sheath depending on the device size. It is essential for fluoroscopy and echocardiography (either transesophageal or intracardiac) to be available during the procedure. These are required for precise sizing and placement of the device. Results with the Amplatzer device have shown very high complete closure rate at 1 year. There are a number of other ASD closure devices currently undergoing clinical trials, which are not yet approved. The primary care physician ought to realize that each device carries special advantages and disadvantages, which are not summarized in this chapter; however, this information is available through the internet or from various pediatric cardiology centers.

Complications of ASD closure thus far are rare. Major complications such as device embolization (migration), erosions, or complete heart block occur in <1% of the cases.

After closure, SBE prophylaxis is required for 6 months. Aspirin is usually given for 6 months to prevent thrombus formation until the device is endothelialized.

Device Closure of Patent Foramen Ovale (PFO)

Indications for PFO closure include: (1) embolic stroke, transient ischemic attack (TIA) or peripheral embolism, with evidence of right to left shunting across a PFO; (2) orthodoxia/platypnea syndrome; and (3) the presence of a PFO in a deep water scuba diver to prevent decompression illness. These indications are rare in the pediatric age group. In the past, closure was surgical and involved cardiac bypass. With the development of closure devices, a PFO can be closed in the cardiac catheterization laboratory. A number of devices are available to perform this; however, all are still undergoing clinical trials at this time. It is anticipated that the devices will be clinically available in the near future.

Device Closure of Ventricular Septal Defects (VSDs)

Closure of VSDs is a more complex procedure than ASD or PDA closure. The location of the VSD may vary in the septum. The current standard method of closure has been via open heart surgery, and may continue to be with complex VSDs such as inlet VSDs associated with an endocardial cushion defect. Closure of a paramembranous VSD remains a relatively uncomplicated surgical procedure. Muscular VSDs remain a problem for the surgeon as they may be multiple and difficult to visualize because of the trabecular meshwork of the right ventricle, from which the surgical closure is performed. In the past, pulmonary artery banding has been performed with the intention of allowing time for spontaneous closure of some of the muscular VSDs. This may simplify the surgical closure while protecting the pulmonary vasculature until the time of surgery. With the recent development of VSD occluder devices to close muscular VSDs, surgical treatment may be further simplified or become unnecessary. Currently, only one device (CardioSEAl) is approved for clinical use, though approval of more devices is expected in the near future. Paramembranous VSD occluder devices are currently undergoing clinical trials. Approval for use is also anticipated in the future.

Endomyocardial Biopsy

This is a technique used to obtain small pieces of myocardial tissue for diagnostic purposes. The diagnosis of myocarditis and monitoring for transplant rejection are the usual indications for endomyocardial biopsy. Patients with cardiomyopathy may also be candidates in order to help determine the cause of the muscle disorder. The amount of tissue obtained with an endomyocardial biopsy is small which is problematic in the diagnosis of the exact etiology of a cardiomyopathy as numerous genetic cell and molecular, and biochemical studies may be needed. In addition, many disease processes do not affect the cardiac muscle in a uniform fashion, which creates the possibility of sampling error.

The technique of obtaining a biopsy varies depending on the age of the patient. In neonates and smaller infants, the biopsy is performed from the femoral vein; however, in older children, it is best performed from the right internal jugular vein. A bioptome with forceps at the end is used to grab "bite" the endomyocardial wall. Five good pieces are usually needed for a good diagnostic test.

Complications of endomyocardial biopsy are the same as with cardiac catheterization with the additional risks of trauma (perforation with tamponade, and/or arrhythmia) from the procedure. These risks are greater in small infants.

Transvenous Dual Chamber Pacemaker

This topic is covered in detail in the electrophysiology chapters.

Foreign Body Retrieval

This is a rare procedure in pediatrics; however, on rare occasions, catheters (umbilical lines) may break, or devices may embolize (migrate) inside the vascular system. In addition, bullets, BBs, and other foreign bodies may enter the vascular system where they may become lodged at any place in the body. Retrieval of such foreign bodies may be performed safely in the pediatric cardiac catheterization laboratory.

Combined Interventional Catheterization with Cardiac Surgery (Hybrid Surgery)

The fusion of transcatheter technology with cardiothoracic surgery is currently allowing more procedures to be performed with the collaboration of interventional cardiologists and cardiac surgeons in hybrid operating rooms/catheterization suites to repair certain defects. Closure of muscular VSDs in small infants is under investigation and may be performed in operating rooms without the need of cardiopulmonary bypass. In this combined approach, using a small chest incision, the right ventricle free wall is punctured with a needle. Through this access, a wire and then a VSD occluder may be guided to the left ventricle using transesophageal echocardiographic guidance. Stent implantation under direct vision can also be performed safely in the operating room.

SUMMARY

In summary, the field of interventional cardiology for congenital heart disease has seen tremendous expansion in the last few years. The goal over the next few years is to repair/palliate many forms of congenital heart disease without the need for cardiac surgery or to use cardiac surgery without the need for cardiopulmonary bypass.

Suggested Readings

Chessa M, Carminati M, Cao QL, et al: Transcatheter closure of congenital and acquired muscular ventricular septal defects using the Amplatzer device. *J Invasive Cardiol* 14:322–332, 2002.

Du ZD, Cao QL, Joseph A, et al: Transcatheter closure of patent foramen ovale in patients with paradoxical embolism: Intermediate-term risk of recurrent neurological events. *Catheter Cardiovasc Intervt* 55:189–194, 2002.

Du ZD, Hijazi ZM, Kleinman CS, et al: Comparison between transcatheter and surgical closure of secundum atrial septal defect in children and adults: results of a multicenter non-randomized trial. *J Am Coll Cardiol* 39:1836–1844, 2002.

Ettinger L, Hijazi ZM, Geggel RL, et al: Peripheral pulmonary artery stenosis: acute and mid-term results of high pressure balloon angioplasty. *J Interven Cardiol* 11:337–344, 1998.

Hijazi ZM, Geggel RL: Results of antegrade transcatheter closure of patent ductus arteriosus using single or multiple gianturco coils. *Am J Cardiol* 74:925–929, 1994.

Hijazi ZM, Hakim F, Haweleh A, et al: Catheter closure of perimembranous ventricular septal defects using the new Amplatzer membranous VSD occluder: Initial clinical experience. *Catheter Cardiovasc Intervt* 56:508–515, 2002.

Hijazi, ZM, Fadley F, Geggel RL, et al: Stent implantation for relief of branch pulmonary artery stenosis: immediate and short-term Results. *Cathet Cardiovasc Diagn* 38:16–23, 1996.

Masura J, Gavora P, Formanek A, Hijazi ZM: Transcatheter closure of secundum atrial septal defects using the new self-centering amplatzer septal occluder: initial human experience. *Cathet Cardiovasc Diagn* 42:388–393, 1997.

Masura J, Walsh KP, Thanopoulos B, et al: Catheter closure of moderate-to large-sized patent ductus arteriosus using the new Amplatzer duct occluder: Immediate and short-term results. *J Am Coll Cardiol* 31:878–882, 1998.

McCrindle BW: Independent predictors of long-term results after balloon valvuloplasty. *Circulation* 89:1751–1759, 1994.

Mullins CE, O'Laughlin MP, Vick CW III, et al: Implantation of balloon expandable intravascular grafts by catheterization in pulmonary arteries and systemic veins. *Circulation* 77:188–199, 1988.

O'Connor BK, Beekman RH, Rocchini AP, et al: Intermediate-term effectiveness of balloon valvuloplasty for congenital aortic stenosis. *Circulation* 84:732–738, 1991.

O'Laughlin MP, Perry SB, Lock JE, Mullins CE: Use of endovascular stents in congenital heart disease. *Circulation* 83:1923–1939, 1991.

Rao PS, Galal O, Smith PA et al: Five to nine year follow up results of balloon angioplasty of native aortic coarctation in infants and children. *J Am Coll Cardiol* 27:462–470, 1996.

Rashkind WJ, Miller WW: Creation of an atrial septal defect without thoracotomy: a palliative approach to complete transposition of the great vessels. *J Am Med Assoc* 196:991–992, 1966.

Suarez de Lezo J, Pan M, Romero M, et al: Balloon expandable stent repair of severe coarctation of the aorta. *Am Heart J* 129:1002–1008, 1995.

Zeevi B, Keane JF, Fellows KE, et al: Balloon dilation of critical pulmonary stenosis in the first week of life. *J Am Coll Cardiol* 11:821–824, 1988.

47

RADIOFREQUENCY CATHETER ABLATION

Frank Zimmerman

INTRODUCTION

Radiofrequency (RF) energy is a method for heating and destroying cardiac tissue for the purpose of controlling or eliminating cardiac arrhythmias. The first radiofrequency ablation procedure was performed in adults in 1988. This was shortly followed thereafter in children in 1989. Since that time, the techniques and equipment have improved allowing for expanded application of RF catheter ablation for a variety of arrhythmias with improved safety and efficacy of the procedure.

INDICATIONS

The indications for RF catheter ablation in children are based on the natural history of specific arrhythmias, the life-long risks of the disease versus control with medical therapy and the safety of the procedure (Table 47-1). These guidelines arise mainly from data from the Pediatric RF Catheter Ablation Registry, which has been ongoing since 1991. Class I indications are those for which there is consistent agreement that ablation is likely to be beneficial. Class IIa indications are those for which there is a

majority of opinion/data in favor of the benefits of the procedure and class IIb indications are those for which there is divergence of opinion/data regarding the benefits of the procedure. Class III conditions are those for which there is agreement that ablation is not indicated. Based on the registry, 54% of ablation procedures in children are performed because of parent or patient preference over alternatives such as chronic medical therapy, 32% are performed because of refractoriness to medical therapy, and 7% are performed because of life-threatening situations. The number of elective ablation procedures has increased as the experience of operators and technologic advances continue.

PROCEDURE

The specific details of the RF catheter ablation procedure may vary depending on the institution at which it is performed. Preprocedure testing usually includes an echocardiogram, ECG, and a chest radiograph depending on the patient's age. A complete blood count and a type and cross may be performed before the procedure or once catheters have been placed. The method of sedation used during

TABLE 47-1

INDICATIONS FOR RF CATHETER ABLATION

Class I
1. WPW syndrome associated with an episode of aborted sudden death
2. WPW syndrome and syncope if there is a rapid antegrade conduction property of the accessory connection (shortest preexcited RR interval during atrial fibrillation or antegrade refractory period of <250 ms during EP testing)
3. Chronic or recurrent supra ventricular tachycardias (SVT) associated with ventricular dysfunction
4. Recurrent VT associated with hemodynamic compromise that is amenable to catheter ablation
Class IIa
1. Recurrent SVT refractory to conventional medical therapy and age >4 years
2. Impending congenital heart surgery when vascular or chamber access will be restricted following surgery
3. Chronic or incessant SVT in the presence of normal ventricular function
4. Chronic or recurrent intraatrial reentrant tachycardia
5. Palpitations with inducible SVT during EP testing
Class IIb
1. Asymptomatic preexcitation, age >5 years and no tachycardia but risks and benefits of the procedure and arrhythmia have been explained
2. SVT, age >5 years, as alternative to effective chronic antiarrhythmic therapy
3. SVT, age <5 years, when antiarrhythmic therapy (including sotalol or amiodarone) are not effective or associated with intolerable side effects
4. Intraatrial reentrant tachycardia occurring 1–3 episodes per year requiring medical intervention
5. AV node ablation and pacemaker insertion as alternative therapy for recurrent or incessant intraatrial reentrant tachycardia
6. A single episode ventricular tachycardia (VT) amenable to ablation and associated with hemodynamic compromise
Class III
1. Asymptomatic WPW, age <5 years
2. SVT controlled with conventional medical therapy, age <5 years
3. Nonsustained, paroxysmal VT not associated with ventricular dysfunction
4. Nonsustained SVT that do not require medical therapy and/or are minimally symptomatic

the procedure also varies with age and institutional preference. While most procedures can be performed with conscious sedation, the length of the procedure and the inherent difficulty in obtaining a stable degree of conscious sedation in pediatric patients has led many centers to use general anesthesia. Once the patient is sedated, the catheters are placed in the femoral veins and occasionally in the femoral artery, internal jugular veins or the subclavian vein to achieve access to the heart (Figure 47-1). The catheters used range in size from 2 to 8 French and have either fixed curves or can be manually deflected for easier manipulation. An electrophysiologic study is performed and a determination is

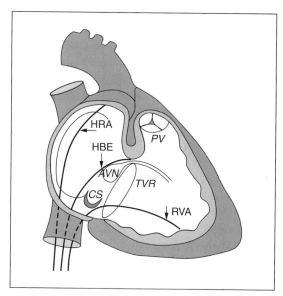

FIGURE 47-1

STANDARD EP CATHETER POSITIONS FOR RF ABLATION

AVN: atrioventricular node; CS: coronary sinus; HBE: his bundle electrogram; HRA: high right atrium; PV: pulmonary valve; RVA: right ventricular apex; TVR: tricuspid valve ring.

responsible for the abnormal rhythm. The catheter is manipulated and guided with fluoroscopy as well as by assessing the electrograms recorded at the tip of the catheter. There are also three-dimensional mapping systems, which can be used to help guide the catheter, thus obviating the need for fluoroscopy and radiation exposure. The use of three-dimensional mapping systems also can help to limit the number of catheters needed for the study. This is particularly useful in young patients with smaller venous structures and limited catheter access. SVT arising from the left side of the heart may be approached retrograde across the aortic valve or antegrade via a transeptal puncture. While both approaches are equally efficacious, the transeptal approach is used more frequently in pediatrics to avoid potential damage to the aortic valve.

The ablation process consists of applying RF energy to the group of cells felt to be the origin of the abnormal rhythm (Figure 47-2). RF energy is similar to microwave energy in that it heats and destroys the cells making them electrically inactive. The area of cells affected by ablation depends on the size of the catheter used, the amount of energy employed, and tissue temperature achieved. The standard ablation catheter has a 4-mm tip and thus the RF application is approximately 4–6 mm in diameter. RF applications can be placed in a single area or a linear series of applications can be created in order to achieve a line of block. This is most

made if the SVT is amenable to RF ablation. Once the electrophysiology study is complete and the type of arrhythmia has been identified, a specialized RF ablation catheter is maneuvered to the area

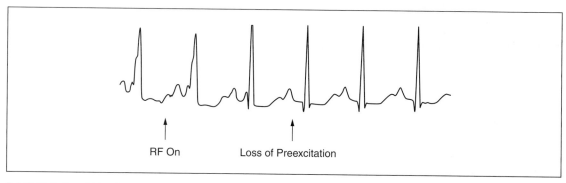

FIGURE 47-2

RHYTHM STRIP SHOWING LOSS OF DELTA WAVE DURING RF ABLATION SIGNIFYING THE DESTRUCTION OF THE ACCESSORY PATHWAY IN WPW

commonly used for reentrant atrial arrhythmias such as atrial flutter or ventricular arrhythmias involving a scar. The RF energy applied is controlled by the power of the generator (50–70 W), and the temperature detected at the tip of the catheter. By limiting the power to maintain a temperature of less than 70°C, there is less risk for cardiac perforation or coagulant formation at the tip of the ablation catheter. In certain instances, RF lesion formation is limited because of poor cooling of the tip resulting in lower energy applied to the tissue. This can result in lower success rates of ablation and is a particular problem in patients with congenital heart disease. Newer technologies such as larger tip RF catheters or cooled tip RF catheters with saline infusion are available to overcome these issues. Alternative sources of ablation energy include cryoablation in which the tissue is cooled rather than heated.

Postprocedure follow-up evaluation includes a visit within 1–3 weeks to assess the catheter sites for healing, at which time an ECG may be performed. Follow-up after that point depends on the patient's history, age, and the results of the catheterization procedure.

RF CATHETER ABLATION

The results of RF catheter ablation differ between patients with and without congenital heart disease. In patients without congenital heart disease, the overall success rates are approximately 92% for ablation of accessory connections. Accessory connections located on the left free wall of the heart have the highest success rate of 96.5% while those on the anteroseptal tricuspid valve annulus have the lowest at 81.1%. Ablation of AV node reentry tachycardia is associated with a 97.4% success rate. Ablation of atrial tachycardias such as ectopic atrial tachycardia and atrial flutter are associated with success rates of 86.7 and 84.8%, respectively. Finally, ablation of idiopathic right ventricular tachycardia is associated with a 79.7% success rate. Young age and small size are not predictors

of failure of ablation but the presence of congenital heart disease decreases the overall success rate to 80%. This is a result of many factors including the variability of anatomy, presence of multiple accessory connections, and limitation of ablation lesions because of low blood flow states. While acute success rates for catheter ablation continue to improve, recurrence of tachycardia remains an issue. This is especially true for right-sided accessory connections where recurrence rates may be as high as 10–20%. Also, intraatrial reentry tachycardia in patients with congenital heart disease may have up to a 50% recurrence rate following acutely successful ablation. Ongoing analysis by the RF Registry and technologic improvements may help to improve these results.

Complications of RF catheter ablation occur in 7.2% of patients undergoing ablation who do not have congenital heart disease. Major complications are defined as those requiring immediate treatment and/or follow-up. The incidence of major complications has decreased from 4.8% in 1991 down to 1.4% in 1997. The most common major complications include complete heart block, cardiac perforation, blood clot formation and embolization, brachial plexus injury, and pneumothorax. The risk of death owing to complications of the ablation procedure was approximately 0.1%. Age less than 4 years or weight less than 15 kg were independent risk factors for complications associated with the procedure. There is currently an ongoing prospective analysis assessing the success rates as well as the recurrence rates and complications of ablation in children.

Specific complications for children immediately following RF catheter ablation procedures are usually bleeding at the sites where the catheters were placed. Therefore, most patients are restricted from vigorous activities for several days to allow for complete healing at these sites following the ablation procedure. Following this time, there are no specific restrictions or precautions although some patients may be placed on aspirin for 4–6 weeks following the procedure to avoid any thrombus formation at the site of the RF ablation.

SUMMARY

RF catheter ablation in children greater than 4 years of age or greater than 15 kg in weight is both safe and effective and in some cases may be considered first-line therapy treatment of arrhythmias. The role of catheter ablation for asymptomatic patients with Wolff-Parkinson-White (WPW) syndrome continues to be debated. Ablation of arrhythmias in patients with congenital heart disease, and in particular atrial flutter or intraatrial reentrant tachycardia, continue to have the lowest success rates and the highest recurrence rates; however, improvement in catheter technology and mapping systems may help to improve the results in this specific population.

Suggested Readings

Friedman RA, Walsh EP, Silka MJ, Calkins H, Stevenson WG, Rhodes LA, Deal BJ, Wolff GS, Demaso DR, Hanisch D, Van Hare GF: NASPE expert conference: radiofrequency catheter ablation in children with and without congenital heart disease. Report of the writing committee. *PACE* 25(6):1000–1017, 2002.

Saul JP: Ablation of accessory pathways, in: Walsh EP, Saul JP, Triedman JK (eds): *Cardiac Arrhythmias in Children and Young Adults with Congenital Heart Disease.* Philadelphia, PA, Lippincott Williams & Wilkins, 2001, pp. 393–425.

Van Hare GF: Indications for radiofrequency ablation in the pediatric population. *J Cardiovasc Electrophysiol* 8:952–962, 1997.

C H A P T E R

48

PEDIATRIC PACEMAKERS AND ICDS

Frank Zimmerman

INTRODUCTION

Pacemaker therapy is rarely indicated in children, accounting for approximately 1% of all pacing in the United States. Children have benefited from advances in technology that have resulted in smaller devices and safer implant techniques. Cardiac pacing in children is primarily used for those with congenital complete heart block. Permanent pacing may be implemented as early as the newborn period. Temporary transvenous or epicardial pacing is frequently used in emergency situations or in the immediate postoperative period following surgery for congenital heart disease. Implantable devices are also available to convert tachycardias and ventricular fibrillation and restore a normal or more stable rhythm.

THE PACEMAKER

Indications

Guidelines for permanent cardiac pacing in children are based on recommendations from ACC/AHA/NASPE in 2002 (Table 48-1).

Class 1 indications are conditions for which there is evidence and/or general agreement that pacing is useful and effective. They include pacing for children if there is the occurrence of symptoms (such as dizziness, fatigue, syncope) in association with documented bradycardia. Bradycardia may be a result of sinus node dysfunction or advanced second-degree or third-degree AV block (complete heart block). Risk factors for sudden death in asymptomatic children with complete heart block include low resting heart rates (less than 50–55 bpm in the infant), a wide complex QRS escape rhythm or prolonged QT interval. The incidence of sudden death in patients with no known risk factors may also be significant, prompting some to recommend elective pacemaker implantation prior to the second or third decade of life in this group. Pacing is also recommended in children with congenital heart disease and complete heart block, as there is a 28% incidence of sudden cardiac death. Complete heart block in the postoperative period that has not resolved within 7 days is associated with an 80–100% incidence of sudden death over a 2-year period and is an indication for permanent pacemaker implantation.

TABLE 48-1

INDICATIONS FOR PACING IN PEDIATRICS

Class 1

1. Advanced second- or third-degree AV block associated with symptomatic bradycardia, ventricular dysfunction, or low cardiac output
2. Sinus node dysfunction with correlation of symptoms during age-inappropriate bradycardia
3. Postoperative advanced second- or third-degree AV block that is not expected to resolve or persists at least 7 days after cardiac surgery
4. Congenital third-degree AV block with a wide QRS escape rhythm, complex ventricular ectopy, or ventricular dysfunction
5. Congenital third-degree AV block in the infant with a ventricular rate less than 50–55 bpm or with congenital heart disease and a ventricular rate less than 70 bpm
6. Sustained pause-dependent VT, with or without prolonged QT, in which the efficacy of pacing is thoroughly documented

Class 2a

1. Bradycardia-tachycardia syndrome with the need for long-term antiarrhythmic treatment other than digitalis
2. Congenital third-degree AV block beyond the first year of life with an average heart rate less than 50 bpm, abrupt pauses in ventricular rate that are two or three times the basic cycle length, or associated with symptoms because of chronotropic incompetence
3. Long QT syndrome with 2:1 AV or third-degree AV block
4. Asymptomatic sinus bradycardia in the child with complex congenital heart disease with resting heart rate less than 40 bpm or pauses in ventricular rate more than 3 s
5. Patients with congenital heart disease and impaired hemodynamics owing to sinus bradycardia or loss of AV synchrony

Class 2b

1. Transient postoperative third-degree AV block that reverts to sinus rhythm with residual bifascicular block
2. Congenital third-degree AV block in the asymptomatic infant, child, adolescent, or young adult with an acceptable rate, narrow QRS complex, and normal ventricular function
3. Asymptomatic sinus bradycardia in the adolescent with congenital heart disease with resting heart rate less than 40 bpm or pauses in ventricular rate more than 3 s
4. Neuromuscular diseases with any degree of AV block (including first-degree AV block), with or without symptoms, because there may be unpredictable progression of AV conduction disease

Class 3

1. Transient postoperative AV block with return of normal AV conduction
2. Asymptomatic postoperative bifascicular block with or without first-degree AV block
3. Asymptomatic type I second-degree AV block
4. Asymptomatic sinus bradycardia in the adolescent when the longest RR interval is <3 s and the minimum heart rate is >40 bpm

Class 2a conditions include those for which the weight of conflicting evidence and/or divergence of opinion are in favor of pacing. Indications include the bradycardia-tachycardia syndrome with need for chronic antiarrhythmic medication and the long QT syndrome with 2:1 heart block. Asymptomatic children with complete heart block and average resting heart rates less than 50 bpm or those with congenital heart disease and sinus bradycardia less than 40 bpm are also included in this group.

Class 2b indications are those for which the usefulness of pacing is less well established. Indications include asymptomatic children with complete heart block and acceptable heart rates, or adolescents with congenital heart disease and heart rates less than 40 bpm. Children with Kearne-Sayre syndrome associated with any conduction abnormality are at risk for the progression to complete heart block thus necessitating early intervention with pacing.

Class 3 indications include conditions for which there is evidence/general agreement that pacing is not useful and in some cases may be harmful. This includes children with return of normal conduction following transient postoperative heart block, those with postoperative bifascicular block (with or without first degree AV block), asymptomatic second-degree (type 1) block, or sinus bradycardia with heart rates greater than 40 bpm.

Temporary cardiac pacing is used in emergency situations or for patients who are ultimately candidates for permanent pacemaker implantation. Conditions necessitating temporary cardiac pacing include sinus node dysfunction or heart block because of medications, metabolic disturbances, and myocardial infarction or in the postoperative period while waiting for recovery. Therapeutic indications for permanent or temporary pacing include antitachycardia pacing for reentrant atrial arrhythmias.

THE DEVICE

Generator

Permanent pacemaker generators usually consist of a metallic can containing the circuitry and lithium iodine battery. They also consist of a plastic header

that connects to the pacemaker leads. The pacemaker generator can usually be placed in a subcutaneous pocket either in the chest or the abdomen. A submuscular pocket may be more appropriate for thin or young patients as this affords more protection to the pacemaker system.

Pacemaker Leads

The pacemaker lead is used to transfer the energy from the pacemaker generator to the myocardium. Transvenous endocardial leads are most commonly used in older patients while epicardial leads are used in younger patients. Transvenous leads usually require less energy to pace the heart and have greater longevity compared to epicardial leads. The concern of the use of transvenous leads in young patients is the risk for venous stenosis or occlusion thus limiting access for placement of subsequent pacing leads. The development of smaller pacing leads has allowed for the use of transvenous approach at younger ages while lowering the risk of venous occlusion; however, the decision of transvenous or epicardial pacing lead placement is dependent on the individual case and institutional preference. Most current leads have a small amount of steroid at the tip in contact with the myocardium in order to prevent scar formation and decrease the overall pacing thresholds.

PACEMAKER PROGRAMMING

Pacemaker Code

The NASPE/BPEG pacemaker code describes the capabilities and programmed functional mode of the pacemaker (Table 48-2). The first letter represents the cardiac chamber that is paced. This can be the atrium, ventricle, both, or neither. The second letter represents the cardiac chamber that is sensed and can represent the atrium, ventricle, both, or neither. The third letter denotes the response of the pacemaker and includes inhibition, triggering, both, or neither. Inhibition occurs when the pacemaker senses intrinsic cardiac activity and withholds pacing. Triggering occurs when the pacemaker senses an

TABLE 48-2

NASPE/BPG PACEMAKER CODE

I	II	III	IV	V
Chamber Paced	Chamber Sensed	Response to Sense	Program/Rate Modulation	Antitachycardia Function
O	O	O	O	O
A	A	T	P(1)	P(2)
V	V	I	M	S
D (A + V)	D (A + V)	D (T + I)	C	D (P + S)
			R	

Abbreviations: A = atrium, C = communicating, D = dual, I = inhibited, M = multiprogrammable, O = none, P(1) = simple programmable, P(2) = antitachyarrhythmia pacing, R = rate modulation, S = shock, T = triggered, V = ventricle.

intrinsic beat and then paces at a programmable interval following that beat. For example, with dual chamber pacing, an atrial sensed beat triggers the ventricle to be paced (tracking of the atrial beats). The fourth letter for permanent pacemakers denotes additional features (e.g., rate response or antitachycardia pacing features). The fifth letter denotes antitachycardia pacing.

COMMON PACEMAKER MODES

AAI pacing is performed in patients with bradycardia but intact intrinsic AV node conduction (sinus node dysfunction, medications, drugs, CNS disease). A rate responsive mode (*AAIR*) can also be programmed in permanent pacemakers in order to achieve increased heart rates when the pacemaker senses increased activity or motion.

VVI pacing is performed for similar reasons as *AAI* pacing but for those in whom atrial pacing cannot be achieved or there is no intrinsic AV conduction. Similarly to the *AAI* mode, *VVI* pacing would be inhibited if the intrinsic ventricular rhythm were greater than the rate limit.

DDD pacing is the most physiologic type of pacing in patients with complete heart block. Intrinsic atrial activity is tracked when between the lower and upper rate limits and ventricular pacing is performed once the programmed AV delay has occurred. Atrial and ventricular pacing can be inhibited if the patient's intrinsic rhythm occurs.

VDI pacing is programmed if atrial pacing is not achievable but atrial sensing is intact. It is also used for special transvenous leads placed in the ventricle that have an electrode for sensing atrial activity.

ANTITACHYCARDIA PACING

Reentrant forms of tachycardia such as atrial flutter or sinus node reentry can often be terminated with atrial pacing. Some forms of ventricular tachycardias have a reentrant mechanism that may also respond to ventricular antitachycardia pacing (usually performed by implantable cardioverter defibrillators (ICD)). Pacemakers with antitachycardia features incorporate antibradycardia pacing with algorithms to automatically detect atrial tachycardia and perform rapid atrial pacing.

The risks of antitachycardia pacing are that a stable reentrant tachycardia may inadvertently be converted into a more unstable type of tachycardia, such as atrial fibrillation with rapid ventricular response or ventricular fibrillation. It is for this reason that antitachycardia pacemakers should be reserved for select patients after careful electrophysiology testing.

OUTPATIENT MANAGEMENT

Outpatient management following pacemaker implantation usually involves frequent clinic visits for the first 2 months after the procedure. If the pacemaker is functioning well, visits can be gradually decreased to 1–2 times per year. Transtelephonic devices can be used to transmit information regarding pacemaker function over the phone. This is usually performed every 1–3 months.

Patients with pacemakers are allowed to participate in many of the daily activities of life. This includes mild to intense levels of exercise as long as contact sports such as hockey or football are avoided. Also, avoidance of exposure to electromagnetic interference such as with magnetic resonance imagings (MRIs) or arc welding is recommended.

Pacemaker generators have a limited battery life and require replacement when battery depletion is detected during pacemaker checks. The estimated battery life can vary greatly based on the amount of energy required to pace the heart, the percent of time paced, and the pacing rate.

IMPLANTABLE CARDIOVERTER DEFIBRILLATOR

The ICD is widely used in the adult population for primary and secondary prevention of sudden death in high-risk patients. It is gaining increasing use in children as the devices and leads are becoming smaller and safer to implant. Conditions for ICD use in children include secondary prevention of sudden death in patients with nonreversible causes of cardiac arrest. Increasing use of ICDs for primary prevention in those with a familial disorder or existing condition at high risk for sudden death (long QT syndrome, cardiomyopathy, arrhythmogenic RV dysplasia) continues as the natural history of such conditions becomes better understood.

ICD BASICS

ICD hardware systems are similar to pacemaker systems and all ICDs can function as pacemakers. In addition, ICDs are capable of delivering a shock internally to the heart if a fast heart rhythm is detected. Most detection algorithms are based on a set rate, above which is labeled as tachycardia. In order to achieve this, the ICD generator is larger than a pacemaker to accommodate larger capacitors. Furthermore, the transvenous ventricular lead is larger to accommodate a shock coil. Epicardial patches placed around the heart in the pericardium can also be used.

FUTURE CONSIDERATIONS

Pacing in children has undergone dramatic changes mainly because of advances in technology that have led to smaller leads and pacemaker generators. As this continues, pacing in children will be safer and may help to overcome issues such as venous stenosis or occlusion. Also, as more patients survive surgery for congenital heart disease, late problems such as sinus node dysfunction requiring intervention with pacing or ventricular arrhythmias requiring ICD implant will become more prevalent. Finally, the possibility of biventricular pacing as adjunctive therapy for heart failure may be applied to select children as it is now gaining widespread use in adults.

Suggested Readings

Bernstein AD, Camm AJ, Fletcher RD, Gold RD, Rickards AF, Smyth NP, Spielman SR, Sutton R: The NASPE/BPEG generic pacemaker code for antibradyarrhythmia and adaptive-rate pacing and antitachyarrhythmia devices. *Pacing Clin Electrophysiol* 10(4 Pt.1):794–799, 1987.

Cazeau S, Leclercq C, Lavergne T, Walker S, Varma C, Linde C, Garrigue S, Kappenberger L, Haywood GA, Santini M, Bailleul C, Daubert JC: Multisite Stimulation in Cardiomyopathies (MUSTIC) Study Investigators. Effects of multisite biventricular pacing in patients with heart failure and intraventricular conduction delay. *N Engl J Med* 344(12):873–880, 2001.

Choo MH, Holmes DR Jr, Gersh BJ, Maloney JD, Merideth J, Pluth JR, Trusty J: Permanent pacemaker infections: characterization and management. *Am J Cardiol* 48(3):559–564, 1981.

Cox J, Krajden M: Cardiovascular manifestations of Lyme disease. *Am Heart J* 122(5):1449–1455, 1991.

Eldar M, Griffin JC, Abbott JA, Benditt D, Bhandari A, Herre JM, Benson DW, Scheinman MM: Permanent cardiac pacing in patients with the long QT syndrome. *J Am Coll Cardiol* 10(3):600–607, 1987.

Esscher E: Congenital complete heart block. *Acta Paediatrica Scandinavica* 70(1):131–136, 1981.

Fukushige J, Porter CB, Hayes DL, McGoon MD, Osborn MJ, Vlietstra RE: Antitachycardia pacemaker treatment of postoperative arrhythmias in pediatric patients. *Pacing Clin Electrophysiol* 14(4 Pt.1): 546–556, 1991.

Furman S, Pannizzo F, Campo I: Comparison of active and passive adhering leads for endocardial pacing. *Pacing Clin Electrophysiol* 2(4):417–427, 1979.

Gillette PC, Edgerton J, Kratz J, Zeigler V: The subpectoral pocket: the preferred implant site for pediatric pacemakers. *Pacing Clin Electrophysiol* 14(7): 1089–1092. 1991.

Gillette PC, Zeigler VL, Case CL, Harold M, Buckles DS: Atrial antitachycardia pacing in children and young adults. *Am Heart J* 122(3Pt.1):844–849, 1991.

Gregoratos G, Cheitlin MD, Conill A, Epstein AE, Fellows C, Ferguson TB Jr, Freedman RA, Hlatky MA, Naccarelli GV, Saksena S, Schlant RC, Silka MJ: ACC/AHA guidelines for implantation of cardiac pacemakers and antiarrhythmia devices: executive summary—a report of the American College of Cardiology/American Heart Association Task Force on Practice Guidelines (Committee on Pacemaker Implantation). *Circulation* 97(13):1325–1335, 1998.

Haskell RJ, French WJ: Optimum AV interval in dual chamber pacemakers. *Pacing Clin Electrophysiol* 9(5):670–675, 1986.

Janosik DL, Pearson AC, Buckingham TA, Labovitz AJ, Redd RM: The hemodynamic benefit of differential atrioventricular delay intervals for sensed and paced atrial events during physiologic pacing. *J Am Coll Cardiol* 14(2):499–507, 1989.

Kertesz N, McQuinn T, Collins E, Friedman R: Surgical atrioventricular block in 888 congenital heart operations: new implications for early implantation of a permanent pacemaker [abstract]. *Pacing Clin Electrophysio* 19:613, 1996.

Lillehei CW, Sellers RD, Bonnanbeau RC, et al: Chronic post-surgical complete heart block. *J Cardiovasc Surg* (Torino) 46:436–456, 1973.

Michaelson M, Engle MA: Congenital complete heart block: an international study of the natural history, in: Brest AN, Engle MA (eds): *Cardiovascular Clinics*. Philadelphia, PA, FA Davis, 1972, pp. 85–101.

Ott DA, Gillette PC, Cooley DA: Atrial pacing via the subxiphoid approach. *Tex Heart Inst J* 9:149–152, 1982.

Parsonnet V, Bernstein AD, Lindsay B: Pacemaker-implantation complication rates: an analysis of some contributing factors. *J Am Coll Cardiol* 13(4): 917–921, 1989.

Pinsky WW, Gillette PC, Garson A Jr, McNamara DG: Diagnosis, management, and long-term results of patients with congenital complete atrioventricular block. *Pediatrics* 69(6):728–733, 1982.

Sholler GF, Walsh EP: Congenital complete heart block in patients without anatomic cardiac defects. *Am Heart J* 118(6):1193–1198, 1989.

St John Sutton MG, Plappert T, Abraham WT, Smith AL, DeLurgio DB, Leon AR, Loh E, Kocovic DZ, Fisher WG, Ellestad M, Messenger J, Kruger K, Hilpisch KE, Hill MR: Multicenter InSync Randomized Clinical Evaluation (MIRACLE) Study Group. Effect of cardiac resynchronization therapy on left ventricular size and function in chronic heart failure. *Circulation* 107(15):1985–1990, 2003.

49

PEDIATRIC CARDIAC SURGERY

Joanne P. Starr and Emile Bacha

INTRODUCTION

Few pediatricians and other primary care providers have patients with congenital or acquired heart abnormalities. Similarly, few primary care providers have ever had the opportunity to observe a congenital heart surgical procedure, especially in the neonate or infant. It is important to have some familiarity with congenital heart defects and the more common surgical interventions to correct or palliate these defects. In this chapter, an overview of congenital cardiac surgery is given, along with some of the major surgical procedures, their risks and benefits. The general postoperative care both early and late will also be discussed. Surgical interventions for specific heart lesions are mentioned in chapters discussing the lesion.

A GENERAL OVERVIEW
OF CONGENITAL HEART SURGERY

The field of pediatric surgery is very different than adult surgery on many levels with the most important difference being that small changes in perioprative management may have significant impact on the patient, some of which can be life threatening. Congenital heart surgery is unique compared to other fields of pediatric surgery because of the hemodynamic effects of the lesions themselves and the use of cardiopulmonary bypass (CPB).

Dr. Robert Gross performed the first congenital heart surgical procedure—ligation of a patent ductus arteriosus (PDA) in a 7-year-old girl in 1938 at Boston Children's Hospital. Shortly thereafter, in 1944 Henry Blalock and Helen Taussig reported their treatment of pulmonic stenosis and pulmonic atresia with a systemic-to-pulmonary shunt in three children (actually pioneered by Vivian Thomas). Open-heart surgical procedures began with the closure of an atrial septal defect using immersion hypothermia and inflow occlusion in 1952 by Dr. John Lewis at the University of Minnesota. In 1953 John Gibbons at Temple University developed the screen oxygenator and this was followed by the closure of a ventricular septal defect using cross-circulation by C. Walton Lillihei at the University of Minnesota, thus marking the beginning of cardiopulmonary bypass. Over the following 30 years, many modifications were made to the cardiopulmonary bypass circuit. In the early 1980s Dr. Aldo Castaneda and Sir Brian Barrett-Boyes introduced deep hypothermic circulatory arrest (DHCA) thereby facilitating the repair of complex lesions in neonates and young infants.

Since 1938, many advances have been made in congenital heart surgery, especially in neonates, with the most significant being the shift from palliative surgery to complete correction. In addition, technical advances have been made with regard to the conduct of cardiopulmonary bypass and postoperative management, which have improved overall morbidity and mortality. With this improvement in overall outcome, there is a new focus being placed on late outcomes, both cardiac as well as neurodevelopmental and psychosocial. As a final result, there is now a growing population of patients (adults) with congenital heart disease.

CLASSIFICATION OF CONGENITAL HEART SURGICAL PROCEDURES

There are many ways to group the different types of congenital heart surgical procedures. They can be subdivided into procedures for excessive pulmonary blood flow, procedures for too little pulmonary blood flow, and procedures to relieve left-sided obstruction. These three groups can further be subdivided into palliative versus complete repair and closed versus open (Figure 49-1) procedures.

Palliative procedures are those procedures, which alter the hemodynamic physiology of the particular defect so that patient can tolerate the defect in order to grow or to withstand another clinical problem (e.g., pulmonary artery banding in a patient with RSV pneumonia). Complete repair are those repairs where the defect is repaired definitively (e.g., closure of a ventricular septal defect) or the last stage in a series is completed (e.g., Fontan in a child with hypoplastic left heart syndrome).

Closed and open procedures are based on whether or not they employ cardiopulmonary bypass (heart-lung pump). Closed procedures do not employ the use of cardiopulmonary bypass and include procedures such as PDA ligation, standard coarctation repair, Blalock-Taussig shunts (BT shunt), or pulmonary artery banding. "Open" or open-heart procedures are those that employ the use of cardiopulmonary bypass with varying degrees of hypothermia. Cardiopulmonary bypass is used to repair intracardiac anomalies (e.g., ventricular septal defects, transposition of the great

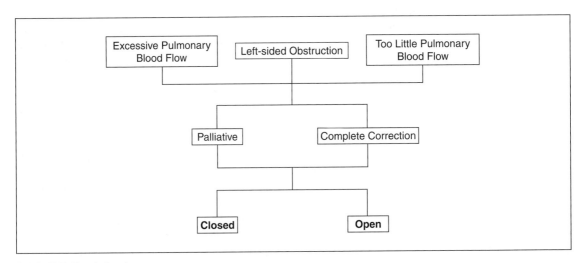

FIGURE 49-1

CONGENITAL HEART SURGICAL PROCEDURES

vessels, atrioventricular canal defects). In addition, cardiopulmonary bypass may be used in special cases for a normally closed procedure such as a BT shunt when the patient's hemodynamic status is compromised (e.g., severe tetralogy of Fallot).

There is a great deal of overlap between these different subgroups. For instance a pulmonary artery banding is a procedure done for excessive pulmonary blood flow. It is palliative and it is usually performed as a closed procedure.

PREOPERATIVE WORKUP

It is important that the patient with congenital heart disease be evaluated completely prior to undergoing surgery. This requires a thorough exam (including neurologic) and evaluation, which is usually orchestrated by the pediatric cardiologist. The evaluation may include some or all of the following: chest radiography, echocardiography, ECG, cardiac catheterization, and appropriate blood tests: complete blood count, electrolytes including blood urea nitrogen (BUN) and creatinine, coagulation profile, +/− liver function tests, thyroid function (especially in the trisomy 21 patients), and chromosomes including FISH, fluorescent in-situ hybridization chromosome test, for DiGeorge syndrome. Other important tests, some of which are more important in the neonate population include a baseline renal evaluation (approximately 3–6% of congenital heart defects are associated with renal defects)[1], a head ultrasound and the identification of any important syndromes. Appropriate evaluation of comorbid conditions needs to be completed as those conditions may affect or be affected by surgery. Social issues need to be identified as they may impact on the child's care. Once the evaluation is completed, the patient's case should be discussed and appropriate management decided. A formal conference, usually held weekly in most large congenital heart programs, is the usual forum for discussion. In these conferences, the patient's data are reviewed in a large group made up of pediatric cardiologists, congenital heart surgeon(s), pediatric anesthesiologists, pediatric intensivists, neonatologists, radiologists, nurses, physician assistants, residents and fellows, and social workers.

CARDIOPULMONARY BYPASS (CPB)

Cardiopulmonary Bypass Circuit

The cardiopulmonary bypass circuit is a form of extracorporeal circulation. It temporarily takes over the job of the heart (pumping) and lungs (gas exchange) while surgery takes place. The circuit consists of a nonpulsatile pump (roller or centrifugal), oxygenator, heat exchanger, venous reservoir, arterial filter, and the arterial and venous cannulae that enter the patient, and various monitors and alarms. The venous cannula (originating in the right atrium, superior or inferior cavae, or femoral vein) returns blood from the patient by gravity or suction to the pump venous reservoir. In addition, there are suction catheters and vents that return blood back to the venous reservoir. The blood then enters the oxygenator where gas exchange occurs. There is a temperature control and monitoring system at the oxygenator to either cool or warm the blood. The blood then leaves the oxygenator and goes through an arterial filter back to the patient (via the aorta, usually, or another major artery). A cardioplegia system is used when it is necessary to arrest the heart.

In order to run the circuit it is imperative to anticoagulate the patient with heparin. Adequate heparinization is monitored with measurement of the ACT (activated clotting time) throughout the period of cardiopulmonary bypass.

Cardiopulmonary bypass time is measured at the moment the patient is placed on pump until the time the patient is separated from the pump. Cross clamp time is the amount of time the heart is ischemic (no blood flow). Circulatory arrest time is that period of time where the body is completely off the pump and is usually referred to as deep hypothermic circulatory arrest (DHCA).

In neonates, infants, and small children (<10 kg) the circuit must be primed with blood. In older children and adults with an adequate hemoglobin or hematocrit, the pump can be primed with crystalloid.

The sequence of events in instituting standard cardiopulmonary bypass is the following:

A median sternotomy is performed, the pericardium opened, and systemic heparinization is carried out. Purse string sutures are placed in the ascending aorta and either right atrium or both caval veins. The aorta is cannulated followed by venous cannulation and the cannulae are attached to the cardiopulmonary bypass circuit. When the ACT is adequate (>400 seconds), the patient is placed on cardiopulmonary bypass and cooled to the desired temperature. The flows are slowly increased and until full flow reached (based on surface area of patient) at which time ventilation is stopped. A cardioplegia cannula is placed either into the ascending aorta or the coronary sinus. Snares are placed around both cavae if cannulated and the aorta is clamped between the aortic cannula and cardioplegia cannula. Cardioplegia (usually cold blood, high potassium) is then infused into the aortic root or coronary sinus and the heart is arrested during diastole. The cardioplegia is stopped and repeat doses are given at various time intervals depending on the length of cross clamp and surgeon preference.

The heart is opened where necessary and the intracardiac work performed. Once the heart is closed (the left ventricle no longer open to air), the heart is deaired and the cross clamp is removed thus marking the ending of the cross clamp time. The heart is allowed to recover adequate function and the patient is rewarmed. Meanwhile any additional right-sided work is completed, then hemostasis, placement of monitoring lines, and pacing wires if necessary.

Once the patient has rewarmed to 36°C, with an adequate repair and function (both visually and by transesophageal or surface echocardiogram), stable rhythm, and ventilation resumed, the patient is separated from cardiopulmonary bypass using inotropic support as needed. Protamine is administered to reverse the heparin followed by decannulation and achievement of hemostasis. Chest tubes are placed for postoperative drainage. When the surgeon is satisfied with hemostasis and adequacy of the repair, the chest is closed. Either heavy absorbable sutures or wires are used to reapproximate the sternum and the fascia, subcutaneous tissue and the skin is closed in layers of absorbable sutures.

Effects of Cardiopulmonary Bypass

The infant or child exposed to cardiopulmonary bypass is different compared to the adult. These differences include the following: smaller circulating blood volume, higher oxygen consumption rates, reactive pulmonary vascular bed, intracardiac and extracardiac shunting, immature organ systems (e.g., renal in the neonate), altered thermoregulation, and poor tolerance to microemboli. Because the infant or child has a much smaller blood volume, there is a large discrepancy between the size of the circuit (priming volume) versus the child's circulating blood volume. This can cause significant hemodilution of blood and coagulation factors. The decrease in circulating coagulation factors leads to a dilutional coagulopathy and increased risk of bleeding. Higher circuit flows are needed to meet the metabolic demands of the neonate and infant (up to 200 cc/kg/min).

Immature organ systems including the pulmonary bed require constant changes in management. The pulmonary bed in the infant has one-tenth the number of alveoli in the adult. The lungs in an infant are very susceptible to pulmonary edema and pulmonary vascular reactivity. The kidneys are immature with the ability to concentrate and dilute, handle sodium and manage acid-base balance limited. The liver's ability to produce vitamin-K-dependent clotting factors is impaired. The immune system is also immature with a low functioning complement system and dysfunctional mononuclear cells. Neurologic effects can be profound especially with prolonged DHCA longer than 30 min.

Global effects of cardiopulmonary bypass include the stress response, systemic inflammation, and endothelial injury.[2] Cardiopulmonary bypass leads to a number of reactions or responses in the body, which can significantly affect the patient postoperatively. These responses are a spectrum from mild to severe depending on the preoperative clinical status, complexity of the actual defect, length of cardiopulmonary bypass, cardiac ischemia, or circulatory arrest.

Systemic Inflammatory Response

One of the most impressive responses of the body to cardiopulmonary bypass is the systemic inflammatory response (SIR). SIR involves a complex interaction of systemic and cellular elements in the body. It begins with the exposure of blood to foreign surfaces (circuit and oxygenator). It is exacerbated by tissue ischemia and reperfusion, hypotension with nonpulsatile perfusion, relative anemia, blood product administration, and the heparin and protamine interaction. The complement system is activated which in turn activates neutrophils and other inflammatory mediators including cytokines, macrophages, and platelets. Neutrophil activation, especially in the pulmonary and neurologic beds can cause direct tissue injury. Overall, the effects of these events lead to endothelial injury. This results in elevation of pulmonary, cerebral, and systemic vascular resistances. Damage to the pulmonary endothelium causes the release of certain substances. The ability of the endothelium to metabolize other substances is impaired. The damage of the endothelium increases capillary permeability with the development of interstitial edema. This damage can be very severe, especially in the neonate.[2]

Myocardial Response

The cardiac effects of cardiopulmonary bypass depend on many factors. Those factors include the anatomical defect and physiology, preoperative function, the age of the patient, length of cardiopulmonary bypass and length if any of cardiac ischemia, and finally the type of myocardial protection. Those patients with long-standing cyanosis and subsequent development of bronchial collaterals are at risk of insufficient myocardial protection. The collaterals can cause increased blood return to the left heart with subsequent warming and washout of cardioplegia. The hypertrophied heart is another example of increased risk because of subendocardial ischemia. The age of the patient is an important factor. The immature myocardium is different structurally and functionally than an adult heart. It is less compliant and has less preload reserve. There is an exaggerated negative inotropic response to anesthetics especially in the neonate, therefore greater doses of inotropes are needed. Glucose and calcium are extremely important in the immature heart as well. Finally, long bypass and cross clamp times are associated with cardiac dysfunction especially when they are greater than 6 and 3 h, respectively.

Endocrine Response

Cardiopulmonary bypass has multiple effects on the endocrine system including native catecholamines, steroids, insulin, glucagons, growth hormone, and thyroid hormones. There is an increase in catecholamine release (greater than expected from surgery alone). This is augmented by peripheral vasoconstriction, lack of pulsatile flow, and acidosis during cardiopulmonary bypass. A surge of catecholamine occurs with reinflation of the lungs and during the rewarming phase postcirculatory arrest. Anesthesia has an important influence on these surges. High dose narcotic induction and maintenance has been shown to decrease the catecholamine response and reduce postoperative complications.[3]

Cortisol increases after induction of anesthesia and surgery. These levels decrease on CPB secondary to hemodilution. After CPB, the level increases for about 24 h, then decreases back to normal in the uncomplicated postoperative cardiac patient. There is a decrease in the level and response of insulin associated with CPB. This results in increases in serum glucose. The levels of insulin then increase after rewarming and reperfusion. As part of the general stress response, glucagon and growth hormone are released. Thyroid hormone changes with CPB has been recently examined.[4,5,6,7] Hemodilution, decreases in thyroid binding globulin and an increase in glucocorticoids are responsible. Very low levels have been associated with poor outcome.[5,8]

Renal

The general stress of surgery causes a decrease in renal blood flow and glomerular filtration. This is primarily a result of the central nervous system release of vasopressin that results in an overall fluid accumulation. The hypothermia during CPB decreases renal perfusion. Cortical blood flow in the kidney is decreased in exchange for medullary flow. Antidiuretic hormone (ADH) elevation in the uncomplicated postoperative patient may last 48–72 h. The renin-angiotensin system is activated thus increasing aldosterone and increased fractional excretion of potassium.

The duration of CPB and preoperative renal dysfunction are risk factors for postoperative renal dysfunction. Temporary renal dysfunction is not uncommon, especially in the neonate. This is usually self-limited unless continued postoperative low cardiac output persists. Some centers prophylactically insert peritoneal dialysis catheters in infants for postoperative dialysis if needed.

Neurologic

The neurologic effects of cardiopulmonary bypass are magnified in the congenital heart patient because of (1) preexisting risks associated with various congenital heart lesions (e.g., Down syndrome), (2) injury induced by CPB, (3) the "vulnerable" period after exposure to CPB.

The risk of abnormal neurologic development in patients with CHD even without correction of the lesion or cardiopulmonary bypass ranges from 2 to 10%. Patients with critical lesions such as hypoplastic left heart syndrome have been shown to have a decrease in cerebral blood flow before CPB, thus stratifying them into a high-risk group. The baseline condition of the patient prior to surgery is important to assess and may influence the neurologic outcome (e.g., episode of severe hypoperfusion and acidosis).

The conduct of CPB and the alterations it produces may affect neurologic injury. For instance, microembolic events are common. The use of membrane oxygenators, arterial filters, and adequate anticoagulation (heparinization) decreases the incidence of microemboli significantly. There is an increased risk of air emboli if the left-sided circulation is exposed.

Hypothermia and its effects on neurologic outcome have been examined closely after early experiences with deep hypothermia (esophageal temperature <10°C) demonstrated significant neurologic (choreoathetosis) and pulmonary injury. Because of this finding, most institutions limit temperatures to 18–20°C. Later studies suggested that it is not the actual temperature, but blood gas management during DHCA, duration of DHCA period (>60 min) and presence of collaterals, which produced these untoward outcomes. Most centers are now using low flow CPB as an alternative to DHCA to improve cerebral blood flow.

IV steroids (usually methylprednisolone) administered at least 8 h prior to CPB have been demonstrated to improve cerebral metabolic response to DHCA. Aprotonin a serine protease inhibitor first used in pancreatitis and now employed in cardiac surgery to decrease bleeding may also be protective. Other drugs under investigation in reducing neurologic injury during CPB include thromboxane A2 inhibitors, platelet activating factor inhibitors, and free radical scavengers.[2]

Pulmonary

The pulmonary parenchyma or vasculature may be affected by cardiopulmonary bypass. Changes in lung compliance occur owing to an increase in lung water from increased ventilatory support. There is also a decrease in the ability of the lung parenchyma to perform gas exchange. An increase in pulmonary vascular resistance is commonly seen. The inflammatory response to CPB is manifested by decreases in functional residual capacity, compliance, gas exchange and increased resistance and pulmonary artery pressures. The decrease in flow to the lungs when a patient is placed on CPB can cause ischemia to the lungs and subsequent pulmonary dysfunction secondary to pulmonary endothelial damage. This damage increases post-CPB pulmonary resistance and pressures, which can be extremely detrimental in certain situations (e.g., hypoplastic left heart syndrome). The use of steroids 8 h prior to bypass and in the circuit reduces lung water accumulation, improves post-CPB compliance and limits pulmonary hypertension post CPB. There is evidence to support the use of modified ultrafiltration post-CPB to improve lung function.[2]

CLOSED-HEART PROCEDURES

Closed-heart procedures are those that do not require the use of cardiopulmonary bypass; however, there are those instances (e.g., BT shunt) when a typical closed-heart procedure may become an open-heart procedure. The procedures and eponyms, their indications and complications are summarized in Tables 49-1–49-3.

Blalock Hanlon Septostomy

In 1950 Blalock and Hanlon reported their first clinical success with surgical creation of an atrial septal defect surgically in a patients with transposition of the great arteries (TGA).[9] An adequate atrial septal defect is necessary in any patient who has critical right ventricular or left ventricular inflow/outflow obstruction. The procedure is done via a right thoracotomy. The pericardium is opened and the pulmonary artery and veins are encircled and snared. A partial occluding clamp is placed so that portions of both the right and left atria are in the clamp. The atria are opened and the fossa ovalis identified and excised. This procedure is rarely done these days because balloon atrial septostomy/blade septectomy either with echo or angiographic guidance is the procedure of choice. If an atrial septectomy is necessary in the operating room, it is usually completed either on bypass or with inflow occlusion.

Brock Procedure

The Brock procedure is a procedure used to treat critical pulmonary stenosis.[10] It is a surgical pulmonary valvotomy without opening the heart. It is common to perform a shunt along with the procedure. A median sternotomy is performed and purse string sutures are placed in the anterior right ventricle. A small incision is made in the right ventricle and serial Hegar dilators are passed through the incision up through the pulmonary valve thus dilating the valve. If the valve is atretic it can be perforated with Brock knives followed by dilators. Surgical valvotomies can also be performed with inflow occlusion as well as with cardiopulmonary bypass. As with the Blalock and Hanlon procedure the Brock procedure is rarely performed today. Balloon angioplasty is usually the procedure of choice. Radiofrequency assisted balloon angioplasty is a newer technique that is being used as well.

Pulmonary Artery Banding

Pulmonary artery (PA) banding was first described in 1952 by Muller and Damman.[11] It served as palliation for children with a large left-to-right shunt such as a VSD or single ventricle to prevent pulmonary overcirculation and thus pulmonary vascular disease. Today it is performed as palliation for pulmonary

TABLE 49-1

CLOSED HEART PROCEDURES

Surgical Procedure	Indication	Complications
Blalock Hanlon	Critical RV/LV inflow/outflow obstruction with no clear palliation	Phrenic nerve injury, bleeding
Brock procedure	Critical pulmonary stenosis	Cardiac perforation
PA band	Pulmonary overcirculation with no other palliation possible	Band too loose or tight PA distortion
Coarctation repairs (see Table 49-2)		
Shunts (see Table 49-3)		

TABLE 49-2

PROCEDURES FOR COARCTATION OF THE AORTA*

Procedure	Advantages	Disadvantages
End-to-end anastamosis	Removes ductal tissue Will grow with patient (no foreign material) Extended to relieve isthmic hyoplasia	Higher recurrence in neonates— especially if not extended Requires extensive dissection/mobilization
Patch angioplasty	Less extensive dissection Allows correction of arch Hypoplasia/isthmus	Patch will not grow with patient Higher risk of aneurysm Foreign material
Subclavian flap	Will grow with patient (no foreign material) Allows enlargement of isthmus	Sacrifice subclavian artery—see limb growth abnormality
Bypass graft	No need for aortic cross clamp Minimal dissection	Does not address all areas of aorta Will not grow (may narrow at surture lines also) Foreign material
Interposition graft	Removes ductal tissue	Does not address arch hyoplasia Does not grow with patient (may narrow at suture lines also) Foreign material

Postoperative Complications Following Coarctation Repair

Complication	Definition	Incidence	Treatment
Paradoxical hypertension	Systemic hypertension— increased catecholamines, derangement of renin- angiotension axis, disrupted baroreceptors	Up to 30% less common in <5 years	Sedation, analgesia B-blockers, nipride, Ace inhibitors
Postcoarctectomy syndrome	Bowel ischemia—mesenteric ischemia, reflex vasoconstriction or reintroduction of pusatile flow and subsequent vessel injury	0-10% More common in older patients	Bowel rest-NPO, NGT decompression, IV fluids
Spinal cord ischemia	Paraplegia—minimal collaterals, intrinsic Anatomy of anterior spinal artery	0.4% Rare in neonates, infants	Treatment limited—evoked potentials, left atrial to left femoral artery bypass in high risk patients
Residual coarctation	Systolic gradient >20 mmHg inadequate repair, ductal remodeling, younger age at repair		Balloon angioplasty/stent or if unsuccessful repeat surgery

*There may be a risk to recurrent laryngeal nerve in any of these.

TABLE 49-3

SHUNTS TO PROVIDE OR INCREASE PULMONARY BLOOD FLOW

Procedure	Advantages	Disadvantages/Complications
Waterston	Easy to place	Uncontrolled pulmonary blood flow—development of pulmonary vascucular disease Distortion of right pulmonary artery
Potts	No real advantage	Uncontrolled pulmonary blood flow—development of pulmonary vascucular disease Distortion of left pulmonary artery Very difficult to take down
Blalock Taussig (Classic)	Controlled pulmonary blood flow Grows with patient	Mild pulmonary artery distortion at site of insertion Sacrifice subclavian artery—limb growth abnormality
(Modified)	Controlled pulmonary blood flow	Mild pulmonary artery distortion at site of insertion Avoids sacrificing subclavian artery Will not grow with patient Thrombosis
Glenn	Will grow with patient	Increased risk of items listed below Cannot be used in neonates, need low PVR

All may be complicated by Horner syndrome, phrenic nerve injury, chylothorax.

overcirculation (cyanotic or acyanotic) when a more definitive procedure cannot be completed, such as a sick infant with large VSD unable to undergo cardiopulmonary bypass. The procedure can be performed either via a left thoracotomy or median sternotomy. Any one of a number of materials can be used for banding (plaited silk, Mersilene, Teflon, Silastic). Care is taken to place the band around the main pulmonary artery and not impinge the right or left pulmonary arteries or the pulmonary valve. The patient should be ventilated on 50% oxygen and the pulmonary artery pressure distal to the band should be approximately half the systemic pressure (gradient across band 30–60 mmHg depending on the lesion) with saturations in the 75–85% range. Once the band is in place, it is secured to the pulmonary artery adventitia so that it does not migrate. Postoperative care of these patients can be quite challenging until the ventricle adjusts to the increased afterload. Postoperatively, patients are followed for increasing hypoxia, ventricular hypertrophy, and subvalvar stenosis. Debanding is performed at the

next stage. Once the band is removed the pulmonary artery usually requires arterioplasty either with native tissue or with a patch of pericardium or prosthetic material. Any associated branch stenosis is addressed at the same time.

Recently, bilateral pulmonary artery banding and stenting of the ductus in hypoplastic left heart syndrome patients has been performed in some centers as an alternative to a Stage I Norwood procedure. The reconstruction of the aorta is then performed at the time of the bidirectional Glenn. In addition, there is ongoing development of an of internal adjustable pulmonary artery band which can be placed during cardiac catheterization.

Shunts

Shunts are created to provide or increase pulmonary blood flow. Blalock and Taussig first reported the use of a systemic-to-pulmonary artery shunt in three patients with pulmonary stenosis or atresia in 1945. The classic BT shunt is created by division of the subclavian artery (left or right) and anastomosis to the ipsilateral pulmonary artery (end to side). Today, most BT shunts are performed using a prosthetic graft made out of Gore-Tex (modified BT shunt, sizes ranging from 3.5 to 5.0 mm for a newborn). Both classic and modified shunts are performed either through a thoracotomy or median sternotomy and are a type of peripheral arterial shunt. Cardiopulmonary bypass may be necessary in the unstable patient. Closure of the modified or classic BT shunt is performed with either suture or hemaclip ligation and subsequent division.

A Potts shunt is a central arterial shunt created between the left pulmonary artery and descending aorta. It is performed through a left thoracotomy. Distortion of the pulmonary artery is common. It is much more difficult to take down than the BT shunt in that a short period of circulatory arrest is usually needed with iliac or femoral arterial cannulation. It is rarely used today.

Like the Potts shunt a Waterson shunt is also a central arterial shunt and is rarely performed today in the classic sense. It is created between the right pulmonary artery and ascending aorta and can be performed via a right thoracotomy or median sternotomy on or off bypass. Today, it is usually performed using a Gore-Tex graft and is referred to as a "central shunt" and is between the ascending aorta and either the left or right pulmonary artery. As with the Potts shunt the classic Waterson can cause distortion of the pulmonary artery but it is less difficult to take down especially when performed using a Gore-Tex tube graft.

An important complication of shunts is thrombosis. It is a life-threatening event if there is no other source of pulmonary blood flow. The standard resuscitation protocol of ABCs (airway, breathing, circulation) should be carried out. This is the one time 100% oxygen can be given to a patient with a shunt. Heparin should be started. If the ductus is not ligated or divided and the child is less than 6 weeks old a prostaglandin E infusion should be started immediately. If feasible, an urgent cardiac catheterization should be performed with possible urgent surgical intervention. Catheter interventions (balloon angioplasty and instillation of thrombolytics) have been reported to restore flow in these shunts. It is not uncommon to begin prophylactic anticoagulation, either low dose heparin or low molecular weight heparin (Lovenox) with transition to aspirin. If a thrombosis occurs, workup for a coagulation disorder is indicated.

Other early postoperative complications include infection, bleeding, chylothorax, and nerve damage (recurrent, phrenic, and sympathetic ganglion leading to Horner syndrome). The overall mortality for shunts is low and influenced by the clinical status, congenital lesion, and type of shunt.

The long-term effects of shunts will vary according to whether they are central or peripheral. Both types have the potential to cause pulmonary overcirculation. This is especially true in as the pulmonary vascular resistance decreases after the newborn period. It is more common to see this overcirculation with central shunts. This tends to lessen with time as the size of the systemic bed increases relative to the fixed size of the shunt.

Pulmonary artery stenosis is another complication of shunts. Complete discontinuity of the pulmonary arteries is not uncommonly seen. As the ductus involutes it can affect the area of the bifurcation of the branch pulmonary arteries and cause complete discontinuity. Cardiac catheterization is performed prior to subsequent surgeries not only to assess the pulmonary artery pressures but also the pulmonary artery anatomy to rule out stenosis. If there is significant stenosis it can be addressed at the next stage of surgery.

Finally, the Glenn shunt[12] is a venous-to-arterial shunt and is an end to side anastomosis of the divided superior vena cava (SVC) to the distal end of the divided right pulmonary artery with closure of the superior veno-cavoatrial junction. In 1972, Azzolina described a modification of this cavopulmonary shunt and named it a bidirectional Glenn.[13] In this procedure, the end of the divided SVC is anastomosed to the side of the RPA. The branch pulmonary artery continuity is preserved, thus the term "bidirectional (Figure 49-2)." Both of these procedures are usually performed via a median sternotomy but can also be performed via a right thoracotomy. The classic Glenn is rarely performed today. Postoperative issues after a Glenn include narrowing of the anastomosis, bradycardia and sinus node injury, elevated SVC and intracranial pressure

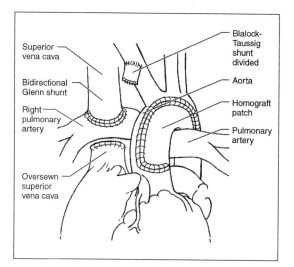

FIGURE 49-2

BIDIRECTIONAL GLENN SHUNT SUPERIOR CAVA TO PULMONARY ARTERY (CAVA PULMONARY SHUNT)

Source: Reitz B, Yuh D. *Congenital Cardiac Surgery.* New York: McGraw-Hill; 2001.

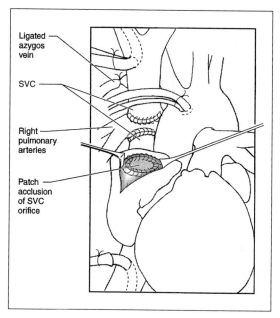

FIGURE 49-3
HEMI-FONTAN PROCEDURE

Bidirectional Glenn-cardiac end of transected SVC is anastomosed to inferior surface of right pulmonary artery. Through a right atriotomy a Gore-Tex patch is sewn over SVC-right atrial oriface.

Source: Reitz B, Yuh D. *Congenital Cardiac Surgery.* New York: McGraw-Hill; 2001.

(owing to increased pulmonary vascular resistance), hypoxemia, and chylothorax. Long term, aorto-pulmonary collaterals can occur. This is thought to be secondary to lack of hepatic factor in the lungs, as the inferior vena cava (IVC) flow does not go to the lungs. Prerequisites for a successful Glenn are a patent and adequate size SVC, adequate pulmonary vessels, and low pulmonary vascular resistance. In the presence of elevated pulmonary resistance or anatomical obstruction, there will be obstruction to forward flow and subsequent elevation of superior central venous and intracranial pressures.

The Hemi-Fontan is a variant of the Glenn. At the time of the Glenn, both the cranial and cardiac ends of the transected SVC are anastomosed to the superior and inferior surfaces of the right pulmonary artery, respectively, and then a patch closure of the SVC-right atrial connection is performed (Figure 49-3). At the Fontan procedure (lateral tunnel modification) the patch is removed and the lateral tunnel is constructed, thereby eliminating one suture line. The Hemi-Fontan is now also being performed in preparation for a percutaneous Fontan done in the cardiac catheterization lab.

Coarctation of Aorta

Surgical correction of coarctation of the aorta is usually performed via a left thoracotomy. In cases where the patient is unstable or if there are other cardiac lesions such as VSD or hypoplastic left heart, a median sternotomy is performed. Various surgical repairs have been described. Today the most commonly used repairs are the end-to-end repair or subclavian flap repair. Table 49-2 outlines surgical procedures employed for repair of coarctation of the aorta and the advantages and disadvantages. Complications after coarctation repair (in addition to the standard infection and bleeding) include paradoxic hypertension, postcoarctectomy syndrome, spinal cord ischemia, residual coarctation, low cardiac output, chylothorax, and injury to surrounding structures (i.e., recurrent laryngeal, phrenic, Horner's syndrome-stellate ganglion-sympathetic injury).

TABLE 49-4
OPEN HEART PROCEDURES

Procedure	Indication	Special Pros/Cons
Ross	Aortic valve disease	Need to replace pulmonary homograft Long-term potential of neo-aortic valve unknown Risk of heart block
Konno	Aortic valve hypoplasia Sub AS	Need a prosthetic aortic valve Risk of heart block
Damus	Aortic arch hypoplasia D-TGA/VSD, sub AS	Aortic valve problems Coronary ischemia
Fontan	Single ventricle	Baffle obstruction Thrombus Effusions, PLE
Norwood	HLHS, single ventricles	Three surgeries, risks are for the components of each surgery

OPEN-HEART PROCEDURES

There are many different types of open-heart procedures. These procedures are discussed in individual chapters with heart defects. Some of these procedures have associated eponyms, which are discussed below and summarized in Tables 49-4 and 49-5.

Ross Procedure (Pulmonary Autograft)

In 1962, Donald Ross reported in *Lancet* on the first successful aortic valve replacement with an

TABLE 49-5
OPEN HEART PROCEDURES—FOR TGA

Procedure	Advantages	Disadvantages
Jatene (ASO)	Should grow with patient Restores normal physiology	Coronary artery distortion—early Pulmonary artery narrowing of distortion—late Technically challenging

Rastelli	Allows appropriate ventricles	May develop LV to aortic baffle
		  obstruction—does not grow
		Need to replace RV to PA
		  conduit

Senning	Senning or Mustard may be combined
	  with Rastelli for the "double switch"
	  procedure for corrected transposition
		Systemic ventricle is the RV
		  Atrial dysrhythmia
		  Baffle problems

Mustard	Senning or Mustard may be combined
	  with Rastelli for the "double switch"
	  procedure for corrected transposition
		Systemic ventricle is the RV Atrial
		  dysrhythmia Baffle problems

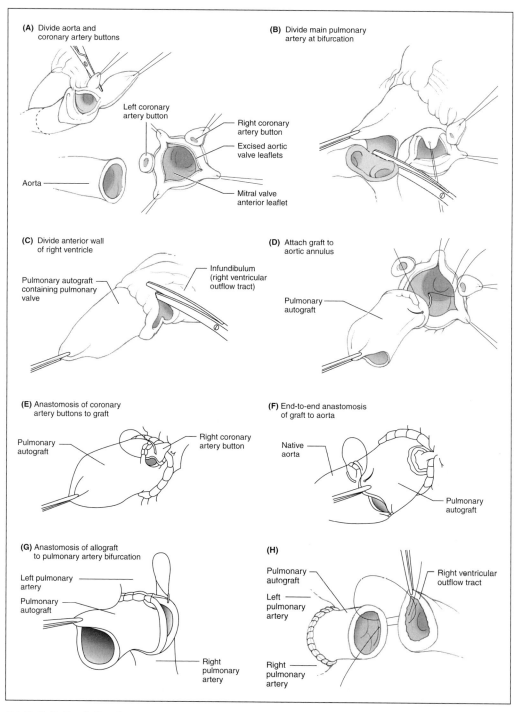

(A) Divide aorta and coronary artery buttons

Left coronary artery button

Right coronary artery button

Excised aortic valve leaflets

Aorta

Mitral valve anterior leaflet

(B) Divide main pulmonary artery at bifurcation

(C) Divide anterior wall of right ventricle

Pulmonary autograft containing pulmonary valve

Infundibulum (right ventricular outflow tract)

(D) Attach graft to aortic annulus

Pulmonary autograft

(E) Anastomosis of coronary artery buttons to graft

Pulmonary autograft

Right coronary artery button

(F) End-to-end anastomosis of graft to aorta

Native aorta

Pulmonary autograft

(G) Anastomosis of allograft to pulmonary artery bifurcation

Left pulmonary artery

Pulmonary autograft

Right pulmonary artery

(H)

Pulmonary autograft

Left pulmonary artery

Right pulmonary artery

Right ventricular outflow tract

F I G U R E   4 9 - 4

ROSS PROCEDURE

Source: Reitz B, Yuh D. *Congenital Cardiac Surgery.* New York: McGraw-Hill; 2001.

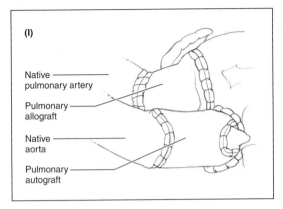

(I)

Native pulmonary artery

Pulmonary allograft

Native aorta

Pulmonary autograft

FIGURE 49-4

(Continued)

aortic valve homograft.[14] Five years later, he described the technique of aortic valve replacement with a pulmonary autograft, now known as the Ross procedure.[15] The Ross procedure is the replacement of aortic valve with the patient's native pulmonary valve and subsequent replacement of the patient's pulmonary valve with a homograft (pulmonary or aortic). (Figure 49-4). It is a technically challenging procedure; however, it has excellent hemodynamic performance, avoids anticoagulation and allows somatic growth. In children it may be preferred because of its potential to grow with the patient and the fact that anticoagulation is not necessary. It is also a good option for the young active adult, the childbearing female, or the adult less than 50 years. Contraindications to the use of the pulmonary autograft include significant pulmonic regurgitation or pathology, Marfan syndrome or any other collagen disorder. Relative contraindications include significant size discrepancy between native pulmonic and aortic valves and multivalvular rheumatic disease.

Operative mortality is low and comparable with that of mechanical or bioprosthetic valves. Long-term survival (20 years) is 80% or greater.[16] Risk of late valve failure requiring reoperation for either autograft valve or homograft valve is low. The

reported freedom from autograft replacement is 85% at 20 years and freedom from all related events of 70% at 20 years. More recent data reports 89% actuarial freedom from reintervention for both autograft and homograft at 5 years and 92% for the autograft alone.[17,18,19] Complications include bleeding, coronary ischemia, aortic insufficiency, ventricular dysfunction, and early replacement of the pulmonary homograft.

A "double Ross" procedure is where the pulmonary autograft used to replace the aortic valve as in a standard Ross, but the native aortic valve is removed, reconstructed, and then used in the pulmonary location.

Konno-Rastan Procedure (Aortoventriculoplasty)

A Konno procedure is performed in patients with a small or hypoplastic aortic valve annulus or subvalvar obstruction. A longitudinal incision is made in the aorta and continued across the aortic annulus into the ventricular septum (Figure 49-5). A diamond-shaped patch (pericardium, Dacron, or Gore-Tex) is used to close the septal incision across the annulus to the aorta thereby enlarging the aortic annulus. The aortic valve-autograft (Ross-Konno), homograft, or prosthetic valve is then sutured to the patch as well as the remainder of the circumference of the aortic annulus. Another patch is then used to close the right ventriculotomy. Complications include bleeding, injury to the conduction system, coronary ostia injury, myocardial infarction from division of the first septal perforator, and patch dehiscence. These complications are reduced in the hands of experienced surgeons.[20]

DAMUS-KAYE-STANSEL (DKS)

The DKS procedure was first described for repair of d-TGA/VSD with subpulmonic stenosis. The pulmonary artery is transected above the valve and the proximal end is anastomosed to the side of

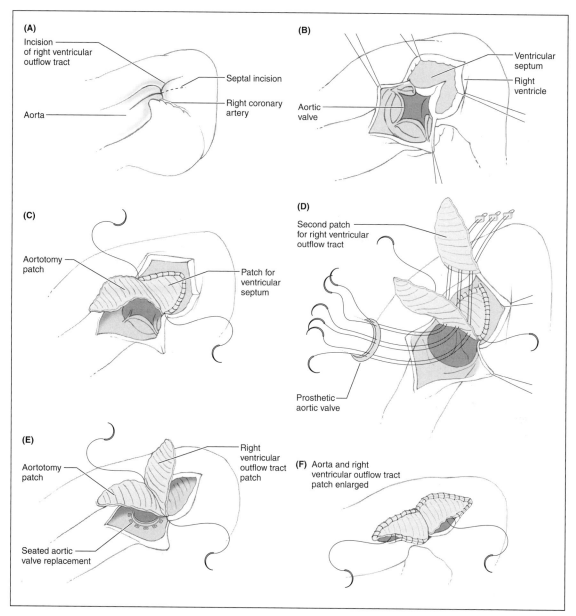

FIGURE 49-5

KONNO-RASTAN AORTOVENTRICULOPLASTY AND AORTIC VALVE REPLACEMENT

Source: Reitz B, Yuh D. *Congenital Cardiac Surgery.* New York: McGraw-Hill; 2001.

ascending aorta (Figure 49-6). In TGA, the aortic valve is closed and an external conduit is placed from a right ventriculotomy to the distal pulmonary artery. Modifications of the original procedure are now used in those patients with single ventricles and TGA. It allows both great vessels and semilunar valves to provide unobstructed flow to the body. The DKS is part of the Norwood Stage I

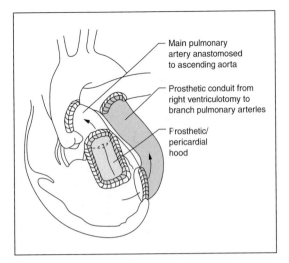

FIGURE 49-6

Damus Kaye Stansel (DKS) and Right Ventricle to Pulmonary artery conduit for d-TGA/VSD and Subpulmonic stenosis.

Source: Reitz B, Yuh D. *Congenital Cardiac Surgery.* New York: McGraw-Hill; 2001.

procedure. The transected pulmonary artery anastomosed to the aorta in combination with the reconstructed aortic arch and descending aorta provides flow from the single ventricle to the body (Figure 49-7). Pulmonary blood flow in the Norwood procedure is established with a RV-PA conduit or BT shunt. Disadvantages include aortic valve regurgitation and thrombus formation, coronary ischemia, and periodic conduit changes when a conduit is used.

Norwood Procedure

The Norwood procedure was first described by William Norwood in 1983 as the first stage procedure for hypoplastic left heart syndrome.[21] It is now applied for most single ventricle lesions (anatomic or physiologic). The purpose of the procedure is to provide reliable, unobstructed flow to both the systemic and pulmonary beds. The procedure includes ligation and division of the ductus arteriosus and transection of the main pulmonary artery proximal to the bifurcation. The pulmonary artery bifurcation is usually closed with an autologous pericar-

dial patch. The proximal main pulmonary artery is anastomosed to the aorta and the aorta is reconstructed using a homograft thus addressing the hypoplasia/ atresia and coarctation. Pulmonary blood flow is reestablished with either a BT shunt/central shunt or a RV to PA conduit. In addition, an atrial septectomy is performed to ensure unobstructed pulmonary venous flow, unless an ASD is already present. The surgery is usually completed with deep hypothermic circulatory arrest; however, it is becoming more common to use low flow hypothermic cardiopulmonary bypass or even beating heart bypass.

The care of these patients postoperatively can be one of the more challenging aspects of congenital heart surgery. Maintenance of balanced pulmonary and systemic blood flow in light of labile pulmonary artery pressures can be difficult. Globally depressed cardiac function is not uncommon postoperatively. Sudden death can occur from significant coronary ischemia or pulmonary hypertensive crisis.

The next stage of surgery is usually the bidirectional Glenn as described above. This is completed anywhere from 3–4 to 8 months of age depending on the patient.

Fontan Procedure

Fontan described this procedure in patients with tricuspid atresia in 1971.[22] This is a total cavopulmonary connection—all systemic venous return is directed to the pulmonary bed thus bypassing the right atrium. There have been multiple modifications of this procedure over the last two decades including conduits, atriopulmonary connections, intermediate cavopulmonary connections extracardiac conduits, and fenestrations. In addition, improved patient selection and postoperative management have contributed to reducing the operative mortality to less than 10%. Focus is now on decreasing the morbidity associated with the procedure and potential long-term durability of the procedure.[23]

The most commonly employed modifications of the Fontan procedure are the lateral tunnel and extracardiac techniques. Both techniques can be done with or without a fenestration. The lateral

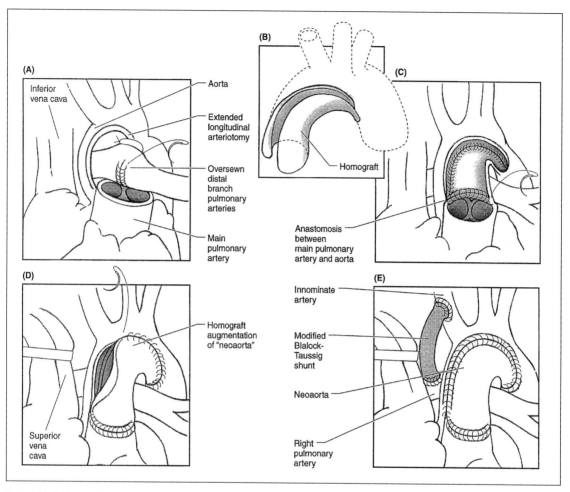

FIGURE 49-7

Norwood Stage I for hypoplastic left heart syndrome. (C) DKS portion—anastomosis between main pulmonary artery and aorta.

Source: Reitz B, Yuh D. *Congenital Cardiac Surgery.* New York: McGraw-Hill; 2001.

tunnel is completed via a right atriotomy and is made usually from Gore-Tex. The tunnel directs/baffles the systemic venous return to the already established Glenn circuit (Figure 49-8). The tunnel may be fenestrated to allow blood to shunt right to left to assure adequate cardiac output (e.g., high pulmonary pressures).

The extracardiac modification is performed using a valveless homograft, Gore-Tex tube graft, or autologous pericardium. It is performed by

transection of the IVC from the right atrium and anastomosis of the proximal end to the tube graft. The cephalic end of the tube graft is then anastomosed to the Glenn. As with the lateral tunnel modification a fenestration may or may not be performed (Figure 49-9).

Criteria for a successful Fontan include (1) adequate cardiac function of the single ventricle, (2) sinus rhythm, (3) normal pulmonary artery resistance and pressures, (4) good pulmonary

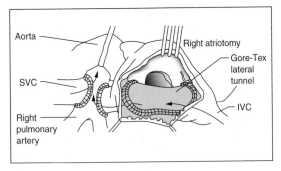

FIGURE 49-8

MODIFIED FONTAN—INTRACARDIAC LATERAL
TUNNEL TECHNIQUE

Source: Reitz B, Yuh D. *Congenital Cardiac Surgery.*
New York: McGraw-Hill; 2001.

artery anatomy, (5) minimal to no AV valve regurgitation, and (6) no obstruction to systemic outflow (e.g., residual coarctation). The procedure is usually performed any where from 18 months to 2 or 3 years of age. The fenestration, if present, is usually electively closed in the cardiac catheterization lab.

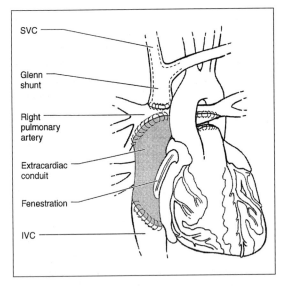

FIGURE 49-9

MODIFIED FONTAN—EXTRACARDIAC TECHNIQUE
TUNNEL

Source: Reitz B, Yuh D. *Congenital Cardiac Surgery.*
New York: McGraw-Hill; 2001.

Early postoperative complications include arrhythmias, low cardiac output, pulmonary hypertension, thrombosis, and persistent pleural effusions/chylothorax (less so with fenestrated Fontans). Late complications include Fontan obstruction, thrombosis, protein losing enteropathy, and arrhythmias.

PROCEDURES FOR D-TRANSPOSITION OF THE GREAT ARTERIES

Mustard, Senning, Arterial Switch, Rastelli

Surgical treatment of d-TGA can be divided into atrial, ventricular and arterial level switch operations. The Senning (1959) and Mustard (1964) procedures preceded and essentially have been replaced by Jatene's arterial switch (1975).[24,25,26]

Both the Senning and Mustard are atrial level switch operations. In other words, they direct the systemic venous return to the left side (mitral valve, LV, and PA) and the pulmonary venous return to the right side (tricuspid valve, RV, and aorta) thus physiologically correcting the transposition. The Mustard procedure uses pericardium or prosthetic material (Gore-Tex or Dacron) to baffle the systemic and the pulmonary venous systems to their appropriate AV valve and ventricle. The Senning directs the appropriate venous flow using the native (autologous) atrium. Initial results were favorable with the Mustard and Senning; however, many late complications have been observed. These include the following: atrial arrhythmias, AV valve regurgitation especially tricuspid, and baffle obstruction and leaks. The most important and significant long-term complication is morphologic right ventricular failure (10% incidence over 10 years). The right ventricle becomes the systemic ventricle and is prone to early failure.

Because of complications seen with the Mustard and Senning procedures, the Jatene arterial switch operation (ASO) has become the preferred surgical treatment for d-TGA in most cardiac centers. This procedure switches the great arteries and transfers the coronaries, thus keeping the left ventricle as the systemic ventricle. It is important that the procedure be done within the first 2 months of life to prevent deconditioning of the left ventricle and postoperative failure. Patients presenting with d-TGA later usually will undergo pulmonary artery banding to "condition" the LV prior to undergoing the arterial switch. Early complications seen after arterial switch include ischemia (coronary injury) and poor LV compliance. Late complications include coronary issues and supravalvar pulmonic stenosis and branch pulmonary artery stenosis. The overall early and late results for the arterial switch are quite good.

The Rastelli procedure (1969) was developed initially to anatomically correct d-TGA associated with a ventricular septal defect and pulmonary stenosis (valvar or subvalvar).[27] The ventricular septal defect becomes the left ventricular outflow tract via a patch baffle to the aorta. The pulmonary artery is divided and the stenotic valve is closed. A conduit, usually a homograft, is brought from the RV to the divided pulmonary artery. Initial results with the Rastelli were quite poor but have improved significantly. A restrictive VSD or anomalous connections of the tricuspid valve to the infundibular septum are relative contraindications to the procedure. Enlargement of the VSD is possible. Postoperative complications similar to other complex repairs include: residual VSD, arrhythmias, and myocardial dysfunction. In the long term, the conduit requires replacement as the child grows, and there may be obstruction of the internal baffle.

POSTOPERATIVE CARE

Postoperative problems associated with congenital heart surgery are in part related to preoperative anatomy, patient risk variables (associated problems such as renal failure, lung disease, and poor nutritional state) as well from the effects of CPB on an already compromised heart. Complications from specific procedures are as noted above. Special problems include postpericardiotomy syndrome or infection.

The postoperative care of the congenital heart surgery patient is one of the more demanding and time consuming jobs in the pediatric surgery subspecialty arena and can be quite challenging to even the most expert of physicians. It can be performed by the surgeon, a critical care physician or more recently by a cardiac intensivist (cardiologist with intensive care specialization). Alternatively, a multidisciplinary team of the above specialists may provide the care. A pediatric cardiac surgeon is always on call, as there are certain procedures that can be performed only by a surgeon (e.g., extracorporeal membrane oxygenation (ECMO) or emergent cardiotomy). In addition to the physicians, there are additional staff that are required to complete the team. These include specialized ICU nurses, preferably with training in the care of congenital heart surgery patients, respiratory therapists, pharmacologists, nutritionists, social workers, as well as availability of speech, occupational and physical therapists.

It is important that the cardiac ICU have available the necessary environment and equipment that is necessary to care for this group of patients including the very small neonate to the older child. This includes proximity to the operating rooms and cardiac catheterization laboratory. Equipment such as cardiac monitoring capability, external pacemaker, echocardiography, surgical cart, rapid access to ECMO circuit, and delivery and monitoring system for nitric oxide.

There are basic care guidelines for all pediatric cardiac surgical patients; however, each lesion carries with it specific problems that are seen postoperatively and is beyond the scope of this chapter. In the following section we will review specifics.

Successful postoperative care includes knowledge of the following:

1. Precise anatomic diagnosis of the patient's cardiac defect(s).
2. Pathophysiologic effects of the defect(s) on the cardiovascular system and other organs prior to surgery.
3. Comorbid factors, preoperative medications.
4. Anesthesia issues in the operating room—intubation, medications, and so forth.
5. Details of the operative events including cardiopulmonary bypass time, circulatory arrest time, and ischemic time; type of repair—palliative or complete repair; residual defects; technical issues or complications (bleeding, dysrhythmias, air embolism, and so forth).

6. Evaluation of data from physical exam, echo, hemodynamic monitoring, cardiac catheterization (if necessary).

7. General ICU management including: ventilator management, anesthetic and sedation medications, antimicrobials, and parenteral nutrition.

8. Pharmacology of drugs that affect the cardiovascular system, which include inotropes, vasodilators, diuretics, and antiarrhythmics.

9. Indications for the select procedures: pacing, pericardiocentesis, and mechanical support of the failing heart—ECMO or ventricular assist device.[28]

Low Cardiac Output

Low cardiac output is one of the most frequently occurring problems seen in the postoperative pediatric cardiac surgery patient. The etiology of low cardiac output in any patient can be separated into five categories—preload, afterload, contractility, rhythm, and ventilation/oxygenation. These five categories are the same that are evaluated in the operating room prior to separating from the cardiopulmonary bypass circuit. In addition there are specific factors which may influence cardiac output in the postoperative cardiac patient include: residual and undiagnosed lesions, inflammatory response associated with CPB, myocardial ischemia from aortic cross clamping or circulatory arrest, hypothermia, reperfusion injury (RI), inadequate myocardial protection, and ventriculotomy (when performed).[29] Treatment of low cardiac output should begin with identifying which one or more of the five above categories (etiologies) is responsible. Once the etiology(s) is(are) identified treatment can be targeted appropriately.

A decrease in cardiac output is commonly observed at about 6 h postoperatively[30] and is usually responsive to volume infusion and an increase in inotropic support. Appropriate anticipation of this decrease in cardiac output will help to avoid significant morbidity and mortality. Postoperative cardiac tamponade should always be kept in the differential. It is usually seen in the patient who comes out of the operating room with generous chest tube output that suddenly decreases or stops.

The patient is usually tachycardic, and hypotensive with a decreased urine output and elevated central pressures, and a decreased response to volume administration. If suspected and time permits, a cardiac echocardiogram will confirm the diagnosis. Prompt decompression is indicated with identification of surgical bleeding and correction of coagulation abnormalities. Surgical decompression is usually accomplished at the bedside.

The different interventions that can be employed in treating low cardiac output states are given in Table 49-6. It is important to realize that there is a great deal of overlap and interaction among these categories.

If a continued low cardiac output state continues it may be necessary to employ mechanical support such as ECMO or a ventricular assist device.

TABLE 49-6

TREATMENT OF LOW CARDIAC OUTPUT STATES

Factor	Treatment
Preload	Increase volume, decrease in positive end-expiratory pressure, decrease RV afterload
Afterload	Afterload reducing agents-milrinone, nitroprusside, Ca+ channel blockers, angiotensin-converting enzyme (ACE) inhibitors, sedation, pain control
Contractility	Inotropic agents, pacing
Rhythm	Pacing, chronotropic agents, antiarrhythmics, sedation
Ventilation/ oxygenation	Appropriate management of ventilators, r/o pneumothorax, effusion; nitric oxide
Cardiac tamponade	Urgent decompression
Right-to-left shunting	Support RV, reduce RV afterload, lower pulmonary vascular resistance

Pulmonary Hypertension

Pulmonary hypertension is a commonly seen problem in the pediatric cardiac surgical unit and can significantly affect the peri and postoperative course. Pulmonary hypertension can be a result of the pathophysiology of the congenital heart lesion itself as well as factors related to the use of cardiopulmonary bypass.[31–34] It can be a result of reactive pulmonary vascular resistance (the majority) or fixed. Neonates typically have reactive pulmonary vascular resistance without necessarily having significant cardiac issues. Pulmonary vascular resistance issues occur commonly in those patients with long-term large left-to-right shunts and patients with pulmonary venous obstruction (e.g., TAPVR). In addition, it is important to rule out any postoperative mechanical obstruction to pulmonary blood flow such as pulmonary venous or arterial obstruction, significantly elevated left atrial pressure, or residual defects causing a large left-to-right shunt as management of these is surgical.

Early correction of congenital heart defects can help to prevent irreversible pulmonary vascular disease. Pharmacologic treatment (pulmonary vasodilators) of pulmonary vascular disease includes tolazine, prostaglandin E1, and prostacyclin, all with some efficacy. The most successfully and frequently employed pharmacologic treatment has been nitric oxide. A reaction between L-arginine and molecular oxygen that is catalyzed by NO synthase in the pulmonary endothelium forms nitric oxide. The nitric oxide induces a vasodilatory effect via a cyclic guanosine monophosphate-dependent pathway. As a gas it is delivered by inhalation to the alveoli and the blood vessels close to the ventilated lung. It is rapidly inactivated by hemoglobin so it does not cause the systemic vasodilatation and increase in intrapulmonary shunting that many of the other pulmonary vasodilators do. When it is effective, it will quickly lower pulmonary vascular resistance without systemic hypotension, especially in a patient with pulmonary hypertensive crisis. Patients with severe left ventricular dysfunction and pulmonary hypertension should be placed on NO cautiously because of the possibility of augmenting preload in the already stressed left ventricle as seen in the adult heart failure patients. When employed at therapeutic levels (1-80 ppm) accumulation of methemoglobin may increase so it is important to check methemoglobin levels while using NO. This increase in methemoglobin may be accentuated by concomitant use of nipride or nitroglycerin. Possible toxicities of NO include methemoglobinemia, cytotoxic effects in the lung from free radical formation, excess nitrogen dioxide development, peroxynitrite production, or injury to pulmonary surfactant system.[35] Weaning from NO should be carried out slowly as an abrupt withdrawal can be associated with rebound pulmonary hypertension. In those patients difficult to wean, the type V phophodiesterase inhibitor, sildenafil (Viagra) may be useful in transitioning off NO.[36]

Pulmonary Issues

Postoperative management of the ventilation/oxygenation depends on whether the patient is intubated or extubated. The perioperative course (CPB time), ease of intubation, type of repair, age and size of the child and comorbid factors will influence early versus late extubation. Most closed cases and noncomplex cases are extubated early. Early extubation is becoming more common. It is not uncommon to see a VSD or ASD repair extubated in the operating room. If extubated, it is important to monitor the child closely for grunting, tachypnea, apnea, and stridor. Pain management, while important, may also cause underventilation. Postoperative chest radiography is performed routinely on all patients.

A number of patients are kept intubated postoperatively. This removes the work of breathing, uncertainty of gas exchange in the extubated patient, and decreases the stress on overall cardiopulmonary function. Various ventilator modes are employed and are dependent on age and size of patient. Higher tidal volumes may be used because of pulmonary edema and decreased compliance. Measures are taken to avoid pulmonary edema, atelectasis, pleural effusion, pneumothorax, and pulmonary hypertensive events. Continuous O_2 sat monitoring and periodic blood gases and chest radiography are used for optimal management.

Intubation/reintubation of the patient with borderline ventricular function or the nonsedated neonate/infant with congenital heart disease may cause major hemodynamic and metabolic derangements. Both appropriate personnel expert in intubation and appropriate dosing of anesthetic and muscle relaxants are essential in the postoperative pediatric cardiac surgical patient. Periodic nasotracheal (rather than orotracheal) suctioning is important in the extubated patient who is having difficulty clearing secretions as well as pulmonary toilet. In the neonate/young infant or the patient with labile pulmonary vascular resistance, suctioning can precipitate a pulmonary hypertensive crisis especially in the first 24–48 h postop. A narcotic bolus (e.g., fentanyl) or extended anesthetic period (paralysis and deep sedation) will help to blunt this response.

Extubation is indicated when hemostasis is complete, hemodynamics are satisfactorily stable, there is no evidence of airway edema, no evidence of a metabolic acidosis, the core temperature <38°C, no evidence of seizures, or significant endotracheal secretions. In the long-term intubated patient, adequate strength and nutrition are equally important. In this group of patients, preextubation steroids may be used. Diaphragmatic and vocal cord paralysis or paresis should be ruled out, especially in the patient who fails extubation.

Fluids, Electrolytes, and Renal Issues

There are significant imbalances in the postoperative pediatric cardiac patient that occur in the total fluid balance, electrolytes, Ca^+ and Mg^+ homeostasis and renal function. These imbalances are magnified in those patients who undergo CPB especially longer CPB times and circulatory arrest, and in neonates and young infants. Significant fluid shifts occur operatively because of large priming volumes needed for the CPB pump. There is an increase in total body water and salt overload.

There is a generalized capillary leak from damaged endothelium caused by the CPB pump and ischemia reperfusion. This is magnified with a longer CPB time and circulatory arrest and in neonates. Interventions employed to treat the capillary leak syndrome include perioperative ultrafiltration either during or post-CPB, prophylactic placement of peritoneal dialysis catheter for use of drainage or

dialysis postoperatively, selective inhibition of adhesion molecules and preoperative steroids.

Management of fluid and electrolyte balance postoperatively requires a urinary catheter for measuring hourly urine output, especially in complex postoperative patients. Periodic physical examinations, continuous monitoring of systemic blood pressure, heart rate and central venous pressures; daily weights and 24-h strict ins and outs; routine laboratory work to include electrolytes, BUN/creatinine, hemoglobin, albumin, and urine analysis all aid in the management of fluid and electrolyte balance in the postoperative cardiac patient.

An early postoperative diuresis may be observed secondary to the intraoperative fluid intake and a subsequent osmotic diuresis secondary to hyperglycemia from the cardioplegia solution, stress and steroid and/or mannitol administration. Maintenance fluids (amount and type) depend on the institution, the type of surgery, and age of the patient and can range from 50 to 120% of normal maintenance, and fluid type again dependent on the institution, the age of the patient. Two to six hours postoperatively, the urine output decreases coinciding frequently with a lower systemic blood pressure and CVP if measured. Patients are usually intravascularly dry despite the presence of total body edema and may require volume replacement in the form of colloid-PRBC or albumin. This continues for the next 12–48 h depending on the patient. ADH secretion beginning with the stress of the surgery continues and when decreased will result in an increase in urine output and a mobilization of fluid from the extravascular to intravascular space. Diuretics and renal dose dopamine (3 μg/kg/min) are used frequently to augment this mobilization and possibly lessen the duration of mechanical ventilation and ICU stay. Diuretics are not usually started until 12–24 h postoperatively; however, the response may be suboptimal until the ADH levels actually decrease. Neonates who inherently have a decreased GFR because of their age may require more time to mobilize and excrete the excess fluid. The decrease in GFR will also affect their ability to metabolize certain drugs. Diuretics employed include loop diuretics such as furosemide, thiazides such as chlorathiazides or metolazone. Continuous furosemide or Bumex is especially helpful in those patients who are hemodynamically labile. Treatment of renal insufficiency or failure in the postoperative period should start with optimization of cardiac output, including ECMO or ventricular assist if needed. Renal ultrasonography should be performed if not obtained preoperatively because of the association of congenital heart disease and renal defects. A trial of high dose diuretic administration can be attempted in the patient with renal insufficiency or failure who is oliguric. Dosages of drugs eliminated renally ought to be adjusted based on serum creatinine. Electro-lytes, with particular attention to potassium, calcium, sodium, and magnesium should be monitored and frequently corrected if abnormal. Options for dialysis in the neonate are limited to peritoneal dialysis, ECMO with CVAVH/D and continuous veno-veno/veno-arterial hemodialysis (not well tolerated in the <10 kg child). In the older child (>10 kg) CVVH/CAVH ± D or standard hemodialysis (if hemodynamically stable) may also be employed.

Gastrointestinal/Nutritional Issues

Pediatric cardiac surgical patients are particularly susceptible to GI disturbances such as gastric distention, prolonged gastric emptying, ileus, hyperamylesemia, pancreatitis, GI bleeding, and constipation. Necrotizing enterocolitis (NEC) and feeding difficulties (e.g., reflux, oral aversion) can occur in neonates and young infants. Specific subgroups of patients have a higher incidence of gastrointestinal complications and include Fontan patients—protein losing enteropathy, coarctation repair—mesenteric enteritis, Norwood procedure—reduced gut perfusion, and ischemia. These patients need more careful assessment for enteral feeding and use of more elemental feeds.

In the early postoperative phase, decompression of the stomach may be indicated to avoid aspiration and optimize ventilation. Postpump hyperamylesemia/pancreatitis is not uncommonly seen in the adult postcardiac surgical patient and on occasion may be seen in the child/young adult. Appropriate treatment including holding enteral feeds, gastric decompression, monitoring for abscess formation, as well as monitoring of serum amylase, lipase, liver function, glucose, calcium, and white blood count is indicated.

Routine postoperative prophylaxis with H_2 blockers ranitidine or famotidine is usually given until patients are extubated and tolerating feeds. Constipation is frequent because of narcotics used. Glycerin suppositories are used to treat this in the neonate/young infant, and laxatives or colace in the older child/young adult.

Necrotizing enterocolitis is not infrequently seen in the neonate.[37] Factors associated with an elevated risk of NEC in infants with heart disease include premature birth, hypoplastic left heart syndrome, truncus arteriosus, and episodes of poor systemic perfusion or shock. A heightened level of suspicion is warranted in these groups.[37] Appropriate treatment of suspected NEC should include abdominal imaging, bowel rest, and antibiotic therapy.

Nutrition (enteral or parenteral) ought to be started in the postoperative period as soon as possible to minimize the catabolic effects that occur in the intensive care setting, especially in the chronically ill cardiac surgical patient. Positive nitrogen balance is the goal for wound healing. A goal of 120–150 kcal/kg/day may be necessary in the postoperative period. Enteral feeding is preferred because it can allow for complete nutritional support with minimal complications and prevent translocation of bacteria. Enteral feeds may be given via naso/oro-gastric/jejunal routes. Total parenteral nutrition (TPN) may be necessary in those patients who have prolonged ileus, gut ischemia, malabsorption, or a primary intestinal disorder. TPN is a formula containing amino acids, glucose, trace minerals and vitamins, and intralipids. It can be administered either peripherally or centrally but must be given centrally if the glucose concentration is >12.5%. Complications include line infections, hypertriglyceridemia, hepatic steatosis, and increased work of breathing because of excess glucose administration.

Feeding difficulties are common in the neonate/ young infant after complex cardiac surgery. This is because of the lack of any or optimal feeding preoperatively and neurodevelopmental immaturity. In addition, oral feeding is an increased physical demand for infants and thus may be best to begin via a continuous nasogastric (NG) route after a safe period post extubation. Once the patient is tolerating continuous feeds at full strength, then bolus feeds can be attempted. The next step is to try oral feeding prior to the bolus feed through the NGT transitioning to full oral feeding. If there is difficulty with either tolerating NGT feeds or oral feeding a speech/swallow consult and GI consult should be sought. Nutritional goals for most cardiac babies should be 120 kcal/kg/day. The volume needed to achieve this depends on the calories/oz. Increasing the caloric density to 24-27 kcal may be necessary in those infants who need volume restriction (e.g., left-to-right shunts).

Breastfed babies should initially be fed either nasogastrically or by bottle first to assure that they obtain adequate nutrition. After achieving this, they can be switched to breastfeeding while monitoring closely. If the patient is taking breast milk and more calories are needed, the breast milk can be fortified.

Metabolic/Endocrine Issues

Steroids

It is common to administer steroids to patients prior to bypass and in the pump prime to help blunt the systemic inflammatory response. The role of steroids postoperatively is not well studied. In the hemodynamically unstable patient not responsive to usual therapy, adrenal insufficiency should be considered in the differential. A cortisol level should be sent and treated with stress doses of steroids if it is low. ACTH should also be sent to rule out a central etiology. Patients who have been on recent steroids should receive prophylactic stress doses in the perioperative period.

Thyroid hormones have both inotropic and vasoactive effects.[38] Studies in adult and pediatric cardiac surgery patients have reported alterations in thyroid hormone metabolism.[4,5,6] In children, the half-life of serum T3 after heart surgery has been shown to be markedly decreased.[7] A low serum T3 level in children after cardiac surgery was a predictor of adverse outcome and T3 treatment significantly improved cardiac function.[5,8] Another study did not show this positive result though there were no ill effects of T3 administration; however, in the newborns there was a tendency for a positive therapeutic response to T3

treatment. This study suggested that there might be some therapeutic benefit to T3 infusion to normalize serum T3 levels in newborns undergoing operations for complex congenital heart disease.[39] Trisomy 21 patients should always be screened for hypothyroidism since it is commonly seen in this genetic defect.

Lactate

Serial blood lactate levels in some centers are followed closely starting prebypass and continuing well into the postoperative period. Prospective studies have demonstrated a positive correlation between rising serum lactate and increased morbidity and mortality especially in the neonatal population.[40,41]

Neurologic Issues

Preoperative Status

It is important to have a good neurologic assessment in all patients preoperatively because congenital heart disease poses an increased risk of neurologic impairment from a wide spectrum of causes. Other congenital defects should be identified such as brain dysgenesis, the prevalence of which can be 10–29% in congenital heart disease patients.[42,43,44] Infants with CHD are also at increased risk for acquired and antenatal and perinatal brain injury.[45] Issues such as chronic cyanosis, polycythemia, and right-to-left shunts can be responsible for neurologic injury. Early, complete repairs that are now being performed in most centers have alleviated some of the increased risk from these above-mentioned issues. In order to perform these early repairs, the use of intraoperative techniques such as hypothermic circulatory arrest have been employed, which itself is a risk for neurologic impairment. Outcome measurements are being evaluated which include neurodevelopmental status. Early studies suggest that those patients undergoing DHCA for complex repairs such as HLHS are scoring within the normal limits on neurodevelopmental tests; however, the scores are lower than normal.[46–49] More studies are necessary to further clarify the effects on neurodevelopmental outcome in congenital heart surgery patients.

IVH-Neonates

One of the more common neurologic issues facing neonates is intraventricular hemorrhage. The CHD patient is at even higher risk because of significant hemodynamic changes which may occur at or shortly after birth, especially in the undiagnosed patient with a significant congenital heart defect such as hypoplastic left heart syndrome, transposition, or obstructed total anomalous pulmonary venous return. For this reason, accurate prenatal diagnosis of a congenital heart defect is preferable so that the birth of the child can occur at an appropriate center equipped to deal with the problems associated with congenital heart disease.

Routine head ultrasound should be performed in all neonates diagnosed with congenital heart disease as a baseline study and further studies as necessary. If an abnormality is identified, then a neurologic consultation/evaluation should be obtained prior to surgery. When the patient has had a significant bleed the timing of cardiac repair or palliation becomes important, especially if CPB is necessary. There are no prospective studies examining this issue in the pediatric population. The defect and its severity, complexity of the surgery, and the severity of the hemorrhage should all be taken into account when making the decision to proceed with surgery.

Intraoperative Neurologic Injury

The etiology of intraoperative neurologic injury is multifactorial. The use of the cardiopulmonary bypass itself increases the risk of neurologic injury during operation in both children and adults. Devastating air embolism is prevented by vigilance of the surgical team. The incidence of air embolism has decreased with the increased use of multiple alarms along the cardiopulmonary bypass circuit.[50] More commonly seen and more difficult to detect during the operative period is hypoxia-ischemia/reperfusion injury (H-I/RI). Neuroprotective strategies to reduce the risk of H-I/RI are currently being employed. Preemptive suppression of cerebral metabolism with hypothermia and drugs (e.g., barbiturates) in anticipation of decreased cerebral oxygen supply is one strategy to reduce the risk of intraoperative neurologic injury. There is a trend toward the decreased use of DHCA, especially of long duration, because of data, which has shown a greater incidence of perioperative neurologic dysfunction (seizures and delayed psychomotor development) at 1 year of age in those infants undergoing arterial switch operation.[51] Acid-base management strategies during DHCA were shown not to affect early neurodevelopmental outcomes.[52] Future neuroprotective strategies are under investigation as are better tools for the intraoperative monitoring of cerebral blood flow.

Postoperative Issues

A recent multicenter survey found that up to 20% of children undergoing cardiac surgery will present with neurologic dysfunction during the early postoperative period.[53,54] The etiology of this injury is multifactorial: intraoperative events, postoperative hemodynamic instability, and impairment of cerebrovascular autoregulation. Thorough postoperative neurologic assessment ought to occur as the patient enters the ICU, and reevaluated throughout the postoperative period.

One of the more common neurologic events that occur postoperatively is seizure. The frequency of clinical seizures following CPB ranges from 4 to 15%. The identification of seizures in children can be subtle, especially neonates and young infants and patients who are paralyzed and sedated. Sudden increases in systemic blood pressure, heart rate, or acidosis (increasing lactate) should be suspect as well as the more classic signs of clinical seizures. Management of seizures should include treatment with anticonvulsants. Many of the anticonvulsants are myocardial and respiratory depressants and therefore, they should be administered with close hemodynamic monitoring. Assessment and treatment of any disturbances in acid-base status, glucose, calcium, and magnesium should be treated. A neurologic consultation should be requested as well as an EEG, head ultrasound (neonate), or CT scan/MRI, if necessary. The etiology of seizures includes, metabolic disturbances, ischemic injury, cerebrovascular accident (embolic or thrombotic), and less likely an infectious cause. Stroke can occur intraoperatively or postoperatively and not be appreciated in the patient who is paralyzed and sedated. As with seizures, the etiology of stroke is multifactorial. Prior to the shift from palliation to early corrective surgery for congenital heart defects, chronic hypoxia and polycythemia were risk factors for stroke especially in the older patient. Early corrective surgery has lead to a decrease risk of stroke because of the reduced number of surgeries, and avoidance of long-term exposure to chronic hypoxia and polycythemia. Embolic phenomena (particulate or gaseous) can occur in and out of the operating room. New innovations in CPB circuit have helped to decrease the incidence of embolic stroke. It is especially important to make sure any IV infusion is free of air to avoid air embolus. Postoperatively there are several factors which make the patient high risk for stroke including, stasis, altered vascular surfaces, coagulation abnormalities, low flow states, prosthetic material, and right-to-left shunts.

Pain Management

Postoperative pain management depends on whether the patient is extubated or intubated. Patients who are clinically stable and extubated soon after surgery can usually be managed with judicious use of opioids (e.g., morphine) while monitoring for respiratory depression. In children with agitation or restlessness that may interfere with the safety of intravenous/arterial lines and chest tubes, it may be necessary to use sedation in the form of benzodiazepenes or chloral hydrate. A patient planned for a long intubation period is best managed with a continuous IV infusion of Fentanyl, Dilaudid or morphine with or without a benzodiazepine like Versed. Of note is that narcotics and benzodiazepenes can be myocardial depressants. If paralysis is necessary, either intermittent or continuous infusions of muscle relaxants can be used. Patients with limited myocardial reserve; labile pulmonary hypertension, complex repairs or bleeding should be managed with continuous infusions of both narcotics with or without benzodiazepines and paralytics. For those patients who receive long-term narcotics, withdrawal is managed with a methadone wean. For bedside procedures, the combination of ketamine or Fentanyl, benzodiazepines with or without paralytics are useful. Nonsteroidal anti-inflammatory agents such as ketorolac (Toradol) and ibuprofen (Motrin) are useful in the older patient population. In the later postoperative period, after extubation, and nearing discharge to the floor or home, acetaminophen (Tylenol), ibuprofen, or acetaminophen with codeine are usually used for pain control.

Hematologic Issues

Postoperative hematologic issues can be separated into two phases—acute and chronic. In the immediate postoperative phase bleeding can be significant. It is important to distinguish surgical versus post-CPB coagulopathy. Information from the surgeon regarding surgical concerns and the appearance of the operative field is important to obtain to guide management. Once surgical bleeding has been ruled out, then post-CPB effects on coagulation factors and platelets and replacement of losses is addressed. A baseline CBC with platelets and coagulation studies (PT, PTT, INR, and fibrinogen) should be obtained on arrival to the ICU. These should be used as guideline, with appropriate correction if the patient is bleeding. If the patient has significant bleeding, systemic blood pressure control, intubation, and sedation/paralysis are achieved as hypertension and agitation will exacerbate the bleeding. Other interventions include administration of protamine if the PTT or ACT is elevated, continuation of either Amicar or Aprotonin begun in the OR, and giving Factor 7 (NOVA 7), a new product used for significant postoperative bleeding. The possibility of cardiac tamponade should always be kept in mind when a patient has significant bleeding. Calcium replacement is important when giving large amounts of blood products, especially in neonates.

After the acute phase, further administration of blood products depends on the patient. Some patients require special considerations. The first are those with mixing lesions (cyanotic, single ventricle, shunted patients), where it is important to keep the hemoglobin elevated (12–14) for optimal oxygen carrying capacity. The second are those with chylothorax or large amounts of serous chest tube drainage as they lose an enormous amount of protein and albumin, including coagulation factors which should be replaced. Fresh frozen plasma is usually used to replace those factors. Careful monitoring of coagulation factors should be carried out. Recently, a mixed group of patients has been identified with clotting disorders either acquired or congenital. The presentation is usually a clotted shunt or obstructed access site (femoral vein, internal jugular, and so forth.) The management of these patients should include base line hematologic studies, hematology consultation and appropriate treatment.

Infectious Disease Issues

Perioperative antibiotics are a standard of care with a well-established efficacy of their use. A previous history of resistant organisms is an important presurgical historical factor as it may alter the choice of antibiotics. Similarly, long preop hospitalization, or patients with tracheostomies or gastric tubes, will have different normal flora and an increased risk of developing resistant organisms. Despite antibiotics and sterile technique, sternal wound infections continue to occur and require thorough inspection of the wound for any erythema, warmth, drainage, or chest instability, which may indicate the presence of infection. Prompt treatment is indicated and includes antibiotics and possible open debridement.

Inflammatory Issues

Postpericardiotomy syndrome is an inflammation of the pericardium that may occur 2–4 weeks after pericardial injury such as cardiac surgery in which the pericardium was incised. It begins as a flu-like illness (low-grade fever, poor appetite, vomiting, myalgia) and may be mistaken for such; however, a pericardial effusion may develop and progress to cause cardiac tamponade. Symptoms to suggest a worsening pericardial effusion include tachycardia, tachypnea, pallor or frank signs and symptoms of shock. The primary care provider ought to be aware of this entity in a postoperative patient. Management includes confirmation of the diagnosis with echocardiography, followed by anti-inflammatory therapy (steroids or aspirin). Pericardiocentesis and/or surgical drainage may be indicated if there is impending tamponade.

WOUND CARE

Surgical wound care recommendations vary among surgeons. Most incisions have been closed with absorbable sutures. The incisions require very little care other than keeping the wound clean and dry. A bath or shower may be taken 24–48 h after any wires, lines, or when nonabsorbable external stitches have been removed, but the chest area should not be soaked. This timing usually correlates with discharge to home in most uncomplicated cases. Clothing with buttons or zippers should be avoided in the early postoperative period. Lotions and powders should not be used on the incision for 3–4 weeks. Antibiotic ointment can be applied twice a day to alleviate pruritis associated with wound healing. The possibility of a wound infection will exist for approximately 6–8 weeks following surgery. The primary care provider may be the first person to note a possible wound infection during a routine examination. Potential infection may manifest as redness, drainage, instability of the sternum, or dehiscence of the incision; however, it is important to know that the absorbable subcutaneous stitches that are frequently used to close the surgical incision will break down over the next 1–3 months and occasionally will cause localized erythema and drainage of and from the incision. The surgeon should be notified of *any* change in the incision, regardless. The risk of sunburn is great up to 6 months or 1 year following surgery, thus sun protection (clothing, sunscreen/block or sun avoidance) is indicated. Patients are generally allowed to return to school in 2 weeks while avoiding physical education and sports for 6–8 weeks and bike riding or swimming for 4 weeks. Driving is avoided for 4 weeks. In older children, collision sports or activities (e.g., football) ought to be withheld until there is complete healing of the sternum.

PSYCHOSOCIAL ISSUES

Psychosocial issues in the postoperative congenital heart surgery patient are a very broad topic, far beyond the scope of this chapter. There are many complex interrelating factors surrounding a child with congenital heart disease. The many psychosocial needs of both the patient and the family can be met by careful assessment, open and informative communication with the ICU team, maintenance of an open avenue for the patient and the family to express their concerns and reactions. A social worker can help to guide the ICU team (MDs, nurses, and so forth) in carrying out the above mentioned. It is important to provide close and regular communication, cooperation and mutual support between ICU team and social workers, childcare, teaching, psychiatric/psychologic staff, and clergy.

References

1   Greenwood RD, Rosenthal A, Parisi L, et al: Extracardiac abnormalities in infants with congenital heart disease. *Pediatrics* 55:485–492, 1975.

2   Jaggers J, Ungerleider RM: Cardiopulmonary bypass in infants and children, in: Williams WG (ed): *Seminars in Thoracic and Cardiovascular Surgery, Pediatric Cardiac Surgery Annals 2000*, Philadelphia, PA, WB Saunders, 2000, pp. 82–109.

3   Anand KJS, Hickey PR: Halothane-morphine compared with high dose Sufentanil for anesthesia and post-operative analgesia in neonatal heart surgery. *N Engl J Med* 326:1–9, 1992.

4   Chowdhury D, Parnell VA, Ojamaa K, Boxer R, Cooper R, Klein I: Usefulness of tri-iodothyronine (T3) treatment after surgery for complex congenital heart disease in infants and children. *Am J Cardiol* 84:1107–1109, 1999.

5   Bettendorf M, Schmidt KG, Grulich-Henn J, Ulmer HE, Henrich UE: Tri-iodothyronine treatment in children after cardiac surgery: a double blind, randomized, placebo-controlled study. *Lancet* 356:529–534, 2000.

6   Mainwaring RD, Capparelli E, Schell K, Acosta M, Nelson JC: Pharmacokinetic evaluation of tri-iodothyronine supplementation in children after modified Fontan procedure. *Circulation* 101:1423–1429, 2000.

7   Portman MA, Fearneyhough C, Ning XH, et al: Tri-iodothyronine repletion in infants during cardiopulmonary bypass for congenital heart disease. *J Thorac Cardiovasc Surg* 120:604–608, 2000.

8   Bettendorf M, Schmidt KG, Tiefenbasher, et al: Transient secondary hypothyroidism in children after cardiac surgery. *Pediatr Res* 41:375–379, 1997.

9   Blalock A, Hanlon CR: Interatrial septal defect: its experimental production under direct vision without the interruption of the circulation. *Surg Gynecol Obstet* 87:183, 1983.

10 Brock RC: Pulmonary valvotomy for the relief of congenital pulmonary stenosis. Report of three cases. *Br Med J* 1:1121, 1948.

11 Muller WH, Damman JF: The treatment of certain congenital malformations of the heart by the creation of pulmonic stenosis to reduce pulmonary hypertension and excessive pulmonary blood flow. *Surg Gynecol Obstet* 95:213, 1952.

12 Glenn WWL: Circulatory bypass of the right side of the heart. IV. Shunt between superior vena cava and distal right pulmonary artery—report of clinical application. *N Eng J Med* 259:117, 1958.

13 Azzolina G, Eufrate S, Pensa P: Tricuspid atresia: experience in surgical management with a modified cavopulmonary anastomosis. *Thorax* 17:11, 1972.

14 Ross DN: Homograft replacement of the aortic valve. *Lancet* 2:487, 1962.

15 Ross DN: Replacement of aortic and mitral valves with a pulmonary autograft. *Lancet* 2:956, 1967.

16 Ross DN, Jackson M, Davies J: The pulmonary autograft-a permanent aortic valve. *Eur J Cardiothorac Surg* 6:113, 1992.

17 Ross DN, Jackson M, Davies J: Pulmonary autograft aortic valve replacement: Long-term results. *J Cardiac Surg* 6:529, 1997.

18 Kouchoukos NT, Davila-Roman VG, Spray TL, et al: Replacement of the aortic root with a pulmonary autograft in children and young adults with aortic valve disease. *N Engl J Med* 330:1, 1994.

19 Elkins RC, Lane MM, McCue C: Pulmonary autograft reoperation: incidence and management. *Ann Thorac Surg* 62:450, 1996.

20 Rastan H, Abu-Aishah N, Rastan D, et al: Results of Aortoventriculoplasty in 21 consecutive patients with left ventricular outflow obstruction. *J Thorac Cardiovasc Surg* 775:659, 1978.

21 Norwood WI, Lang P, Hansen DD: Physiologic repair of aortic atresia-hypoplastic left heart syndrome. *N Engl J Med* 308:23, 1983.

22 Fontan F, Baudet E: Surgical repair of tricuspid atresia. *Thorax* 26:240, 1971.

23 Wernovsky G: Single ventricle lesions, in: Chang AC, Hanley FL, Wernovsky G, Wessel DL (eds): *Pediatric Cardiac Intensive Care.* Baltimore, MD, Williams & Wilkins, 1998, p. 281.

24 Senning A: Surgical correction of transposition of the great vessels. *Surgery* 45:966, 1959.

25 Mustard WT: Successful two-stage correction of transposition of the great vessels. *Surgery* 55:469, 1964.

26 Jatene AD, Fontes VF, Paulista PP, et al: Anatomic correction of transposition of the great vessels. *J Thorac Cardiovasc Surg* 72:364, 1976.

27 Rastelli GC, McGoon DC, Wallace RB: Anatomic correction of transposition of the great arteries with ventricular septal defect and subpulmonary stenosis. *J Thorac Cardiovasc Surg* 58:545–552, 1969.

28 Roth SJ: Postoperative care, in: Chang AC, Hanley FL, Wernovsky G, Wessel DL (eds): *Pediatric Cardiac Intensive Care.* Baltimore, MD, Williams & Wilkins, 1998, p. 163.

29 Wessel DL: Managing low cardiac output syndrome after congenital heart surgery. *Crit Care Med* 29(Suppl. 10);S220–S230, 2001.

30 Wernovsky G, Wypij D, Jonas R, et al: Postoperative course and hemodynamic profile after the arterial switch operation in neonates and infants. A comparison of low-flow cardiopulmonary bypass and circulatory arrest. *Circulation* 92:2226–2235, 1995.

31 Hickey PR, Hansen DD: pulmonary hypertension in infants: postoperative management, in: Yacoub M (ed): *Annual of Cardiac Surgery.* London, Current Science, 1989, pp. 16–22.

32 Kirklin JW, Barratt-Boyes BG: *Cardiac Surgery.* New York, NY, Wiley Medical Publishers, 1986, pp. 29–82.

33 Koul B, Willen H, Sjoberg T, et al: Pulmonary sequelae of prolonged total venoarterial bypass: Evaluation with a new experimental model. *Ann Thorac Surg* 51:794–799, 1991.

34 Koul B, Wollmer P, Willen H, et al: Venoarterial extracorporeal membrane oxygenation: How safe is it? *J Thorac Cardiovasc Surg* 104:579–584, 1992.

35 Hallman M, Bry K, Lappalainen U: A mechanism of nitric oxide-induced surfactant dysfunction. *J Appl Physiol* 80:2035–2043, 1996.

36 Atz AM, Wessel DL: Sildenafil ameliorates effects of inhaled nitric oxide withdrawal. *Anesthesiology* 91:307–310, 1999.

37 McElhinney D, Hedrick H, Bush D, et al: Necrotizing enterocolitis in neonates with congenital heart disease: risk factors and outcomes. *Pediatrics* 106(5):1080–1087, 2000.

38 Klein I, Ojamaa K: Mechanisms of disease: thyroid hormone and the cardiovascular system. *N Engl J Med* 344:501–509, 2001.

39 Chowdhury D, Ojama K, Parnell V, et al: A prospective randomized clinical study of thyroid hormone treatment after operations for complex congenital heart disease. *J Thorac Cardiovasc Surg* 122:1023–1025, 2001.

40 Charpie JR, Dekeon MK, Goldberg CS, et al: Serial blood lactate measurements predict early outcome after neonatal repair or palliation for complex congenital heart disease. *J Thorac Cardiovasc Surg* 120(1):73–80, 2000.

41 Munoz R, Laussen PC, Palacio G, et al: Changes in whole blood lactate levels during cardiopulmonary bypass for surgery for congenital cardiac disease: An early indicator of morbidity and mortality. *J Thorac Cardiovasc Surg* 119(1):155–162, 2000.

42 Terplan K: Patterns of brain damage in infants and children with congenital heart disease: association with catheterization and surgical procedures. *Am J Dis Child* 125:175–185, 1973.

43 Jones M: Anomalies of the brain and congenital heart disease: a study of 52 necropsy cases. *Pediatr Pathol Lab Med* 11:721–736, 1991.

44 Glauser T, Rorke L, Weinberg P, et al: Congenital brain anomalies associated with hypoplastic left heart syndrome. *Pediatrics* 85(6):984–990, 1990.

45 van Houten J, Rothman A, Bejar R: Echoencephalographic (ECHO) findings in infants with congenital heart disease (CHD). *Pediatr Res* 33(4):376A, 1993.

46 Wernovsky G, Stiles K, Gauvreau K, et al. Cognitive development after the Fontan operation. *Circulation* 102:883–889, 2000.

47 Mahle W, Clancy R, Moss E, et al: Neurodevelopmental outcome and lifestyle assessment in school age and adolescent children with hypoplastic left heart syndrome. *Pediatrics* 105:1082–1089, 2000.

48 Forbess J, Visconti K, Hancock-Friesen C, et al: Neurodevelopmental outcome after congenital heart surgery: Results from an institutional registry. *Circulation* 106[Suppl. I]:I-95–I-102, 2002.

49 del Nido PJ: Developmental and neurologic outcomes late after neonatal corrective surgery. *J Thorac Cardiovasc Surg* 124;3, 2002.

50 Sadel S: Safety and management of perturbations during cardiopulmonary bypass, in: Mora CT (ed): *Cardiopulmonary Bypass-Principles and Techniques of Extracorporeal Circulation.* New York, NY, Springer-Verlag, 1995, p. 301.

51 Newberger J, Jonas R, Wernovsky G, et al: A comparison of the perioperative neurologic effects of hypothermic circulatory arrest versus low-flow cardiopulmonary bypass in infant heart surgery. *N Engl J Med* 329:1057–1064, 1993.

52 Bellinger DC, Wypij D, du Plessis AJ, et al: Developmental and neurologic effects of alpha-stat versus ph-stat for deep hypothermic cardiopulmonary bypass in infants. *J Thorac Cardiovasc Surg* 121:374–383, 2001.

53 Ferry P: Neurologic sequelae of cardiac surgery in children. *Am J Dis Child* 141:309–312, 1987.

54 Ferry P: Neurologic sequelae of open-heart surgery in children; an irritating question. *Am J Dis Child* 144:369–373, 1990.

C H A P T E R

50

SPORTS RESTRICTIONS AND ADOLESCENTS

David G. Ruschhaupt

INTRODUCTION

Exercise is a natural event in the lives of most people. Routine levels of activity are exceeded by individuals who are interested in recreational or competitive athletic activities. Questions arise as to what can be considered an appropriate level of exercise for any individual, and whether exercise, even if thought to be beneficial, can indeed be harmful. The sudden, unexpected death of a presumed healthy youngster occurring during an exercise activity is a major tragedy. Prevention of such events is at the heart of medical screening programs, both for general health maintenance as well as for athletic participation. The possibility for short-term or long-term adverse effects of exercise on the hearts of individuals known to have existing cardiac conditions is also a potential concern. This chapter reviews the issues of exercise in the presumed healthy child as well as the population of

children and adolescents with known cardiac abnormalities.

PERSPECTIVE

Athletic training for excellence and competition with others requires systematic aerobic and anaerobic exercise training. In addition to professional and collegiate athletes, an estimate of at least 4 million competitive high school age athletes, and larger numbers of younger children participate in organized athletic programs. Estimates of athletic field deaths in this group suggest an incidence of 1:100,000. The incidence of death during participation in athletics, therefore, is low in the presumed healthy child. Fortunately, children with known or corrected heart defects also have a low risk of death during exercise. Even though there is only a small number of participants at risk of cardiac death, screening programs that may establish the risk for the young athlete are desirable.

APPROACH TO SCREENING

Effective medical screening for unrecognized cardiac abnormalities requires knowledge of the common possible abnormalities (Table 50-1) that may cause sudden cardiac death. While there is no universal recommendation or format, the athletic exam should include a medical history that inquires about palpitations and exercise associated chest pain, syncope or unexpected dyspnea; and ascertains if there is a family history of sudden death or disability from heart disease. At-risk patients may not answer these questions positively, but a positive response will alert the examiner to search for underlying problems. Parents should be responsible for answering these questions as the student athlete may not have knowledge of family members. The cardiovascular examination should include right brachial artery blood pressure determination, auscultation of the heart at rest (in the supine and standing positions), and after mild exercise such as sit-ups on the exam table to identify dynamic obstruction of left ventricular outflow, aortic valve or pulmonary valve stenosis, or mitral valve insufficiency. Femoral pulses should be palpated to exclude coarctation of the aorta, particularly if hypertension is present. Recognition of the physical stigmata of Marfan syndrome is important, particularly in the group of tall athletes who aspire to play basketball or volleyball. If an abnormality is suspected from the screening history or

TABLE 50-1

CAUSES OF UNEXPECTED CARDIAC DEATH

Hypertrophic cardiomyopathy
Anomalous left coronary artery
   Origin and course
Marfan's syndrome
   Aortic rupture
Myocarditis/dilated cardiomyopathy
Prolonged QT syndrome

TABLE 50-2

CARDIOVASCULAR SCREENING FOR ATHLETES

History
   Chest pain with exercise
   Syncope with exercise
   Unexpected shortness of breath
   Family history of sudden death
   Palpitations
Blood pressure, right brachial artery
Palpation of femoral pulses
Auscultation of the heart

examination, the athlete should be referred to a cardiovascular specialist for evaluation or confirmation of the diagnosis (Table 50-2). Because of the large number of potential participants and the low incidence of sudden death, routine screening electrocardiograms or echocardiograms are not recommended. These studies should be reserved for individuals whose screening exam has suggested a possible abnormality.

RECOMMENDATIONS

A universal exercise recommendation for all individuals and conditions would be presumptive and unworkable. Healthy individuals will be guided by their athletic abilities and interests. For those with known cardiac conditions, knowledge of the defect, information about past and possible future surgical operations, and results of exercise testing are helpful in structuring a realistic recommendation for exercise activity. Final recommendations for exercise activity should be based on the natural history of the cardiac defect, the attitude of the individual and demonstrated exercise capacity. For the specific individual, consideration should be made for affects of possible dehydration, reduction of blood volume, collision, and work-load intensity. Dynamic (aerobic) activity such as distance running or cross country skiing may be associated with increased left ventricular size. Static (anaerobic or isometric) activity such as power weight lifting or gymnastics may disproportionately increase blood pressure and be associated with concentric ventricular hypertrophy (Table 50-3); however, there is no definitive data to suggest what effect strenuous exertion may have on the natural history of the defect or if it will lead to premature death in any given individual. It is likewise not known if withdrawal from competitive athletics will necessarily prolong life. Given these uncertainties, a consensus statement was derived in 1994. The results of this conference are summarized within the discussion below (and Table 50-4).

TABLE 50-3

CLASSIFICATION OF SPORTS (BASED ON PEAK DYNAMIC AND STATIC COMPONENTS DURING COMPETITION)

	Low Dynamic	*Moderate Dynamic*	*High Dynamic*
Low static	Billiards Bowling Cricket Curling Golf Riflery	Baseball Softball Table tennis Tennis (doubles) Volleyball	Badminton X-Country skiing (classic style) Field hockey* Orienteering Race walking Racquetball Running (long distance) Soccer* Squash Tennis (singles)
Moderate static	Archery*,† Auto racing*,† Diving*,† Equestrian*,† Motorcycling*,†	Fencing Field events (jumping) Figure skating* Football (American)* Rodeoing*,† Rugby* Running (sprint) Surfing*,† Synchronized swimming*,†	Basketball* Ice hockey* X-Country skiing (skating) Football (Australian)* Lacrosse* Running (middle distance) Swimming Team handball
High static	Bobsledding*,† Field events (throwing) Gymnastics*,† Karate/judo* Luge*,† Sailing Rock Climbing Waterskiing*,† Weight lifting*,† Windsurfing*,†	Body building*,† Downhill skiing*,† Wrestling*	Boxing* Canoeing/kayaking Cycling*,† Decathlon Rowing Speed skating

*Danger of bodily collision.

†Increased risk if syncope occurs.

Source: Recommendations for Determining Eligibility for Competition in Athletes with Cardiovascular Abnormalities. *JACC.* 1994; 24:845–899.

TABLE 50-4

RECOMMENDED EXERCISE ACTIVITY FOR SPECIFIC CHD

Diagnosis	Type of Activity	Testing		
		Echo	Exercise	EKG
Aortic valve stenosis				
Mild <20 mm gradient	Normal	Yes	No	Yes
Moderate 20–40 mm gradient	Moderate	Yes	Yes	Yes
Severe >40 mmHg gradient	Low	Yes	Yes	Yes
Aortic insufficiency				
Mild—no cardiomegaly	Normal	Yes	Optional	Yes
Moderate to severe	Moderate to low	Yes	Optional	Yes
Atrial septal defect	Normal	No	No	No
Cardiomyopathy	Low	Yes	Yes	Yes
Coarctation of aorta				
Normal BP; gradient <20	Normal	Yes	Yes	No
Hypertension	Normal	Yes	Yes	Yes
Dilated ascending aorta	Moderate to low	Yes	Yes	Yes
Kawasaki's disease				
No coronary involvement	Normal	Yes	Yes	Yes
Minor coronary involvement	Moderate to low	Yes	Yes	Yes
Large aneurysm; stenosis	Low	Yes	Yes	Yes
Marfan's syndrome				
All categories of aortic root				
Dilatation and mitral valve	Low			
Insufficiency	Noncollision	Yes	No	No
Mitral insufficiency				
Mild; no cardiomegaly	Normal	Yes	No	No
Moderate; mild cardiomegaly	Moderate	Yes	Yes	No
Severe; cardiomegaly	Low	Yes	Yes	Yes
Myocarditis				
Acute	None	Yes	No	Yes
Chronic	None to low	Yes	Yes	Yes
Recovered; normal LV	Normal	Yes	Yes	Yes
Patent ductus arteriosus				
Small; normal LV	Normal	No	No	No
Closed	Normal	No	No	No
Pulmonary valve stenosis				
Mild; RV <40 mmHg	Normal	No	No	No
Moderate, RV 40–70 mmHg	Normal	Yes	Yes	No
Severe; RV >70 mmHg	Moderate to low	Yes	Yes	Yes
Pulmonary insufficiency				
Mild; normal RV pressure and volume	Normal	Yes	No	Yes

Source: Recommendations for Determining Eligibility for Competition in Athletes with Cardiovascular Abnormalities. *JACC.* 1994; 24:845–899.

TABLE 50-4 (continued)
RECOMMENDED EXERCISE ACTIVITY FOR SPECIFIC CHD

Diagnosis	Type of Activity	Testing		
		Echo	Exercise	EKG
Moderate; RV dilated, nl septum	Normal	Yes	Yes	Yes
Severe; RV dilated, abnl septum	Moderate	Yes	Yes	Yes
Tetralogy of Fallot				
(repaired)	Normal	No	No	No
Normal RV pressure; no shunt	Normal	No	No	No
RV pressure >50 mmHg,	Moderate	Yes	Yes	Yes
Pulmonary insufficiency and/or ventricular arrhythmia	Moderate to low	Yes	Yes	Yes
D-Transposition (switch repair)				
No "aortic" insufficiency, normal RV pressure	Normal	Yes	Yes	Yes
Significant "aortic" insufficiency, RV pressure >50 mmHg	Moderate to low	Yes	Yes	Yes
D-Transposition (atrial repair)				
All categories and depending on presence of arrhythmia and results of exercise testing	Moderate to low	Yes	Yes	Yes
L-Transposition				
Normal right ventricular function, minimal AV valve insufficiency, sinus rhythm	Moderate	Yes	Yes	Yes
Ventricular septal defect				
Small defect, no AI moderate defect, mild LV	Normal	No	No	No
Dilatation, normal RV pressure large defect, dilated LV, some	Normal	Yes	Optional	Yes
Elevation of RV pressure	Moderate to low	Yes	Yes	Yes

TYPES OF CONGENITAL HEART DEFECTS

Shunting Defects

Athletic restrictions for patients with an atrial septal defect (ASD), ventricular septal defect (VSD) or patent ductus arteriosus (PDA) are rare since moderate to large defects meet criteria for intervention and are completely repaired. If the shunts are small or if the defect has been repaired and there is normal pulmonary artery pressure, no restriction in physical activity is recommended. The rare patient with a large, unrepaired defect with pulmonary vascular disease (Eisenmenger syndrome) ought to be restricted from competitive sports; however, these patients will universally have low exercise tolerance making this restriction moot.

Valve Defects

Pulmonary Valve Stenosis

Recommendations for activity are based on the severity of the obstruction. Patients with mild obstruction (transvalvular gradient less than 40 mmHg) need no limitation in their physical activity. A transvalvular pressure gradient of 40–70 mmHg is considered moderate obstruction and a gradient greater than 70 mmHg is severe. Most patients with a gradient of more that 50 mmHg will undergo balloon valvuloplasty. Once the peak gradient is less than 50 mmHg and right ventricular function is normal, full athletic participation may resume. If pulmonary valve insufficiency develops, individual assessment of right ventricular function will be necessary before recommending an activity level.

Aortic Valve Stenosis

Task force recommendations for aortic stenosis are different than those made for clinical management because of the known association of sudden death and exercise; however, sudden death in aortic stenosis patients is limited to those with severe obstruction and T-wave abnormalities at rest or during exercise testing. Patients with mild aortic stenosis, defined here as a peak systolic gradient less than 20 mmHg, are allowed athletic participation if the electrocardiogram is normal and there are no symptoms of exercise related chest pain, arrhythmia, or syncope. Modified dynamic or static activities are allowed for athletes with moderate obstruction, defined as a peak systolic gradient between 20 and 50 mmHg. Preparticipation evaluation should include an electrocardiogram with only mild left ventricular hypertrophy and absence of "strain" and a normal exercise test with no evidence for ischemia and with normal exercise endurance and blood pressure response. Athletes with severe stenosis should be excluded from sports participation and managed as outlined in the aortic stenosis chapter of this book.

Subaortic Membrane

Eligibility for athletic participation in patients with discrete membranous suboartic stenosis should be determined using the same criteria as for aortic valve stenosis.

Aortic Valve Insufficiency

Insufficiency of the aortic valve may be related to a congenital bicuspid valve or rheumatic inflammation. Unless there is active inflammation from the rheumatic process, the etiology of the regurgitation does not affect the athletic recommendation. Patients with mild regurgitation have no symptoms, no peripheral signs of insufficiency, and no evidence for enlargement of the left ventricle by electrocardiogram and echocardiography. Normal athletic activity is permitted. An exercise test to evaluate exercise capacity is optional. Moderate aortic insufficiency is associated with peripheral signs and increase of left ventricular size by electrocardiogram and echocardiogram. The distinction between moderate and severe aortic insufficiency may be difficult; however, severe regurgitation will be associated with significant left ventricular dilatation by echo as well as marked reversal of Doppler blood flow in the aorta. Recommendations for medical and surgical management detailed elsewhere in this book should be followed. If athletic activity is contemplated, exercise testing up to the level of proposed activity (oxygen consumption) should be performed to exclude the presence of arrhythmia or ischemic EKG changes; however, only modified activity should be allowed in the moderate and severe group of aortic insufficiency patients.

Mitral Valve Insufficiency

Mitral insufficiency may be rheumatic, related to mitral valve prolapse or associated with endocardial cushion defects. In the absence of active inflammation, the etiology of the regurgitation does not affect the recommendation for athletic activity. Patients with mild insufficiency, verified by echocardiographic measurement of normal left ventricular size, may be allowed unrestricted exercise activity. Patients with moderate or severe mitral insufficiency will have increased diastolic volume of the left ventricle. Exercise, particularly isometric activity, may increase the regurgitation and increase left atrial and pulmonary venous pressure. Therefore, athletic activity should be modified. Exercise testing may be useful in documenting an endurance range that is comfortable. Medical and surgical recommendations mentioned elsewhere in this book should be followed.

Tricuspid Valve Insufficiency

Significant tricuspid insufficiency is most often associated with Ebstein's malformation. Athletic activity may be permitted if the right ventricular size is normal or nearly normal, if cyanosis is absent at rest and during exercise testing, and if there are no documented arrhythmias. Moderate and severe cases are associated with physical disability and possible sudden death. Athletic activity should not be recommended. Surgical repair of the tricuspid valve may reverse much of the disability. Exercise testing may be useful in assessing endurance level and risk for arrhythmia during exercise activity.

Cardiomyopathy

Hypertrophic Cardiomyopathy

Hypertrophic cardiomyopathy is an inherited, autosomal dominant, abnormality of cardiac muscle manifested by increased thickness as measured by echocardiography. The relative individual risk for athletic participation is unknown. The risk for sudden cardiac death in this disorder is variable. Tragically, however, many young athletes have died suddenly before the diagnosis was made clinically. Therefore, athletes with an unequivocal diagnosis of hypertrophic cardiomyopathy, with or without evidence of obstruction, should not participate in most competitive sports. A possible exception for activity type may be low intensity sports such as bowling or golf.

Myocarditis

Myocarditis may be present with no associated signs or symptoms. Alternatively, there may be signs and symptoms of inflammation of cardiac muscle along with signs and symptoms of a dilated cardiomyopathy such as congestive heart failure, arrhythmias, syncope, electrocardiographic changes, and reduced left ventricular function by echocardiogram. It is currently recommended that athletic activity be prohibited for at least 6 months. Normal activity may be resumed if left ventricular function returns to normal and if there is no evidence for ventricular arrhythmias by holter monitor and exercise testing.

Dilated Cardiomyopathy

Dilated cardiomyopathy may occur as the end stage of acute myocarditis or be related to metabolic

illnesses. Most likely, athletic participation will be self-limited by symptoms of reduced cardiac output. Exercise testing will establish levels of cardiac endurance and will identify exercise-induced arrhythmias. Under most circumstances, very low levels of physical activity are tolerated or recommended.

Cyanotic Heart Defects

The most common cyanotic congenital heart defect is tetralogy of Fallot. D-transposition of the great arteries, truncus arteriosus, hypoplastic left heart complex and tricuspid valve/pulmonary valve atresia are also frequent cyanotic defects. Surgical intervention has improved the natural outcome of these defects. Patients with good surgical results can be allowed athletic participation.

Tetralogy of Fallot

Full participation in competitive sports should be allowed if the right ventricular pressure is normal or near normal and if there is only mild right ventricular volume overload from pulmonary valve insufficiency, no or very minimal residual left-to-right shunting and absence of arrhythmia with exercise testing. Patients with significant right ventricular volume overload and/or right ventricular hypertension greater than 50 mmHg or rhythm abnormalities should have restricted athletic activity.

D-transposition of the Great Arteries

Patients who have had the arterial switch operation have a very low incidence of ventricular dysfunction, arrhythmia, or hemodynamic abnormality with the exception of pulmonary artery stenosis at the anastomotic site or branch pulmonary artery stenosis. Exercise testing should be performed to assess for T-wave abnormalities which would be a sign of an underlying coronary artery abnormality. If a patient has a normal echocardiogram and exercise test, athletic participation should be permitted. High levels of static exercise, however, should be limited because the neo-aortic valve is the original pulmonary valve and it may theoretically be prone to developing insufficiency.

Patients with atrial repair of transposition may have significant hemodynamic abnormalities even if they are clinically well. The right ventricle is now the systemic ventricle. Right ventricular function may not be normal. Tricuspid valve insufficiency, atrial arrhythmias, left ventricular outflow tract obstruction, or systemic venous obstruction may all be present. Exercise testing usually shows reduced exercise indurance. For these reasons, athletic activity should be restricted to low or moderate level activities.

Postoperative Fontan Operation

The Fontan procedure creates a direct communication between the systemic veins and the pulmonary artery. This operation is used as a long-term palliation of pulmonary/tricuspid atresia, hypoplastic left ventricle and other complex congenital heart defects. In the young patient, exercise endurance is good but not to the level of competitive athletes. Sports participation should be based on patient desire, endurance as demonstrated by exercise testing, and freedom from significant arrhythmia.

Congenitally Corrected Transposition

Congenitally corrected transposition of the great arteries, also known as L-transposition of the great arteries or ventricular inversion, uses the right ventricle as the systemic ventricle. Frequently the systemic atrioventricular (AV) valve has an Ebstein's malformation that may create significant "mitral" insufficiency. There is also the potential for heart block. If the ventricular size and function are normal, there is no significant insufficiency of the systemic AV valve and the heart rhythm is sinus, then normal athletic participation may be considered. Annual follow-up is required regarding AV valve competence, ventricular function and cardiac rhythm. Exercise testing is critical for assessment of exercise endurance and to be certain that exercise-induced heart block does not occur.

Marfan Syndrome

The cardiovascular manifestations of Marfan syndrome are mitral valve prolapse and aortic root dilatation. Aortic root dissection may cause rupture of the aorta and sudden death. Therefore, athletic activity should be limited to low intensity, noncollision sports. If the patient is participating in regular athletic activity, the aortic root dimension should be checked every 6–9 months by echocardiography.

Coarctation of the Aorta

Patients who have had a repair of coarctation of the aorta without residual hypertension, aortic valve problems or dilatation of the ascending aorta may have normal athletic activity. Patients with mild residual coarctation (gradient less than 20 mmHg) and a peak exercise blood pressure less than 230 mmHg are generally allowed competitive sports, again if the aortic valve and ascending aorta are normal. If balloon angioplasty or Gore-Tex patch repair have been performed, MRI studies should be performed to exclude the presence of aortic aneurysms before permitting athletic activity. If the above pressure criteria are not met, therapeutic considerations should be made before granting unlimited exercise.

Kawasaki's Disease

Coronary artery aneurysm occurs in 20% of untreated children with Kawasaki disease. Some of these will regress. Others persist as large aneurysms, of which some have associated coronary artery stenosis. Guidelines from a 1994 conference dealing with sports eligibility have recommended participation in all competitive sports be allowed for those athletes who have never had any coronary involvement. There is a cautionary note for long-term follow-up. This is important because myocardial perfusion defects have been reported with exercise in patients not thought to have coronary involvement. Athletes with minor abnormalities should have exercise tests and probably perfusion scans before permitting exercise activity. They should be restricted to low static or low to moderate dynamic activity. Patients with large aneurysms or coronary artery stenosis should be considered at increased risk and should be limited to low intensity activities.

Contact sports should also be limited for those patients receiving anticoagulation (warfarin) or taking aspirin as part of their medical management program.

Arrhythmias

Irregularities of the heart rhythm are not uncommon in the pediatric and adolescent population. Isolated sinus arrhythmia, sinus bradycardia, ectopic atrial rhythm, premature atrial beats, and premature junctional beats with narrow QRS complex are all considered benign. Normal athletic participation is recommended.

Atrial Flutter/Atrial Fibrillation

Atrial flutter is more common than atrial fibrillation in pediatric patients. Neither is very common in children unless there is a recognized congenital heart defect or previous cardiac surgery. These patients should have a thorough electrophysiologic investigation. If there are no anatomic or conduction abnormalities such as an accessory bypass tract, and exercise testing is normal in terms of endurance and heart rate response, normal athletic participation should be permitted.

Ventricular Preexcitation (AV reciprocating tachycardia)

Normal cardiac structure should be verified. Athletes may be at risk if their accessory connection has a short refractory period. Therefore, electrophysiologic testing with atrial pacing or transesophageal pacing is recommended. Athletes with normal cardiac structure and who are without syncope and have had electrophysiologic evaluation may participate normally. Athletes with successful radiofrequency may also compete.

Premature Ventricular Contraction (PVC)

PVCs occur commonly in people with otherwise normal hearts. Most often, exercise suppresses these beats. If a 24-h holter recording and exercise testing exclude ventricular tachycardia, normal athletic participation is allowed.

Ventricular Tachycardia

Nonsustained or sustained monomorphic or polymorphic ventricular tachycardia is always a potentially serious event. Participation in sports should be prohibited for at least 6 months past the most recent episode. The task force indicates an exception to this recommendation. If the athlete is asymptomatic with brief (less than 8 consecutive ventricular beats) episodes of nonsustained monomorphic ventricular tachycardia at a rate less than 150 beats/min, there does not appear to be a risk of sudden death. Sports participation is permitted.

Atrioventricular Block

AV Block

First degree AV block that does not worsen with exercise should not prevent normal athletic participation. Type I, second degree AV block (Wenckebach) may be normally present in well-trained athletes. If the AV block does not worsen or even improves with exercise, normal athletic activity is allowed. If the AV block increases with activity, further evaluation for the possible need of a pacemaker is warranted. Type II, second degree AV block (Mobitz) should be managed in a manner similar to acquired heart block, which means that a permanent pacemaker should be implanted and contact sports prohibited.

Congenital Complete Heart Block

Athletes with congenital heart block but an otherwise normal heart may be permitted normal athletic activity if it is documented that their heart rate increases with activity; however, consideration should be given to the effect that the activity will have on an already dilated heart. AV synchronous pacing should be considered.

Bundle Branch Block

Patients with either left or right bundle branch block may participate normally if it is documented that they do not develop AV block with exercise.

Congenital Long QT Syndrome

A corrected QT (QTc) interval of 450 ms or more is considered abnormal, particularly if there is a family history of sudden death. Athletes with the prolonged QTc interval are at risk for sudden death with activity and therefore should be prohibited from competitive sports.

Suggested Readings

AHA medical/scientific statements: cardiovascular participation screening of competitive athletes. *Circulation* 94:850–856, 1996.

26th Bethesda Conference. Recommendations for determining eligibility for competition in athletes with cardiovascular abnormalities. *J Am Coll Cardiol* 24(4): 845, 1994.

Fredriksen PM, Veldtman G, Hechter S, Therrien J, Chen A, Warsi MA, Freeman M, Liu P, Siu S, Thaulow E, Webb G: Aerobic capacity in adults with various congenital heart diseases. *Am J Cardiol* 87: 310–314, 2001.

Mahle WT, McBride MG, Paridon SM: Exercise performance after the arterial switch operation for D-transposition of the great arteries. *Am J Cardiol* 87:753–758, 2001.

Minamisawa S, Nakazawa M, Momma K, Imai Y, Satomi G: Effect of aerobic training on exercise performance in patients after the Fontan operation. *Am J Cardiol* 88 September15, 2001:695–698.

Paridon SM, Galiato FM, Vincent JA Tomassoni TL, Sullivan NM, Bricker JT: Exercise capacity and incidence of myocardial perfusion defects after Kawasaki disease in children and adolescents. *J Am Cill Cardiol* 25(6):1420–1424, 1995.

Strong WB, Steed D: Cardiovascular evaluation of the young athlete. *Pediatr Clin North Am* 29(6): 1325–1339, 1982.

Yetman AT, Lee KJ, Hamilton R, Morrow WR, McCrindle BW: Exercise capacity after repair of tetralogy of Fallot in infancy. *Am J Cardiol* 87:1021–1023, 2001.

Yetman AT, King S, Bornemeier RA, Fasules J: Comparison of exercise performance in patients after pulmonary valvulotomy for pulmonary stenosis and tetralogy of Fallot. *Am J Cardiol* 90:1412–1414, 2002.

51

TELEMEDICINE

Andrew S. Bensky

Telemedicine can be broadly defined as the transmission of medical information across distances. In its simplest form, it can be the telephone consultation between two physicians discussing patient management. With advances in technology, these interactions have become more sophisticated. Telemedicine is becoming widely used in pediatric cardiology. One of more commonly used examples involves the facsimile transmission of electrocardiograms for physician interpretation. Although some centers have experimented with remote auscultation using electronic stethoscopes,[1] provision of cardiology consultations across distances is not widespread at the present time.

Transmission of medical images is a natural extension of telecommunications systems developed to provide teleconferencing to industry and government. Transmission of static radiographic images across standard telephone systems was one of the first applications in this area.[2] With advances in image processing technology and the development of broadband telecommunications systems, the transmission of moving images became feasible. This is the type of telemedicine application with the greatest current appeal to pediatric cardiologists.

Tele-echocardiography typically involves the transfer of echocardiographic images and sound from a remote location to a center able to provide the specialized interpretive services not available at the remote location. Because of the relatively small number of pediatric cardiologists and the tendency of these specialists to practice in larger cities; tele-echocardiography is a logical extension of the practice of pediatric cardiology. The type of pediatric patient most likely to benefit from tele-echocardiography is the newborn with suspected congenital heart disease. The prompt identification of infants with congenital lesions that require specialized treatment should have a positive impact on the morbidity of these lesions, by allowing for the prompt institution of medications such as prostaglandin E1 and early transfer to a tertiary care center before symptoms worsen. Conversely, those infants without heart disease, or those with less acute need for specialized care, could be spared the expense and inconvenience of transfer to a tertiary care center, as well as the possible separation from their mothers. There are also potential cost savings in the appropriate triage of these newborns.

TELE-ECHOCARDIOGRAPHY SYSTEM DESIGN

The design of a tele-echocardiography system depends on several variables. It must be decided whether the studies will be sent in real-time or stored for later off-line transmission. Another factor is whether the transmitted images are intended to provide the basis for a complete diagnostic study and interpretation, or serve as a screening examination with the complete study being sent by traditional methods for interpretation at a later time. In addition, it must be determined whether an analog video signal, digitized video stream, or digital cine-loops and still frames will provide the basis for the transmitted study. The decision regarding the type of signal source mirrors the discussion involving conversion of pediatric echocardiography laboratories from analog video recordings to a digital acquisition and storage system. Adult laboratories have shown that diagnostic accuracy was maintained when a series of digital still frames and cine-loops were compared to fully videotaped studies.[3,4] In pediatric echocardiography, however, complex anatomy is often better visualized by sweeping the transducer across multiple planes than by viewing a series of standard imaging planes. Mathewson et al. reported that a pediatric digital protocol that incorporated multiplane digital sweeps in addition to cine-loops of standard views provided complete diagnostic information in nearly all cases.[5] While acquisition of loops and multiplane sweeps is technically possible with most equipment, the proper selection of images may require more training and experience than some sonographers at smaller centers have received.

Centers that have not converted to a digital system for their echocardiography laboratories use the analog video and audio signal from their echocardiographic equipment as the source for their tele-echocardiography transmissions. Several vendors are marketing the hardware and software needed to provide telemedicine using these analog signals. The basic components of such systems include a CODEC (coder-decoder) to process the analog video and audio output signal from the echocardiography machine. These signals are converted to a digital format compliant with the H.320 protocol. The H.320 protocol specifies requirements for processing audio and video information, and allows multimedia terminals to use communications links and synchronize their audio and video signals.[6] Digital conversion also allows for a compression algorithm to be applied to the signal to allow for a more manageable file size. Systems that use the Internet or wide-area networks for data transmission use a similar protocol, H.323. Computers are often used to store, prepare, and view the digital data files transferred using telemedicine. It is also possible to use the CODEC to return the digital file to its original analog form for storage on videotape. Routers and switches are used to interface the digital data stream and the telecommunications system being used for transmission.

Echocardiography laboratories that have made the conversion to digital image acquisition and storage have different options when performing telemedicine. Many echocardiography vendors have made their digital image files compliant with an industry accepted standard. A joint committee created by the American College of Radiology (ACR) and the National Electrical Manufacturers Association (NEMA) in 1983 initially proposed the format currently used. These groups recognized the need for a standard method for transferring images and associated information between devices manufactured by various vendors to avoid the production of a variety of incompatible digital image formats. The current version of these standards is designated Digital Imaging and Communications in Medicine (DICOM) Version 3.0.[7] After the digital studies are acquired and stored in a DICOM-compatible format, the digital files can be transmitted over a telecommunications link using routers and switches. Once received at the central site, the digital files can be viewed by a variety of DICOM-compatible viewers. It is also possible to store the digital files on a secured network server at the remote site, where they can be accessed using a wide-area network or over the Internet.

COMPRESSION

Each 640×480 pixel frame of digitized video contains approximately 1 Mb of information. A study recorded at the broadcast standard of 30 frames per second would require 1.8 Gb per minute to store, or about 25 Gb for a 15-min study. Even with current storage technology and high-speed telecommunications equipment, it is not feasible to process and transfer such large files in a reasonable amount of time. For this reason, some form of compression must be applied to the studies.

Clinical compression is applied by the sonographer at the remote site. In traditional analog echocardiography laboratories, the sonographer compresses the amount of data acquired by only taping certain portions of the study for later review. This same approach can be applied in store and forward telemedicine systems that use a digitized video stream. With digital image acquisition, clinical compression is achieved by storing cine-loops and still frames of selected views for analysis. Since telemedicine studies at remote centers are often performed by sonographers with less experience than those at the receiving centers, performing any form of clinical compression may decrease the diagnostic yield.

Digital compression involves the application of different mathematic algorithms to the digital video and audio streams, shrinking the file size considerably. JPEG is a commonly used image compression mechanism. JPEG stands for Joint Photographic Experts Group, the original name of the committee that wrote the standard.[6] JPEG is designed for compressing either full-color or gray-scale images. JPEG is designed for still images, but echocardiography systems treat the digitized cine-loops as a series of still images and apply JPEG compression. JPEG is "lossy," meaning that the decompressed image isn't exactly the same as the original. There are lossless image compression algorithms, but JPEG achieves much greater compression than is possible with lossless methods. An important property of JPEG is that the degree of compression can be varied by adjusting software parameters. This means that a system can trade off file size against output image quality. Current digital echocardiography machines allow the user to select the degree of JPEG compression that will be applied. Studies have shown that digital cardiac image loops compressed to ratios of 10:1 and 20:1 are virtually indistinguishable from uncompressed loops,[7] and that compression ratios of less than 30:1 provide image quality superior or equal to videotape.[8]

Since JPEG compression is optimized for still images, telemedicine programs that use real-time video streaming for their telemedicine applications often rely on other compression modalities. MPEG is an abbreviation for the Moving Pictures Experts Group, which defines the protocols. MPEG compression transforms a stream of moving images, exploiting the fact that much of the information in a moving image is unchanged from frame to frame. As with JPEG, the MPEG standard is being revised and updated to keep pace with advances in technology. MPEG-2 is the standard used to develop such technologies as digital television and DVDs. MPEG-4 has expanded the protocol to allow for the seamless integration of digital media across the Internet, multimedia graphics applications, and the digital television spectrum.[8] Systems using MPEG compression of streaming video content are available for use today, though it should be pointed out that MPEG is not currently supported by the DICOM standard.

BANDWIDTH

Bandwidth refers to the speed at which telecommunications systems can transmit information. Given the large size of the data files containing digitized video and audio information, bandwidth is critical for any telemedicine system. Table 51-1 shows the approximate transfer times for a 30 Mb file using several different transmission modalities. Another important concept to understand is that the speed of any telecommunications system is limited by the slowest link in the circuit. For this reason, the specialized transmission lines used in real-time telemedicine systems must be present

TABLE 51-1

APPROXIMATE TRANSMISSION TIMES FOR A 30 MB STUDY

56.6 kbps modem	1 h 10 min
384 kbps ISDN line	10 min
768 kbps SDSL line	5.2 min
1.54 Mbps T1 line	3 min
622 Mbps ATM line	0.4 s

from the bedside at the remote location into the reading room at the receiving end. The expenses associated with provision of the relatively large bandwidth required for telemedicine applications represent the largest ongoing costs of such activities.

POTS (PLAIN OLD TELEPHONE SERVICE)

The advantages of POTS are its universal availability and the ability to connect to any other user (i.e., it is a switched system). In addition, POTS is the least expensive transmission modality currently available. Modems using POTS are currently limited by a data transfer rate of about 56.6 kbps, making them impractical for most forms of tele-echocardiography.

ISDN (INTEGRATED SERVICES DIGITAL NETWORK)

Integrated services digital network is a standard that allows for the transfer of digital information at high speed across existing copper telephone lines. Each ISDN line consists of three independent channels, two for carrying the digital data at rates of 64 kbps each and a third channel to carry information about the network connection. Many current videoconferencing systems use an aggregate connection of three ISDN lines, giving a data transfer capacity of 384 kbps. The advantages of ISDN service include data transfer rates much faster than POTS and widespread availability. Like POTS, ISDN service is provided over a switched network, allowing users to connect with anyone else having comparable service. This allows a tertiary care center to connect to a variety of remote sites using the same ISDN lines.

T1

T1 is a term for a standard adopted for the transfer of digital information across a high-speed network using fiber-optic lines. A full T1 line provides data transfer rates of 1.544 Mbps. These services are usually provided by a line leased from a telecommunications provider. Some companies provide service at a fraction of the full T1 transfer rate, for example 1/4 T1 service provides a 384 kbps transfer rate comparable to three ISDN lines. T1 service is usually provided on a point-to-point basis, meaning that a dedicated service is created between two points. Though more stable than ISDN service, this means that the circuit will sit unused for much of the day. In addition, connecting one center to multiple remote sites may require the creation of multiple circuits, with the resulting increases in cost.

DSL (DIGITAL SUBSCRIBER LINE)

Digital subscriber line technology allows for the transmission of digital information at high speeds across existing copper phone lines. The residential application of this technology is typically ADSL, or asymmetric DSL, which allows for faster downloading than uploading. This is not ideal for telemedicine since the transfer would be limited by the relatively slower upload speeds. SDSL, or symmetric DSL, is more commonly used by business users and provides equal upload and download speeds. The actual transfer rates vary, and may depend on the distance between the telephone company's central office and the site served.

ATM (ASYNCHRONOUS TRANSFER MODE)

Asynchronous transfer mode is the protocol used by telecommunications providers to transfer data between their large switching centers. Transfer rates of 622 Mbps to 2.3 Gbps are possible over these fiber optic networks. ATM will provide the backbone for the next generation Internet, or Internet 2. Some universities and government sites are experimenting with these systems today. Delivery of this bandwidth to end-users is not widespread at present, and is currently too expensive for most clinical applications in telemedicine.

REAL-TIME VERSUS STORE AND FORWARD

Real-time tele-echocardiography offers the advantages of direct supervision of the performance of the study at the remote site and the fastest provision of an interpretation. The use of this type of system will insure that all necessary diagnostic views are obtained before the study is completed, insuring that all interpretations are complete and that an additional study will not be necessary to provide missing views. There is also the opportunity for ongoing continuing education of the sonographers at the remote site, with immediate feedback on the quality of images and the ability to interact in real-time with the specialists at the receiving end.

Disadvantages of real-time systems include the high bandwidth requirements, and their associated high ongoing costs, and the need to bring the telecommunications equipment and specialized communication lines into the clinical settings such as the neonatal intensive care unit. Other concerns include the time commitment needed to insure availability of an interpreting physician at the receiving end at the time the remote site is able to perform the study. Since there is no ability to provide clinical compression with a live study, there will be a larger time commitment for the physician on the receiving end than there would be in review of videotaped studies or digitized cine-loops.

Store and forward telemedicine systems are the most widely used for the transfer of medical images, including echocardiography. With these systems, the study is acquired at the remote site and stored on either videotape or digital media such as an optical disk. The images are brought to the telecommunications equipment and are prepared for transmission. At the receiving site, the incoming digital signals can be stored on the appropriate media, or it can be converted back to an analog video signal and recorded into videotape. When the interpreting physician is ready to review the images, the appropriate files can be accessed.

The advantages of store and forward technology include the ability to use a wider range of transmission protocols, since the images do not need to be reviewed in real-time. Larger files needed to provide images with less compression can take as much time as is needed for transmission. Study times are shorter in a store and forward approach, since clinical compression can be applied at the remote site. Since the studies can be stored at the receiving site for later review, the interpreting physician can read the studies when his or her schedule allows. Disadvantages of the store and forward approach include the inability to provide feedback to less experienced sonographers at the remote sites, raising the possibility of incomplete studies requiring the acquisition of additional images at a later time. The longer time necessary to transmit and interpret these studies will also delay provision of an interpretation.

CLINICAL EXPERIENCE

Many centers around the world have described their clinical experience with tele-echocardiography. Finley et al. described the use of a broadband dial-up system to perform real-time tele-echocardiography between a general hospital and a children's hospital in Canada in 1989.[9] Eighteen studies were transmitted, with a complete segmental diagnosis made in 16 patients. Two patients required additional imaging at a later date. Sobczyk et al. reported on the use of a store and forward system using limited digitized cine-loops over standard telephone lines in 1993.[10] Of 47 studies transmitted, 83% were felt to provide accurate diagnostic impressions compared to later review of videotape. Sable et al. published their telemedicine experience using three multiplexed ISDN lines between rural sites and a tertiary hospital in 1999.[11] Sixty studies were transmitted with a diagnostic accuracy of 100% when compared to videotape, and an average time from request to interpretation of 43 minutes at a distance of 200 mi. The same year, Randolph et al. reported on the use of dedicated T1 lines to perform real-time tele-echocardiography on 133 patients from Grand Forks, North Dakota to Rochester, Minnesota.[12,15] All studies were felt to be diagnostic, and 59% of the interactions resulted in a change in medical management or timing of cardiology follow-up. Bensky et al. described their experience in performing real-time echocardiography using a high-speed ATM network protocol in North Carolina.[13,16] Over 3 years, more than 1300 studies were successfully transmitted from an intensive care nursery at a community hospital to the tertiary care hospital. Fifty-four percent of the studies ordered to exclude congenital heart disease were positive, and 77% of those with congenital heart disease were found to have lesions that could be managed at the community hospital.

FUTURE DIRECTIONS

Although experience over the past 10 years has clearly proven the feasibility of tele-echocardiography, there have been significant costs involved in the provision of these services. Several centers have postulated that despite their relatively high initial and ongoing costs, tele-echocardiography actually saves money by avoiding unnecessary transfers.[14,17,18] At this time, however, reimbursement for telemedicine services is not standardized. Advances in telecommunications technology and image compression should lead to lower ongoing costs for even faster data transmission rates in the future. In addition, although the feasibility of tele-echocardiography has been demonstrated it has not been proven to lead to a clinically significant improvement in the long-term outcome for infants with congenital heart disease. These data should be available as the clinical expedience grows.

Laws and regulations governing medicine need to keep pace with advances in technology. State medical licensing laws vary in how they deal with the provision of interpretive services by out of state physicians. Since telemedicine is not constrained by state borders, providers need to understand the laws in other states when they set up their programs. Recent changes in medical privacy laws also impact telemedicine programs. Confidentiality must be protected when medical images are stored on servers with remote access, and images are transmitted across public telecommunications systems. Despite these concerns, it is reasonable to

foresee a time when high quality cardiac images can be quickly shared among specialists across the world, improving the quality of care for children with heart disease everywhere.

References

1   Belmont JM, Mattioli LF, Goertz KK, Ardinger RH Jr, Thomas CM: Evaluation of remote stethoscopy for pediatric telecardiology. *Telemed J* 1(2):133–149, 1995.

2   Gayler BW, Gitlin JN, Rappaport W, Skinner FL, Cerva J: Teleradiology: an evaluation of a microcomputer-based system. *Radiology* 140(2):355–360, 1981.

3   Mobarek SK, Gilliland YE, Bernal A, Murgo JP, Cheirif J: Is a full digital echocardiography laboratory feasible for routine daily use? *Echocardiography* 13(5):473–482, 1996.

4   Segar DS, Skolnick D, Sawada SG, Fitch G, Wagner D, Adams D, Feigenbaum H: A comparison of the interpretation of digitized and videotape recorded echocardiograms. *J Am Soc Echocardiogr* 12(9):714–719, 1999.

5   Mathewson JW, Perry JC, Maginot KR, Cocalis M: Pediatric digital echocardiography: a study of the analog-to-digital transition. *J Am Soc Echocardiogr* 13(6):561–562, 2000.

6   *Recommendation H.320.* Geneva, Switzerland, International Telecommunication Union, 1999.

7   Digital Imaging and Communications in Medicine (DICOM) Standard, version 3.0. Washington, DC, National Electrical Manufacturers Association (NEMA), parts 1–9 (1993), parts 10–12 (1994).

8   Cavigioli C: JPEG compression: spelling out the options. *Adv Imaging* 6:44–48, 1991.

9   Karson TH, Zepp RC, Chandra S, Morehead A, Thomas JD: Digital storage of echocardiograms offers superior image quality to analog storage, even with 20:1 digital compression: results of the Digital Echo Record Access Study. *J Am Soc Echocardiogr* 9(6):769–778, 1996.

10 Soble JS, Yurow G, Brar R, Stamos T, Neumann A, Garcia M, Stoddard MF, Cherian PK, Bhamb B, Thomas JD: Comparison of MPEG digital video with super VHS tape for diagnostic echocardiographic readings. *J Am Soc Echocardiogr* 11(8):819–825, 1998.

11 MPEG protocols. Geneva, Switzerland: International Organization for Standards (ISO)/International Electrotechnical Commission (IEC).

12 Finley JP, Human DG, Nanton MA, Roy DL, Macdonald RG, Marr DR, Chiasson H: Echocardiography by telephone—evaluation of pediatric heart disease at a distance. *Am J Cardiol* 63(20):1475–1477, 1989.

13 Sobczyk WL, Solinger RE, Rees AH, Elbl F: Transtelephonic echocardiography: successful use in a tertiary pediatric referral center. *J Pediatr* 122(6):S84–S88, 1993.

14 Sable C, Roca T, Gold J, Gutierrez A, Gulotta E, Culpepper W. Live transmission of neonatal echocardiograms from underserved areas: accuracy, patient care, and cost. *Telemed J* 5(4):339–347, 1999.

15 Randolph GR, Hagler DJ, Khandheria BK, Lunn ER, Cook WJ, Seward JB, O'Leary PW: Remote telemedical interpretation of neonatal echocardiograms: impact on clinical management in a primary care setting. *J Am Coll Cardiol* 34(1):241–245, 1999.

16 Bensky AS, Covitz W, Chimiak WJ: Realtime paediatric echocardiography using ATM: three-year experience. *J Telemed Telecare* 5(3):208–210, 1999.

17 Rendina MC, Long WA, deBliek R: Effect size and experimental power analysis in a paediatric cardiology telemedicine system. *J Telemed Telecare* 3 (Suppl. 1) :56–57, 1997.

18 Finley JP, Sharratt GP, Nanton MA, Chen RP, Bryan P, Wolstenholme J, MacDonald C. Paediatric echocardiography by telemedicine—nine years' experience. *J Telemed Telecare* 3(4):200–204, 1997.

52

OFFICE EMERGENCIES AND TRANSPORT

Joel T. Hardin

INTRODUCTION

Pediatric cardiac emergencies in the office setting or community hospital emergency department are relatively rare occurrences for family physicians, pediatricians, and emergency medicine specialists. Examples include cyanotic newborns presenting after nursery discharge and infants or older children presenting with cardiac arrhythmia. In addition, there are potentially life-threatening complications related to the postoperative pediatric cardiac surgical patient that may initially present in the outpatient setting (e.g., cardiac tamponade from pericardial effusion).

Prevalence and incidence rates relative to outpatient pediatric cardiac emergencies are difficult to estimate. One recent study identified a prevalence of children presenting with severe respiratory distress or cardiac arrest at approximately 4% of primary care office practices.[1] Depending on how an emergency is defined, several studies report incidence of office-based emergencies ranging between 1 and 5 cases per week to as infrequently as one case per month. The incidence is higher in community hospital emergency departments. Finally,

the impact of recent national trends toward earlier neonatal discharge, and triage of managed-care patients to the outpatient setting for initial evaluation has not been fully evaluated.

Regardless of the infrequent nature of pediatric outpatient emergencies, it is widely held that all children deserve access to high-quality emergency medical services and that primary care office and community hospital preparedness can be raised in a cost-effective manner. The Committee on Pediatric Emergency Medicine of the American Academy of Pediatrics has published a reference source of guidelines in this regard,[2] focusing on emergency preparedness at the level of the individual practitioner, primary care office, community EMS capability, and specialized pediatric transport teams.

In this chapter, common outpatient pediatric cardiac emergencies will be reviewed, with a focus on preparedness and stabilization prior to transport to a neonatal or pediatric intensive care unit. In addition, the potential impact of regionalization of pediatric cardiac care, and emerging technology such as remote diagnosis of heart disease via telemedicine and tele-echocardiography will be discussed.

The reader should consult other chapters in this text for in-depth discussion of the pathophysiology and management of the specific cardiac conditions discussed in this review.

PREPAREDNESS

The best resuscitation results are derived from practitioners and support staff who have dedicated special effort toward continuing education in neonatal and pediatric advanced life support, and from facilities that have made advanced preparations to care for critically ill children. Resuscitation skills are refined through systematic and repetitive training with so often called "mock codes" that enlist participation of all staff likely to be called on in an emergency.

Preparedness included maintaining an appropriate inventory of resuscitation equipment, supplies, and medications. Table 52-1 lists resuscitation equipment and supplies that should be maintained in the outpatient office, and Table 52-2 expands this inventory for the community hospital emergency department. Office supply items or medications are further prioritized as essential versus desirable or optional. In most cases, optional equipment and medications in the office can be supplied by rapid-response emergency medical personnel.

Ideally, each point of pediatric emergency care delivery has, *in advance*, an identified point of next (higher echelon) contact. For the office practitioner, points of contact for local EMS resources, nearby community hospitals, and the regional children's hospital(s) should all be recorded and periodically updated.

Community hospitals should establish consulting arrangements with pediatricians and pediatric specialists within or near their locale (e.g., neonatology, pediatric critical care, and pediatric cardiology). In addition, the community hospital should maintain contact information for primary and back-up team support. There is now little argument against establishing regionalized centers of excellence as it relates to the treatment of congenital heart disease. When neonatal and pediatric transport

TABLE 52-1

EMERGENCY EQUIPMENT AND SUPPLIES FOR THE OFFICE

General
- *Preprinted age/weight specific pediatric resuscitation guidelines (e.g., Broselow Tape)*
- *Gowns, gloves, goggles (for universal precautions)*
- *Warm blankets*
- *Neonatal and pediatric blood pressure cuffs*
- *Pulse oximeter*
- ECG monitor
- Cardioverter-defibrillator or automated external defibrillator
- Nasogastric tubes

Airway and Breathing
- *Suction device and suction catheters/tips*
- *Oxygen*
- *Ambu-bag with variety of face mask sizes*
- *Nasal cannula and oxygen masks (neonatal, pediatric, and adult sizes)*
- Laryngoscope
- Endotracheal tubes and stylets

Vascular Access
- *Tourniquets*
- *Arm boards*
- *Butterfly and intraosseus needles*
- Intravenous catheters
- *Syringes*
- *IV tubing*
- *Tape*
- *Isotonic intravenous fluids (e.g., normal saline)*

Medications
- *Atropine*
- *Epinephrine*
- *Dextrose (25 and 10% solutions)*
- *Sodium bicarbonate*

Note: Essential inventory is italicized. Note that these recommendations are intended to only address the needs of the infant or child with a likely cardiac emergency. The inventory of supplies and medications to adequately prepare for the broader spectrum of all common pediatric emergencies (e.g., trauma, near-drowning, sepsis, airway obstruction, and poisoning) will of necessity be much larger.

TABLE 52-2

EMERGENCY EQUIPMENT AND SUPPLIES FOR THE COMMUNITY HOSPITAL EMERGENCY DEPARTMENT

General
- Pediatric Resuscitation Cart to house pediatric resuscitation inventory
- Preprinted age/weight specific pediatric resuscitation guidelines (e.g., Broselow Tape)
- Gowns, gloves, goggles (for universal precautions)
- Warm blankets
- Radiant warmer bed
- Infant scale
- Neonatal and pediatric blood pressure cuffs
- Pulse oximeter
- ECG monitor
- Cardioverter-defibrillator
- Nasogastric tubes
- Foley catheters

Airway and Breathing
- Suction device and suction catheters/tips
- Oxygen
- Ambu-bag with variety of face mask sizes
- Nasal cannula and oxygen masks (neonatal, pediatric, and adult sizes)
- Laryngoscope
- Endotracheal tubes and stylets
- Oral and nasopharyngeal airways

Vascular Access
- Tourniquets
- Arm boards
- Butterfly and intraosseus needles
- Intravenous catheters
- Central venous catheter kits (4–5 French catheter sizes, 5–15 cm lengths)
- Umbilical vessel catheters
- Syringes
- IV tubing
- T-connectors
- Tape
- Isotonic intravenous fluids (e.g., normal saline, Ringer's lactate, 5% albumin)

Medications
- Atropine
- Epinephrine
- Dextrose (25 and 10% solutions)
- Sodium bicarbonate
- Calcium chloride

(continued)

TABLE 52-2 (continued)

EMERGENCY EQUIPMENT AND SUPPLIES FOR THE COMMUNITY HOSPITAL EMERGENCY DEPARTMENT

Medications
- Lidocaine
- Magnesium sulfate
- Dopamine
- Dobutamine
- Adenosine
- Amiodarone
- Prostaglandin E1 (optional if nearby regional children's hospital can rapidly supply this drug)

Note: These recommendations are intended to only address the needs of the infant or child with a likely cardiac emergency. The inventory of supplies and medications to adequately prepare for the broader spectrum of all common pediatric emergencies (e.g., trauma, near-drowning, sepsis, airway obstruction, and poisoning) will of necessity be much larger.

teams from such regional centers are made integral to the transport process, there is a greater likelihood of stabilization prior to transport, safety is enhanced during transport, and perioperative outcomes are optimized after admittance to the tertiary care facility.[3]

Advances in telemedicine, specifically high-band width transmission of real-time echocardiograms, are also shaping how pediatric cardiac patients are triaged for transport. Remotely directed and interpreted pediatric echocardiograms can accurately diagnose critical congenital heart defects at risk for severe hypoxemia or cardiogenic shock, and help guide patient-specific recommendations for stabilization during transport. Conversely, telemedicine can convincingly reassure a referring physician that an infant or child with noncritical disease need not be urgently transferred to a distant tertiary care center, providing additional cost-effectiveness merit to this emerging technology.[4]

OUTPATIENT PEDIATRIC CARDIAC EMERGENCY SCENARIOS

Neonate with Cyanosis or Cardiogenic Shock

Compared to older children with congenital heart disease, neonates have a greater tendency toward presentation with acutely life-threatening disease. Furthermore, the trend toward earlier neonatal hospital discharge has shifted the likelihood of presentation with important heart disease from the inpatient nursery to the outpatient office or emergency department. Ductal-dependent cardiac defects such as hypoplastic left heart syndrome, severe coarctation of the aorta, or severe tetralogy of Fallot represent examples of congenital heart disease which may present as a life-threatening event as the ductus arteriosus constricts over the first few days of life.

Most of these infants will present with obvious cyanosis, respiratory distress, and signs of poor circulation. Clinical recognition of cyanotic congenital heart disease can be further facilitated by routine noninvasive pulse oximetry oxygen in these situations. Although there is an important differential diagnosis for a cyanotic or newborn in shock (e.g., sepsis, pneumonia, inborn error of metabolism), a definitive clinical and laboratory diagnosis may take several hours to days after the initial outpatient presentation. Priority in the outpatient setting should therefore be placed on fundamentals of neonatal resuscitation and early contact with the regional neonatal transport team, rather than extensive laboratory testing that may delay urgently needed medical and/or surgical intervention.

In neonates with severe hypoxemia (PaO_2 <40 mmHg or pulse oximetry saturation <80%), and in those with cardiogenic shock (Chapter 8), maintaining or reestablishing patency of the ductus arteriosus is the greatest priority. There is a prerequisite for stable vascular access in this regard, and every effort should be made to gain or preserve future access to the umbilical vessels. Prostaglandin E1 can be infused through peripheral venous or central venous catheters, as well as through an umbilical artery catheter. The initial infusion rate is generally between 0.05 and 0.1 $\mu g/kg/min$. Potential side effects of prostaglandin E1 include hypotension, apnea, fever, and platelet dysfunction. Hypotension is generally amenable to treatment with isotonic fluid bolus, and is a dose-related side effect. When it occurs, apnea usually develops within the first few hours of prostaglandin E1 infusion. Given that endotracheal intubation can be more difficult while en route between the referring hospital and tertiary care center, many transport teams recommend elective endotracheal intubation as a safety measure prior to transport.

The decision whether or not to give supplemental oxygen in a neonate with suspected critical congenital heart disease prior to obtaining a definitive diagnosis by echocardiography can have important consequences. With ductal-dependent univentricular heart disease, supplemental oxygen can induce pulmonary arterial vasodilation and subsequent steal of cardiac output from the systemic circulation. This decision-making is facilitated by remotely directed and interpreted tele-echocardiography, where available. In lieu of this capacity, the stabilizing physician should cautiously titrate supplemental oxygen to clinical endpoints of improved circulation and acid-base status. It is generally unnecessary to target "normal" PaO_2 or pulse oximetry saturation when stabilizing infants with suspected heart disease. PaO_2 >40 mmHg or pulse oximetry saturation >80% represent reasonable and safe target values pending a complete cardiology and echocardiography evaluation at the tertiary care center.

The one major caveat to the approach to supplemental oxygen treatment outlined above relates to treating infants with primary pulmonary hypertension or secondarily raised pulmonary vascular resistance, in whom oxygenation and hemodynamics may be quite labile. It is precisely this lability that should weigh decision-making in favor of higher concentrations of supplemental oxygen, and higher target PaO_2 and pulse oximetry saturation values.

After priorities of vascular access, prostaglandin E1 infusion, assessment regarding control of the airway, and decisions regarding supplemental oxygen treatment have been made, only a few additional considerations remain. For example, infants with critical heart disease often present with hypoglycemia. For this reason, rapid (bedside) determination of serum glucose should be routine in these cases. Hypoglycemia is treated with 0.5–1 g/kg IV glucose bolus.

Conotruncal heart defects frequently coexist with chromosome 22 deletions (i.e., monosomy 22q11), which form the basis for the velocardiofacial syndrome and the DiGeorge sequence. The latter in turn carries a risk for immunodeficiency and neonatal hypocalcemia secondary to hypoparathyroidism. Thus, any transfused blood products should be irradiated to mitigate the risk of graft versus host disease in the recipient, and serum calcium levels should be closely monitored during stabilization and transport. When possible, a peripheral blood lymphocyte specimen should also be collected for cytogenetic karyotype analysis before blood transfusion therapy.

Measures such as sedation, neuromuscular relaxation, assisted ventilation, and prompt antipyretic treatment of fever can optimize cardiac output and tissue oxygen delivery in the patient at risk for decompensated cardiogenic shock (Chapter 8).

Cardiac Arrhythmia

Most pediatric cardiac arrhythmias do not represent true emergencies, and typically relate to diagnoses such as atrial or ventricular premature depolarizations or asymptomatic ECG abnormalities (e.g., ventricular preexcitation of Wolff-Parkinson-White syndrome). Clinically evident compromised cardiac output dictates emergency treatment. Since cardiac output can be defined as the product of heart rate and stroke volume, it should be apparent that significant bradyarrhythmia and tachyarrhythmia (via reduced diastolic filling time) can both generate reduced cardiac output (Chapter 8).

While it is possible to generate a focused differential diagnosis related to cardiac arrhythmia solely on the basis of clinical evidence, ECG monitoring and recording capability enhances the diagnostic capability and affords the opportunity for highly focused treatment. Additional desirable equipment capabilities include synchronized cardioversion and defibrillation, with patch or paddle connections appropriate to infants and small pediatric patients. New guidelines on the use of automated external defibrillators in pediatric patients as young as 1 year old have recently been published.[5] Automated external defibrillators may now be used for children 1–8 years of age who have no signs of circulation. Ideally the device should be capable of selective programming that can deliver a defibrillating energy dose for a child.

The most common destabilizing cardiac arrhythmia in pediatric patients is sustained and rapid supraventricular tachycardia (SVT). Infants, children with severe developmental disabilities, and those with palliated univentricular heart disease are at greatest risk from SVT. In general, faster tachycardia rates and increasing duration in tachycardia are associated with higher risks of cardiogenic shock. Infants can have unrecognized tachycardia for hours to days, and often present with shock owing to SVT.

Most pediatric patients with SVT have otherwise structurally normal hearts. There are, however, congenital heart defects that predispose to SVT such as Ebstein's anomaly. In addition, atrial arrhythmias can complicate postoperative congenital heart disease such as transposition of the great arteries treated with Mustard or Senning procedures, or univentricular heart disease palliated with modifications of the Fontan procedure.

When outpatient or emergency treatment for SVT is planned (i.e., when there are signs of cardiogenic shock), there should be immediate access to equipment and supplies for vascular access, medications such as adenosine, and an ECG monitor with cardioversion-defibrillation capability. Recorded documentation of the original arrhythmia is often omitted in the rush to treatment, which is unfortunate given that such a record is often invaluable to the cardiology and cardiac electrophysiology consultant who will eventually take charge of these patients.

Intravenous rapid administration of adenosine at an initial dose of 0.1 mg/kg (maximum single-dose 12 mg) is the drug of first choice in treating SVT in symptomatic infants and children. The dose of adenosine can be doubled if the initial treatment is unsuccessful. If vascular access cannot be rapidly obtained, electrical synchronized cardioversion should not be delayed in an unstable patient. The initial energy dose for synchronized cardioversion is 0.5 J/kg, and this dose can be doubled if the initial cardioversion is unsuccessful. Nonpharmacologic measures (Valsalva, diving reflex, other vagal reflexes) can be attempted in stable patients, but are frequently either not effective or only transiently effective.

Ventricular arrhythmias, by comparison, are much less common than SVT in pediatric patients. The majority of children with ventricular arrhythmia have underlying congenital heart disease or the long QT syndrome. Secondary ventricular arrhythmias may follow hypoxic ischemic injury, severe electrolyte abnormalities (e.g., hyperkalemia), or poisoning (e.g., tricyclic antidepressant medication). As with decision-making related to SVT management, appropriate ECG monitoring and cardioverter-defibrillator equipment should be in place before initiating treatment. Lidocaine (1 mg/kg IV or endotracheal bolus; followed by continuous IV infusion 20–50 μg/kg/min) and amiodarone (2.5–5 mg/kg IV bolus) are standard drugs used in ventricular arrhythmia management. Magnesium sulfate (50 mg/kg IV) is the treatment of choice for torsade de pointes in patients suspected of having long QT syndrome. As with SVT, cardioversion or defibrillation (the latter for patients without a palpable pulse; 2–4 J/kg) should not be delayed while awaiting vascular access in an unstable patient.

SUMMARY

Outpatient pediatric cardiac emergencies are rare, most commonly involving neonates with critical hypoxemia or cardiogenic shock secondary to ductal-dependent congenital heart disease, and cardiac arrhythmias in older children. Specific measures to improve practitioner and facility preparedness include continuing education on pediatric resuscitation, maintaining appropriate equipment and supply inventory, and affiliation with a regional pediatric tertiary care center capable of specialized neonatal and pediatric transport.

Effective management of the neonate with critical congenital heart disease is facilitated by telemedicine connections between the referring hospital and tertiary care center. High priorities on maintaining ductal patency and judicious use of supplemental oxygen will minimize morbidity during stabilization and transport of these infants.

The most common cardiac arrhythmias to present with cardiogenic shock in the pediatric population are SVT and ventricular arrhythmias. Preparedness for these emergencies involves having immediate access to ECG monitoring and cardioverter-defibrillator equipment, along with a limited inventory of useful antiarrhythmic medications.

References

1 Mansfield CJ, Price J, Frush KS, Dallara J: Pediatric emergencies in the office: are family physicians as prepared as pediatricians? *J Fam Pract* 50(9): 757–761, 2001.

2 American Academy of Pediatrics, Committee on pediatric emergency medicine, in: Seidel JS, Knapp JF (eds): *Childhood Emergencies in the Office, Hospital, and Community: Organizing Systems of Care.* Elk Grove Village, IL, American Academy of Pediatrics, 2000.

3 Hellstrom-Westas L, Hanseus K, Jogi P, Lundstrom NR, Svenningsen N: Long-distance transports of newborn infants with congenital heart disease *Pediatr Cardiol* 22(5):380–384, 2001.

4 Sable CA, Cummings SD, Pearson GD, Schratz LM, Cross RC, Quivers ES, Rudra H, Martin GR: Impact of telemedicine on the practice of pediatric cardiology in community hospitals. *Pediatrics* 109(1):E3, 2002.

5 Samson RA, Berg RA, Bingham R, Biarent D, Coovadia A, Hazinski MF, Hickey RW, Nadkarni V, Nichol G, Tibballs J, Reis AG, Tse S, Zideman D, Potts J, Uzark K, Atkin D: Use of automated external defibrillators for children: an update: an advisory statement from the pediatric advanced life support task force, international liaison committee on resuscitation. *Circulation* 107:3250–3255, 2003.

53

ANESTHETIC ISSUES IN THE PEDIATRIC CARDIAC PATIENT

Suanne Daves

INTRODUCTION

When a child with congenital heart disease is scheduled to undergo a surgical procedure, it is often the pediatrician who fields the family's initial questions about the anesthetic. Can I be with my child until he is asleep? Are there risks to anesthesia? Is it okay for my child to have an anesthetic if she has a cold? Is the child "cleared" for surgery? The anesthesiologist should and will discuss these topics in detail before the procedure; however, the family may initially approach the pediatrician with these questions. The pediatrician also may be aware, long before the anesthesiologist, of concurrent illnesses or issues that can change the timing or conduct of an anesthetic.

Consequently, the intent of this chapter is several-fold. First, we hope to address the anesthetic issues that are pertinent to the pediatrician, such as behavioral changes in a child postoperatively and the impact of upper respiratory infections on anesthetic risk. These conditions are likely to be managed by the pediatrician, and knowledge of the anesthetic literature will assist in clinical decision-making and in discussions with parents. Second, we will address the issue of parent-child separation and the factors that influence an anesthesiologist's decision to allow parents to be present during induction. This is an important issue for both parent and child and one in which the pediatrician can help establish realistic expectations. Third, we hope to educate the pediatrician about the overall risk of anesthesia and the factors that influence risk, including the anesthesiologist's level of expertise with patients who have congenital heart disease. Lastly, we hope to define "surgical clearance" in terms of its applicability to pediatric patients with congenital heart disease. We hope that after considering these topics, a pediatrician will be better equipped to educate the family and to coordinate the child's care during a complex and stressful period.

POSTOPERATIVE BEHAVIOR PROBLEMS

Negative postoperative emotional and behavioral changes, such as nightmares, may occur in up to 54% of children who have undergone general anesthesia and surgery.[1-3] In a study of 91 children from 1 to 7 years of age who had elective ambulatory surgery, common negative behaviors were bad dreams, waking up crying, disobeying parents, separation anxiety, and temper tantrums.[2] A child undergoing surgery is exposed to many stressors that might influence subsequent behavior. The impact of these stressors on behavior may depend on the personality characteristics of the child. Among potential predictors of postoperative negative behavior in children are age less than 4 years, few or no siblings, and preoperative anxiety in the child and mother.[3] Young age, pain, and a previous bad experience with health care have also predicted negative behavioral changes postoperatively.[1] These changes dissipate with time and fewer than 10% persist at 1-year follow-up.[3] Aggressively controlling pain, establishing a good rapport with the child, and using various strategies to alleviate anxiety perioperatively may lower the incidence of postoperative behavioral changes. Informing the parents of the possibility that their child may exhibit these behaviors is prudent.

UPPER RESPIRATORY INFECTIONS

A common dilemma faced by pediatric anesthesiologists is whether to proceed with an anesthetic in a child with an upper respiratory tract infection (URI). Studies of adverse anesthetic events associated with URIs have yielded conflicting results. URI is not defined uniformly in the literature, and a comparison of study results is difficult because anesthetic techniques and airway management (intubation vs. mask anesthetic) vary. Two studies in the late 1980s failed to show that the incidence of adverse respiratory events increased in pediatric patients with active URIs who underwent surgery and general anesthesia.[4,5] One of these investigations, a retrospective study of 3585 patients, may

have unintentionally preselected patients with minor symptoms since those with severe symptoms may have had their surgery cancelled.[4] The other investigation, a prospective study of 489 patients who had bilateral placement of myringotomy tubes, found no differences in complication rates among patients with an active URI, recent URI, or no URI. The patients in the study, however, were not intubated.[5] In a recent prospective study of 1078 children aged 1 month to 18 years who had elective surgery, incidence of major arterial oxygen desaturation and overall adverse respiratory events was significantly higher in children with active or recent URIs than in children with no URIs. Independent risk factors for adverse respiratory events were presence of copious secretions; intubation in a child less than 5 years of age; history of prematurity, nasal congestion, reactive airway disease, parental smoking, and surgery involving the airway.[6] In other studies, incidence of laryngospasm increased in unintubated patients and bronchospasm increased in intubated patients with current or recent URIs undergoing general anesthesia.[7-10] In all of these studies cited, no adverse event led to significant morbidity. The anesthesiologist is well equipped to handle bronchospasm, laryngospasm, and hypoxemia in the operating room, and serious sequelae after these events are unusual.

It is important to note that the studies described above included children who were often not clinically "ill," who did not have significant cardiopulmonary comorbidities, and who rarely underwent major surgical procedures. Pediatric patients with cardiac disease, however, are susceptible to complications associated with respiratory infections, particularly if they have pulmonary hypertension.[11,12] Altman et al. examined the effect of infection with respiratory syncytial virus (RSV) on the postoperative course of children who had cardiac surgery. Patients with RSV infections had a longer hospital stay (by a factor of 2.1), required prolonged intensive care and prolonged mechanical ventilation compared with age-matched controls. The average total hospital charges were 2.6 times greater for the patient with RSV. RSV disease was occasionally subclinical at the time of a child's admission for surgery, and by implementing routine preoperative screening for RSV antigen during the late fall and winter months, the incidence of postoperative infections decreased.[13] In general, it is common practice to delay surgery in pediatric patients with fever, purulent rhinitis, a productive cough, or abnormal findings on chest auscultation (rales, wheezing, rhonchi). Mild URI symptoms (clear rhinitis, nasal congestion, dry cough) or ill contacts during RSV season, prompt screening for RSV.

How long should surgery be delayed following resolution of a URI? Spirometry and airway hyper-reactivity may remain abnormal up to 7 weeks after a URI.[14,15] In one study the incidence of adverse respiratory events was similar when children with a URI were compared with those who had had a URI recently. Similarity persisted for at least 4 weeks after resolution of symptoms.[6] Since children contract an average of 3–8 URIs a year[16], very little "well" time remains for elective surgery if the wait to reschedule is more than 4 weeks. In other words, how long to delay surgery after resolution of a URI is unclear. Other factors such as the urgency of surgery and scheduling issues affect the timing of general anesthesia and surgery following a URI. Common practice[17], is to reschedule 2–4 weeks after URI symptoms abate.

PARENTAL PRESENCE AT INDUCTION

Parental presence at induction of a child's anesthetic is a common practice in Great Britain that is slowly gaining popularity in the United States. A 1997 survey found that 84% of U.K. respondents allowed parents to be present in more than 75% of their cases; in contrast, 59% of U.S. respondents never allowed parents to be present during induction.[18] Different induction practices (intravenous (IV) vs. mask, induction room vs. operating room), medicolegal atmosphere, or parental expectations and demands may account for the variance.

The decision to allow parental presence at a child's induction is made by the anesthesiologist after the preoperative visit. There are several factors that influence this decision. One of the most challenging aspects of anesthetizing children is coping with their anxiety over strangers and separation from their parents. This anxiety can occur as early as 9 months of age. One method of lessening the anxiety is to allow parent/s to be present until their child is anesthetized. Potential advantages of parental presence at induction are alleviating the anxiety of child and parent, avoiding increased airway secretions that accompany crying, facilitating a smooth induction, and avoiding an unpleasant experience that may negatively affect the child and future anesthetics. There are also disadvantages of parental presence at induction. The induction of anesthesia in a pediatric patient is a period fraught with potential complications including laryngospasm, hypoxia, arrhythmias, and even cardiac arrest. A parent's presence during a crisis can distract the staff who must stay focused on the child. Not all parents are good candidates for presence at induction. Their level of anxiety may heighten that of the child, the OR staff, and the anesthesia team. Some parents agree to be present even though they are highly uncomfortable doing so and prefer to remain in the waiting area. Many non-premedicated children are inconsolable even by their parent. In a study that examined the anxiolytic effect of parental presence at induction, anxiety was reduced only if a child was older than 4 years of age, the parent had a low trait anxiety score, or the child had a low baseline activity level as measured by a temperament scale.[19]

The benefits of parental presence at induction may be achieved by other means. Preoperative education through child-life services, videotapes, and play therapy can often ease child and parent's discomfort with separation. A number of sedatives and anxiolytics can be given to ease separation, and can be orally administered, since most anesthesiologists avoid an intramuscular injection whenever possible. If an IV is in place, administering an anxiolytic is atraumatic and rapid and can easily attenuate separation anxiety.

In summary, the anesthesiologist determines whether a parent will be present on induction based on several factors: the child's age, the demeanor of the parents, the presence or absence of an IV, the likelihood of successful administration of oral pre-medication, assessment of the potential difficulty or risk of induction, and personal level of comfort with parental presence.

THE REAL RISKS OF ANESTHESIA

Serious anesthetic complications are rare across all patient ages but several studies have found that perioperative risk is higher in younger patients.[20–25] In a review of more than 29,000 cases at Winnipeg's Children's Hospital, major adverse events were found in approximately 4% of children versus 0.5% of adults and were more likely in infants less than 1 month of age. Mortality for neonates was 83 per 10,000 anesthetics and for infants was 8 per 10,000 anesthetics.[21] In a retrospective study of 250,543 anesthetics at the Karolinska Hospital in Stockholm, the highest incidence of cardiac arrest was found in patients less than 1 year of age. Incidence of cardiac arrest in infants was 17 per 10,000 anesthetics versus 4.6 per 10,000 in all age groups combined.[25] In another large study of complications associated with 198,103 anesthetics performed in 460 public and private facilities in France, the rate of complications was higher in children under 1 year of age (3.5 per 10,000 anesthetics) than in other pediatric age groups and in adults up to 65 years of age.[24] In a retrospective study of bradycardia during anesthesia in children 0–4 years of age, the incidence was much more frequent in the first year of life.[20]

In 1994 under the auspices of the Committee on Professional Liability of the American Society of Anesthesiologists and the American Academy of Pediatrics Section on Anesthesiology, the Pediatric Perioperative Cardiac Arrest (POCA) Registry was formed to investigate the causes of cardiac arrest in anesthetized children. Data from this registry estimated the mean overall incidence of anesthesia-related cardiac arrest at 1.4 ± 0.45 per 10,000 anesthetics per year. Of the first 150 cases reported to the POCA Registry, 55% were in children less than 1 year of age. Of these 150 cases of arrest, 26% of children died, 6% suffered permanent injury, and 68% had temporary or no injury. Emergency surgery and a higher acuity of coexisting disease, not age, were independent predictors of mortality. A disproportionate number of children who suffered cardiac arrest had coexisting cardiac disease.[22]

Who is best equipped to provide anesthetic care for the pediatric patient with congenital heart disease? Parents of these children often ask health care professionals about their expertise and training in pediatrics and specifically in pediatric congenital heart disease. In pediatric hospitals, anesthesiologists undoubtedly have experience and a special interest in caring for children. In institutions where both adults and children are cared for, however, most groups have anesthesiologists with a special interest in the pediatric population, but some anesthesia groups have individuals who care for both types of patients. Whether a pediatric anesthesiologist influences outcomes in children more than a "generalist" does is a controversial topic in the anesthesia community. Some would argue that residency training provides adequate experience with the pediatric patient; others believe that additional training or experience is required. The Accreditation Council for Graduate Medical Education (ACGME) has set minimum requirements for pediatric experience during the 4-year residency training in anesthesiology. Among the requirements for residency training are providing anesthesia for 100 children under the age of 12 years, including 15 infants less than 1 year of age and infants less than 45 weeks postconceptual age.[26] In 1997, the ACGME recognized subspecialty training in pediatric anesthesiology. Currently there are 41 accredited training programs in pediatric anesthesiology in the United States,[27] but there is no board examination for a certificate in pediatric anesthesia approved by the American Board of Medical Subspecialties.

In two retrospective studies, Keenan et al., concluded that the number of cardiac arrests and bradycardic episodes was reduced when a pediatric anesthesia subspecialist provided care.[20,28] In these studies, the pediatric subspecialist was an anesthesiologist with pediatric anesthesia fellowship training, or the equivalent clinical experience, who was a recognized member of the department's pediatric anesthesia service. In a French postal survey of pediatric anesthetic complications relative to volume of pediatric anesthetics conducted at each reporting institution, rate of complications was significantly higher in the groups that performed fewer than 200 pediatric anesthetics a year.[29]

The right facility and level of expertise must be available for the child with complex congenital heart disease who undergoes an anesthetic. To ensure an appropriate referral, the pediatrician must consider the possibility that the necessary level of expertise may not be found in community hospitals and ambulatory surgical centers. Anesthetics, including those used for sedation, can have profoundly detrimental effects on the cardiopulmonary system of the healthiest child. Anesthesia for a seemingly simple placement of a myringotomy tube becomes a potentially hazardous anesthetic in a child with complex cardiac anomalies. Anesthesia providers caring for such infants and children must have a good working knowledge of congenital cardiac lesions, their pathophysiology, and their anesthetic implications. Table 53-1 lists the congenital cardiac anomalies that require the involvement of an anesthesiologist experienced in managing patients with congenital heart disease. In general, patients with simple congenital heart disease and good ventricular function or those with more complex disease who have had a good biventricular repair may not need a special level of care; however, a child whose congenital heart disease has been repaired may still present a challenge to the anesthesiologist. Even in an asymptomatic, well appearing child, the stress of anesthesia and surgery may unmask cardiac pathophysiology such as arrhythmias and hypoxemia.

Many pediatricians provide sedation for children undergoing procedures outside of the operating room. Pediatric patients with complex congenital heart disease may be particularly prone to the myocardial and respiratory depressant effects of commonly used sedatives. Children who have undergone several operative cardiac procedures or who have had prolonged postoperative courses may require general anesthesia because they are tolerant of narcotics and difficult to sedate. All practitioners who sedate patients must be able to rescue the airway of a child who has crossed the thin boundary between sedation and general anesthesia. Skill and facility with airway management is paramount. Oxygen reserves are often critically low and decrements in oxygen delivery are poorly tolerated. On the other hand, infants with single ventricular physiology may decompensate with the administration of oxygen. Practitioners must know the complex pathophysiology of these children and how it alters the pharmacodynamics and pharmacokinetics of various sedatives. As with operative procedures, sedation in children with cardiac disease who undergo nonoperative procedures should be relegated to practitioners with expertise in congenital heart disease.

TABLE 53-1

CARDIAC ANOMALIES IN CHILDREN WHO REQUIRE AN ANESTHESIOLOGIST WITH EXPERTISE IN PEDIATRIC CONGENITAL HEART DISEASE

Single right or left ventricle
Complete atrioventricular canal
Tetralogy of Fallot with cyanotic episodes
Severe pulmonary or aortic stenosis
Severe Ebstein anomaly
Pulmonary atresia
Persistent truncus arteriosus
Interrupted aortic arch
Uncorrected transposition
Cavopulmonary circulation (Glenn or Fontan)
History of significant dysrhythmias

SURGICAL CLEARANCE—WHOSE RESPONSIBILITY IS IT?

The pediatrician, the pediatric cardiologist, or the anesthesiologist is frequently asked to "clear" a patient for surgery. The word "clearance" is frequently misunderstood. From an anesthesiologist's perspective, "clearing" a patient for an anesthetic means determining the relative risks and benefits of proceeding versus delaying an anesthetic. The surgical and anesthetic risks are usually interwoven such that the anesthesiology consultant clearing the patient must have a thorough working knowledge of the surgical procedure as well as the impact of an anesthetic on the patient's physiology. From the surgeon's point of view, "clearance" implies the decision of whether or not to operate based on the relative benefits of surgical intervention versus the risk of doing so or delaying the procedure. This takes into account the risks of anesthesia as well.

The pediatrician has an important role in preoperative evaluation. In the case of a newly noted murmur or arrhythmia, frequent causes of referral to a pediatric cardiologist, the role of the primary care physician is to evaluate the condition and to decide if a pediatric cardiology consultation is required. The pediatrician should then relay the information from the preoperative evaluation and consultation to the anesthesiologist for determination of anesthetic and surgical eligibility. Ideally, this process is performed well before the time of the surgery so that testing or interventions can be scheduled and unnecessary delays avoided. In cases of known heart disease, or other abnormalities, it is the primary care physician's role to provide this information to the anesthesiologist and surgeon.

In the case of a patient with known congenital heart disease, it is the pediatric cardiologist's responsibility to communicate relevant information (anatomic, electrophysiologic, hemodynamic) to the anesthesiologist, for both cardiac and noncardiac surgeries. In most pediatric cardiac centers, cardiologists, anesthesiologists, and surgeons meet in conference to discuss all upcoming surgeries and their management. Such conferences eliminate lapses in communication and potential sources of error.

In conclusion, it is the combined responsibility of the pediatrician, the anesthesiologist, the surgeon, and the pediatric cardiologist to communicate patient information and concerns to one another and arrive at consensus over the relative risk and benefit of proceeding with a planned surgical procedure. Only then can informed consent be obtained.

SUMMARY

In summary, children with congenital heart disease can benefit only if pediatricians and anesthesiologists collaborate in their perioperative care. Care of these children can be complex, particularly in the perioperative setting. The pediatrician who is familiar with the literature on URIs and anesthesia will know when a patient is at increased risk and can facilitate the timing of elective procedures. The pediatrician who appreciates the frequency and nature of postoperative behavioral problems is better prepared to recognize and treat them. Finally, physicians who are expert in the anesthetic care of the child with complex congenital heart disease should be responsible for administering general anesthesia or sedation, even for relatively simple procedures (noncardiac included). The pediatrician who is informed about anesthetic practices, techniques, and concerns and who is familiar with institutional or community resources is able to align resources and expertise when an anesthetic is indicated.

References

1   Kotiniemi LH, Ryhanen PT, Moilanen IK: Behavioural changes in children following day-case surgery: a 4-week follow-up of 551 children. *Anaesthesia* 52:970, 1997.

2   Kain ZN, Wang SM, Mayes LC, et al: Distress during the induction of anesthesia and postoperative behavioral outcomes. *Anesth Analg* 88:1042, 1999.

3   Kain ZN, Mayes LC, O'Connor TZ, et al: Preoperative anxiety in children. Predictors and outcomes. *Arch Pediatr Adolesc Med* 150:1238, 1996.

4   Tait AR, Knight PR: Intraoperative respiratory complications in patients with upper respiratory tract infections. *Can J Anaesth* 34(3(Pt.1)):300, 1987.

5   Tait AR, Knight PR: The effects of general anesthesia on upper respiratory tract infections in children. *Anesthesiology* 67:930, 1987.

6   Tait AR, Malviya S, Voepel-Lewis T, et al: Risk factors for perioperative adverse respiratory events in children with upper respiratory tract infections. *Anesthesiology* 95:299, 2001.

7   Olsson GL, Hallen B: Laryngospasm during anaesthesia. A computer-aided incidence study in 136,929 patients. *Acta Anaesthesiol Scand* 28:567, 1984.

8   Olsson GL: Bronchospasm during anaesthesia. A computer-aided incidence study of 136,929 patients. *Acta Anaesthesiol Scand* 31:244, 1987.

9   Cohen MM, Cameron CB: Should you cancel the operation when a child has an upper respiratory tract infection? *Anesth Analg* 72:282, 1991.

10 Schreiner MS, O'Hara I, Markakis DA, et al: Do children who experience laryngospasm have an increased risk of upper respiratory tract infection? *Anesthesiology* 85:475, 1996.

11 Moler FW, Khan AS, Meliones JN, et al: Respiratory syncytial virus morbidity and mortality estimates in congenital heart disease patients: a recent experience. *Crit Care Med* 20:1406, 1992.

12 MacDonald NE, Hall CB, Suffin SC, et al: Respiratory syncytial viral infection in infants with congenital heart disease. *N Engl J Med* 307:397, 1982.

13 Altman CA, Englund JA, Demmler G, et al: Respiratory syncytial virus in patients with congenital heart disease: a contemporary look at epidemiology and success of preoperative screening. *Pediatr Cardiol* 21:433, 2000.

14 Empey DW, Laitinen LA, Jacobs L, et al: Mechanisms of bronchial hyperreactivity in normal subjects after upper respiratory tract infection. *Am Rev Respir Dis* 113:131, 1976.

15 Collier AM, Pimmel RL, Hasselblad V, et al: Spirometric changes in normal children with upper respiratory infections. *Am Rev Respir Dis* 117:47, 1978.

16 Herendeen N, Szilagy P: Infections of the upper respiratory tract, in: Behrman R, Kliegman R, Jenson H (eds): *Textbook of Pediatrics*, 16th ed. Philadelphia, PA, WB Saunders, 2000, p. 1261.

17 Cote CJ, Todres ID, Ryan JF, et al: Preoperative evaluation of pediatric patients, in: Cote CJ, Todres ID, Ryan JF, et al. (eds): *A Practice of Anesthesia for Infants and Children*, 3rd ed. Philadelphia, PA, WB Saunders, 2001, p. 37.

18 Kain ZN, Ferris CA, Mayes LC, et al: Parental presence during induction of anaesthesia: practice differences between the United States and Great Britain. *Paediatr Anaesth* 6:187, 1996.

19 Kain ZN, Mayes LC, Caramico LA, et al: Parental presence during induction of anesthesia. A randomized controlled trial. *Anesthesiology* 84:1060, 1996.

20 Keenan RL, Shapiro JH, Kane FR, et al: Bradycardia during anesthesia in infants. An epidemiologic study. *Anesthesiology* 80:976, 1994.

21 Cohen MM, Cameron CB, Duncan PG: Pediatric anesthesia morbidity and mortality in the perioperative period. *Anesth Analg* 70:160, 1990.

22 Morray JP, Geiduschek JM, Ramamoorthy C, et al: Anesthesia-related cardiac arrest in children: initial findings of the Pediatric Perioperative Cardiac Arrest (POCA) Registry. *Anesthesiology* 93:6, 2000.

23 NCEPOD and perioperative deaths of children. *Lancet* 335(8704):1498, 1990.

24 Tiret L, Desmonts JM, Hatton F, et al: Complications associated with anaesthesia—a prospective survey in France. *Can Anaesth Soc J* 33(3 Pt.1):336, 1986.

25 Olsson GL, Hallen B: Cardiac arrest during anaesthesia. A computer-aided study in 250,543 anaesthetics. *Acta Anaesthesiol Scand* 32:653, 1988.

26 *Program Requirements for Residency Education in Anesthesiology*. The Accreditation Council for Graduate Medical Education, 2000. (Accessed November 3rd, 2002, at http://www.acgme.org/)

27 List of programs within pediatric anesthesiology for current academic year and those newly accredited programs with future effective dates (year ending June 30, 2003). The Accreditation Council for Graduate Medical Education, 1997. (Accessed November 3, 2002, at http://www.acgme.org/adspublic/)

28 Keenan RL, Shapiro JH, Dawson K: Frequency of anesthetic cardiac arrests in infants: effect of pediatric anesthesiologists. *J Clin Anesth* 3:433, 1991.

29 Auroy Y, Ecoffey C, Messiah A, et al: Relationship between complications of pediatric anesthesia and volume of pediatric anesthetics. *Anesth Analg* 84:234, 1997.

54

HEART TRANSPLANTATION

David J. Waight

INTRODUCTION

Pediatric heart transplant has been an effective therapeutic option for children and adolescents with end-stage heart disease or severe congenital heart disease since the early 1980s. Successful pediatric transplantation followed successful adult heart transplantation after the introduction of effective immunosuppression with the use of cyclosporin.

PRETRANSPLANT ISSUES

Transplant Indications

General indication for heart transplantation is an expected survival of less than 1–2 years with medical therapy or unacceptable quality of life. Conditions that are usually considered are:

1. No acceptable surgical alternative.
2. High mortality expected with medical therapy alone.
3. Failed surgical palliation.

4. Failed transplantation.
5. Unacceptable morbidity or quality of life expected with surgical palliation or medical therapy.

Specific indications include: congenital heart disease, cardiomyopathy, failed transplantation, coronary artery disease, valvular lesions, and other rare indications. Another category includes various uncontrolled arrhythmias despite antiarrhythmic therapy (pharmacologic therapy, radiofrequency ablation or antiarrhythmic device/implantable cardiac defibrillator/pacemaker therapy). Many congenital heart defects as listed in Table 54-1 may be treated with heart transplantation. These defects include those in which there is no effective palliation or the palliative procedures have a higher morbidity and mortality than would be expected with cardiac transplantation.

Indications for heart transplant change with advancing age. Under a year of age, congenital heart defects are the major indication with cardiomyopathy being a secondary indication. As patients reach the second decade of life, cardiomyopathy becomes the primary indication with a decreased rate of congenital heart disease as an indication.

TABLE 54-1

CONGENITAL HEART DEFECTS IN WHICH HEART TRANSPLANTATION MAY BE INDICATED

1. HLHS
2. Critical Shone's Complex
3. Complex single ventricle with outflow obstruction
4. Interrupted aortic arch and sub-aortic stenosis
5. Critical AS and fibroelastosis
6. Neoplasm—obstructive
7. Failed palliation
8. Severe cardiomyopathy
9. Pulmonary atresia with coronary sinusoids
10. AV valve insufficiency with ventricular dysfunction
11. TGA and straddling of tensor apparatus
12. Unbalanced AV canal variant
13. Truncus arteriosus with valve abnormalities
14. Ebstein's anomaly in a symptomatic newborn

TABLE 54-2

TESTS USED IN PRETRANSPLANT WORKUP

Tests (age and Dx dependent)
ECG
CXR AP, Lat
Cardiac catheterization
Exercise stress test
Pulmonary function testing
PPD

Laboratory Tests (patient dependent)
Type and screen
CBC w Diff, Plts
Basic metabolic panel, Ca, Mg, Phos
Cholesterol
Triglycerides
PT/PTT, INR
ABG
UA
HSV titers
CMV titers and Cx (buffy coat) urine for CVM Cx
EBV titers
Toxoplasmosis titers
HIV (need to send signed consent w/sample)
Hep B, Hep B core Ab, Hep B surface antigen
Hep C
Bld Cx and urine Cx at time of TX
Panel reactive antigen (measures presence of preformed antibodies to HLA antigens)

Evaluation for Heart Transplantation

Patients are referred for evaluation for heart transplantation for the above indications when it is felt that the risk of death from their disease is greater than the risk of death from transplant or when their quality of life is unacceptable to the patients or the parents. The evaluation of the pretransplant patient varies amongst institutions, but generally includes a complete cardiac evaluation, pulmonary evaluation, and evaluation for infectious disease processes. Neurologic and psychiatric evaluations are performed for appropriate patients. The patient's support system must also be evaluated as children cannot be responsible for their own medical care and heart transplantation recipients require constant medical supervision and continued supervision until they reach adulthood. The extent of the evaluation will depend on the clinical condition and age of the patient. Commonly performed diagnostic and laboratory tests are listed in Table 54-2.

Listing for Transplantation

In the United States, all cardiac transplantation organ distribution is performed through the United Network of Organ Sharing, abbreviated as UNOS. This service matches potential donors with potential recipients on a nationwide basis organized by Geographic Region and Listing Status. The current listing status is 1A, 1B, 2, and 7.

Patients that are inactive (meaning they would not currently accept an organ because of an acute infection or other reason) but remain on the list are status 7. Status 2 patients are all patients listed for transplant who do not meet the criteria for status 1. Status 1B patients are on low-dose inotropic support, have an expected survival of less than 6 months, or have growth failure (at or less than the 5th percentile on the growth curve or a loss of 1.5 standard deviations on the growth curve). Status 1A patients are ventilated, undergoing mechanical assist of their circulation with an Extracorporeal-Membrane Oxygenation (ECMO) circuit, or ventricular assist device (balloon assist pump). They are on high-dose inotropic support and have a less than 14-day survival or a <6-month survival in the presence of pulmonary hypertension. Listing status is presented in Table 54-3.

Status 1A patients are the first to be matched for a prospective donor, then 1B, and then status 2 patients. Status 7 patients remain with the system, but are not actively being matched for prospective donors. As patients are on the list for a longer period of time, they will move toward the top of the list as the patients at the top of the list are transplanted or die. Minimal listing criteria includes name, age, weight, and blood type. The patients can be listed for a prospective crossmatch, which means only donors who lack specific HLA antigens would be

acceptable. Prospective crossmatch requires donor blood to be crossmatched with the recipient's blood, which can be a relatively lengthy procedure. This may further limit the geographic area in which a donor can come from, as there is a limited time after the heart becomes available, when it can be effectively transplanted into a recipient.

Organ Selection

Blood group matching is performed with the recipients receiving heart transplant donors with the same blood type, i.e., a recipient blood type A receives a heart from a donor with blood type A. Rh positivity or negativity is not an important consideration. Recipients are also matched by weight. Transplanted organs may come from donors that are up to two to three times the size of the recipient. This is evaluated on an individual basis. In general, the donor heart should have no congenital heart defects other than a small atrial septal defect, PDA, or small VSD, which can be surgically closed at the time of transplant. Donors who are on low-dose inotropic support are usually acceptable. Five to six hours of cold ischemia time is generally acceptable. Cold ischemia time is the time from when the donor heart has no coronary perfusion during the explantation, to the time that heart is placed into the chest of the recipient and coronary perfusion is restored. The surgical procedure of explantation of the donor heart varies in technique depending on the recipient's need. Specifically, patients with aortic arch abnormalities, severe pulmonary abnormalities, or abnormal pulmonary venous return require additional tissue from the donor to provide adequate tissue for reimplantation because of the recipient's complex anatomy.

Surgical Procedure

Orthotopic heart transplantation (OHT) is performed with two standard techniques. The first involves removal of the ventricles and a portion of the atria of the recipient leaving the superior vena cava (SVC), inferior vena cava (IVC), and a cuff of right atrial tissue and a significant portion of the left

TABLE 54-3

TRANSPLANT LIST STATUS CLASSIFICATION

Status 1A
a. Ventilated
b. Mechanical assist/ECMO/balloon pump
d. <6 month survival and pulmonary hypertension
e. High-dose inotropic support
f. <14-day survival
Status 1B
a. Low-dose inotropic support
b. <6-month survival
c. Growth failure, <5%, lose 1.5 SD
Status 2
All others
Status 7
Inactive

atrium including all the pulmonary veins and a block of atrium. The donor heart is then anastomosed with a right atrial and left atrial anastomosis and aortic and pulmonary artery anastomosis. The second technique is a total technique or often referred to as a bicaval anastomosis. In this procedure, the recipient's heart is removed leaving only the SVC, IVC, main pulmonary artery, ascending aorta, and a cuff of tissue around both the left and right pulmonary veins where the pulmonary venous blood returns to the left atrium. The donor heart is then sewn in at the SVC, IVC, main PA, ascending aorta, and around both pulmonary vein cuffs into the recipient's left atrium.

Contraindications to cardiac transplant are relative and vary amongst institutions, and over time. Prior contraindications have now been proven to be surmountable and have become relative contraindications. There are no absolute anatomical contraindications to cardiac transplantation. There are some anomalies, which may require the addition of lung transplantation with cardiac transplantation to achieve acceptable physiology including hypoplastic lungs, pulmonary venous stenosis, severe diffuse branch pulmonary artery stenosis, multiple pulmonary arteriovenous malformations, and severe pulmonary vascular disease. The presence of ECMO support may increase the morbidity and mortality prior to transplant but has not proven to be a risk factor for posttransplant mortality. Chromosomal abnormalities are a relative contraindication to cardiac transplantation, but are generally considered on a case-by-case basis. Psychosocial dysfunction can be a relative contraindication to transplantation as it may have a severe affect on the posttransplant medical care. This is a very important and life-long consideration. Contraindications are listed in Table 54-4.

Results

The success of pediatric transplant has improved since its introduction in the 1980s. From 1982 to 2001, the ISHLT (International Society for Heart and Lung Transplant) has collected data indicating a 1-year survival of 78% and a 60% survival at 9 years. The expected half-life for patient survival

TABLE 54-4

CONTRAINDICATIONS TO HEART TRANSPLANTATION

1. PVR >5 Wood units, TPG >15 mmHg
2. Malignancy
   <1 year disease free
   <5 year, relative because of recurrence
3. HIV, hepatitis C with active liver disease, hepatitis C alone (controversial) (HIV may change)
4. Active infection, uncontrolled
5. Retransplant
6. Chronic systemic disease
7. Chromosomal abnormality
8. Obesity—>140% IBW (adult, relative in a child)
9. Psychosocial: all relative
   a. Dysfunctional family
   b. Poor parenting—care taker skills
   c. Inability to read
   d. Language barriers
   e. Poor problem solving—coping
   f. Noncompliance, inability to work with team
   g. Adolescents with noncompliance, drug use
10. Anatomic—no true absolute contraindications, only relative

is quoted as 12.4 years. This has improved by approximately 5 years over the last 7 years of data collection. Fifty percent of the mortality occurs in the first year post transplant. Patients who have survived the first year have an annual mortality less than 3%. The improved current survival is felt to be related to better organ preservation, improved preoperative care, and increased experience with immunosuppression.

There is a 30–40% mortality rate after being listed for transplant for older teens and adults, and an approximately 10% mortality for infants and children while waiting for an acceptable donor heart. A high-risk subgroup of infants are those with hypoplastic left heart syndrome (HLHS). Approximately 30% of infants with aortic atresia and HLHS die waiting for transplant. Although cardiac transplantation is an effective therapy for patients born with hypoplastic left heart syndrome, there are adequate donors to transplant only approximately 10% of these infants.

Most infants and children are in good health with no significant disabilities following transplantation. Fifty percent of patients do not require rehospitalization within the first posttransplant year. Ninety-seven percent of transplant recipients are without any limitations at 1-year follow-up. Almost all children are in New York Heart Association Class 1 following transplantation, meaning they have no restrictions and no exercise difficulty. These children can participate in all normal childhood activities once their chest wound has healed.

POSTTRANSPLANT ISSUES

Transplant recipients have the same immediate postoperative concerns as any other patient who has undergone open-heart surgery. Specific transplant related issues include:

1. Rejection
2. Infection
3. Coronary artery disease
4. Lymphoproliferative disease
5. Other complications

Rejection

Rejection is the body's normal immunologic response to what is perceived as a foreign body. The transplanted heart is generally perceived as a foreign body and the recipient's immune system attempts to destroy the transplanted heart with both cellular, T-cell mediated activity, and possibly humoral or antibody mediated activity. Cellular rejection is most commonly evaluated by the use of endomyocardial biopsy in which small pieces of right ventricular muscle are evaluated by microscopy for lymphocyte infiltrates and necrosis of myocardial cells. Acute rejection accounts for greater than 10% of the mortality in the first 3 years posttransplantation, which decreases to less than 10% after

the third year. Rejection is thought to be associated with the development of transplant coronary artery disease, which limits long-term survival of the heart grafts. Prevention of rejection is achieved with immunosuppression of the heart recipient. Standard immunosuppression includes triple drug therapy mentioned below.

1. Steroids: Solu-Medrol or prednisone
2. Calcineurin inhibitor: cyclosporin or FK506/tacrolimus/Prograf
3. Antiproliferative agent: azathioprine (Imuran) or Mycophenolate Mofetil (MMF)/CellCept

Acute episodes of cellular mediated rejection (the most frequent form of rejection) are often treated with a short course of high-dose steroids. Additional immunosupression may include cytolytic therapy with antithymocyte globulin (ATGAM or thymoglobulin), T-cell monoclonal antibody (OKT-3), or methotrexate. Humoral, or antibody mediated, rejection can also be treated with a steroid pulse, plasmapheresis, and/or IVIG. Rejection is a life-long risk for transplantation recipients and is difficult to accurately diagnose. Up to a third of patients develop severe rejection 2 years after transplantation. The symptoms of rejection are somewhat ambiguous. In general, irritability, low-grade fever, nausea, decreased appetite, fatigue, and general malaise can be seen. Specific signs include arrhythmias, tachycardia, and an S3 or S4 gallop. Fluid retention or signs of poor cardiac output may be noted with possible pulmonary edema or an enlarged heart on the chest radiograph. ECG abnormalities including tachycardia with low voltages can be seen with acute rejection. Echocardiographic evaluation may demonstrate poor systolic ventricular function or abnormal diastolic function. A new pericardial effusion may be noted. Multiple protocols for evaluating rejection noninvasively have been proposed but surveillance endomyocardial biopsy is still the most common method of diagnosing rejection.

Infection

Patients who are immunosuppressed are at increased risk for infection. This is a life-long risk but is significantly higher in the first 6 months following transplantation. Infection accounts for approximately 12% of early death at less than 30 days of age, approximately 25% of deaths from 30 days to 1 year, and it accounts for less than 10% of the long-term mortality. Cytomegalovirus (CMV) is a concerning infection as it is associated with increased risk of development of transplant coronary artery disease. Epstein-Barr virus (EBV) has been associated with development of lymphoproliferative disorder. Because of the risk of infection, infection prophylaxis is generally given to patients for at least the first 6 months following transplantation. Antiviral agents such as acyclovir or ganciclovir are used to prevent recurrence of a new infection with CMV or herpes viruses. Bactrim is commonly given as prophylaxis for pneumocystis pneumonia. Nystatin is used for prophylaxis of oral fungal infections. The risk of acute infection falls after approximately 6 months after transplant and these prophylactic medicines are typically discontinued.

Transplant Coronary Artery Disease

The coronary vasculature of the transplanted heart is at risk for developing accelerated allograft coronary vasculopathy also termed heart graft vasculopathy, transplant vasculopathy, or posttransplant coronary artery disease. This is believed to be related to an immune reaction and it is felt that there is an association with episodes of acute and chronic rejection. There is a strong correlation between the incidence of coronary disease and acute CMV infection.

Transplant coronary artery disease is responsible for the majority of late, i.e., after 1-year, mortality. This process is the most significant limiting factor to long-term graft survival. The incidence is approximately 4–8% at 3 years in adult studies as assessed via angiography. A more sensitive test is the use of intracoronary ultrasound, which detects a much higher incidence of mild disease. This disease consists of diffuse circumferential intimal proliferation. This intimal proliferation reduces the lumen for effective blood flow in multiple areas throughout the coronary artery distribution. The lesions can be proximal or more distal. Often one significant lesion is associated with multiple other abnormal areas. It is important to remember that patients with a transplanted heart have a denervated heart, and generally experience no chest pain even during periods of severe ischemia or infarction of their transplanted heart.

Significant transplant coronary artery disease is generally considered an indication for retransplantation in children. Balloon angioplasty or stenting has been used, but only with limited and transient success. Bypass surgery has been performed, but it is only useful for proximal lesions without distal disease. Prevention of transplant coronary artery disease is the holy grail in the world of cardiac transplantation.

Lymphoproliferative Disease

Posttransplant lymphoproliferative disease (PTLD) is a significant complication of immunosuppression with antirejection medications. It accounts for less than 5% of posttransplant mortality. It consists of proliferation of B-lymphocytes and can produce a range of illnesses from a mild mononucleosis-type illness to a monomorphic B-cell lymphoma. The symptoms of lymphoproliferative disease include fever, fatigue, anorexia, or respiratory difficulty. On examination, patients are generally ill appearing and will have significant adenopathy. The adenopathy is the one sign that is significantly different than patients with acute rejection who may present with similar symptoms but do not have adenopathy. Lymphoproliferative disease is associated with EBV infections. A primary infection of EBV posttransplant places the patient at higher risk for lymphoproliferative disease. The patients who are EBV positive at the time of transplant do not appear to develop PTLD.

Complications

Transplant patients can develop significant complications secondary to the medications used for immunosuppression. Major complications include hypertension, hyperlipidemia, diabetes, malignancy, and renal dysfunction. The incidence of complications is listed in Tables 54-5 and 54-6.

TABLE 54-5

COMPLICATIONS OF HEART TRANSPLANTATION

Follow-up	1 year Percent	3 years Percent
Hypertension	45.1	35.0
Hyperlipidemia	7.1	10.6
Diabetes	3.0	2.8
Malignancy	1.3	1.6
Renal dysfunction	2.8	4.1
Cr >2.5	1.5	0.7
Chronic dialysis	0.1	0.0

Cyclosporin has the highest incidence of side effects of all the immunosuppressive medicines. It still remains the most commonly used medication owing to its long history of use and effective immunosuppression. Pediatric patients are generally treated with a medication called Neoral, which is a special formulation of cyclosporin with an improved and consistent absorption. Cyclosporin produces renal disease, hypertension, hirsutism, gingival hyperplasia, osteoporosis, facial bone changes, and seizures at higher serum levels.

Prograf or tacrolimus is an alternative calcineurin inhibitor to cyclosporin with a slightly

TABLE 54-6

SIDE EFFECTS OF IMMUNOSUPPRESSION

Cyclosporin (CSA)—renal, hypertension (HTN), hirsutism, gingival hyperplasia, osteoporosis, facial bone changes, seizures with high levels
Prednisone—cushingoid habitus, behavioral problems, glucose intolerance, hypercholesterolemia, HTN, cataract, ulcers, osteoporosis, poor growth
FK506—neurologic, renal, anemia, insulin secretion decrease, hyperkalemia, GI
Azathioprine/MMF—myelosuppression

decreased incidence of side effects that include neurologic complications (seizures), renal disease, anemia, decreased insulin secretion, hyperkalemia, and gastrointestinal abnormalities. Prograf does not cause hirsutism, gingival hyperplasia, osteoporosis or facial bone changes.

Prednisone is a commonly used immunosuppressant early after transplant, but has significant side effects including a cushingoid habitus, behavioral problems, glucose intolerance, hypercholesterolemia, hypertension, cataracts, ulcers, osteoporosis, and poor growth. Many transplant physicians attempt to wean patients from steroids within the first year of posttransplantation.

The antiproliferative medications including azathioprine or MMF/CellCept can produce myelosuppression with low white blood cell counts placing the patient at increased risk for infection. Myelosuppression is dose-dependent and generally recovers with a reduction or brief cessation of the medication.

Follow-up

Heart transplant patients require vigilant long-term follow-up with their physicians and other caretakers. Early after transplant, patients are seen at least weekly and have surveillance for acute rejection. There is a decreasing frequency of follow-up over the course of the first year. After the first year, most patients require less frequent visits. This varies between 1 and 3 months with blood draws for evaluation of their immunosuppressive drug levels and monitoring for infectious diseases. The caretakers of these patients must be vigilant as the symptoms of rejection and lymphoproliferative disorder are similar to symptoms of common childhood illnesses. Transplant patients are also at risk for more severe responses to the typical illnesses of childhood. When these patients present with symptoms of general malaise, GI symptoms of nausea, vomiting or anorexia, difficulty with exercise or respiratory difficulty they should be evaluated promptly and have their care discussed with their transplant cardiologist. This is essential as severe acute rejection can present with these mild symptoms and progress to life-threatening, hemodynamically significant rejection within a short period of time. The primary pediatrician or physician must also be vigilant for symptoms that may be related to immunosupression or infection. The other common complications of renal disease, hypertension, glucose intolerance, and neurologic changes may also present first to the primary caretaker who can then make the appropriate diagnosis and appropriate referrals to the transplant cardiologist, neurologist, endocrinologist, or nephrologist.

Immunizations

Immunizations are generally delayed 3–6 months following cardiac transplantation because of the initial high level of immunosuppression after transplantation. After this delay, they should receive routine immunizations using recombinant formulations or killed vaccine. *Transplant patients should not receive live vaccines!* Polio should be a killed vaccine given to the patient and the patient's family. Measles, mumps, and Rubella should be given to the family members only, not to the patient. Varicella vaccine should be given to family members only, not to the patient. Diphtheria, tetanus, pertussis, haemophilus influenza B (HIB), and hepatitis, should be given to the patient and the family. Influenza A and B vaccine may be given to the patient. Hepatitis B vaccine should be given to the patient. If the patient is accidentally given a measles, mumps, or Rubella vaccine or varicella vaccine, the patient should receive IVIG or varicella immune globulin within the first 72 h to prevent activation of the disease. Future vaccines or combination vaccines should not include any live vaccines.

The Older
Pediatric Transplantation Patient

The field of pediatric transplantation is complicated because of the need for the caretaker being responsible for the patient's medications. In infants and children, this is routinely assumed to be the parent's responsibility. As children grow and become more independent in the teenage years, many family members assume that these patients will become responsible for their own medication administration. Unfortunately, teenagers and young adults often engage in high-risk activities, which include skipping or discontinuing their medications. In most chronic diseases, this may make the patient ill, with eventual recovery once properly treated. Unfortunately, after heart transplantation, failure to continue immunosuppressant medications universally leads to acute rejection. This acute rejection can be severe and life threatening. Noncompliance is a major cause of graft failure and death in the teenage transplant population. The transplant patient and their parents will have heard of the incredible importance of proper compliance for their long-term survival multiple times after their transplantation. The only guarantee in pediatric heart transplantation is that patients who do not receive proper immunosuppression will develop fatal rejection. Significant noncompliance by the patient and their caretakers can lead to the patient not being considered for retransplantation. The common issues of adolescence also apply to the transplant population with an additional concern of the risk of sexually transmitted disease because of their immunosuppressed state and the risk of complications with pregnancy. Transplant patients who become pregnant may have severe problems with their immunosuppression medications or with their pregnancy. These concerns need to be discussed with the patient and their family as patients begin to enter their second decade of life.

SUMMARY

Cardiac transplantation is an effective last resort therapy for patients with congenital or acquired heart disease. Survival of up to 80% at 5 years has been reported and continues to improve. New immunosuppressive regimens are continually being developed and evaluated and reduce both the incidence of rejection and the complications associated with immunosuppressant medications. Transplant patients generally lead normal lives with few limitations. As pediatric heart transplantation is a relatively new procedure, long-term results will continue to be evaluated as patients enter their second, third, and hopefully fourth, fifth, and sixth decades of life.

Suggested Readings

Boucek MM, Edwards LB, Keck BM, et al: The Registry of the International Society for Heart and Lung Transplantation: Sixth Official Pediatric Report-2003. *J Heart Lung Transplant* 22:636–652, 2003.

Boucek MM, Faro A, Novick RJ, Bennett LE, Keck BM, Hosenpud JD: The Registry of the International Society for Heart and Lung Transplantation: Fourth Official Pediatric Report-2000. *J Heart Lung Transplant* 20:39–52, 2001.

Fricker FJ, Addonizio L, Berstein D, et al: Heart transplantation in children: Indications. *Pediatr Transplant* 3:333–342, 1999.

Fricker FJ, Armitage JM: *Heart and heart-lung transplantation in children and adolescents*, in: *Heart Disease in Infants, Children, and Adolescents*, 5th ed. Baltimore, MD, Williams & Wilkins, 1995.

Gajarski RJ, Rosenblatt H, Frazier OH: Pediatric cardiac transplantation. in: *The Science and Practice of Pediatric Cardiology*, 2nd ed. Baltimore, MD, Williams & Wilkins, 1998.

Webber SA: The current state of, and future prospects for, cardiac transplantation in children. *Cardiol Young* 13:64–83, 2003.

55

SYSTEMIC DISEASES AND THE HEART

William Bonney and Ra-id Abdulla

INTRODUCTION

The heart may be affected by many systemic diseases. Many genetic syndromes are known to include congenital heart disease. It is not clear why certain congenital heart diseases, although frequently associated with congenital heart disease, may not be present consistently. It is thought that there may be multifactorial genetic or environmental factors which eventually participate in congenital heart disease. Table 55-1 lists common cardiac findings for congenital syndromes.

TABLE 55-1

CONGENITAL SYNDROMES WITH ASSOCIATED HEART DEFECTS

Syndrome Name/Characteristic Features	Common Cardiac Findings	Notes
Down Syndrome		
Trisomy 21 or unbalanced translocation. Mental impairment, hypotonia, epicanthic folds, flat nasal bridge, small ears, transverse palmar crease.	Atrioventricular canal, VSD, ASD, PDA, TOF. Pulmonary vascular disease. Mitral valve prolapse.	Fifty percent will have some form of congenital heart disease. AV canal, when present, is usually complete. American Academy of Pediatrics recommends echocardiography for all newborns with Down syndrome.

(continued)

Syndrome Name/Characteristic Features	Common Cardiac Findings	Notes
Chromosome 22 Microdeletion Syndromes • DiGeorge • Velo-cardio-facial • CATCH22 *Microdeletion in short arm of chromosome 22.* Hypoplastic or aplastic thymus, hypocalcemia secondary to parathyroid hypofunction. Bulbous nose, anteverted palpebral fissures, small or low-set ears, cleft palate, and small stature.	Conotruncal malformations: truncus arteriosus, double outlet right ventricle, interrupted aortic arch, right aortic arch, coarctation of the aorta, and tetralogy of Fallot. Also PDA, VSD, and others	FISH will detect up to 80% of cases. One in 32 infants with a cardiac malformation will have a chromosome 22 microdeletion.
Turner Syndrome *Complete or partial absence of one X chromosome.* Mental impairment, ambiguous genitalia, short stature, webbed neck, broad chest with widely spaced nipples. Edema of the hands and feet in neonates. Risk of gonadal malignancy.	Coarctation of the aorta (20%), bicuspid aortic valve (35%). Anomalous pulmonary venous connection, hypoplastic left heart syndrome, mitral valve abnormalities, and aortic aneurysm occur rarely.	Clinical appearance may be confused with Noonan syndrome, but in general, cardiac defects do not overlap.
Noonan's Syndrome *Normal chromosomes, autosomal dominant inheritance.* Short stature, hypertelorism, low-set ears, ptosis.	Valvular pulmonary stenosis (39%), hypertrophic cardiomyopathy (10%), ASD (8%), tetralogy of Fallot (4%), coarctation of the aorta (9%), mitral valve anomalies (6%). Atrioventricular canal (15%).	ECG usually shows superiorly oriented QRS axis. Ventricular tachycardia and hypertrophic cardiomyopathy may occur. Pulmonary stenosis may involve thickened dysplastic valve leaflets. AV canal, when present, is usually partial.
Marfan Syndrome *Autosomal dominant inheritance with clinical variability.* Connective tissue defect resulting from mutation in fibrillin gene. Kyphoscoliosis, pectus carinatum, arachnodactyly, high-arched palate, loose joints, and lens dislocation.	Progressive aortic root dilatation leading to aortic dissection. Mitral valve prolapse.	High risk of aortic dissection with pregnancy. Treatment with beta-blockers may slow aortic dilation and delay the need for surgical repair.

Syndrome Name/Characteristic Features	Common Cardiac Findings	Notes
Williams Syndrome *May be a 7q deletion or autosomal dominant 6;7 translocation.* Connective tissue disorder with deletion of elastin gene. Characterized by elfin facies, mental impairment, gregarious "cocktail" personality.	Supravalvular aortic stenosis (66%), supravalvular pulmonic stenosis, VSD, PDA, and systemic hypertension. Diffuse arterial wall thickening involves coronary arteries. Renal artery stenosis and parenchymal dysgenesis may cause systemic hypertension.	Cardiac defects are often undetected until developmental delay is discovered at school age. Characteristic facial appearance may become more striking with age.
Ehler Danlos Syndrome Type IV *Autosomal dominant connective tissue disorder.* Defect in type III collagen. Hyperextensibility of the skin and hypermobility of the joints.	Mitral valve prolapse is common. Aortic root dilatation is less common. Spontaneous rupture of large and medium caliber arteries may occur. Elective vascular surgery is not advised because arteries hold sutures poorly.	May present as aortic rupture, bowel rupture, or uterine rupture during pregnancy. Pregnancy is not advised. Skin fibroblast culture is used to make the diagnosis.
Holt-Oram Syndrome *Deletion in HOS1 gene with autosomal dominant transmission.* Upper limb defects.	ASD, VSD, atrioventricular septal defect, TOF, and conduction abnormalities.	
VACTERL Association Vertebral anomalies, anal atresia, cardiac disease, tracheo-esophageal fistula, renal anomalies, limb anomalies (radial agenesis).	VSD	
Wolf-Hirschhorn Syndrome *Caused by 4p deletion.* Characteristic facial dysmorphia, severe growth and mental retardation, microcephaly, hypotonia, and weak suck.	VSD, ASD, PDA, pulmonary stenosis. Overall prevalence of CHD is 50%	
Cri-du-Chat Syndrome *Associated with 5q deletion.* Striking craniofacial dysmorphia, "cat-like" cry, low birth weight, failure to thrive, and developmental delay.	VSD, ASD, bicuspid aortic valve, TOF, and PDA	

(continued)

Syndrome Name/Characteristic Features	Common Cardiac Findings	Notes
Fetal Alcohol Syndrome *In utero alcohol exposure.* Characteristic facial anomalies, growth retardation and low birth weight, microcephaly, neurologic signs, behavioral abnormalities.	ASD, VSD, TOF	15–40% will be associated with CHD.

Abbreviations: ASD (atrial septal defect), VSD (ventricular septal defect), PDA (patent ductus arteriosus), TOF (tetralogy of Fallot), FISH (fluorescence in situ hybridization), CHD (Congenital Heart Disease).

CARDIAC MANIFESTATIONS OF HIV AND AIDS

1. Up to 20% incidence of heart failure. At least 6–7% of HIV+ adults and children will have cardiac morbidity. At least 1–3% will die of cardiac complications.
2. *Left ventricular dysfunction*: Twenty-nine percent of HIV-infected children had reduced LV shortening on echo. Depressed contractility with reduced LV performance is seen.
3. *Congestive heart failure*: It affects 10–20% of patients. Coinfection with EBV was the strongest predictor of chronic congestive heart failure and may identify children at particularly high risk.
4. *Vascular disease*: Coronary arteries and cerebral arteries are affected by a variety of abnormalities including vasculitis and aneurysmal dilation.
5. *Autonomic dysfunction*: Case reports describe autonomic insufficiency presenting with orthostatic hypotension, diarrhea, syncopal reactions, and fatal arrhythmias.
6. *Arrhythmias and ECG findings*: Tachycardia (49–70%), ventricular hypertrophy, ST- and T-wave changes. Also marked sinus arrhythmia, atrial ectopy, and ventricular arrhythmias. Remember that HIV infected infants are more frequently exposed to illicit drugs in utero, and

this alone is associated with a twelve-fold increase in cardiac arrhythmias.

7. *Cardiac tumors*: The heart may be the site of a primary or disseminated lymphoma. Kaposi sarcoma may affect the heart in disseminated disease.
8. *Pericarditis and myocarditis*: There is a high prevalence of lymphocytic infiltration into the myocardium. Infectious organisms include cytomegalovirus (CMV), fungal infections (cryptococcus, candida, histoplasma, coccidioides), tuberculosis, protozoans (*P. carinii*, toxoplasmosis). The heart is no. 1 site of extracerebral toxoplasmosis infection.
9. *HIV-associated primary pulmonary hypertension*: May be a consequence of LV dysfunction, repeated respiratory infections, or thromboembolic disease, but occasionally may be a primary process with no discernable cause; affects 0.5% of hospitalized AIDS patients.

Common Findings

1. Physical exam may show signs of congestive heart failure (CHF) (hepatomegaly, sinus tachycardia, gallop rhythm, tachypnea).
2. The ECG, as noted above, commonly shows sinus tachycardia, and less commonly demonstrates arrhythmias.

Suggested Diagnostic Studies and Periodic Screening

Children with asymptomatic HIV infection should receive a baseline cardiac evaluation, including ECG and echocardiogram at diagnosis. Routine follow-up including echocardiography and holter monitoring is recommended every 6–12 months, or as clinically indicated. This should be done more frequently in children with symptoms. The screening is not only for cardiac involvement of the HIV infection, but also for any side effects of drug therapy.

INFANT OF A DIABETIC MOTHER

In order to compensate for high maternal glucose levels, the fetus produces excessive insulin. This combination of high insulin and glucose will cause excessive growth of fetal organs (macrosomia). The myocardium exhibits this with hypertrophy of the ventricles, particularly that of the ventricular septum resulting in an asymmetrical ventricular septal hypertrophy, which may cause left ventricular outflow tract obstruction. Infants of diabetic mothers are also known to have higher incidence of transposition of the great arteries (TGA), VSD, and coarctation of the aorta. For this reason, maternal diabetes is an indication for fetal echocardiography to assess for these anomalies. Hypertrophic cardiomyopathy may occur late in gestation (beyond 30 weeks) therefore, assessment at later stage of gestation may be needed to assess for hypertrophy of the ventricular septum.

Hypertrophic cardiomyopathy secondary to maternal diabetes tends to progressively improve after birth as the levels of glucose and insulin decrease; however, it cannot be assumed that this will occur. Therefore, once diagnosed, follow-up of the hypertrophic cardiomyopathy is indicated to demonstrate resolution and thus differentiate it form a primary hypertrophic cardiomyopathy. Secondary hypertrophic cardiomyopathy usually resolves within the first few months after birth (usually by 6 months).

PEDIATRIC OBESITY AND HEART DISEASE

Obesity is a common cause for hypertension in older children. This typically resolves with proper weight control. Hyperlipidemia can lead to coronary artery disease in adulthood. Obstructive sleep apnea is also associated with obesity and may result in chronic elevation of CO_2 levels causing pulmonary hypertension. Management of hypertension and hyperlipidemia are discussed in Chapters 10 and 57. Cardiac evaluation is an adjunct to the management of the primary illness and may indirectly demonstrate the severity of the disorder by demonstrating right ventricular hypertrophy (RVH) (if obstructive sleep apnea and cor pulmonale are present) or left ventricular hypertrophy (LVH) in the presence of hypertension, however, management is rarely changed after cardiac evaluation. If cardiac involvement is not present, the risk of future involvement is present and therefore weight loss is indicated. If cardiac involvement is noted, then weight loss is indicated to reverse the cardiac findings. In either case, weight loss is the primary goal.

FETAL COMPLICATIONS OF MATERNAL SYSTEMIC LUPUS ERYTHEMATOSUS (SLE)

Mothers with systemic lupus erythematosus produce antibodies, which are capable of crossing the placenta into the fetus. These antibodies may result in damage of the atrioventricular conduction system, causing complete atrioventricular heart block. Damage to the fetal myocardium by these antibodies may cause dilated cardiomyopathy. Furthermore, children with maternal SLE are at a higher risk, for unknown reasons to develop corrected transposition of the great arteries (l-TGA). Fetal echocardiography is indicated in all mothers with SLE to assess for these anomalies. Steroid and immunoglobulin therapy have been proposed as means to prevent complete atrioventricular block and cardiomyopathy. Results of this therapy are controversial as experience is mostly anecdotal.

Workup of an infant born to a mother with SLE consists of an ECG to document the absence of heart block. Further testing is indicated as per the physical and historical findings. The infant is still at risk for heart block after birth. Therefore, future examinations should be performed assessing for this. A repeat ECG is indicated if there is an inappropriately low heart rate or dysrhythmia. In the absence of these, a repeat ECG at 1 year of age may be helpful, though the yield may be low in the absence of clinical findings.

CARDIAC FINDINGS IN OTHER COLLAGEN VASCULAR DISEASES

Other collagen vascular diseases such as juvenile rheumatoid arthritis, dermatomyositis, polyarteritis nodosa (PAN), Takayasu arteritis may also involve the cardiovascular system. The latter two cause an arteritis, though PAN may also have direct cardiac involvement. The collagen vascular disease may also cause pulmonary hypertension. A general concept of all the collagen vascular diseases is that they may cause pericarditis, myocarditis, or valvulitis. Treatment of the primary inflammatory disease is also treatment for the cardiac involvement, though recognition of possible cardiac involvement is important in order to provide supportive care if needed. The signs and symptoms of pericarditis, myocarditis, and valvulitis are discussed in the appropriate respective chapters. Myocardial involvement may also cause conduction abnormalities and arrhythmias, which should be recognized as well.

CARDIAC ABNORMALITIES IN SICKLE CELL ANEMIA

Anemia because of sickle cell may result in the following:

1. Compensate for anemia with increased cardiac output
2. Increased stroke volume and volume overload
3. Impaired myocardial diastolic function
4. 72–100% will have a heart murmur
5. ECG abnormalities—such as voltage criterion for left and right ventricular hypertrophy
6. Microinfarction
7. Pulmonary hypertension has been described in adults with SCA

CARDIAC FINDINGS IN ONCOLOGICAL DISEASES

It is well recognized that chemotherapeutic agents cause myocardial damage, which may result in a dilated cardiomyopathy. The myocardial damage may be reversible or persist. The major agents felt to be responsible for causing a cardiomyopathy are the anthracyclines, especially a total cumulative dose of 550 mg/m^2; however, lower doses have been reported to cause cardiomyopathy, and other drugs or combinations have been implicated as well. Therefore, the clinical suspicion of cardiomyopathy is an important aspect of the care of patients with oncologic disorders. Routine cardiac surveillance through echocardiography is indicated. At many institutions, yearly echocardiography is performed as part of the surveillance, with additional calculations made to predict the early development of myocardial dysfunction (e.g., wall stress indices).

LUNG DISEASE

Severe lung disease may result in pulmonary vascular pathology, which will eventually cause pulmonary vascular obstructive disease. The elevation of pulmonary vascular resistance, if sustained, may result in right-sided heart failure. Electrocardiography and echocardiography may demonstrate right ventricular hypertrophy. Right ventricular thickness may be measured directly via echocardiography, and the pulmonary artery systolic pressure can be estimated via Doppler echocardiography. These are useful tools in the assessment of the degree of lung disease in conditions such as bronchopulmonary dysplasia (BPD), asthma (chronic reactive airways disease), as well as other conditions such as upper airways obstruction. Although cardiac evaluation is useful, the manner in which it influences clinical decision making, and the type and frequency of evaluation (i.e., echocardiography) are areas which require further clinical investigation. In addition to evaluation of the cardiac sequelae to the primary lung disease, the heart may be affected by the drugs used to treat the disease (e.g., arrhythmias with asthma medications, hypertension with steroid use). This ought to be recognized, especially in the management of a patient with concurrent cardiac abnormalities.

RENAL DISEASE

Chronic renal parenchymal disease or reno-vascular disease may lead to hypertension. This may cause left ventricular hypertrophy and left heart failure. In addition, renal failure and uremia may lead to a uremic cardiomyopathy as well as a pericardial effusion. All of these cardiac manifestations of underlying renal disease can be assessed clinically, and via echocardiography. The correlation of increased voltage on an ECG and LVH is poor. Thus, there is probably no role for electrocardiography in the serial evaluation of cardiac changes in renal disease. An echocardiogram is both a sensitive and specific modality to evaluate these changes, though the frequency for routine surveillance for LVH or other changes because of renal failure is not agreed upon. Echocardiography is indicated in the presence of clinical findings, but the indications are less clear in an asymptomatic individual. Many clinicians evaluate cardiac thickness and function on an annual basis.

PSYCHIATRIC ILLNESSES—PSYCHOTROPIC DRUGS

Cardiologists are frequently asked to "clear" a patient for the administration of various psychotropic medications. Similar to surgical "clearance," the role of the cardiologist is to provide an evaluation for any underlying cardiac abnormalities and an estimation of the risk for use of these drugs. The decision to use these drugs is made by the primary care provider after consideration of the risks and benefits of their use. Guidelines for the cardiovascular monitoring of psychotropic drugs in children and adolescents were published by the American Heart Association in 1999. The major untoward cardiac side effect of these drugs is their effect on the conduction system and the induction of dysrhythmias. Generalizations can be made based on drug classes. Stimulants such as methylphenidate can cause tachycardias and palpitations, with no specific monitoring indicated. Tricyclic antidepressants can cause prolongation of the corrected QT (QTc), PR, and QRS intervals as well as sinus tachycardia. This may lead to an increased risk of sudden death. They also may interact with other drugs. Because of these side effects, baseline evaluation with a history and physical examination as well as a baseline ECG is indicated. Thereafter, a follow-up evaluation is indicated, including an ECG, after a stable dose of the drug is achieved. Serotonin uptake inhibitors used in the treatment of depression (fluoxetine—Prozac, sertraline—Zoloft, and paroxetine—Paxil) are not associated with any significant cardiac side effects other than tachycardia, and thus, there is no specific cardiac monitoring indicated. Other antidepressants, such as lithium are associated with arrhythmia and T-wave changes, though no specific monitoring is indicated. Clonidine and Guanfacine are associated with hypotension and rebound hypertension, which ought to be monitored with a change in dose, or discontinuing therapy. The antipsychotic medications, phenothiazines, butyrophenones, diphenylbutylpiperidine, are all associated with prolongation of the QTc. They may cause tachycardia as well. Therefore, a baseline history and physical as well as ECG is indicated with a follow-up after a stable dose of the drug is achieved. Many of the medications may interact with other medications; therefore, this requires investigation during the baseline evaluation. In addition, some medications such as lithium are teratogenic and may cause cardiac defects in utero.

Specific recommendations are:

1. Baseline history and physical with inquiry of symptoms such as palpitations and syncope or lightheadedness. Any ongoing medication or

drug use ought to be determined. Determination of the family medical history (sudden death, or any features to suggest long QTc) is also indicated. A baseline ECG is indicated as stated above. Any positive responses or findings ought to be investigated further with consideration of consultation.

2. Follow-up visits should repeat the above to assess for interim changes.

3. With TCA, or antipsychotic medication treatment, any symptoms such as palpitations, syncope or lightheadedness, or ECG changes (HR >130, PR >200 ms, QRS >120 ms, or QTc >460 ms) should prompt the consideration of an alternate therapy and/or pediatric cardiology consultation.

4. Always be aware of interactions with other drugs.

Suggested Readings

Cunniff C, et al: American Academy of Pediatrics. Health supervision for children with Down syndrome. *Pediatrics* 107(2):442–449, 2001.

Freeman S, Taft L, Dooley K, Allran K, Sherman S, Hassold T, et al: Population-based study of congenital heart defects in Down syndrome. *Am J Med Genet* 80:213–217, 1998.

Geggel RL, O'Brien JE, Feingold M: Development of valve dysfunction in adolescents and young adults with Down syndrome and no known congenital heart disease. *J Pediatric* 122:821–823, 1993.

Gutgesell H, Atkins D, Barst R, et al: Cardiovascular monitoring of children and adolescents receiving psychotropic drugs. A statement for health care professionals from the committee on congenital heart defects, council on cardiovascular disease in the young, American Heart Association. *Circulation* 99:979–982, 1999.

Johnson WH, Moller JH: *Pediatric Cardiology*. Baltimore, MD, Lippincott Williams & Wilkins, 2001.

Khan A, Abdulla R: *Genetic and Metabolic Testing in Congenital Heart Disease*. Rush Children's Heart Center Home Page (http://www.rchc.rush.edu/genetic.htm).

Lipschultz SE, Bancroft EA, Boller AM: Cardiovascular manifestation of HIV infection in children, in Garson A, Bricker JT, Fisher DJ, et al. (eds): *The Science of Pediatric Cardiology*, Baltimore, MD, Lippincott Williams & Wilkins, 1998.

Marino B, Digilio MC, et al: Congenital heart diseases in children with Noonan syndrome: an expanded cardiac spectrum with high prevalence of atrioventricular canal. *J Pediatr* 135(6), 1999.

Suzuki K, Yamaki S, et al: Pulmonary vascular disease in Down syndrome with complete atrioventricular septal defect. *Am J Cardiol* 86:434–437, 2000.

Thackray HM, Tifft C: Fetal Alcohol Syndrome. *Pediatr Rev* 22(2), 2001.

56

ROUTINE PEDIATRIC COMPLAINTS IN THE PEDIATRIC CARDIAC PATIENT

Joel Schwab, Laura Schwab, and Patricia Smith

INTRODUCTION

Congenital heart disease (CHD) affects 8 in 1000 live births. In 1998, 29,000 infants in the United States were born with congenital heart disease. With the recent changes in managed care and the changing health care environment, greater aspects of medical care of the pediatric patient with heart disease will be the responsibility of the general pediatrician who must be familiar with the problems that may arise. The pediatric population as a whole now encompasses a more acutely ill group of children. As advances are being made in correcting congenital heart disease, the patients are living longer. The pediatrician's role should be to address the routine health care needs of cardiac patients, and to be vigilant in the management of

health issues that arise. It is important for the pediatrician to know about current cardiac interventions, as well as the baseline status of the cardiac patients he/she cares for. This includes their baseline oxygen saturation, medications, and radiographs.

Pediatricians should work in conjunction with the patient's cardiologist to manage the patient. It is often assumed that the patient and family with complex heart disease would prefer a cardiologist to manage most of their health needs; however, in a recent study in Pediatrics, the majority of parents of teenagers with congenital heart disease prefer their primary care physician for routine health care maintenance and for many of their cardiac health needs. With these attitudes, it is important to address the many routine issues that arise in these patients (Table 56-1).

TABLE 56-1

CHECKLIST FOR ROUTINE HEALTH CARE OF A PATIENT WITH CHD

1. Review cardiac history
    a. Make sure chart is updated with the most recent letters and reports from consultants
    b. Review medications and compliance and compare with consultant letters
2. Check vital signs and growth
3. Routine H and P or focused visit
4. Communicate any new findings with the cardiologist

HEALTH CARE MAINTENANCE

Blood Pressure

At every routine health care visit, all patients over 3 should have their blood pressure measured. Abnormalities in blood pressure can signify new onset cardiac disease or problems with preexisting heart disease.

Certain medications may lead to an increase in blood pressure. These include steroids, oral contraceptives, decongestants, cold preparations, illicit drugs (cocaine, amphetamines, phencyclidine), rebound after discontinuing antihypertensives, beta-agonists, theophylline, caffeine, and nicotine. Other causes of an acute increase in blood pressure may be volume overload, anxiety, and pain. Once this acute increase in blood pressure is noted, any underlying cardiac disease must be evaluated, a relevant history elicited, and proper intervention taken.

Chronic increases in blood pressure may also be seen at repeated visits in a patient with cardiac disease. Coarctation of the aorta, William's syndrome and vasculitis may manifest with increases in blood pressure. Certain medications as well may lead to chronic increases such as steroids, erythromycin, cyclosporine, tacrolimus, and oral contraceptives.

Any change in blood pressure should be considered significant in a cardiac patient. Routine follow-up of the patient is important, inciting medications should be discontinued, and the cardiologist should be made aware of these changes.

Growth

The pediatrician should evaluate the growth of all patients at every visit. Most children with congenital heart disease are undernourished, irrespective of the cardiac defect and the presence or absence of cyanosis. The cause of this is multifactorial, including decreased caloric intake, increased energy requirements, and malabsorption. Children with severe cardiac defects are often hypermetabolic from increased cardiac effort, decreased splanchnic blood flow, tissue hypoxia, and frequent infections. Children with congenital heart disease may need as much as 50% more calories than normal children to achieve normal growth.

There is a large range of growth disturbances, from mild malnutrition to failure to thrive. Acyanotic lesions tend to affect weight gain rather than height; cyanotic lesions tend to affect both height and weight. For both entities, the growth impairment is directly proportional to the severity of the hemodynamic disturbance. A recent study looked at four patient groups, with and without cyanosis, and with and without pulmonary hypertension. Of the 89 patients, 65.2% were less than 5th percentile for weight, 41.6% were less than the 5th percentile for weight and height, and 27% were less than 80% of ideal body weight.

Other factors may affect the growth of cardiac patients. Children with congenital heart disease are often born at a lower birth weight. Up to 30% of infants with congenital heart disease have features of various genetic syndromes. Their caloric requirement may be increased, and they may have concomitant musculoskeletal, central nervous system, renal, and gastrointestinal problems. Since these cardiac patients have the propensity for malnutrition, the pediatrician must optimize their nutritional status.

Careful screening and monitoring of all growth parameters must be performed. Flattening or falling off the growth curve requires evaluation, and intervention may be indicated. Nutritional

TABLE 56-2

RECONSTITUTION OF STANDARD INFANT FORMULA—POWDER

Caloric Density	Water		Level Scoopfuls	Approximate Yield	
kcal/fluid oz	fluid oz	mL		Fluid oz	mL
20 (standard mixture)	2	60	1	2	60
22	3.5	105	2	4	120
24	5	150	3	6	180
27	4.25	128	3	5	150

intervention should include increasing the volume of the feedings, increasing the caloric density of the formula (Tables 56-2–56-4), and offering smaller and more frequent feedings. Oral feeding is optimal, but patients may need to begin enteral feedings in order to increase the caloric intake without compromising the metabolic effort. The severity of cardiac disease does not predict the ability to breastfeed, and all attempts as well as encouragement of breastfeeding should be offered.

Immunizations

Immunization of infants is critical to the health and well-being of the individual as well as the population as a whole. Every attempt should be made to adhere to the current recommended immunization schedule; however, there are certain children in whom special consideration needs to be taken in order to optimize overall outcomes. These are children with certain congenital abnormalities or chronic illnesses, who may require hospitalization, surgery, transfusions, or immune globulins. As the age for surgical intervention has decreased in children with congenital heart defects (CHD), potential problems exist in the scheduling of surgical interventions and maintaining the recommended immunization schedule. The concerns involve immunization side effects complicating the identification of preoperative and postoperative problems, potential exposure of immunocompromised patients during hospitalization of a recently immunized child, and problems with adequate

TABLE 56-3

RECONSTITUTION OF STANDARD INFANT CONCENTRATED LIQUID FORMULA

Caloric Density	Water		Concentrated Liquid		Yield	
kcal/fluid oz	fluid oz	mL	fluid oz	mL	fluid oz	mL
20 (standard mixture)	1	30	1	30	2	60
22	2	60	2.5	75	4.5	135
24	2	60	3	90	5	150
27	1	30	2	60	3	90

TABLE 56-4

INFANT FORMULA RECIPES—CONCENTRATE

kcal/oz	kcal/cc	Amount of Concentrate (oz can)	Amount of Sterile Water (oz)	Total Volume (oz)	By Bottle
20	0.67	13	13	26	1 oz concentrate to 1 oz water
24	0.8	13	9	22	3 oz concentrate to 2 oz water
27	0.9	13	6.5	18.5	2 oz concentrate to 1 oz water
30	1.0	13	4.5	17.5	3 oz concentrate to 1 oz water

seroconversion following cardiopulmonary bypass and transfusion of blood products.

Vaccines can have adverse effects (Table 56-5), including fever, rash, joint pain, and neurologic sequelae. There are rare, more severe adverse effects that can be detrimental to children with an already compromised health status. Live-virus vaccines can cause the disease being immunized against. Measles vaccine has been shown to cause a six-fold increase in the rate of thrombocytopenia,

TABLE 56-5

EXPECTED TIME FRAME FOR MOST ADVERSE REACTIONS

	DTP	DTaP	OPV[a]	IPV	Measles (MMR)	Hib	HBV	Varivax[c]	PCV 7
Fever	24–72 h	Occurs less			7–12 days, lasts 1–5 days	Rare	Slight	1–42 days	24–48 h
Rash					7–12 days			5–26 days	
Joint pain					Onset 7–21 days (Rubella)				
Thrombo-cytopenia					2–3 weeks, up to 2 months				
Neurologic/seizures	1–7 days				15 days				
Illness			4–6 weeks (VAPP)		6 months	7 days		4–6 weeks	
Viral shedding			4–6 weeks (VAPP)		—[b]			4–6 weeks with rash	

[a]Especially with first dose, no longer recommended in the United States.
[b]No transmission of vaccine-strain virus.
[c]No salicylates for 6 weeks.
Source: Adapted from—Committee on Infectious Diseases (2003) in Redbook, 26th ed. p. 423.

which would be detrimental to a child having open-heart surgery.

Congenital heart disease (except following heart transplantation) is not a contraindication to maintaining the recommended immunization schedule. Children with CHD should receive additional immunizations such as influenza according to standard recommendations. Standard practice at this time is to retain the immunization schedule using a full dose vaccine and to use prophylactic acetaminophen to prevent fever, which may not be tolerated in some children with CHD. Surgical interventions for CHD are now being scheduled at earlier ages than in the past, during the same period of time that most immunizations are being given. Although it is important to avoid any barriers to immunization, there may be adequate reason to alter the recommended schedule in order to optimize surgical and immunization outcomes.

Surgery for congenital heart defects requires hospitalization, the use of cardiopulmonary bypass, the need for blood component transfusion, and has the potential for postoperative infection or neurologic and other organ sequelae. These factors present a number of concerns. Potential exposure of immunocompromised patients can occur during hospitalization, if there is active viral shedding or disease develops, such as with oral polio (which is no longer recommended, but may still be available in certain settings) and varicella vaccines. Potential exacerbation of an illness from the vaccine itself or related to the alteration of the immune system by cardiopulmonary bypass can complicate the postoperative course in a mild to severe degree. Cardiopulmonary bypass significantly effects platelet count and function, which may be compounded by any vaccine-induced thrombocytopenia. Transfusion of blood products, which appears to have significant immunomodulatory effects for 4 or more weeks may effect the immune response to all vaccines (Table 56-6). Specific blood products diminish the body's capacity to mount an active response to live virus vaccines over varying periods of time. This can create a situation in which there may be a false sense of safety, unless immunizations are postponed, children are reimmunized, or titers are checked. There is the potential need to

TABLE 56-6

IMMUNIZATION INTERVAL FOLLOWING TRANSFUSION[a]

	Measles (MMR)[b]	Varivax[b]
Washed RBCs	None	None
RBCs	3 months	3 months
Packed RBCs	5 months	5 months
FFP	7 months	7 months
Platelets	7 months	7 months
Whole blood	6 months	6 months
Immunoglobulin		
Kawasaki	11 months	11 months
VZIG	5 months	5 months
Palivizumab (Synagis)	None	None

Table 56-6 illustrates the time frame from blood transfusion that effects seroconversion. These parameters should be taken into consideration when scheduling either the immunizations or elective surgical procedures. If the PCP and the subspecialist coordinate plans with this information in mind, surgeries will not be cancelled and immunizations will be most effective.

[a]Time for decrease in passive antibodies to allow for adequate response to vaccine.

[b]Immunization within 2 weeks before transfusion may effect response.

Source: Adapted from—Committee on Infectious Diseases (2003) in Redbook, 26th ed, p. 423.

use salicylates (which are not recommended for 6 weeks following varicella vaccine administration) to control postoperative inflammatory responses or for platelet inhibition. The more common adverse reactions—fever, rash, joint pain—which pose little risk to healthy infants, can mask the presence of postoperative infection or postpericardiotomy syndrome.

Respiratory syncytial virus (RSV) can cause serious lower airway infections that are extremely detrimental to infants with hemodynamically significant CHD. In the past the only preventive treatment was RSV-IVIG, given monthly; however, serious adverse reactions were noted in children with cyanotic heart disease and its use was suspended. Recently a monoclonal antibody, Palivizumab (Synagis), was developed and approved for use in high-risk children following a double-blinded, placebo controlled study. The use in children with cyanotic and acyanotic heart disease was studied over a four-year period of time with the conclusion that "Palivizumab given IM monthly during the RSV season is safe for children with serious CHD and effective in reducing RSV hospitalization in this high-risk population." The American Academy of Pediatrics (2003) recommends the use of Palivizumab in children less than 24 months of age with hemodynamically significant cyanotic and acyanotic heart disease, depending on the degree of compromise. The Food and Drug Administration has also approved this medication as indicated and safe for use in hemodynamically significant CHD. Those children requiring medications for the management of congestive heart failure, moderate/ severe pulmonary hypertension, or cyanosis are candidates for this vaccine. Injections should be started in October and be given once a month. The Centers for Disease Control publishes information by region stating the month to end palivizumab (Synagis) administration. Cardiopulmonary bypass has been noted to decrease serum concentrations of Palivizumab, a postoperative dose should be administered as soon as the child is medically stable.

Reyes syndrome has been associated with aspirin use and influenza. Therefore, it is recommended that all children >6 months to 18 years of age requiring long-term aspirin therapy (e.g., Kawasaki disease) be immunized with influenza vaccine.

Dental Care

Dental care in children with CHD is an important consideration when their first tooth erupts, because of the risk of bacterial endocarditis (BE) (Chapter 33). Transient bacteremia occurs frequently during dental procedures with instrumentation, therefore, preventive dental care, including good oral hygiene and regular dental visits, is especially important in a child with CHD. Dental visits every 6–12 months starting at 2–3 years of age are important. Fluoride treatments are necessary in areas where the community water supply is not fluoridated. The best BE prophylaxis is meticulous oral hygiene. Poor oral hygiene and plaque accumulation

are major causes of periodontal disease, which can result in bacteremia from normal chewing or brushing the teeth. The incidence and severity of bacteremia is directly proportional to the degree of oral inflammation and infection. In children, special risks for BE include baby-bottle caries as well as chipped or damaged teeth. These should be extracted if darkened, indicating pulp involvement and the increased potential for bacteremia.

Specific dental considerations important in the care of a child with CHD include the following:

- 20% of children with cyanotic CHD may have delayed formation or eruption of primary teeth.
- Use of pulsating water-type cleaning devices is not recommended.
- Digoxin elixir contains 30% sucrose, which can be cariogenic (cavity-producing) in selected individuals.
- Gingival bleeding and bleeding from dental procedures is increased in patients on anticoagulants or with a hematocrit >60.*
- A dental examination 1–2 months preoperatively allows time for treatment of any abnormalities, which should decrease the risk of postoperative infection. Dental treatment also should be completed before heart transplant, if possible.
- Elective dental procedures should be postponed for 4–6 months following cardiac surgery.

Bacterial Endocarditis Prophylaxis

Recommendations for prophylactic antibiotics (Table 56-7) to prevent bacterial endocarditis (BE) (Chapter 33) are based on general principles including the possibility of bacteremia and cardiac risk factors. A procedure (Table 56-8) causing bacteremia that is not treated with antibiotics prodives a source of bacteria which can cause infection. Cardiac risk factors (Table 56-9) are due to any lesion which produces a high velocity jet or turbulent blood flow. If a patient is already on antibiotics or on chronic antibiotic treatment,

---

*Gingival hyperplasia, which increases the risk of infection, is a common side effect of Cyclosporin A (immunosuppressant), in the transplant patient, and phenylhydantoin (Dilantin), which is sometimes used in the treatment of arrhythmias.

TABLE 56-7

RECOMMENDED ANTIBIOTIC TREATMENT FOR THE PROPHYLAXIS OF BACTERIAL ENDOCARDITIS

Prophylactic Regimens for Dental, Oral, Respiratory Tract, or Esophageal Procedures. (Follow-up Dose No Longer Recommended.) Total Children's Dose Should Not Exceed Adult Dose

I. Standard General Prophylaxis for Patients at Risk

Amoxicillin: Adults, 2.0 g (children, 50 mg/kg) given orally 1 hour before procedure

II. Unable to Take Oral Medications

Ampicillin: Adults, 2.0 g (children 50 mg/kg) given IM or IV within 30 min before procedure

III. Amoxicillin/Ampicillin/Penicillin Allergic Patients

Clindamycin: Adults, 600 mg (children 20 mg/kg) given orally 1 h before procedure. -OR-
Cephalexin[a] or Cefadroxil[a]: Adults, 2.0 g (children 50 mg/kg) orally 1 h before procedure. -OR-
Azithromycin or Clarithromycin: Adults, 500 mg (children 15 mg/kg) orally 1 h before procedure

IV. Amoxicillin/Ampicillin/Penicillin Allergic Patients Unable to Take Oral Medications

Clindamycin: Adults, 600 mg (children 20 mg/kg) IV within 30 min before procedure. -OR-
Cefazolin[a]: Adults, 1.0 g (children 25 mg/kg) IM or IV within 30 min before procedure

Prophylactic Regimens for Genitourinary/Gastrointestinal Procedures

I. High-Risk Patients

Ampicillin plus gentamicin: Ampicillin (adults, 2.0 g; children 50 mg/kg) plus gentamicin 1.5 mg/kg (for both adults and children, not to exceed 120 mg) IM or IV within 30 minutes before starting procedure. Six hours later, ampicillin (adults, 1.0 g; children, 25 mg/kg) IM or IV, or amoxicillin (adults, 1.0 g; children, 25 mg/kg) orally

II. High-Risk Patients Allergic to Ampicillin/Amoxicillin

Vancomycin plus gentamicin: Vancomycin (adults, 1.0 g; children, 20 mg/kg) IV over 1–2 h plus gentamicin 1.5 mg/kg (for both adults and children, not to exceed 120 mg) IM or IV. Complete injection/infusion within 30 min before starting procedure

III. Moderate-Risk Patients

Amoxicillin: Adults, 2.0 g (children 50 mg/kg) orally 1 h before procedure -OR-
Ampicillin: Adults, 2.0 g (children 50 mg/kg) IM or IV within 30 min before starting procedure

IV. Moderate-Risk Patients Allergic to Ampicillin/Amoxicillin

Vancomycin: Adults, 1.0 g (children 20 mg/kg) IV over 1–2 h. Complete infusion within 30 minutes of starting the procedure

[a]Cephalosporins should not be used in patients with immediate-type hypersensitivity reaction to penicillins.
Source: Adapted from *Prevention of Bacterial Endocarditis: Recommendations by the American Heart Association* by the Committee on Rheumatic Fever, Endocarditis, and Kawasaki Disease. *JAMA* 1997, 277:1794–1801, *Circulation* 1997, 96:358–366, and *JADA* 1997, 128:1142–1150.

TABLE 56-8

PROCEDURES CAUSING BACTEREMIA, AND THEREFORE INCREASING THE RISK OF BE IN SUSCEPTIBLE INDIVIDUALS

Dental Procedures for which Endocarditis Prophylaxis is Recommended[a]

- Dental extractions
- Periodontal procedures including surgery, scaling, and root planing, probing, and recall maintenance
- Endodontic (root canal) instrumentation or surgery only beyond the apex
- Subgingival placement of antibiotic fibers or strips
- Initial placement of orthodontic bands but not brackets
- Intraligamentary local anesthetic injections
- Prophylactic cleaning of teeth or implants where bleeding is anticipated

Other Procedures for which Endocarditis Prophylaxis is Recommended

Respiratory tract

- Tonsillectomy and/or adenoidectomy
- Surgical operations that involve respiratory mucosa
- Bronchoscopy with a rigid bronchoscope

Gastrointestinal tract[b]

- Sclerotherapy for esophageal varices
- Esophageal stricture dilation
  Endoscopic retrograde cholangiography with biliary obstruction
- Biliary tract surgery
- Surgical operations that involve intestinal mucosa

Genitourinary tract

- Prostatic surgery
- Cystoscopy
- Urethral dilation

[a]Prophylaxis is recommended for patients with high- and moderate-risk cardiac conditions.
[b]Prophylaxis is recommended for high-risk patients; it is optional for medium-risk patients.
Source: Adapted from *Prevention of Bacterial Endocarditis: Recommendations by the American Heart Association* by the Committee on Rheumatic Fever, Endocarditis, and Kawasaki Disease. *JAMA* 1997, 277:1794–1801, *Circulation* 1997, 96:358–366, and *JADA* 1997, 128:1142–1150.

another type of antibiotic is recommended for BE prophylaxis to cover the possibility of resistant organisms.

COMMON COMPLAINTS AND DISEASES

Colds

One of the most common complaints in a pediatrician's office is the common cold. The pediatrician must differentiate the presence of lower versus upper respiratory tract infection. With a lower respiratory tract infection, the pediatrician must be aware that lung disease may affect cardiac function (especially in a patient with a cardiac abnormality), and that lung and heart disease may be confused (Table 56-10). It is prudent for any patient with underlying heart disease presenting with increased work of breathing, tachypnea, or retractions to have a chest radiograph. This may reveal changes from previous films, which may

T A B L E   5 6 - 9

PATIENTS WITH AN INCREASED RISK OF BE OWING TO THE FOLLOWING UNDERLYING CONGENITAL HEART DEFECTS

Cardiac Conditions Associated with Endocarditis
High-Risk Category
• Prosthetic cardiac valves, including bioprosthetic and homograft valves
• Previous bacterial endocarditis
• Complex cyanotic congenital heart disease (e.g., single ventricle states, transposition of the great arteries, tetralogy of Fallot)
• Surgically constructed systemic pulmonary shunts or conduits
Moderate-Risk Category
• Most other congenital cardiac malformations (other than above)
• Acquired valvar dysfunction (e.g., rheumatic heart disease)
• Hypertrophic cardiomyopathy
Mitral valve prolapse with valvar regurgitation and/or thickened leaflets

Source: Adapted from *Prevention of Bacterial Endocarditis: Recommendations by the American Heart Association* by the Committee on Rheumatic Fever, Endocarditis, and Kawasaki Disease. *JAMA* 1997, 277:1794–1801, *Circulation* 1997, 96:358–366, and *JADA* 1997, 128:1142–1150.

T A B L E   5 6 - 1 0

LUNG VS. CARDIAC DISEASE

Lung Disease	*Heart Disease*
History	**History**
Fever more likely	Fever less likely
Dyspnea	Dyspnea
Cough more likely	Cough less likely
Exercise intolerance less likely	Exercise intolerance more likely
PMH pulmonary disease	Weight gain, decreased urine output
	PMH heart disease
Physical Exam	**Physical Exam**
Increased RR/HR, nl BP	Increased RR, HR, BP may be abnormal
Abnormal lung exam—lower tract	May have abnormal lung exam—lower tract
Normal cardiac exam	Abnormal cardiac exam pathologic murmurs, S3, S4
"Enlarged" liver possible because of hyperinflation	Enlarged liver—truly enlarged
No edema	Peripheral edema
Laboratory Studies	**Laboratory Studies**
Normal heart size on chest radiograph (CXR)	Abnormal heart size on CXR
Normal vascularity on CXR	Venous congestion on chest film
ECG usually normal	Possible abnormal ECG

TABLE 56-11

LOWER VS. UPPER TRACT RESPIRATORY INFECTION

	Upper Tract—Glottic/Supraglottic	
Lower Tract—Subglottic	Periglottic	Pharyngeal/Nasopharyngeal
Increased work of breathing (WOB)	Increased WOB	Rhinorrhea, cough
	Tachypnea	Nasal congestion
Cough	Retractions	Unlabored breathing
Tachypnea	Stridor	Normal lung exam
Retractions	Normal lung exam	
Flaring		
Gasping respirations		
Abnormal lung exam	Cardiac disease (vascular rings or	Cardiac disease, if present,
Wheezing	tracheal compression) possible	not related to symptoms
Crackles/rales		
Decreased breath sounds		
Egophany		
Abnormal percussion		
Cardiac disease a possibility		

indicate worsening heart failure (new or worsening cardiomegaly), pleural or pericardial effusions, or other manifestations of CHD. In order to interpret these results, baseline chest radiographs must be available for comparison, and all findings need to be placed in context of the clinical picture. When differentiating between upper and lower respiratory disease, the importance of knowing the child's baseline oxygen saturation, respiratory rate, work of breathing, and color is underscored (Table 56-11).

Many patients wish to ignore the pediatrician's advice that upper respiratory infections only require symptomatic treatment. They often seek antibiotics and over-the-counter medications. Many of the over-the-counter cold remedies contain ingredients such as sympathomimetics, caffeine, and pseudoephedrine, that can alter blood pressure and cause arrhythmias, and in turn affect cardiac status. Thus, the pediatrician must be strict in advising to refrain from the tempting drug-store marketing.

Treating viral upper respiratory infections with antibiotics may mask underlying bacteremia or lead to resistant organisms.

Fever

Fever in a cardiac patient may be a mild viral infection; however, fever may also signify serious illness. As children with congenital heart disease survive longer and the incidence of rheumatic heart disease decreases, congenital heart disease has become the predominant underlying condition for infective endocarditis for children over 2 years old in developed countries. Postoperative infective endocarditis is a long-term risk in patients after correction of complex congenital heart disease.

The presentation of infective endocarditis is often indolent. The patient may have a prolonged low-grade fever, somatic complaints consisting of fatigue, weight loss, weakness, arthralgias, myalgias, anorexia, and diaphoresis. These symptoms are nonspecific, and can be the result of a simple viral infection. However, careful evaluation, including blood cultures and referral to a cardiologist if positive, is necessary. Blood cultures are indicated in all patients with fever without localization and a history of cardiac disease. A blood culture should be drawn in patients at risk for BE prior to starting antibiotics.

The treatment of a fever must also be considered carefully. Pediatricians often start nonsteroidal anti-inflammatory drugs (NSAIDS) for patients with fever. Certain NSAIDS may alter the effectiveness of beta-blockers, furosemide, and angiotensin-converting enzyme inhibitors. Thus, acetaminophen is the drug of choice, unless the pediatrician can be certain that the patient is on no medication that will interfere with the NSAIDS. A small number of cardiac patients are unable to tolerate a fever, though it may cause increased cyanosis in patients with right-to-left shunts, and may accentuate any underlying tachycardia or tachypnea.

In summary, fever is treated slightly different in a patient with CHD. Stronger suspicion for endocarditis should be present and antipyretics and other medications ought to be used judiciously.

Anemia

The pediatrician must evaluate the hematologic status of the cardiac patient to avoid anemia. This becomes even more important with cyanotic heart disease. Children with cyanotic heart disease do not tolerate a decreased hemoglobin and oxygen carrying capacity. To compensate, they will have higher than normal hematocrits and hemoglobins to enhance oxygen carrying ability. With values in the normal range for acyanotic patients, these children may actually be anemic and may require iron supplementation. Other indices such as mean corpuscular volume, ferritin, and red cell distribution width may need to be checked. Microcystosis in a cyanotic patient implies iron deficiency despite a normal hemoglobin or hematocrit value. The pediatrician must recommend diets that are high in iron to avoid anemia.

Headaches

Many children present to their pediatrician with the chief complaint of headache. Changes in blood pressure can present with a headache. Care must be taken to elicit a complete history of all medications. Children with right-to-left shunts are more prone to thromboembolic episodes. Paradoxic emboli, produced by air or a thrombus within the venous circulation may travel to the systemic circulation and subsequently to the cerebral arteries. The emboli can also become a nidus for bacteria, leading to an abscess. Presenting complaints of a brain abscess are headache, fever, focal neurologic signs, and seizures. Thus, a headache in a cardiac patient must be evaluated with caution. The physical examination should include assessment of blood pressure and a more detailed neurologic examination to help to exclude hypertension or a neurologic lesion as the underlying cause of headache.

Syncope

There are many reasons why a cardiac patient may suffer from syncope. Vasovagal or neurocardiogenic syncope are the most common causes of fainting in children and adolescents. In the presence of underlying cardiac pathology, syncope can be caused by arrhythmogenic conditions or structural heart defects. Structural defects causing outflow obstruction and decreased cardiac output are a rare cause of syncope and usually have other symptoms and signs of low cardiac output (fatigue, dyspnea, edema, poor perfusion, murmur of obstruction, hepatomegaly, and so forth). Arrhythmias are a more common cause, which can be either transient or permanent. Although, an isolated primary arrhythmia may be present, an arrhythmia secondary to congenital heart disease or as a sequelae of surgical repair of congenital heart disease is more common. Complete heart block may be seen in complex congenital heart disease. Since, any surgical repair of congenital heart disease involving the ventricular septum may lead to heart block, the presenting complain of syncope must be taken seriously and the heart must be closely evaluated. Pediatricians should be familiar with medications that may cause syncope in their cardiac and non-cardiac patients. The pediatrician should notify the cardiologist of any new onset syncope in a patient with CHD because of the seriousness of the above diagnoses.

Asthma

Patients with asthma and congenital heart disease must be evaluated carefully. The baseline respiratory effort and respiratory rate should be recorded; this allows for the pediatrician to not overreact to symptoms that may be a result of the cardiac lesion as opposed to asthma. Because albuterol is the mainstay of therapy for an acute asthma exacerbation, the beta-agonist affect on the heart must be monitored carefully. In addition, some patients should not use albuterol or other beta-agonists for prophylaxis. Tachycardia may not be tolerated well in a cardiac patient. The effects of hypoxia that may occur with asthma are also less well tolerated. For a routine asthmatic, many pediatricians use 93% oxygen saturation as a minimum saturation; however, this may be too low or too high for a cardiac patient. In general, patients with CHD who have had complete repair should have normal oxygen saturations and should be treated like other patients with reactive airways disease keeping in mind the possibility of arrhythmia and cardiac dysfunction. Patients who have had palliations such as a BT shunt, Glenn shunt or Fontan procedure may have abnormal resting oxygen saturations, thus these should be compared to baseline. With the latter procedures, and other types of complex CHD, the cardiologist must be made aware of the new physical findings and may be able to provide guidance in the treatment.

In addition, congestive heart failure presents with such symptoms as cough, shortness of breath, exercise intolerance, crackles, and wheezing. This can often be confused with reactive airway disease. The pediatrician must be able to differentiate a cardiac versus pulmonary etiology (Table 56-10). Chest radiography should be ordered more routinely in patients with CHD and asthma in order to help in this process. Once this differentiation is made, the drugs used to treat asthma should be used with appropriate caution. Albuterol, ipratropium,

theophylline, and other drugs that are used to treat asthma can be dangerous in patients with underlying cardiac disease and should be prescribed on an individual basis.

Bronchiolitis

Respiratory syncytial virus (RSV) is the most common pathogen causing upper and lower respiratory tract infection in children. RSV infections are often much more severe in patients with underlying cardiac disease. The management of lower tract RSV disease is supportive care only; hence, the goal for patients with cardiac disease is prevention of the illness. Since RSV is spread by contact with secretions, intensive contact precautions and hand washing are necessary to protect patients.

Patients with cyanotic and significant acyanotic congenital heart disease (most often PDA or VSD), chronic lung disease, or are less than or equal to 32 weeks gestation are candidates for Synagis (the monoclonal antibody). This is given monthly during the RSV season.

It is the role of the pediatrician to identify the subset of patients who are candidates for Synagis. If a patient does not fit the criteria, then the pediatrician must guide the parents in supportive treatment strategies of this often devastating illness. These guidelines are in current debate, thus the pediatrician remains current in the knowledge of the most recent literature.

Vomiting and Diarrhea

Patients with underlying cardiac disease do not have a higher incidence of acute gastrointestinal illnesses. They are at risk for problems if their hemodynamic state is altered by dehydration secondary to vomiting and diarrhea. In addition, alterations in serum sodium, potassium, and acidosis may affect cardiac function and should be carefully monitored during the acute illness. Aggressive fluid management and electrolyte replacement may need to be performed in some children with cardiac disease, especially those with hypertrophic obstructive cardiomyopathy in whom dehydration is poorly tolerated. One must remember that volume overloading some patients may be detrimental, such as patients with dilated cardiomyopathy or left-to-right shunts.

SUMMARY

The general pediatrician can perform many aspects of the care of pediatric patients with cardiac disease. The pediatrician can be considered the "eyes and hands" of the cardiologist. He/she must maintain an open dialogue with the cardiologist and the cardiologists should send them frequent reports of the child's progress. The pediatrician must monitor normal changes and detect any deviations that may be related to underlying heart disease. With this partnership between the general pediatrician and the cardiologist, the specialist will be grateful for the help, and the pediatrician will have a rewarding experience.

Suggested Readings

American Academy of Pediatrics. Pickering LD, ed. *Red Book 2003: Report of the Committee on Infectious Disease*, 20th ed. Elk Grove Village, IL, 2003.

Baren JM: Contemporary approach to the emergency department management of pediatric asthma. *Emerg Med Clin North Am* 20(1):115–138, 2002.

Blecker U: Nutritional problems in patients who have chronic disease. *Pediatr Rev* 21(1):29–32, 2000.

Braunwald E: *Heart Disease: A Textbook of Cardoavascular Medicine*, 6th ed. Philadelphia, PA: WB Saunders, 2001, pp. 1520–1527, 1616.

Devine S, Anisman P, Robinson B: A basic guide to cyanotic congenital heart disease. *Contemp Pediatr*, 15(10):133–163, 1998.

Ferrieri P, et al: Unique features of infective endocarditis in childhood. *Pediatrics* 109(5):931–943, 2002.

Lauer RM, Saunders SP: Results of expert meetings: conducting pediatric cardiovascular trials—pediatric issues and diseases. *Am Heart J* 142:224–228, 2001.

Malhotra A: Influenza and RSV. Update on infection, management, and prevention. *Pediatr Clin North Am* 47(2):353–372, vi–vii, 2000.

Maxwell LG: Perioperative management issues in pediatric patients. *Anesthesiol Clin North Am* 18(3):601–632, 2000.

Miller MR: Parental preference for primary and specialty care collaboration in the management of teenagers with congenital heart disease. *Pediatrics* 106(2 Pt. 1): 264–269, 2000.

Mitchell IM, Logan RW, Pollock JC, Jamieson MP: Nutritional status of children with congenital heart disease. *Br Heart J* 73(3):277–283, 1995.

Narchi H: The child who passes out. *Pediatr Rev* 21(11): 2000.

Norwood VF: Hypertension. *Pediatr Rev* 23(8):197–209, 2002.

Prevention of Bacterial Endocarditis: Recommendations by the American Heart Association by the committee on rheumatic fever, endocarditis, and Kawasaki's disease. *JAMA* 277:1794–1801, 1997; *Circulation* 96:358–366, 1997; and *JADA* 128:1142–1150, 1997.

Prober CG: Advances in prevention of respiratory syncytial virus infections. *J Pediatr* 135(5):546–558, 1999.

Saenz RB, Beebe DK, Triplett LC: Caring for infants with congenital heart disease. *Am Fam Physician* 01-Apr-1999; 59(7):1857–1868.

Smith P: Primary care in children with congenital heart disease. *J Pediatr Nurs* 16(5):308–319, 2001.

Strom BL, Abrutyn E, Berlin JA, Kinman JL, Feldman RS, Stolley PD, Levison ME, Korzeniowski OM, Kaye D: Dental and cardiac risk factors for infective endocarditis. A population-based, case-control study. *Ann Intern Med* 129(10):761–769, 1998.

Varan B, Tokel K, Yilmaz G: Malnutrition and growth failure in cyanotic and acyanotic congenital heart disease with and without pulmonary hypertension. *Arch Dis Child* 81:49–52, 1999.

57

HYPERLIPIDEMIA AND PREVENTATIVE CARDIOLOGY

Margaret M. Samyn

ATHEROSCLEROSIS

Introduction

Coronary heart disease (CHD) is prevalent, afflicting more than 60 million Americans.[1] Having a good understanding of the underlying biology will allow clinicians to recognize the usefulness of soluble biomarkers for assessing pediatric patients "at-risk" for CHD. Traditional risk factors for development of atherosclerosis are listed in Table 57-1.[2] Addressing these risk factors will enable clinicians to target and treat patients with asymptomatic atherosclerosis who are ripe for prevention efforts, and to monitor successful treatment regimens, ultimately leading to plaque regression and event reduction. Such preventive cardiology efforts should even begin in childhood.[2–9]

ANATOMY AND HISTOPATHOLOGY

The Tunica Intima

The tunica intima[10] is the innermost layer of the arterial wall, comprised of the crucial endothelial cell layer which interfaces with the vessel lumen and maintains contact with liquid blood. This structure is much more complex and heterogeneous than the simple monolayer often depicted in diagrams. It plays an intimate role in vascular homeostasis and is at the crux of the pathobiology of developing coronary artery disease (CAD), also referred to as CHD. Through heparin sulfate proteoglycan molecules that serve as cofactors for antithrombin III (inactivating thrombin) and through thrombomodulin which binds thrombin activating protein C and S, blood is in contact with the endothelial layer in a liquid, unclotted state. Clot formation is normally

**RISK FACTOR ASSESSMENT FOR
CORONARY HEART DISEASE (CHD)**

- Lipids: ⇑ LDL, ⇑ triglycerides, or ⇓ HDL
- Hypertension (HTN)
- Diabetes
- Smoking
- Family history
- Obesity (>95% for wt.)
- Physical inactivity
- Age

Source: National Cholesterol Education Program Report of the Expert Panel on Blood Cholesterol Levels in Children and Adolescents. *Pediatrics* (Suppl.) Vol. 89, No. 3, Pt. 2, March 1992.

obliterated by surface fibrinolytic mechanisms (specifically tissue and urokinase plasminogen activation) catabolizing plasminogen to plasmin, the natural fibrinolytic.

With aging, human arteries develop a more complex intima containing arterial smooth muscle cells and fibrillin forms of interstitial collagen (types I and III). This process is known as *diffuse intimal thickening* and does not necessarily occur coincident with pathologic lipid accumulation. The internal elastic membrane serves as the boundary between the intima and the next layer, the media (Figure 57-1).

The Tunica Media

The tunica media[10] varies depending on whether it is present in a large elastic artery (like the aorta) or in a smaller muscular artery. In the former, it is comprised of concentric layers of smooth muscle cells and elastic rich extracellular matrix. The organization is less rigid in the smaller vessels with smooth muscle cells arranged in a continuous rather than in a lamellar array. Such smooth muscle cells and extracellular matrix are normally rather quiescent, or dormant, with regard to cell growth and turnover. The organization of the vessels continues, as the external elastic lamina separates the media from the adventitia.

The Adventitia

The adventitia[10] of arteries has a loose architecture, being comprised of collagen fibrils, the vaso vasorum, and nerve endings. A few mast cells and fibroblasts may exist in this layer too.

THE PATHOGENESIS OF ATHEROSCLEROSIS

The theories of the initiation of atherosclerosis[10] arise from animal experimentation, and epidemiologic research from cohorts of children (Bogalusa Heart Study and Muscatine Heart Study).[11,12,13] In a cohort of biracial children from Louisiana, studied in the latter part of the twentieth century, autopsies were performed on young people (ages 2–39 years), dying from noncardiac causes, revealed striking levels of early atherosclerotic lesions, especially fatty streaks, that could be correlated with cardiovascular risk factors, especially body mass index, systolic and diastolic BP, and serum lipid levels (i.e., most notably, increased total cholesterol, triglycerides, and low density lipoprotein (LDL) cholesterol and decreased high density lipoprotein (HDL) levels). In fact, the extent of fatty streaks and fibrous plaques in the aorta and coronary arteries increase with age (Figure 57-2).[11]

Accumulation of lipoprotein particles (especially LDL) in the intima is thought to be the inciting event for atherosclerosis development. Lipoprotein particles bind intimal proteoglycan and can reside in the intimal layer for a long time.[14,15] Such bound particles seem to be more susceptible to oxidation and chemical modification caused by interacting leukocytes and vascular cells.[16]

Leukocyte Recruitment and Transformation into Foam Cells

Leukocyte recruitment, in fact, is thought to play a very significant role in the pathobiology and "maturation" of the atherosclerotic plaque. Leukocyte adherence to endothelial cells, something that is generally "taboo" in vessels with healthy endothelium, occurs routinely in the hyperlipidemic vessel.

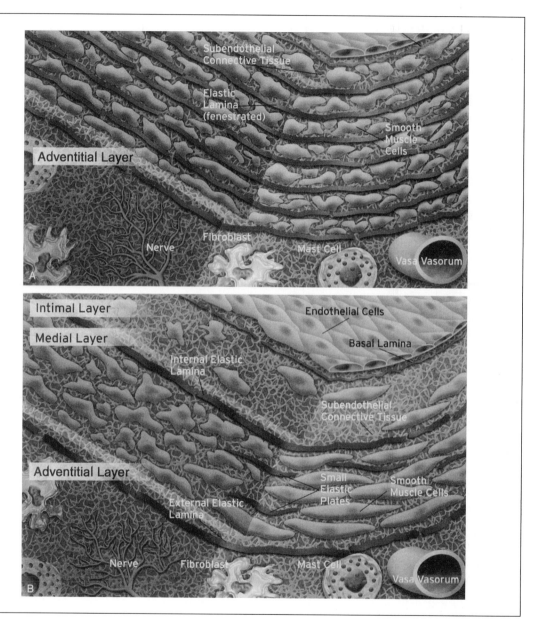

F I G U R E   5 7 - 1

NORMAL ARTERY ANATOMY

Source: Libby P. *The Vascular Biology of Atherosclerosis Heart Disease: A Textbook of Cardiovascular Medicine*, 6th ed. Philadelphia, WB Saunders, 2001, Vol. 1, Chap. 30.

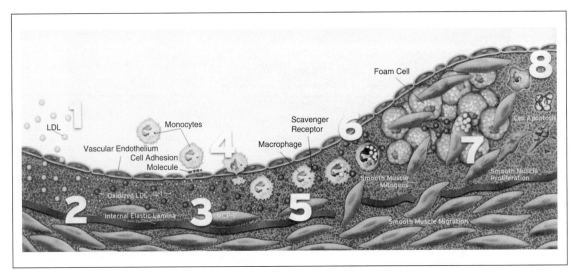

FIGURE 57-2

THE INITIATION OF ATHEROSCLEROSIS

Source: Libby P. *The Vascular Biology of Atherosclerosis. Heart Disease: A Textbook of Cardiovascular Medicine*, 6th ed. Philadelphia, WB Saunders, 2001, Vol. 1, Chap. 30.

Leukocytes can be seen by electron microscopy intercalating (undergoing diapedesis) through gap junctions into the tunica intima where, by accumulating lipids, they are transformed into foam cells.[17] Both monocytes and T lymphocytes participate in this activity. Two groups of chemokines attract white blood cells into the developing atheroma. The first is monocyte chemoattractant protein-1 (MCP-1), produced by endothelium as a result of lipoprotein oxidation or stimulation by inflammatory mediators. The second is a trio of chemoattractant chemokines—consisting of interferon—inducible protein 10 (IP-10) and T cell alpha chemoattractant (I-TAC), as well as monokine induced by interferon gamma (MIG). MCP-1 is unique in its selectivity for macrophage influx while the "trio" attracts lymphocytes.[18,19]

Next endothelial cell leukocyte attractant molecules (like vascular cell adhesion molecule (VCAM-1), intercellular adhesion molecule-1 (ICAM-1), E selectin, P selectin, and L-selectin) variously bind white blood cells (monocytes, lym-

phocytes, and granulocytes) increasing the growth of the emerging atheroma. Clinicians should be familiar with these factors, as various clinical trials with adult patients are looking at these as possible soluble markers present in the "at-risk" patient. Likewise, new pharmaceuticals may influence/target these markers.

The transformation of the lipid laden macrophage, or foam cell, into the more mature atheroma involves continual lipid uptake by "scavenger receptors" on monocytes/macrophages. These transformed cells also may replicate and, in fact, are stimulated to do so by macrophage colony stimulating factor (M-CSF). The cells eventually coalesce into the visible fatty streak which characterizes atherosclerotic lesions in the early second decade (Bogalusa Heart Study).[11] Results from numerous animal and adult studies suggest that dietary modifications may reverse these lesions, giving hope to practicing clinicians who are attempting preventive measures for cardiovascular risk factor modification in "at-risk" children.[5,20]

Smooth Muscle Cell Incorporation

Beyond the fatty streak, smooth muscle cells begin to become incorporated into the architecture of the developing atheroma. The atheroma is now thought to be "maturing." A complex cascade of events occurs. Chemoattractants, such as platelet derived growth factor (PDGF) secreted by macrophages, cause smooth muscle cells of the media to migrate into the intima. Such muscle cells also divide spontaneously, or in response to a stress (most commonly to plaque rupture and exposure to thrombus). Variable periods of smooth muscle proliferation and programmed cell death occur during the gradual maturation of atherosclerotic plaque. It appears the T lymphocytes, acting via inflammatory cytokines, may be involved in apoptosis. Additionally, the smooth muscle cells increase the extracellular matrix component of the maturing plaque. The smooth muscle cells produce interstitial collagen, proteoglycans, and elastin fibers. Matrix metalloproteinases, catabolic enzymes typically involved in remodeling processes, also are present in the maturing plaque, contributing to the transformation of plaque burden. While plaque initially grows outward into the media, causing a paradoxic enlargement of the vessel lumen (Glagov's principle), luminal stenosis begins to occur after the plaque burden exceeds 40% of the cross-sectional area of the artery.[21] (Plaque burden is a term used by many adult cardiologists and pharmaceutical researchers referring to the amount of plaque, its volume and extent in a particular vascular bed.) This phenomenon is important for practicing clinicians to understand, because it serves as the basis for the increased emphasis on lesion assessment by intravascular ultrasound (IVUS) and magnetic resonance imaging (MRI) of vessels. These two imaging modalities (IVUS and MRI) allow a look at the full extent of plaque burden (i.e., the amount of plaque extending deep into the media in addition to the amount impinging on the vessel's lumen). Much of this was heretofore hidden via conventional angiographic assessments. Cardiologists should no longer simply look at the dimensions of the lumen, but should understand the extent of plaque.[21] While once the gold standard for assessing coronary artery

disease, quantitative coronary angiography (QCA) is increasingly viewed as a study of "lumenology," somewhat incomplete in its depiction of the extent of atherosclerotic disease that extends into the vessel wall.[22]

Angiogenesis

As the plaque's complexity increases, not only do smooth muscle cells divide, but endothelial cells also replicate—producing a plexus of micro vessels— in response to two chief angiogenic factors: basic fibroblast growth factor (bFGF) and vascular endothelial growth factor (VEGF). This extensive plaque microcirculation enhances the plaque by allowing additional leukocyte migration and oxygen and nutrient diffusion into the vital plaque milieu. The friable micro vessels, are also part of the advancing pathology, because they are known to rupture. This produces local hemorrhage, thrombosis, which results in continued smooth muscle cell proliferation. A viscous circle ensues. Lastly, sequestration of calcium may occur as the plaque evolves—yet another feature that clinicians might take advantage of during the CAD risk assessment of patients.[23] Electron beam computerized tomography (EBCT) can be used in conjunction with the Framingham risk assessment for adult patients with subclinical atherosclerosis[24] (see Figure 57-3).[25]

From Fatty Streak to Stenotic Lesion

The process of atherosclerosis begins in childhood with lipid accumulation and monocyte transformation into lipid laden foam cells comprising the fatty streaks that can be seen as early as the second decade of life. Yet, most of the patients that pediatric cardiologists will see are asymptomatic. After the encroachment of plaque on the medial layer of the vessel wall, described by Glagov, the atheroma begins to impinge on the lumen and may cause symptoms. Stenosis develops and can impair normal blood flow, especially when lumen dimension decreases by greater than 60% from baseline. Symptoms of chronic stable angina are typical of such advanced coronary lesions and are rare in

Estimate of 10-Year Risk for Men

(Framingham Point Scores)

Age	Points
20–34	–9
35–39	–4
40–44	0
45–49	3
50–54	6
55–59	8
60–64	10
65–69	11
70–74	12
75–79	13

Total Cholesterol	Points				
	Age 20–39	Age 40–49	Age 50–59	Age 60–69	Age 70–79
<160	0	0	0	0	0
160–199	4	3	2	1	0
200–239	7	5	3	1	0
240–279	9	6	4	2	1
≥280	11	8	5	3	1

	Points				
	Age 20–39	Age 40–49	Age 50–59	Age 60–69	Age 70–79
Nonsmoker	0	0	0	0	0
Smoker	8	5	3	1	1

HDL (mg/dL)	Points
≥60	–1
50–59	0
40–49	1
<40	2

Systolic BP (mmHg)	If Untreated	If Treated
<120	0	0
120–129	0	1
130–139	1	2
140–159	1	2
≥160	2	3

Point Total	10-Year Risk %
<0	<1
0	1
1	1
2	1
3	1
4	1
5	2
6	2
7	3
8	4
9	5
10	6
11	8
12	10
13	12
14	16
15	20
16	25
≥17	≥30

10-Year risk _____ %

Estimate of 10-Year Risk for Women

(Framingham Point Scores)

Age	Points
20–34	–7
35–39	–3
40–44	0
45–49	3
50–54	6
55–59	8
60–64	10
65–69	12
70–74	14
75–79	16

Total Cholesterol	Points				
	Age 20–39	Age 40–49	Age 50–59	Age 60–69	Age 70–79
<160	0	0	0	0	0
160–199	4	3	2	1	1
200–239	8	6	4	2	1
240–279	11	8	5	3	2
≥280	13	10	7	4	2

	Points				
	Age 20–39	Age 40–49	Age 50–59	Age 60–69	Age 70–79
Nonsmoker	0	0	0	0	0
Smoker	9	7	4	2	1

HDL (mg/dL)	Points
≥60	–1
50–59	0
40–49	1
<40	2

Systolic BP (mmHg)	If Untreated	If Treated
<120	0	0
120–129	1	3
130–139	2	4
140–159	3	5
≥160	4	6

Point Total	10-Year Risk %
<9	<1
9	1
10	1
11	1
12	1
13	2
14	2
15	3
16	4
17	5
18	6
19	8
20	11
21	14
22	17
23	22
24	27
≥25	≥30

10-Year risk _____ %

U.S. DEPARTMENT OF HEALTH AND HUMAN SERVICES
Public Health Service
National Institutes of Health
National Heart, Lung, and Blood Institute

NIH Publication No. 01-3305
May 2001

FIGURE 57-3

FRAMINGHAM RISK SCORES

Source: Adult Treatment Panel III—ATP III: Executive Summary. NIH Publication No. 01-3670, May 2001.

pediatric patients. In adult patients, most acute myocardial infarctions (AMI), the event pediatric cardiologists are targeting with preventive therapy, actually occur from lesions that do not produce critical stenoses and limited coronary flow. Only 15% of myocardial infarctions in four studies occurred in subjects where stenoses were greater than 60%; most others occurred in vessels with stenoses of less than 50%.[26,27] While it is true that critical stenoses cause AMI, the nonocclusive lesions actually cause more AMI through plaque rupture and thrombosis. The reason for this is that more such nonocclusive lesions exist.

Thrombosis and the Vulnerable Plaque[26,28,29]

It is now understood that plaque rupture and subsequent thrombosis are at the root of most cases of unstable angina (UA) and AMI. Two-thirds of the time it is believed that acute rupture of a thinned fibrous cap is the ominous inciting event, while superficial erosion underlies most of the remaining cases. Determining which plaques are "at-risk" is the crucial question and the subject of much feverish research. The so-called "vulnerable plaque" is characterized by a thinning fibrous cap with the following:

- Decreased collagen content because of reduced collagen synthesis and increased collagen degradation
- Decreased smooth muscle content resulting from programmed apoptosis invoked by T lymphocyte-stimulated inflammatory markers
- Increased lipid pool and increased macrophage accumulation especially at "shoulder regions" of the plaque—contributing to increased susceptibility of this region to shear stress

The progression of atherosclerosis, a gradual process beginning in childhood and teen-age years with the foam cell rich fatty streaks and progressing to the complex smooth muscle cell and calcium rich plaques, involves a complex interplay of lipoprotein mediated and inflammatory mediated mechanisms. Understanding this complex pathophysiology allows clinicians/scientists to fathom many possible ways to identify "at-risk" patients, for both non-pharmaceutical and pharmaceutical treatment of disease, and for imaging and biomarker assessment of disease regression.

LIPID BIOCHEMISTRY

Prevention efforts for atherosclerosis have concentrated on altering cardiovascular risk factors—especially hyperlipidemia, hypertension, obesity, insulin resistance and diabetes, sedentary life style, and smoking habits.[30] The pathophysiology of atherosclerotic plaque development indicates that a key risk factor to address is hyperlipidemia. It is estimated that ~41.3 million Americans suffer from hyperlipidemia.[1] Less complete epidemiologic data are available for pediatric patients. The National Cholesterol Education Program's Report of the Expert Panel,[2] however, points to several facts when describing the rationale for pediatric screening of fasting cholesterol profiles. First, because high cholesterol plays a role in the development of coronary artery disease in adults and numerous studies have clearly demonstrated that the atherosclerotic process begins in childhood, it is best to target youngsters "at-risk." Next, compared to most other countries, children and teens in the United States of America, like U.S. adults, have higher blood cholesterol values and additionally, higher intake of saturated fatty acids and cholesterol. American adults also have higher morbidity and mortality from CAD than people in other parts of the world. Finally, cholesterol values tend to track from childhood into adulthood, as children with high cholesterol levels are more likely, than the average child, to have high cholesterol values as adults. Studies have shown that as little as a 1% reduction in cholesterol levels leads to a 2% reduction in CAD, while an increase of HDL by 1% decreases CAD by 4%.[31,32]

A brief review of lipid biochemistry is important as a foundation for later understanding of the mechanism of action of new pharmaceuticals used to treat dyslipidemias. Not all cholesterol is detrimental to health; in fact, cholesterol comprises a necessary component of cell membranes, especially contributing to myelination of neurons. It is also important for hormone synthesis. Lipoproteins are spherical particles with a surface composed of free cholesterol, phospholipids, and protein and a core containing predominantly cholesterol esters and triglycerides. Lipoproteins are classified based on their relative density, composition, and electrophoretic mobility: chylomicrons, very-low density lipoproteins (VLDL), LDL, and HDL (Figure 57-4).[5,33]

Chylomicrons are produced in the intestine from dietary fats. They are large particles rich in triglycerides. They are transported via the lymphatics from the gastrointestinal tract through the thoracic duct to the venous system.

Very-low density lipoproteins particles are synthesized in the liver and to a minor extent in the intestine. They, too, are rich in triglycerides, transporting this to adipose tissue. VLDL particles are gradually metabolized to intermediate-density lipoprotein particles (IDL) and then to (LDL) by the enzymatic action of lipoprotein lipase and hepatic lipase.

High density lipoproteins particles are produced in both the intestine and the liver from chylomicrons and VLDL catabolism. They serve to remove cholesterol from tissues, and as such, have been colloquially deemed "good cholesterol." Apoproteins A-I and A-II are prominent proteins comprising the HDL particles surface and may serve as soluble biomarkers in assessing patients' likelihood of CAD.

Low density lipoproteins cholesterol particles, the focus of much research and therapy efforts, are the major cholesterol carrying particle in plasma. Apoprotein B-100, prominent on LDL particles, is capable of binding to LDL receptors on hepatic and peripheral cells, allowing metabolism and use of LDL cholesterol. These particles, more than any other, have been associated with premature coronary artery disease.

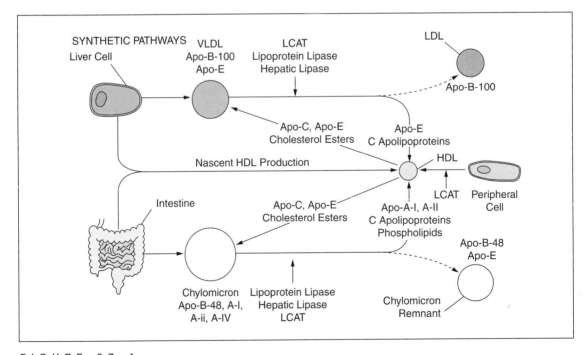

FIGURE   57-4

LIPID BIOCHEMISTRY

Source: Newberger JW: *Dyslipidemia in Childhood and Adolescence. Nadas' Pediatric Cardiology.* Mosby Yearbook, 1991, Chap. 20.

DETECTION OF PEDIATRIC PATIENTS "AT-RISK" FOR PREMATURE ATHEROSCLEROSIS: REVIEW OF THE NATIONAL CHOLESTEROL EDUCATION PROGRAM (NCEP) GUIDELINES

Screening Recommendations: NCEP and ATP III Guidelines

The National Cholesterol Education Program (NCEP) Guidelines set forth a series of recommendations for screening the pediatric patient.[2] Screening is recommended for all children over the age of 2 years if any of the situations listed in Table 57-2 exist. Using fasting plasma samples (obtained after a minimum of 10–12-h fast), an accurate assessment of the lipid composition can be obtained. The classic formula, the Friedwald Formula,[5] shows the breakdown:

$$LDL = Total\ cholesterol - HDL - TG/5$$

Most laboratories today do not need to rely on the calculated LDL cholesterol values provided by this equation, but can (if necessary) directly measure LDL from the plasma sample. In fact, while most often the calculated value is part of the lab results reviewed by clinicians, if the triglyceride value is >400 mg/dL, then this calculated value is inaccurate and not useful. Variations might be seen for lipid measurements even during the fasting state and are related to biologic variation, acute illness, ongoing weight loss, pregnancy, and occasionally to specific medications (like Accutane or birth control pills). Also, elevated triglyceride values >200 mg/dL should cause clinicians to question whether the sample was taken after a complete 10–12-h fast. Repeating the profile can be useful before making the diagnosis. Shaefer describes how even posture and stasis might affect cholesterol values.[34] This can be mitigated if the sample is drawn after a subject has been sitting quietly for a minimum of 5 minutes with the tourniquet applied just prior to venipuncture. Screening is recommended for all youngsters over the age of 2 years (children and teens) if any of these situations exist.[2]

Finally, the NCEP Guidelines recommend that all adults over 20 years have their total cholesterol measured every 5 years.[2] Furthermore, the recently published Third Report of the Expert Panel on Detection, Evaluation, and Treatment of High Blood Cholesterol in Adults [Adult Treatment Panel (ATP) III] emphasizes a more intensive approach to LDL lowering with a keen focus on primary prevention of CAD in patients with multiple risk factors. Guidelines (both pediatric and adult) are summarized in Tables 57-2 to 57-8.

TABLE 57-2

PEDIATRIC CHOLESTEROL SCREENING RECOMMENDATIONS

Draw a fasting total cholesterol if:

- Either of the youngster's parents have high total blood cholesterol (≥240 mg/dL)

If the child's or adolescent's total cholesterol is high (>200 mg/dL), then draw a fasting lipoprotein analysis (cholesterol profile)

Draw a fasting lipoprotein analysis (cholesterol profile) as the initial screening test if:

- The parents or grandparents, at age 55 years or less, underwent a diagnostic coronary angiography and were found to have CAD [± angioplasty or stent placement or coronary artery bypass grafting (CABG) procedure]
- The parents or grandparents, at age 55 years or less, suffered a documented myocardial infarction, angina pectoris, peripheral vascular disease (PVD), cerebral vascular disease, or sudden cardiac death
- The parental or grandparental history is unobtainable, especially if the child has other cardiovascular risk factors (e.g., obesity, hypertension, diabetes or insulin resistance, sedentary lifestyle, or smoking habit)

Source: National Cholesterol Education Program Report of the Expert Panel on Blood Cholesterol Levels in Children and Adolescents. *Pediatrics* (Suppl.) Vol. 89, No. 3, Pt. 2, March 1992.

See also Figure 57-5 and 57-6.

TABLE 57-3

CHOLESTEROL GUIDELINES FOR PEDIATRIC PATIENTS

	Total Cholesterol (mg/dL)	LDL – C (mg/dL)
Desired	<170	<110
Borderline	170–199	110–129
High	≥200	≥130

Source: The National Cholesteral Education Program Report of the Expert Panel on Blood Cholesterol Levels in Children and Adolescents. Pediatrics (Suppl.) Vol. 89, No. 3, Pt. 2, March 1991.

These are important because pediatric cardiologists are treating older teens and young adults, especially as they follow youngsters with repaired congenital heart disease into adulthood.[25,35] Of note, is the fact that in many medical centers, pediatric patients with hyperlipidemia are not seen by pediatric cardiologists, but rather by pediatric gastroenterologists or endocrinologists. The primary care provider should, therefore, become familiar with

TABLE 57-4

ATP III CLASSIFICATION CHOLESTEROL FOR ADULTS

Total Cholesterol (mg/dL)	
<200	Desirable
200–239	Borderline high
≥240	High
LDL Cholesterol (mg/dL)	
<100	Optimal
100–129	Near optimal/ above optimal
130–159	Borderline high
160–189	High
≥190	Very high
HDL Cholesterol (mg/dL)	
<40	Low
≥60	High

Source: ATP III: Executive Summary. NIH Publication No. 01-3670, May 2001.

TABLE 57-5

THREE CATEGORIES OF RISK THAT MODIFY ADULT LDL CHOLESTEROL GOALS

Risk Category*	LDL Goal (mg/dL)	Risk of Event in 10 years
I. CHD and CHD risk equivalents	<100	>20%
II. Multiple (2+) risk factors*	<130	≤20%
III. Zero to one risk factor	<160	<10%

*CHD risk equivalents and risk factors that modify the overall risk category are listed in Tables 57-6 and 57-7.
Source: ATP III: Executive Summary. NIH Publication No. 01-3670, May 2001.

what services are provided by the specialists in his/her community. The ideal goal of multidisciplinary clinics, with exercise physiologists and registered dieticians, is not always possible in every community.

Additional Work-up for "At-Risk" Pediatric Patients

Dyslipidemia most often results from a combination of genetic and environmental factors, especially diet and exercise habits; however, clinicians ought to rule out secondary causes of dyslipidemia (see

TABLE 57-6

CHD RISK EQUIVALENTS

Clinical forms of atherosclerosis
- Peripheral arterial disease, abdominal aortic aneurysm, symptomatic carotid artery disease
- Diabetes
- Multiple risk factors (from Table 57-8) conferring a 10-year risk for CHD of >20%.

Source: ATP III: Executive Summary. NIH Publication No. 01-3670, May 2001.

TABLE 57-7

MAJOR RISK FACTORS MODIFYING ADULT LDL GOALS

- Cigarette smoking
- Hypertension (BP >140/90 mmHg or on any anti-hypertensive medications)
- Low HDL cholesterol (<40 mg/dL)
- Family history of premature coronary heart disease (CHD)
  (CHD in male first degree relative <55 years old or female first degree relative <65 years old)
- Age (men >45 years and women >55 years)

Note: In ATP III, diabetes is regarded as a coronary heart disease equivalent (see Table 57-6).
Source: ATP III: Executive Summary. NIH Publication No. 01-3670, May 2001.

TABLE 57-9

CAUSES OF SECONDARY HYPERCHOLESTEROLEMIA

Hypothyroidism
Nephrotic syndrome
Chronic liver disease (mainly biliary cirrhosis)
Dysglobulinemia
Cushing's syndrome
Hyperparathyroidism
Acute intermittent porphyria
Medications

Source: Gotto AM: Lipid and Lipoprotein Disorders, in: *Primer in Preventive Cardiology*. American Heart Association, 1994, pp. 107–130.

Tables 57-9 to 57-11). Usually a good history and physical examination serve as the foundation for this determination and can guide more selective, pertinent laboratory evaluations. Common secondary causes of dyslipidemia include diabetes mellitus, hypothyroidism, nephrotic syndrome, chronic renal failure, obstructive liver disease, alcohol abuse, and use of certain medications including birth control pills (especially related to estrogens), steroids, some antihypertensive medications, and antiacne medications (e.g., Accutane). Such diagnoses and therapies, while less prevalent in pediatric populations, but should be considered during the initial screening and evaluation of children.

TABLE 57-8

ATP III-LDL THERAPY FOR DIFFERENT RISK CATEGORIES (ADULTS)

Risk Category	LDL Goal (mg/dL)	LDL Level at which to Initiate TLC[a] (mg/dL)	LDL Level at which to Consider Drug Therapy (mg/dL)
CHD or CHD risk equivalents (10-year risk >20%)	<100	≥100	• ≥130 • If 100–129, LDL lowering drug optional
>2 risk factors (10-year risk <20%)	<130	≥130	• If 10-year risk 10–20%, then ≥130 • If 10-year risk <10% then ≥160
0–1 risk factor	<160	≥160	• >190 • If 160–189, then LDL lowering drug optional

[a]TLC = Therapeutic Lifestyle Changes.
Source: ATP III: Executive Summary. NIH Publication No. 01-3670, May 2001.

TABLE 57-10

CAUSES OF HYPERTRIGLYCERIDEMIA

*Nonfasting profile	Hypopituitarism	Glucocorticoid use
*Obesity	Hypothyroidism	B-blocker use
Alcoholism	Pancreatitis	Diuretic use
DM	Dysglobulinemia	Estrogen use
CRF	Glycogen storage disease	Stress
Acute intermittent porphyria	Lipodystrophy	Pregnancy
Uremia	Cushing's syndrome	

*Common causes of hepertriglyceridemia.

Source: Gotto AM: Lipid and Lipoprotein Disorders, in: *Primer in Preventive Cardiology*, American Heart Association, 1994, pp.107–130.

Secondary causes of hypercholesterolemia are listed in Table 57-9 and causes of elevated triglycerides in Table 57-10.[33] Finally, reasons for low HDL, an independent risk factor for coronary artery disease include elevated triglycerides, obesity, physical inactivity, type II diabetes, cigarette smoking, very high carbohydrate intake (>60% of energy sources), and certain drugs (especially beta-blockers, anabolic steroids, and progestational agents) (see Table 57-11).[36,37,38]

Once a patient's fasting total cholesterol exceeds 170 mg/dL on two occasions, a fasting cholesterol profile is obtained (see Figure 57-5). If this fasting profile is abnormal, then *ideally*, the patient should be referred to a specialist. In some communities, this is the pediatric cardiologist; in others it is the pediatric gastroenterologist or endocrinologist. Preferably, this specialist works in a multidiscipli-

nary clinic where access to a registered dietician and exercise physiologist is possible. In this setting, further risk assessment can be performed in conjunction with a repeated fasting lipoprotein analysis.[30] Referring physicians should be aware that such multidisciplinary teams are not always available. Therefore, the workup need to be done locally, with dietary and exercise counseling provided with aid of materials from the National Institutes of Health (NIH), National Lung, Heart, and Blood Institute (NHLBI), and American Heart Association (AHA). The guidelines given in Figures 57-6 and 7, and in Tables 57-2, 3, and 12, may assist with patient management in the event that referral is not possible.

Familiarization with the Fredrickson Classification[33] of dyslipidemias is important to practicing pediatric cardiologists (Table 57-13). The most common phenotypes seen in pediatrics are familial hyperlipidemia (FH), especially type IIa and somewhat less commonly, type IIb.

Type IIa dyslipidemia (FH) is related to the absence of functional LDL receptors. This autosomal dominant disorder results in increased LDL-C de-tectable at birth or shortly thereafter. Individuals with heterozygous FH will have total cholesterol values of 300–500 mg/dL and coronary artery disease by the fourth or fifth decade, while individuals with homozygous FH are much more severely affected often with total cholesterol values of 700–1200 mg/dL and LDL-C of >400 mg/dL. The premature coronary artery disease can occur very early in the second or third decade of life. Therapy here

TABLE 57-11

CAUSES OF LOW HDL

- Elevated triglycerides
- Overweight status and obesity
- Physical inactivity
- Type 2 diabetes
- Cigarette smoking
- Very high carbohydrate intake (>60% of energy)
- Certain drugs: B-blockers, anabolic steroids, progestational agents

Source: Pasternak R: AJC, Mar 2002.

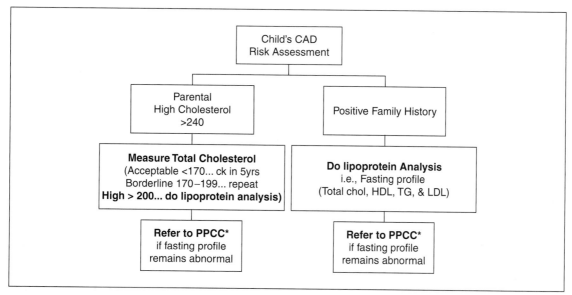

FIGURE 57-5

REFERRING PRIMARY CARE PHYSICIANS' INITIAL SCREENING

PPCC: Pediatric Preventive Cardiology Clinic or equivalent specialist with multidisciplinary clinic, if possible.

Source: Goldberg CS, Samyn MM: A method for preventive cardiology in children. *Progress in Pediatric Cardiology* 12(2001):155–160.

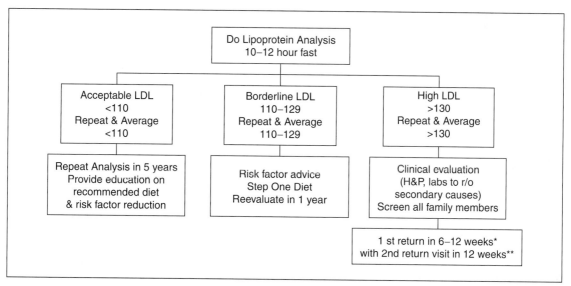

FIGURE 57-6

GUIDELINE FOR EVALUATION BY PEDIATRIC CARDIOLOGISTS

PPCC: Pediatric Preventive Cardiology Clinic or equivalent specialist with multidisciplinary clinic, if possible.

Source: Goldberg CS. Samyn MM: A method for preventive cardiology in children. *Progress in Pediatric Cardiology* 12(2001): 155–160.

TABLE 57-12

INITIAL "WORKUP" OF HYPERLIPIDEMIC PEDIATRIC PATIENTS: RULE OUT SECONDARY DISEASES

Fasting cholesterol profile

Electrolytes including calcium

BUN/creatinine

Fasting glucose

Urinalysis

Total protein and albumin

Liver function tests

Thyroid stimulating hormone (TSH)

should be aggressive. Sometimes pharmaceutical therapy, including statins, may be ineffective in homozygous patients—necessitating extreme treatment regimens including apheresis or liver transplantation.

Hypertriglyceridemia often occurs in conjunction with low HDL. Extreme cases (type V) are often first diagnosed when a patient presents to the Emergency Department with abdominal pain and vomiting, symptoms akin to pancreatitis. It is important to look for secondary causes of hypertriglyceridemia too, which can commonly be a result of medications or total parenteral nutrition. Premature coronary artery disease can be seen in some patients with familial endogenous hypertriglyceridemia, but not in others.

Lastly, familial HDL deficiencies do not receive a Fredrickson classification, but have been increasingly recognized.[39] Premature CAD is characteristic of familial Apo A-1/C-III deficiency, Apo A-1/C-III A-IV deficiency and some forms of isolated Apo A-1 deficiency. Moreover, the Framingham risk assessment identifies low HDL as an independent risk factor for coronary artery

TABLE 57-13

FREDRICKSON CLASSIFICATION OF HYPERLIPIDEMIAS

Phenotype	Lipoprotein Elevated	Serum Cholesterol	Serum Triglyceride	Atherogenicity	Associated with Genetic Disorders
I	Chylomicrons	Normal to ⇑	⇑ ⇑ ⇑ ⇑	None seen	Familial lipoprotein lipase deficiency; apoprotein CII deficiency
IIa	LDL	⇑ ⇑	Normal	+ + +	Familial hypercholesterolemia—LDL receptor abnormal; familial combined hyperlipidemia; polygenic hypercholesterolemia
IIb	LDL and VLDL	⇑ ⇑	⇑ ⇑	+ + +	Familial hypercholesterolemia; familial combined hyperlipidemia
III	IDL	⇑ ⇑	⇑ ⇑ ⇑	+ + +	Familial dysbetalipoproteinemia
IV	VLDL	Normal to ⇑	⇑ ⇑	+	Familial hypertriglyceridemia; familial combined hyperlipidemia
V	VLDL and chylomicrons	Normal to ⇑	⇑ ⇑ ⇑ ⇑	+	Familial hypertriglyceridemia; familial multiple lipoprotein type hyperlipidemia

Source: Gotto, AM Lipid and Lipoprotein Disorders in: *Primer in Preventive Cardiology*, American Heart Association, 1994, pp. 107–130,

disease and so too do the Bogalusa and Muscatine Studies of children.

Metabolic Syndrome

Primary care providers also ought to consider a constellation of signs and laboratory values that mimic metabolic syndrome, an adult diagnosis receiving increased attention from research and pharmaceutical companies.[40] The US prevalence of metabolic syndrome in adults is between 20 and 25%.[41] The syndrome is defined by the ATP III Guidelines as having ≥3 of the following features:

- Waist circumference >102 cm in men or >88 cm in women
- Serum triglycerides >150 mg/dL
- HDL <40 mg/dL (men) or <50 mg/dL (women)
- BP of at least 130/85 or more (borderline hypertension)
- Fasting serum glucose of >110 mg/dL

A similar retrospective survey of pediatric subjects referred to the University of Michigan Prevention clinic illustrates a similar prevalence for "metabolic syndrome-like" characteristics in children (~25%).[42] Metabolic syndrome, previously called Syndrome X, causes people to be at increased risk of developing overt diabetes mellitus and cardiovascular disease, as well as increased mortality from cardiovascular disease and all causes.[40–45]

OBESITY

Definition and Prevalence

One of the key components of metabolic syndrome, contributing to the insulin resistance, hypertension, and lipid disorders seen, is obesity. Obesity, a challenging clinical diagnosis to treat and a cause of hypertension, is increasing in prevalence in the United States.[46] According to the American Heart Association's Scientific Statement on Cardiovascular Health in Children, recent epidemiologic data indicate a 2–4-fold increase in obesity in the past two decades. The highest rates of obesity are among African American and Latino youths.[9] More than one of five children are now overweight or at-risk for true obesity.[47] This represents a growth in prevalence by 5–11% from the 1960s to the 1990s.[48] This complex problem is a public health issue as it has many important long-term implications for physical and emotional health.[50] It is estimated that >80% of obese children have either elevated systolic or diastolic blood pressure. Approximately 97% have four or more cardiovascular risk factors (increased total cholesterol, elevated triglyceride, decreased HDL-C, increased systolic or diastolic blood pressure, decreased maximal work capacity, type II diabetes, and a strong family history of coronary artery disease).[9,50]

Obesity has been variously defined, but most would agree with the American Heart Association's briefing: Obesity is ". . . a level of overweight that is associated with adverse physical or psychologic health problems."[9] Body mass index (BMI) has been recommended for clinical assessment of obesity. BMI is calculated as weight (in kilograms) divided by the square of the height (in meters). The Centers for Disease Control have recently published age and sex-specific BMI norms for the United States population.[51] The 85th percentile is the cut-off used to identify those who are mildly to moderately overweight (and thus at increased risk of obesity), while being greater than the 95% identifies those with frank obesity. This corresponds with being at 130% of the ideal weight percentile (or 30% overweight). The clinician should regularly calculate the BMI for any child whose height or weight exceeds the 75 percentile for age. Children crossing BMI percentiles at consecutive health maintenance office visits are at-risk of becoming obese.[9]

Obesity is a result of a combination of genetic and environmental features. Key secondary causes, that the clinician ought to rule out by physical examination and selected laboratory evaluations, are hypothyroidism and hyperinsulinism, as well as syndromes such as Prader Willi (marked by mental retardation and short stature). All obese children (>95% for weight) should, according to the recent AHA policy statement, undergo blood pressure assessment and fasting lipoprotein, insulin, and glucose measurement. Additionally, special care should be taken to evaluate for co-existing psychologic disorders (like depression, bulimia nervosa, and binge-eating disorder), all of which might warrant referral to a specialized care giver (child psychologist or psychiatrist).[9]

Obesity Hypertension

A very strong association has been made over the years for all races and ages between obesity and increased blood pressure. Two large studies show a high correlation coefficients for these two diseases. The largest study, by Rosner et al.,[51a] pooled data from eight large U.S. epidemiology studies ($N =$ 47,000 children). Irrespective of race, gender, or age, the risk of elevated blood pressure was shown to be significantly higher for children in the upper compared with the lower decile of BMI (with odds ratio of systolic hypertension ranging from 2.5 to 3.7). The results of the landmark Bogalusa Heart study in Lousiana are similar with an odds ratio of 4.5 for increased systolic blood pressure and 2.4 for increased diastolic blood pressure.[48] "Obesity hypertension" initially is characterized by isolated systolic hypertension—a very strong risk factor correlated with cardiovascular morbidity and mortality in later adult years.

Accurate blood pressure assessment is very difficult in the obese child because of a very large arm girth. It is important to choose the appropriate BP cuff size, in line with the AHA recommendations. The cuff's bladder width should cover at least 40% of the arm circumference midway between the elbow's olecrenon process and the acromion process of the shoulder. Additionally, the cuff should extend two-thirds of the distance from the antecubital fossa to the shoulder.[52] Manual assessment of blood pressure, with either stethoscope auscultation or doppler assessment of the brachial artery, should be performed after the youngster has been seated comfortably for 3–5 minutes. The right arm is best used, so that comparisons can be made with normal values that have recently been updated.[53] After inflating the BP cuff 20–30 mmHg above the suspected systolic BP, the first appear-

ance of the tapping noise is noted, as the cuff pressure is gradually released (i.e., the 1st Korotkoff sound, marking the systolic BP). Next, the disappearance of sound (i.e., the 5th Korotkoff sound, marking the diastolic BP) is noted. The 1996 NHLBI Working Group on High Blood Pressure resolved the discrepancy between pediatric and adult blood pressure assessment. Its policy statement indicates that the 5th Korotkoff sound (disappearance of tapping) is the most appropriate for the diastolic blood pressure regardless of age. This eliminates the confusion when previous recommendations for children differed from adult recommendations, focusing on the muffling of sound (4th Korotkoff sound) as the diastolic BP, especially in children less than 13 years old. If the sound is audible through 0 mmHg, then the NHLBI Working Group indicates that this effectively rules out diastolic hypertension. A cuff that is too small for the large arm girth of the obese patient may falsely identify elevated blood pressure, when the *actual* BP may be normal. Large blood pressure cuffs do not, in general, underestimate the BP.[9,52]

Normal blood pressure is defined for all youngsters as an average systolic *and* diastolic blood pressure less than the 90th percentile for age, sex, and height. High normal, or borderline elevated blood pressure, is defined as the average systolic *or* diastolic BP between the 90 and 95th percentile for age, sex, and height. "True" hypertension is defined as an average systolic *or* diastolic BP of >95% after the blood pressure has been measured on three separate occasions. Usually, children and teens are referred to a pediatric specialist (a cardiologist or, in some institutions, a nephrologist) if, after three separate office visits, the BP measurements remain in the borderline or hypertensive range. Occasionally, severely hypertensive pediatric patients are referred appropriately after a single office visit shows a dramatically elevated blood pressure.[54] After identification, with/without referral, the workup for secondary causes and possible early end organ damage owing to hypertension can begin.

The strategy for treating hypertensive obese children is similar to treating nonhypertensive obese children (or hyperlipidemic children), as exercise and dietary plans are central to the nonpharmacologic therapy. For chronically hypertensive children (who are not experiencing severe elevations in BP which would constitute an emergency), the initial goal for a given pediatric patient is to reduce the BP to less than the 95% for age, sex, and height.

TREATMENT

Primary Prevention of Dyslipidemia

The United States population of infants, children, and teens was about 70 million at the turn of the millennium (1999–2000).[55] The great majority of children are healthy; yet, many have "silent" cardiovascular risk factors which, although not causing overt symptoms, contribute to disease in adulthood. Despite advances in modern medicine, heart disease remains the number one cause of morbidity and mortality for the US adult population. Local campaigns exist at the state level and much federal attention has been placed on smoking cessation as a way to address a key risk factor for atherosclerosis. Treatment of hypertension is covered in Chapter 10. Appropriate therapies for the common forms of dyslipidemia are discussed below.

Diet and Exercise

The initial therapy for hyperlipidemia addresses dietary and exercise habits. Balanced diets are sought, such that nutritional requirements are met with a wide variety of foods.[2] Caloric intake should be sufficient to support appropriate growth and development. Children under the age of 2 years should not be placed on special diets low in fats, as adequate fat intake is necessary for good neurologic development during this period of rapid growth. To be successful, prevention efforts should ideally involve nutritionists who can appropriately address dietary questions.[30] Also, in the present environment of dual career families and alternative day care arrangements, it is best if both father and mother (or any other primary care giver) are present for dietary discussions. Child-friendly literature is available from the National Heart, Lung, and Blood Institute for distribution to pediatric patients and their families. Dietary therapy is best prescribed in two steps (outlined in Table 57-14) with the Step One Diet being that which all in the general population should consume. The NCEP Guidelines call for three months of good compliance with the Step One Dietary recommendations prior to proceeding to the more restrictive Step Two Diet. Meal plans, in line with Step Two, can be prepared by registered dieticians working with the families. As compliance can be an issue at various times for all families, ongoing dietary guidance is ideal; it is important to ensure that though lower in fat, each patient's diet contains adequate nutrition. Changes in cholesterol profiles can often be seen after the initial 3 months of dietary modifications if compliance is

TABLE 57-14

AMERICAN HEART ASSOCIATION DIETS[a]

Step One Diet	Total fat ≤30%	Saturated fat 8–10% (<10% polyunsaturated fats)	Cholesterol <300 mg/dL
Step Two Diet	Total fat ≤30%	Saturated fat <7% (<10% polyunsaturated fats)	Cholesterol <200 mg/dL

Source: National Cholesterol Education Program, NHLBI Publication No. 91-2731, 1991. *Pediatrics* (Suppl.) Vol. 89, No. 3, Pt. 2, March 1992.

[a]No restriction of fat or cholesterol if youngsters are <2 years old. Advance to Step Two Diet, if no significant results in 3 months

rigorous; thus, generally return visits are scheduled within 6–12 weeks of the first appointment to enable reassessment of the fasting cholesterol profile.[2,30]

Regular physical activity is less common today than in the past. In the recent report from the Surgeon General,[56] the following statistics were noted:

- Approximately 14% of children/teens do *not* participate in light, moderate, or vigorous physical activity.
- Nearly 50% of teens do not participate in regular physical activity at all.
- Daily physical education class attendance declined from 42% in 1991 to 25% in 1995.
- Children's/adolescents' participation in physical activity declines with age.
- Female adolescents were less active than male adolescents, and black females were less active than white females.

Many have noted, not only the decline of physical education classes in schools, but also the popularity of video games, as reasons for children and teens today to be spending less time engaged in aerobic activities than their counterparts were years ago.[57] Regular aerobic exercise, if fun, may not only engage/entertain children, but also have healthy consequences such as raising HDL cholesterol, enhancing weight loss, lowering blood pressure, and reducing atherosclerotic risk.[30] Such involvement also sets a pattern of exercise which might well be carried into adult years. In ideal preventive cardiology settings, involving trained exercise physiologists can benefit pediatric patients and their families—educating them on the proper ways to exercise, lift weights, and assess heart rate response to exercise, while motivating youngsters to find enjoyable activities. Exercising aerobically for an average of 30 min per day on most, if not all days of the week, is recommended for everyone.[56,58] Again, family involvement is essential for success.

Physical activity begins at home. Children and adolescents who are physically active usually have parents and other family members who encourage them to participate in physical activity, participate in physical activity with them, watch them play or compete, and provide transportation to physical activity and sports events. Periodic reassessments of activity level, by exercise physiologists or physicians, are essential to success. Self-assessments using exercise diaries can be helpful, because they actively engage the participation of pediatric patients and serve as a starting point for dialogue during follow-up visits. Children and adolescents alike will benefit from an explanation of why physical activity is beneficial and from the positive coaching of health care teams. Young patients need help in setting realistic goals, making plans for change, and reducing barriers (e.g., schedule conflicts) to exercise participation. Once active, they benefit from continued support to prevent a relapse to inactivity.[59]

Pharmacologic Therapy

With very good/excellent compliance with the above dietary and exercise recommendations, clinicians may expect to see, at most, a 10–15% improvement in fasting cholesterol profile. There are some children and adolescents for whom this reduction is enough; others will require a greater improvement in fasting cholesterol profile to prevent coronary heart disease. Table 57-15 shows those for whom prescription medication might be needed.[2]

Generally, for elevated LDL cholesterol, it is recommended that clinicians start with bile acid

TABLE 57-15

CONSIDERATIONS FOR INITIATION OF PHARMACOLOGIC TREATMENT

If the following exist, then consider prescription medication for LDL lowering:
• Children >10 years old
• After 6–12 months of diet/exercise tx
• LDL cholesterol remaining ≥190 mg/dL
• LDL cholesterol ≥160 mg/dL plus:
1. Positive family history (<55 CHD) *or*
2. Child has two risk factors for CHD

Source: National Cholesterol Education Program, NHLBI Publication No. 91-2731, 1991. *Pediatrics* (Suppl.) Vol. 89, No. 3, Pt. 2, March 1992.

TABLE 57-16

PRESCRIPTION MEDICATIONS FOR CHOLESTEROL LOWERING

Drug Class	Examples	Lipid Effects	Potential Side Effects	Monitoring
Bile acid sequestrants	Cholestyramine (Questran) (Prevalite) Colestipol (Cholestid) Colesevelam (WelChol)	Use if: 1. young patient, as first line therapy. 2. low risk for CHD. LDL ⇓ 15–30% HDL ⇑ 3–5% TGs—no change	**Absolutely contraindicated if:** 1. ⇑ TG (>400 mg/dL) 2. Dysbetalipoproteinemia **Relatively if:** 1. TG >200 mg/dL 2. Using certain drugs: digoxin, warfarin, etc. **Side effects:** GI distress, constipation, poor absorption of other medications	**Give multivitamin**
Nicotinic acid	Niacin (Niaspan) (Niacor) (Slo Niacin)	Recommended therapy for elevated triglycerides (TG) TG ⇓ 20–50% LDL ⇓ 5–25% HDL ⇑ 15–35%	**Side effects:** Flushing, ⇑ glucose, ⇑ uric acid (gout), need to ⇑ anti HTN meds, hepatotoxicity *ASA 30 min prior: ⇓ side effects* **Exercise caution with:** 1. Diabetics—⇑ glu 2. Statins—may cause hepatitis and myopathy **Contraindicated if:** Chronic liver disease, severe gout	
Fibric acid	Clofibrate (Atromid) Fenofibrate (Tricor) Gemfibrizol (Lopid)	Recommended therapy for elevated triglycerides (TG) TG ⇓ 20–50% LDL ⇓ 5–20% HDL ⇑ 10–20%	**Side effects:** GI (e.g., dyspepsia, gall stones, pancreatitis), myopathy, mild ⇓ Hgb, Hct, & WBC **Exercise caution with:** 1. Oral anticoagulants— potentiates effect 2. *⇑ TG: LDL may ⇑ 3. Statins **Contraindicated if:** Severe renal/hepatic dz.	Liver function studies Periodic CBC during first year of tx CPK levels if myalgias reported

(continued)

TABLE 57-16 (continued)

PRESCRIPTION MEDICATIONS FOR CHOLESTEROL LOWERING

Drug Class	Examples	Lipid Effects	Potential Side Effects	Monitoring
HMG—CoA reductase inhibitors (statins)	Atorvastatin (Lipitor) Fluvastatin (Lescol) Lovastatin (Mevacor) Pravastatin (Pravachol) Rosuvistatin (Cerivistatin) Simavastatin (Zocor)	On average: LDL ⇓ 18–55% HDL ⇑ 5–15% TG ⇓ 7–30%	**Side effects:** Elevated liver functions Transient myalgias **Exercise caution with:** Nicotinic acid and fibrates **Effective means of birth control essential** **Contraindicated if:** Active or chronic liver disease **Relative contraindication:** Concomitant use of other drugs like: Cyclosporine, macrolide antibiotics, anti fungals, cytochrome P450 inhibitors like fibrates and niacin	Liver functions/CPK should be checked at baseline, 12 weeks, and then q 6 months.

Source: Adapted from *Implementing the NCEP ATP III Guidelines and Primer in Preventive Cardiology.* See *Physician's Desk Reference* for full prescribing information and precautions.

sequestrants (e.g., cholestyramine), which bind to cholesterol in the intestine before absorption. The addition or change (after sufficient time on therapy, 8–12 weeks) to other medications with more complicated mechanisms of action (e.g., fibrates, niacin, and HMG reductase inhibitors, also known as statins) is recommended as needed. Recent federal legislation (FDAMA 1997, Pediatric Rule 1999, and Best Pharmaceuticals for Children Act 2002) has encouraged the conduct of pediatric clinical trials by corporate sponsors.[60,61] As a result, more pharmaceuticals, including cholesterol lowering medications, are being tested in pediatric populations. Some, such as Lipitor (atorvastatin), have recently received approval for use in familial hypercholesterolemia in children ages 10–17 years—thus, obviating the need to extrapolate the adult dose to that appropriate for pediatrics.[62] If primary care providers choose to proceed to pharmacologic

treatment of hyperlipidemia, referral to the appropriate subspecialists is indicated for aid in managing patients. Table 57-16 lists the most frequently used medications with their affects on the lipid profile, most common side effects, and monitoring needs. (Prescription medication therapy of hypertension is discussed elsewhere in this text.)[33,63,64]

SUMMARY

Despite many strides in cardiovascular care, coronary heart disease remains the number one cause of death in the United States at the dawn of the 21st century. Perhaps attacking the problem in its early stages, by identifying and treating pediatric patients at-risk for atherosclerosis, is the key to decreasing the incidence of morbid cardiovascular events such as angina, stroke, and peripheral vascular disease.

Certainly, the risk factors for coronary heart disease are apparent in the youth of America. Through the concerted efforts of health care teams (i.e., primary care givers and specialists, including registered dieticians and qualified exercise physiologists along with schools, communities, and family unit), the message of healthy diet and exercise practices can be taught. Where needed, for the selected "at-risk" pediatric population, appropriate cardiovascular risk factor screening and prescription medication can be adopted.

References

1. American Heart Association. *2002 Heart and Stroke Statistical Update*. Dallas, TX, American Heart Association, 2001.

2. National Cholesterol Education Program Report of the Expert Panel on Blood Cholesterol Levels in Children and Adolescents. Bethesda, MD, US Department of Health and Human Services, Public Health Service, National Institutes of Health, National Heart, Lung, and Blood Institute Publication No. 91-2731, 1991. *Pediatrics* (Suppl.) 89(3), Part 2, 1992: 495–501.

3. Schieken RM: Atherosclerosis. *Moss and Adams Heart Disease in Infants, Children, and Adolescents Including the Fetus and Young Adult*, 5th ed. Baltimore, MD, Williams & Wilkins, 1995, Vol. 2, Chap. 96:1627–1641.

4. Mahoney LT, Lauer RM: *Preventative Cardiology Across the Lifespan: Pediatric Issues. Primer in Preventive Cardiology*. American Heart Association, 1994, pp. 255–260.

5. Newberger JW: *Dyslipidemia in Childhood and Adolescence. Nadas' Pediatric Cardiology*. Mosby-Year Book, 1991, Chap. 20.

6. Muhonen, LE, et al: Coronary risk factors in adolescents related to their knowledge of familial coronary heart disease and hypercholesterolemia: the Muscatine study. *Pediatrics* 93(3), 1994.

7. Lauer RM, Clarke WR: Use of cholesterol measurements in childhood for the prediction of adult hypercholesterolemia: the Muscatine study. *JAMA* 264(23), 1990, 3034–3038.

8. Gidding SS: Preventive pediatric cardiology: tobacco, cholesterol, obesity, and inactivity. *Pediatr Clin North Am* 46(2), 1999.

9. Williams CL, et al: AHA scientific statement: cardiovascular health in childhood: a statement for health professionals from the committee on atherosclerosis, hypertension, and obesity in the young (AHOY) of the council on cardiovascular disease in young. *Circulation* 106(1):143, 2002.

10. Libby P: *The Vascular Biology of Atherosclerosis. Heart Disease: A Textbook of Cardiovascular Medicine*, 6th ed. Philadelphia, PA, WB Saunders, 2001, Vol. 1, Chap. 30.

11. Berenson GS, et al: Association between multiple cardiovascular risk factors and atherosclerosis in children and young adults: the Bogalusa heart study. *N Engl J Med* 338(23):1650–1656, 1998.

12. Clarke WR, et al: Tracking of blood lipids and blood pressures in school age children: the Muscatine study. *Circulation* 58:626–634, 1978.

13. Lauer RM, et al: Coronary heart disease risk factors in school children: the Muscatine study. *J Pediatr* 86(5): 697–706, 1975.

14. Camejo G, et al: Association of apo B lipoproteins with arterial proteoglycans: pathological significance and molecular basis. *Atherosclerosis* 139:205–222, 1998.

15. Williams KJ, Tabas I: The response-to-retention hypothesis of atherosclerosis reinforced. *Curr Opin Lipidol* 9:471–474, 1998.

16. Nievelstein PF, et al: Lipid accumulation in rabbit aortic intima 2 hours after bolus infusion of low density lipoprotein: A deep-etch and immunolocalization study of ultra rapidly frozen tissue. *Arterioscler Thromb* 11:1795–1805, 1991.

17. Faggiotto A, et al: Studies of hypercholesterolemia in the nonhuman primate: changes that lead to fatty streak formation. *Arteriosclerosis* 4:323–340, 1984.

18. Nelken N, et al: Monocyte chemoattractant protein-1 in human atheromatous plaques. *J Clin Invest* 88:1121–1127, 1991.

19. Mach F, et al: Differential expression of three T lymphocytes-activated CXC chemokines by human atheroma-associated cells. *J Clin Invest* 104: 1041–1050, 1999.

20. Willett, WC: *Eat, Drink and Be Healthy: The Harvard Medical School Guide to Healthy Eating*. New York, NY, Simon & Schuster, 2001.

21. Glagov S, et al: Compensatory enlargement of human atherosclerotic coronary arteries. *N Engl J Med* 316:1371–1375,1987.

22. Nissen S: Application of intravascular ultrasound to characterize coronary artery disease and assess the

progression or regression of atherosclerosis. *Am J Cardiol* 89 (Suppl.):24B–31B, 2002.

23. Demer LL: A skeleton in the atherosclerosis closet. *Circulation* 92:2029–2032, 1995.

24. Salazar HP, Raggi P: Usefulness of electron beam computed tomography. *Am J Cardiol* 89(Suppl.): 17B–23B, 2002.

25. Third report of the National Cholesterol Education Program Expert Panel on detection, evaluation, and treatment of high cholesterol in adults (Adult Treatment Panel III) executive summary. NIH Publication 01–3670, May 2001.

26. Falk E, et al: Coronary plaque disruption. *Circulation* 92:657–671, 1995.

27. Smith S Jr: Risk-reduction therapy: the challenge to change. *Circulation* 93:2205–2211, 1996.

28. Farb A, et al: Coronary plaque erosion without rupture into the lipid core: a frequent cause of coronary thrombosis in sudden cardiac death. *Circulation* 93:1354–1363, 1996.

29. Lee R, Libby P: The unstable atheroma. *Arterioscler Thromb Vasc Biol* 17:1859–1867, 1997.

30. Goldberg CS, Samyn MM: A method for preventive cardiology in children. *Prog Pediatr Cardiol* 12:155–160, 2001.

31. Frick MH, et al: Helsinki Heart Study: Primary prevention trial with gemfibrizol in middle-aged men with dyslipidemia. *N Engl J Med* 317:1237–1245, 1987.

32. Lipid Research Clinics Program: The Lipid Research Clinics Coronary Primary Prevention Trial Results II. The relationship of reduction in incidence of coronary heart disease to cholesterol lowering. *JAMA* 251:365–374, 1984.

33. Gotto AM. Lipid and Lipoprotein Disorders. *Primer in Preventive Cardiology.* American Heart Association, 1994, pp.107–130.

34. Shaefer EJ: When and how to treat dyslipidemia. *Hosp Pract* 15:57–72, 1988.

35. Expert panel on detection, evaluation, and treatment of high blood cholesterol in adults. Executive summary of the third report of the National Cholesterol Education Program (NCEP), Adult Treatment Panel III *JAMA*, 2001:285:2486–2497.

36. Pasternak R. Adult Treatment Panel II versus Adult Treatment Panel III: what has changed and why? *Am J Cardiol* 89(5A), 2002.

37. Gordon DJ, et al: High-density lipoprotein cholesterol and cardiovascular disease. Four prospective American studies. *Circulation* 79:8–15, 1989.

38. Gordon DJ, et al: High-density lipoprotein—the clinical implications of recent studies. *N Engl J Med* 321:1311–1316, 1989.

39. Assman G, et. al: Apoliproteinemia A-1 and HDL deficiency. *Curr Opin Lipidol* 1:110–115, 1990.

40. Ford ES, et al: Prevalence of the metabolic syndrome among US adults. *JAMA* 287(3), 2002.

41. Reaven G: Metabolic Syndrome: pathophysiology and implications for management of cardiovascular disease. *Circulation* 286–288, 2002.

42. Samyn MM, et al: Impact of a multidisciplinary pediatric preventative cardiology clinic on precursors of metabolic syndrome. *Pediatrics* (forthcoming).

43. Haffner SM, et al: Prospective analysis of insulin-resistance syndrome (syndrome X) *Diabetes* 41: 715–722, 1992.

44. Isomaa B, et al: Cardiovascular morbidity and mortality associated with the metabolic syndrome. *Diabetes Care* 24:683–689, 2001.

45. Trevisan M, et al: Syndrome X and mortality: a population based study. *Am J Epidemiology* 148: 958–966, 1998.

46. Trowbridge FL, et al: Management of child and adolescent obesity: study design and practitioner characteristics. *Pediatrics* 110(1), 2002.

47. Anderson C, et al: Weight loss and gender: an examination of physician attitudes. *Obes Res* 9:257–263, 2001.

48. Sorof J, Daniels S: Obesity hypertension in children: a problem of epidemic proportions. *Hypertension* 40, 2002.

49. Dietz WH: Health consequences of obesity in youth: childhood predictors of adult disease. *Pediatrics* 101(Suppl.):518–525, 1998.

50. Becque MD, et al: Coronary risk incidence of obese adolescents: reductions of exercise plus diet intervention. *Pediatrics* 81:602–612, 1988.

51a. Rosner B, Prineas R, Daniels SR, Loggie J. Blood pressure differences between blacks and whites in relation to body size among US children and adolescents. *Am J Epidemiol* 2000: 151, 1007–1019.

51. CDC Growth Charts: United States. *Adv Data*, Number 314. Vital Health and Statistics of the Centers for Disease Control and Prevention. National Center for Health Statistics. US Department of Health and Human Services. December 4, 2000.

52. Ingelfinger JR: Systemic arterial hypertension. *Nadas' Pediatric Cardiology.* Mosby-Year Book, 1991, Chap. 21.

53. National Heart, Lung, and Blood Institute: Update on the 1987 Task Force on blood pressure in children

and adolescents: a working group from the national high blood pressure education program. *Pediatrics* 98:649, 1996.

54. Report of the Second Task Force on blood pressure control in children 1987. *Pediatrics* 79:1, 1987.

55. www.childstats.gov

56. CDC, National Center for Chronic Disease Prevention and Health Promotion: President's council on physical fitness and sports. 1996. Physical Activity and Health: A report of the surgeon general. Washington, DC: Centers for Disease Control and Prevention, National Center for Chronic Disease Prevention and Health Promotion: President's council on physical fitness and sports.

57. Francis KT: Status of the year 2000 health goals for physical activity and fitness. *Phys Ther* 79(4): 405–414, 1999.

58. Willett WC: *Eat, Drink, and Be Healthy: The Harvard Medical School Guide to Healthy Eating.* Simon & Schuster, New York, NY, 2001.

59. Patrick K, Spear B, Holt K, Sofka D (eds): *Bright Futures in Practice: Physical Activity.* Arlington, V, National Center for Education in Maternal and Child Health Georgetown University.

60. *The Pediatric Exclusivity Provision: January 2001 Report to Congress.* Department of Health and Human Service and the U.S. Food and Drug Administration.

61. www.fda.gov/opccom/laws/pharmkids.html 107th Congress of the United States. The Best Pharmaceuticals Act for Children, January 2002.

62. Park J: Pfizer medicines receive FDA OKs for pediatric use. Dow Jones Newswires, November 7, 2002.

63. Jones PH, Kinlay S, Mosca LJ: Implementing the NCEP ATP III Guidelines. *CME Notes.* Vol. 1, No. 4, QD Healthcare Group 2001.

64. *Physician's Desk Reference*, 56th ed. Montvale, NJ, Medical Economics, 2002.

58

ETHICS IN PEDIATRIC CARDIOLOGY

Tracy K. Koogler

INTRODUCTION

Significant improvements in congenital heart disease therapy have led to better outcomes and fewer early deaths or "lethal" anomalies. With these advances, new ethical dilemmas arise surrounding these infants and children with life-threatening diseases. Physicians traditionally counseled parents of children with neurologic issues and other medical problems, such as trisomy 18 and Cri-du-Chat to allow their children to die because the burden of surgery outweighed the potential benefits; however, today, many of these procedures are routine and some can even be accomplished in the catheterization lab with only one night stay in the hospital. Parents of children with complex heart disease, such as hypoplastic left heart syndrome (HLHS), that as little as 10 years ago were routinely given the option to do nothing, are increasingly not being given the option to withhold care on their children. As surgery has become more successful, qualified surgeons more available in the United States, and interventional catheterization procedures curing more routine congenital heart disease, medical standards have changed. The question becomes how to apply ethical standards to our new medical knowledge.

BEST INTEREST STANDARD

In the United States, the ethical model of autonomy and privacy allow competent adults to make their own health care decisions in consultation with their physician. Infants and young children lack decision-making ability so therefore a surrogate must make these decisions. In cases, such as pediatrics, where a person has never had decision-making ability, decisions are made using the best interest standard. Historically, parents determine their child's best interests because of the responsibility conferred on parents to care for their children until adulthood. This responsibility gives the parent the right to make all decisions for their child including healthcare, religion, culture, and education. These multiple child-rearing decisions affect the family dynamic and play a role in every decision that the parent makes for her child. The government does not interfere with parent's child rearing unless there is evidence of clear harm to the child.

Physicians contribute to a best interest decision by giving an expert medical opinion about which therapy would provide the maximal medical benefit, i.e., beneficence without causing undue harm, nonmaleficence. Ideally, the decision is medical and does not involve any quality-of-life interpretation; however, physicians seldom think about therapies without considering quality-of-life considerations. They usually interpret quality-of-life and sanctity of life differently based on their ethnic, religious, and personal values. By recognizing that personal values enter into medical decisions then one can try to present information in an unbiased format and accept when families have value systems different from our own. Most physicians examine quality of life as the value that person's life has for other people. The appropriate way to examine quality of life is what is the value of the life for the person who must live it. A severely developmentally delayed child may still get happiness from the love, care, and interaction with her family. Physicians cannot adequately assess these elements without recognizing the belief system of the individual family.

The child's best interests includes what is medically necessary to palliate or cure this child's medical condition, which a physician is best able to determine. A child's best interests may also include religious preferences, family values, and ethnic values that a medical professional is not able to determine. For this reason, parents are given the right and responsibility to make decisions in their child's best interests. Ethical dilemmas arise when there is conflict between the parents and physicians about what constitutes the best interest for a child.

CASES

Case 1

A well-educated Indian couple is expecting their third child. The mother has a prenatal ultrasound, which suggests congenital heart disease so she is referred for prenatal echocardiography. The echocardiogram shows the baby has hypoplastic left heart syndrome. The cardiologist recommends plans be made for the mother to be transferred to a high risk maternal fetal center 2 hours away near the time expected delivery. This is planned so that the child can be delivered and immediately transferred to the children's hospital for care and surgery. The surgeon there has an excellent reputation and excellent results with the Norwood procedure. The family thanks the cardiologist for the advice and makes an appointment with the surgeon. They also search the Internet for options for hypoplastic left heart syndrome. After talking to the surgeon, their respective families, and others in the community the parents decide not to have surgery but plan to take the child home after birth with comfort measures only. They believe that the three surgeries entailed in the palliation for hypoplastic heart syndrome are an unreasonable burden on a small infant, despite a reasonable chance of success. Furthermore, they believe that surgery 2 hours from their home will strain the resources of the family and be detrimental to their other two children. The NICU calls the cardiologist at the time of the delivery and he verifies the diagnosis by echo. What should the cardiologist do now?

Case 2

A family makes a cardiology appointment for their 6-month-old son with trisomy 18 who has a large ventricular septal defect (VSD). On arrival, the family states they were told their child would die shortly after birth and that they took the child home with palliative care. The child has done remarkably well until about 1 month ago when he started having respiratory distress, poor feeding, and diaphoresis. Their pediatrician felt the symptoms were because of heart failure from the VSD. The parents are now asking if the VSD can be repaired. They know their child is significantly handicapped, but he smiles at them and is trying to roll over. They wish to do anything for him which they would do for their other two children. One of the cardiologists in the group has just started closing VSDs in the catheterization lab and there is a very competent surgeon at your hospital. What should the cardiologist do?

DISCUSSION

These two cases exemplify the conflicting issues surrounding a child's best interest. In the first case, the physician may see surgery as in the child's best interest because without surgery the child will certainly die. The child experiences some pain and suffering with the surgeries and other therapies in exchange for a chance at survival. The family recognizes the potential benefit but sees a minimum of three surgeries, daily medication, and several heart catheterizations for a palliative repair resulting in premature death or the need for transplantation in the future. Additionally, the long trip to the children's hospital and the time away from the other children seems prohibitive for this family. They believe there is no cure for hypoplastic left heart syndrome and they do not want their child to suffer and then still likely die an early death. They do not believe their son will experience a normal childhood, since he will require medications, have several hospitalizations, and be unable to participate fully in physical activities.

In the second case, the physician sees congestive heart failure as the way for this neurologically devastated child to die and recommends continuing comfort measures only. The medical decision would be that a VSD is easily correctable with minimal pain and suffering; however, the physician's decision-making is affected by quality-of-life issues. The family recognizes quality-of-life issues also. Their child has been incorporated into the family dynamic and is an interactive member of the family. The child suffers with tachypnea, diaphoresis, and feeding intolerance. The child would feel better if the VSD were repaired. The neurologic devastation does not factor highly in the family's decision at this stage.

The families in both of these cases would disagree with the physician based on their perspective of the child's suffering and the risk/benefit analysis of medical procedures to prolong the child's life. Both families are incorporating quality-of-life judgments into their best interest decisions. Their quality-of-life standards differ from their physicians but that does not make them wrong. Physicians must give the medical opinion and then allow families to incorporate their belief system to best determine what is right for their child. The staged surgical procedure or heart transplantation for HLHS has many obstacles even in the best hands. Prolonged periods in the hospital, daily medications, and risk for significant morbidity and mortality at anytime during the three procedures are all burdens on the child that the family must consider. Many would choose surgery, but for the few that disagree, the choice not to palliate should still rest with the parents. The other family must also consider the burden of minimal intellectual development and an uncertain lifespan but they believe the benefits of life to this child and family outweigh the burdens. Again, when the medical risks are minimal and the procedure straightforward, we should allow the family to choose therapy even in cases where others might choose to do nothing.

The physician who disagrees with the parent and cannot agree to the family's request in either situation must recognize that these views are paternalistic. The physician believes he or she knows the child's best interests better than the child's parents and intentionally overrides their decision. The physician then has three possible choices, which should be examined carefully. First, there can be an attempt to transfer care to another physician willing to respect the family's wishes. The child with trisomy 18 might fall into this category. For personal reasons, the physician does not see the VSD repair as a viable option and is unwilling to perform requested surgery or interventional catheterization. The physician should give the parents names of other qualified cardiologists and/or surgeons in the area for a second opinion.

Second, a physician who disagrees with the parents and believes the child is being neglected or abused can call an ethics consultation. An ethics consult may help to clarify the families understanding of the medical issues and their preferences so that the physician feels the child's interests are being respected appropriately. An impartial examination of the situation might help clarify the issues and allow both parties to come to an amenable solution. Findings of the ethics consultation may also allow a physician to see that the family's choice is in the child's best interests.

However, a cardiologist may pursue surgery as the only option and choose to contact the local child welfare department to take custody of the child. By going to the courts for HLHS, one asks the courts for permission to perform surgery without parental permission. In this case, the parents usually do not lose parental rights for other issues and the child returns to the family home after surgery. This situation would be similar to court requests for blood products for children who are Jehovah Witnesses. If custody is taken only for the surgery, then the family is left with a child who will require daily medication, additional catheterizations and surgery, and possibly tube feedings secondary to the feeding intolerance seen in children with complex congenital heart disease. The physician may feel the child is palliated, but this has left the parents with the daily responsibility to care for the child, in ways, which they may see as burdensome to the child and their family.

When therapy is forced on a child with chronic medical problems, the stakes are higher because either the family must accept the responsibility of this ongoing care or the child must be placed in foster care. Child protective services might need to remove the child from the home for an extended period of time or permanently. Placing a child in foster care dramatically changes the life for that child and his family. This serious situation deserves thought as to whether the child's best interests are truly being ignored by the parents or do the parents have a different value system from the physicians, which should be respected. Additionally, the physician who forces surgery on a family and the child has severe complications, such as an intracranial hemorrhage, must deal with the second guessing as to whether surgery was the right answer. Debates, concerning this scenario are being played out all over the United States. Ten years ago, families were routinely given the option for comfort measures for surgeries such as the Norwood procedure for HLHS. The premier programs in the country now have survival rates exceeding 75% with few neurologic sequelae and the decision is becoming more problematic. Outcomes are not universal, however, and the burdens for individual patients and families can be substantial so choice should still rest with the parents.

ADOLESCENT ISSUES

In the United States, parents are the decision-makers for children until 18 years of age unless the child is an emancipated minor, which is quite rare; however, ethically, it is recognized that adolescents should be involved in their medical decision-making and should be allowed to *assent*, or agree to the therapy for which their parents have *consented*. Adolescents should be included in discussions of their healthcare status, medication regimens, and therapy options. Although, teenagers are not the ultimate decision-makers, their opinion counts. Most people would not allow teenagers to refuse therapy without their parents agreement, but teens should have a chance to express their opinion about treatment options.

On the other hand, parents must recognize teenagers are not adults and still require supervision of their medications and therapies. Commonly, chronically ill teenagers stop taking their medications because they magically think their disease goes away during adolescence and they do not like the side effects of the medications. These children can become quite ill, and it is common to have teens with transplants have severe rejection episodes, sometimes leading to death. Physicians must tell both parents and teens the outcomes of stopping medications and the importance of both parties taking responsibility for compliance issues. For the child with chronic heart disease, compliance can improve long-term survival and delay the need for transplantation. For the transplant patient compliance is necessary for life. Unfortunately, most transplant centers will not retransplant the teen that has stopped taking their immunosuppressive medications because transplants are limited resources, which cannot be wasted on the noncompliant patient, regardless of age. The family and teen must take responsibility for medication compliance.

PALLIATIVE CARE

Despite the numerous advances, we unfortunately still find ourselves with some heart disease that is not curable. Children who are entering the end of their lives deserve the same exceptional care they received early in their disease. Ideally, when a physician recognizes that a child is in the end stages of his disease and heroic measures such as transplant are either not an option or have been rejected by the child and/or family, then he should address issues of do-not-resuscitate, desires for additional ICU care, and desire for palliative care services. It is much easier for families to discuss these issues before the child is critically ill in the ICU without forewarning. Families will have time to plan final trips, see friends and family, and discuss options for care if they are given adequate preparation time. Anger and denial may be normal first responses to these discussions, but once the subject has been introduced, the family can deal with the information at their own pace. Families may never accept a DNR order or wish to discontinue ICU care because it is viewed as "giving up," but they need to be given the option.

Palliative care services can be established for these children and families to help establish pain management and emotional support. Unlike many adult hospice programs, children's programs do not focus on the rule that the child should likely have less than six months to live and many do not require families to choose a DNR or relinquish the ability to enter the hospital or ICU setting. The goal is to get families to recognize aggressive therapy and resuscitation in a terminal child is not in his best interest and many successfully do this through emotional support and counseling; however, palliative care services can be used as a therapy even when the child is receiving intensive care or aggressive therapies. Families are not asked to choose aggressive therapy versus palliative services; therefore, they do not see palliative services as "giving up" on their child. Despite a family's initial reluctance for palliative services, studies have shown that families of children who have died, even those who have spent longer amounts of time in intensive care, feel deserted by healthcare teams, unprepared for the death, and unable to deal with the loss. Palliative care services prepare families and help to provide the necessary emotional support. Palliative care is also an excellent service for families of children with complex congenital disorders, such as trisomy 13 or Cri-du-Chat, who may have chosen to pursue nonaggressive therapy.

Suggested Readings

American Academy of Pediatrics: Palliative care for children. *Pediatrics* 106(2):351–357, 2000.

Beauchamp TL, Childress JF: *Principles of Biomedical Ethics*, 5th ed. Oxford, UK, Oxford University Press, 2001.

Ross LF: *Children, Families and Health Care Decision Making*. Oxford, UK, Oxford University Press, 1998.

59

HEMATOLOGIC ISSUES IN THE PEDIATRIC CARDIOLOGY PATIENT

Ruth Retondo Rudinsky

INTRODUCTION

As advances in treatment of congenital heart disease have improved outcomes, patients with such conditions are achieving prolonged survival. This survival has allowed manifestation of previously unrecognized emerging chronic systemic conditions. Among these conditions, presenting new challenges for therapeutic intervention, are disorders of hematologic parameters. Bleeding disorders, both hypo- and hypercoagulable states, and anemia will be discussed. Erythrocytosis secondary to chronic cyanosis is less prevalent than in previous eras, owing to improved management of underlying cardiac abnormalities. Specific hematologic chronic disease states, such as sickle cell disease, are discussed in the chapter on systemic diseases. A detailed review of hemostasis can be found in many general medical textbooks and will not be discussed in its entirety in this chapter.

BLEEDING DISORDERS

Pathophysiology of Coagulation Disorders

The major factors in determining normal hemostasis are the blood vessel wall, platelets, coagulation factors in the plasma, and the hemodynamics of blood flow. Factors predisposing to thrombogenesis include injury to the vascular endothelium, alterations in blood flow, and alterations in blood properties (hypercoagulability). Active equilibrium results from opposing diatheses of bleeding versus thrombosis. The normal physiologic balance of coagulation activity provides for maintenance of unimpeded vascular channels. The appearance of blood vessel injury requires rapid response to contain bleeding complications while remodeling to meet the needs of tissue perfusion. Patients with persisting cardiovascular abnormalities after intervention to ameliorate either congenital or acquired conditions can have several disturbances of this interactive balance. Their state may subsequently be shifted toward either a bleeding or a clotting tendency.

Platelet Disorders

A common platelet abnormality in patients with congenital/acquired heart disorders is a simple quantitative decrease. Thrombocytopenia may be seen related to physical peripheral destruction of platelets, such as may occur in shear stress from mechanical valves, or owing to sequestration secondary to hepatosplenomegaly. The resultant thrombocytopenia can lead to a bleeding tendency. When chronic cyanosis is present, there is some evidence that qualitative platelet defects occur because of chronic platelet activation; this pathophysiologic state disturbs the system by impairing platelet function while contributing to an increase in both procoagulant and anticoagulant factors in the circulation. Physical platelet damage can occur during cardiopulmonary bypass during surgery. Another platelet disorder related to heart disease and surgery is heparin-induced platelet aggregation. Also described as heparin-induced thrombocytopenia (HIT), this disorder results in mild to moderate thrombocytopenia but is paradoxically associated with venous or arterial thrombosis. Evidence suggests that heparin/platelet factor 4 complexes appear both on platelet and endothelial cell surfaces. These complexes produce an immunogenic antigen which can stimulate antibody production. The IgG antibody response in this setting has been shown to result in two procoagulant scenarios: platelet activation, and endothelial cell damage exposing procoagulant substances such as collagen in the subcellular matrix. The result is a local increase in thrombin production, leading to thrombosis. Treatment has included discontinuation of heparin and use of alternative inactivators of thrombin such as hirudin compounds, or danaparoid sodium (a low-molecular-weight heparinoid). Unfortunately, standard heparin alternatives such as low-molecular-weight heparin (LMWH) and coumadin have caused exacerbation of the thrombosis related to HIT, the former interacting with antibody similarly to heparin and the latter producing lowered levels of the anticoagulant proteins C and S. Finally, primary platelet disorders such as genetic aggregation defects may be influential factors in the management of congenital heart defect (CHD), though are beyond the scope of this discussion.

Disorders in the Vasculature and Blood Flow

Further complicating hemostatic equilibrium, erythrocytosis resulting from erythropoietic response to chronic cyanosis is thought to produce blood hyperviscosity, thus sluggish blood flow, and is associated with an increased likelihood of venous thrombosis. In a similar fashion, sluggish blood flow can be seen in low cardiac output states (cardiomyopathy), venous obstruction, and in patients with a Fontan circulation (passive blood flow from the systemic veins to the pulmonary arteries—see also the chapter on the Fontan operation). Finally, damage to endothelium, such as could occur during acquired vasculitic conditions (e.g., Kawasaki's disease), augments the procoagulant state by triggering interactions of damaged endothelium, platelets, and circulating coagulation factors.

Disorders of Blood Coagulation Properties

Primary coagulation disorders such as hemophilia can influence the management of CHD, but usually are managed in conjunction with consultation by a hematologist. Similarly, the inherited coagulation disorders causing thrombosis (such as protein S/protein C/antithrombin III deficiency, factor V Leiden, and so forth) should prompt consultation. Acquired coagulopathies in CHD include problems related to impaired synthesis of clotting factors, and a decrease in circulating high-molecular-weight multimers of Von Willebrand's factor (the latter is seen in acyanotic conditions such as septal defects). With right-sided heart failure, hepatic production of coagulation factors may be diminished. Right-sided heart failure may also cause malabsorption of vitamin K, which can further exacerbate coagulation abnormalities.

Management of Bleeding Disorders in CHD

Clinical Indications for Anticoagulation in Congenital Heart Disease

Anticoagulation is a therapeutic strategy applied in select clinical situations in pediatric cardiology patients. It is often instituted after certain surgical procedures for congenital heart disease, including systemic-to-pulmonary arterial shunts and prosthetic valve placement (abnormal vessel walls/foreign material), and abnormal flow patterns causing predisposition to thrombosis such as post-Fontan-type surgery or dilated cardiomyopathy. In addition, acquired conditions, including Kawasaki's disease (thrombocytosis/vasculitis) are often managed with long-term anticoagulation. There may be an indication for antithrombotic therapy in other, less commonly encountered situations in pediatric populations, including atrial fibrillation in the setting of a preexisting cardiac malformation, and myocardial infarction. Clinical guidelines for anticoagulation in this heterogeneous group of patients have, in general, been empirically derived; practices vary.

Given the enlarging group of congenital heart disease patients receiving treatment to alter their coagulation status, ongoing prospective therapeutic trials are gathering important data for those who require anticoagulation for extended periods. Guideline revisions will likely ensue, but there is consensus for many currently recommended practices.

Initiation of Antithrombotic Therapy

The decision to begin anticoagulation is generally made in the acute care setting. Decision algorithms are individualized by the Pediatric Cardiology/Cardiac Surgery team. Heparin has been the initial pharmaceutical of choice historically, although trials of LMWH, even for very young and preterm infants, are demonstrating efficacy and safety. The difficult-to-achieve necessity for maintaining intravenous access in order to treat a patient long term with heparin has made the subcutaneous delivery of LMWH particularly attractive as an alternative.

Oral anticoagulation, if indicated, is begun once therapeutic goals have been achieved with heparin or LMWH. Warfarin, often referred to with the brand name coumadin, needs to be given for at least 2–7 days before its full effect is present and dose adjustment can be made to meet target parameters. Heparinization is continued until the desired warfarin effect has been achieved (usually defined as the International Normalized Ratio, or INR, which was adopted in 1982 by the World Health Organization to allow comparisons of clinical trials given the wide variability among clinical laboratory analyses of the prothrombin time). Rarely, a patient undergoing anticoagulation may have a genetic deficiency of the anticoagulants protein C or protein S. Exacerbation of a procoagulant state resulting in thrombosis can occur during the first several days of starting warfarin in such patients (see below), and they should be given a longer heparin overlap period (e.g., 4–5 days instead of 1 or 2). Any patient on warfarin requires frequent initial laboratory evaluation of the anticoagulation status. Intervals between monitoring assays can be increased after a stable therapeutic level of anticoagulation has been achieved, but most pediatric practitioners monitor no less often than every 4 weeks. Adult patients and older adolescents, who have demonstrated a history of good compliance, can be monitored up to every 6 weeks. There are ongoing prospective trials of self-management for children on warfarin, with charts provided to adult caretakers for dose adjustments after home laboratory evaluation. Such a trial program in Denmark includes children as young as 2.2 (to 15.6) years old.

Review of Warfarin Mechanism of Action

Warfarin produces coagulation abnormalities by interfering with interconversion of vitamin K with its 2,3-epoxide. Reduced vitamin K is a necessary cofactor in posttranslation carboxylation modification of vitamin K-dependent proteins in the liver. The result is hepatic production of incompletely carboxylated anticoagulant proteins, which in turn are dysfunctional in coagulation physiologic activity. The affected procoagulant factors are factors II, VII, IX, and

X. Because two anticoagulant factors, proteins C and S, are also dependent on vitamin K-mediated carboxylation for full function, there is a concomitant impairment of anticoagulant physiology during warfarin therapy. Endogenous vitamin K-dependent proteins have different half-lives, which accounts for the length of time required for full efficacy to be achieved during initial oral anticoagulation. In addition, effects on proteins C and S diminish endogenous anticoagulant activity and may produce a thrombotic state early in oral anticoagulation. Clinically, individuals with preexisting protein C or S deficiency are at risk for skin necrosis complications during the initiation of warfarin treatment. Half-lives of the affected proteins are factor II: 60 h; factor VII: 4–7 h; factor IX: 24 h; factor X: 48 h; protein C: 4–7 h; and protein S: 42 h.

Ongoing Management of Patients on Warfarin

Prior to 1994, significant clinical cohort data in managing pediatric oral anticoagulation was not available. In North America, efforts to initiate trials and monitor outcome have been led by investigators such as the pediatric thromboembolic program at Toronto's Hospital for Sick Children. Improved pediatric dosing and monitoring recommendations have resulted. A baseline prothrombin time/INR is established (the target INR varies with the clinical condition being treated; see below). The loading dose of warfarin (after heparinization has been stabilized to a target prolongation of the partial thromboplastin time), is 0.2 mg/kg on day 1 (maximum 10 mg); dosing on days 2–4 is adjusted to the measured INR according to published guidelines; by days 5–7 the target INR should be achievable. INR measurement is generally obtained three times a week until the target value is reached and stable without dose adjustment. Then, the INR is checked once a week for at least 4 weeks, then every 2 weeks for the next 1–2 months. At that time, stable patients can be switched to INR measurement as discussed above for the duration of treatment. Possible events affecting the therapeutic outcome are discussed below, along with the necessary additional measurements and dose adjustments.

Warfarin is quickly and readily absorbed after an oral dose. The maximum blood concentration (in healthy adult volunteers) occurs in about 90 min, and the half-life for elimination is 36–42 h. Metabolism primarily occurs in the liver, and is mediated by the cytochrome P 450 enzyme system. Excretion of metabolites occurs in bile and urine. There is enterohepatic circulation of some metabolites. Once absorbed, warfarin is greater than 99% protein-bound (primarily to albumin). Hence, liver disorders can affect warfarin metabolism on many levels. Since alterations produce complex interactions and prediction is unreliable, frequent monitoring is the best practical tactic. Although renal elimination occurs, this route has little effect on the anticoagulation activity of warfarin, and no dosage adjustment is recommended for individuals with renal disorders.

The target INR is defined for the clinical entity requiring anticoagulation. One common guideline suggests that the INR should be 2.5–3.5 for patients with mechanical valves, and 2.0–3.0 for all others.

Children younger than 12 months old require higher doses of anticoagulants per kilogram than children aged 1–10 years and 11–18 years. Rapid growth periods require increased monitoring. Several clinical scenarios can affect the efficacy of anticoagulation, and are of practical importance. These include breast-feeding versus formula-feeding: infant formula is enriched with vitamin K, and thus affects the INR differently from breast milk. Febrile illnesses, especially acute gastroenteritis, may result in altered absorption of both warfarin and dietary vitamin K. Fluctuating diets during childhood developmental periods may significantly alter oral vitamin K intake. If liver disease appears, warfarin metabolism can change abruptly. The use of antibiotics can either alter hepatic metabolism or affect the vitamin K production of intestinal flora (or both). Recommendations for daily vitamin K intake for adults on warfarin are 70–140 μg per day; pediatric guidelines need to be delineated. Finally, compliance is always an issue with any long-term medical intervention. Complications related to a change in compliance may even affect formerly reliable patients. Assumption of self-responsibility with adulthood, and issues of personal independence, may impact the efficacy of medical treatments for maturing pediatric teenage patients, and may need to be addressed at the appropriate time in each case. A long-term professional relationship can facilitate addressing such issues, and reduce the risk of detrimental behaviors.

Drug Interactions
During Warfarin Therapy

The stability of anticoagulation can be altered by introducing any of several additional medications. Drug interaction analysis should be undertaken whenever new medications are being considered. In addition, if ongoing pharmaceuticals are dose-adjusted or discontinued, the INR may change. Prudent management should include frequent INR monitoring whenever interactions can be expected to affect anticoagulation until a stable therapeutic effect is documented. Even short-term medications, such as antibiotics for intercurrent infections, should prompt consideration of frequent monitoring until after the short-term course has been completed.

Special Concerns
During Ongoing Warfarin Therapy

Some clinical situations warrant mention in that they may be important in patients who are on long-term anticoagulation with warfarin. Use of concomitant nonsteroidal antiinflammatory agents may increase bleeding complications. Use of acetyl salicylate for antiplatelet effect may do the same, and also puts a pediatric patient at risk for Reye's syndrome: vaccinations against varicella (or documented immunity) and influenza are suggested. If pregnancy is possible, the female patient should be aware of the teratogenic potential of warfarin and should be provided with close clinical coordination to provide documentable contraceptive therapy if she is sexually active. Women contemplating pregnancy should be advised to discuss this with their primary clinician so that alternative anticoagulation can be instituted *before conception*. Mothers who have delivered may safely breastfeed their infant while on (resumed) warfarin anticoagulation, since warfarin in breast milk has been altered to an inactive form, and such infants have been shown to have no change in their coagulation profiles.

Ongoing, stable warfarin therapy can unmask a newly developing bleeding source even if dosing and INR have not changed. This is more clinically relevant to older patients who are at increased risk for systemic diseases.

Pediatric immunizations should be administered according to established guidelines. Hematoma formation is less likely for subcutaneous than intramuscular administration. If hematoma formation after immunization is a problem, local treatment with cool packs or pressure dressing may help. The patient's cardiologist may be able to approve lowering the warfarin dose to achieve the lower therapeutic range for the condition being treated.

Finally, there are variations among commercially available warfarin formulations. It is important for patients to be aware that a substitute generic (possibly different) form of warfarin may be provided by their pharmacist. The primary clinician should be alerted if this occurs.

Interruption of Oral Anticoagulation

There are several scenarios during which oral anticoagulation should be altered because of an increased risk of bleeding. These range from minor elective dental or surgical procedures to invasive surgical or diagnostic procedures involving the eye or central nervous system. A case-by-case analysis coordinated among the various clinicians is required.

Some minor procedures can be performed without warfarin discontinuation if the oral surgeon/ surgeon/interventionalist is aware of the need for careful hemostasis. Often, a reduced dose of warfarin with documentation of a lower INR, if approved by the clinician overseeing antithrombotic therapy, may suffice. It may take up to three days on a lower dose to achieve a stable decreased INR. Resumption of the usual dose can be done soon after surgery, with frequent laboratory evaluation until a steady-state is again achieved.

Elective invasive surgical or oral surgical procedures may require discontinuation of warfarin. This should be done at least three days prior to the planned procedure, with documentation of an acceptable INR prior to surgery. If antithrombosis is particularly important in such cases, the use of low-molecular-weight heparin several hours preoperatively (generally 6–12 h) and resumed postoperatively can bridge the time off warfarin until it is safe to resume oral anticoagulation.

Several conditions require discontinuation of warfarin. These include eye surgery, brain/spinal cord surgery, and spinal puncture or epidural anesthesia. Warfarin is often contraindicated for patients with open wounds, skin ulcers, and planned regional block anesthesia (owing to concern about local hematoma formation resulting in tissue damage). Beyond these relatively well-defined clinical situations, warfarin discontinuation should be considered for any procedure associated with a potential for bleeding complications, and in which uncontrolled bleed is judged to be capable of producing significant morbidity.

Reversal of Over-Warfarinization

Nomograms for the reversal of warfarin effect are widely available for adult patients. More recent data from pediatric experience suggest that dosing of vitamin K in a weight-adjusted protocol may be more appropriate for children. The lowest adult dose of 0.5 mg may be too high for young children, and a dose of 30 µg/kg is recommended. Intravenous administration provides the most rapid onset of antiwarfarinization effect, but subcutaneous or oral administration can be used in a stable patient without signs of ongoing bleeding. The use of fresh frozen plasma transfusion is generally not required, and is reserved for patients who are experiencing active bleeding during the interval prior to antiwarfarin effect. In such a setting, if volume administration is a concern, prothrombin complex concentrate may be considered instead of fresh frozen plasma. Activated factor VII holds promise for control of bleeding with fewer adverse effects than prothrombin complex. Finally, children with significant liver disease may require additional doses of vitamin K to achieve adequate reversal.

Heparin

Heparin has been useful for short-term rapid onset anticoagulation in an acute care setting. Heparin functions primarily by activating antithrombin III, with a smaller contribution from facilitation of antithrombin activity of cofactor II. Pediatric dosing/monitoring was initially extrapolated from adult clinical experience; later pediatric trials established current guidelines. Continuous intravenous treatment begins with a loading dose of 50–75 units/kg, followed by 20 units/kg/h, titrated to achieve a partial thromboplastin time of 60–85 seconds. As with warfarin, infants younger than 1 year of age are likely to require higher weight-based doses (maintenance with 28 units/kg/h). Smaller intermittent doses are used in a variety of settings for short-term anticoagulation, such as cardiac catheterization, or for reducing thrombotic complications of intravenous catheters. Over-heparinization can be managed acutely with protamine, 1 mg per 100 units of heparin. Patients with underlying liver or kidney dysfunction may have delayed heparin clearance, and may require adjustments both of heparin dosing and protamine dosing.

Chronic heparin use in pediatrics has not often been instituted. Problems include evidence of poorer outcome with respect to thromboembolic complications compared to oral anticoagulation, the difficulty of maintaining long-term intravenous access, and the late complication of osteopenia. Data on outcome issues of chronic heparin use in pediatrics is limited. The more recent availability of low-molecular-weight heparin offers an option for patients unable to use oral anticoagulation. Although only preliminary data are available, clinical trials have demonstrated at least short-term efficacy and safety of this agent even in very young infants. Much of this information comes from the pediatric thromboembolism program at the Hospital for Sick Children in Toronto. Advantages of LMWH over standard heparin include ease of administration (subcutaneous vs. intravenous), decreased hospitalization requirements, diminished osteopenia effect (preliminary data), and decreased need for phlebotomy to obtain laboratory monitoring.

Antiplatelet Agents

Antiplatelet agents such as acetylsalicylate (aspirin) and dipyridamole have a role in management of adult patients at risk for thromboembolism in a variety of settings. Their use in pediatric thromboembolic prophylaxis is less prevalent, usually limited to adjunct therapy in children with congenital heart disease who have undergone a Blalock-Taussig shunt procedure, or in patients with Kawasaki syndrome. Antiplatelet agents are generally used during the acute phase of Kawasaki syndrome, and are continued in Kawasaki patients who have late-effect coronary artery abnormalities.

Thrombolytic Therapy

A significant thrombotic event can occur in a vessel or shunt, threatening perfusion of a vital structure. If surgery or other intervention is not possible, and initial anticoagulation is ineffective, thrombolysis may be indicated. Currently, recombinant tissue plasminogen activator (t-PA) is used safely for bolus treatment of thrombus occluding central venous catheters, but the use of continuous-infusion t-PA has had only limited application in children; however, it has been used effectively at doses of 0.1–0.6 mg/kg/h in cases of femoral arterial thrombosis after cardiac catheterization. Supplementation with plasminogen (fresh frozen plasma or cryoprecipitate) may assist with clot lysis if response to t-PA alone is judged inadequate. Bleeding from superficial puncture sites is common during continuous-infusion t-PA, but is fortunately usually clinically insignificant. Yet there is a small risk of more serious bleeding, particularly intracranial hemorrhage. Bleeding complications can be minimized by maintaining platelet counts with transfusion and by infusing fibrinogen (cryoprecipitate). Continuous t-PA infusion in pediatric patients has been given for up to 6 h without undue adverse events if close monitoring and supplementation with fibrinogen and platelet transfusion are carefully and promptly performed.

ERYTHROCYTOSIS AND ANEMIA

Erythrocytosis

Chronic cyanosis in congenital heart disease, particularly in the growing population of adults with congenital heart disease, produces an expanded red cell mass to meet physiologic oxygen delivery needs. This erythrocytosis contributes to increased blood viscosity, but there are recent studies which indicate that hematocrit alone is an imperfect indicator of the need for intervention. Historically, phlebotomy in such patients has been recommended to reduce red cell mass/viscosity at given hematocrit levels, such as 65%; however, recent studies of adults with cyanotic congenital heart disease have demonstrated that iron deficiency and a history of repeat phlebotomy are independent risk factors for stroke, while an isolated elevated hematocrit is not. Similar smaller studies in children have correlated iron deficiency with an increased incidence of central venous thrombosis in chronic cyanosis. Iron-deficient red cells are less deformable than those that are iron-replete, and may therefore contribute more effectively to increased blood viscosity. Recommendations have been made to reserve phlebotomy for patients who have adequate iron stores, erythrocytosis, and symptoms of cerebral perfusion abnormalities (dizziness, headache, visual changes, altered mentation including a sense of dissociation, paresthesias, or fatigue). Patients of any age with chronic cyanosis should be monitored for iron deficiency, and correction of this state should be undertaken in order to lower their risk of cerebrovascular events. Care should be taken to monitor erythropoietic response during iron therapy, and to keep the rise in hematocrit from proceeding too quickly (increasing viscosity). Laboratory analysis and monitoring for symptoms listed above should be done frequently (several times a week), and dose of iron decreased if needed. Phlebotomy, when indicated, should be performed with careful follow-up as well. Isovolumic colloid or crystalloid infusion during the phlebotomy may help reduce volume shifts which could adversely affect perfusion.

Anemia

There are many scenarios contributing to the development of anemia in patients with congenital heart disease. As mentioned above, even in the presence of erythrocytosis, iron deficiency "anemia" may occur. Additional causes of anemia in CHD include hemolysis from a shearing effect through abnormal or synthetic valves, or through other cardiovascular defects. In these settings, a pressure gradient usually serves as the force applied to the blood jet. Any patient who has had surgery for congenital heart disease and abnormally darkened urine should be evaluated for the presence of hematuria versus hemoglobinuria, with appropriate evaluation for each. Anemia owing to blood loss may also be seen after cardiac surgery or other interventions, requiring therapy as clinically indicated (transfusion vs. iron supplementation). Finally, transient anemias related to viral infections or adverse effects of medications can occur in patients with CHD, just as in any individual.

The presence of anemia alters hemodynamics in ways which may worsen deleterious effects of CHD. Anemia will result in decreased oxygen carrying capacity. Compensatory increase in cardiac output returns oxygen carrying capacity to normal. This can manifest as an increase in heart rate and/or stroke volume. The latter is seen in patients with chronic anemia such as sickle cell disease. Most of the time, these compensatory measures are adequate and advantageous; however, if there are additional hemodynamic abnormalities such as severe aortic regurgitation, the added increased heart rate and stroke volume may lead to signs of heart failure. Thus, causes of anemia should be addressed, and correction implemented.

In addition to the effects of anemia on oxygen carrying capacity, an altered hemocrit also changes blood viscosity. The development of anemia has been shown to lower blood viscosity in patients with septal defects, and increase the left-to-right shunt to the lungs. Although such effects may be clinically minor, onset of anemia should be detected and treated when managing patients with septal defects.

CONCLUSION

Hematologic abnormalities in patients with congenital heart disease are not unusual. A procoagulant state is often present. Long-term anticoagulation in pediatric cardiology patients continues to be assessed with respect to therapeutic goals, risks, and outcomes. Trials of lower target INR values in selected clinical groups may provide safer treatment while maintaining efficacy. Newer technology to facilitate monitoring using capillary whole blood home PT/INR testing should ease the health care burden for patients and their families. Erythrocytosis and iron deficiency need to be assessed regularly in patients with chronic cyanosis; phlebotomy should be limited to those with symptoms of cerebral perfusion deficits. Management of anemia in the pediatric cardiology patient is important to optimize clinical status.

Suggested Readings

Bolton-Maggs P, Brook L: The use of vitamin K for reversal of over-warfarinization in children. Correspondence. *Br J Haematol* 118(3):924, 2002.

Massicotte P, Adams M, Marzinotto V, Brooker L, Andrew M: Low-molecular-weight heparin in pediatric patients with thrombotic disease: a dose finding study. *J Pediatr* 128(3):313–318, 1996.

Massicotte P, Marzinotto V, Vegh P, Adams M: Andrew M: Home monitoring of warfarin therapy in children with a whole blood prothrombin time monitor. *J Pediatr* 127(3):389–394, 1995.

Perloff JK, Marelli AJ, Miner PD: Risk of stroke in adults with cyanotic congenital heart disease. *Circulation* 87(6), 1993.

Reller MD: Congenital heart disease: current indications for antithrombotic therapy in pediatric patients. *Curr Cardiol Rep* 3:90–95, 2001.

Streif W, Andrew M, Marzinotto P, Chan AKC, Julian JA, Mitchell L: Analysis of warfarin therapy in pediatric patients: a prospective cohort study of 319 patients. *Blood* 94(9):3007–3014, 1999.

Thorne SA: Management of polycythemia in adults with cyanotic congenital heart disease. Editorial. *Heart* 79(4):315–316, 1998.

Van Doorn C, Yates R, Tunstill A, Elliott M: Quality of life in children following mitral valve replacement. *Heart* 84(6):643–647, 2000.

60

FETAL CARDIOLOGY

Ernerio Alboliras

Congenital heart defects are seen in approximately 8 per 1000 live births, making them among the most common major congenital malformations seen in newborns. Heart defects are frequently seen in abortuses, are associated with perinatal mortalities and morbidities, are the primary causes of mortality in newborns with major chromosomal anomalies, and may be observed in fetuses of mothers with comorbidity or with a history of a heart defect. With the presence of new technologies allowing antenatal diagnosis of cardiac malformations and fetal arrhythmias, and with the emerging understanding of prenatal and postnatal natural histories of various cardiac malformations, fetal cardiology has become a unique field of pediatric cardiology. Fetal cardiology requires the special ability to perform echocardiographic studies of the fetal heart, diagnose fetal heart defects and, in many instances, treat fetal cardiac disease. Because of the interplay of the fetus with the pregnant mother, the field necessitates appreciation of various maternal, obstetrical, and other medical conditions. A close working relationship with the perinatologist/obstetrician is crucial in facilitating optimal care for the mother and her unborn child. In addition, cooperation with the geneticist, neonatologist and cardiovascular surgeon will provide the comprehensive care of the fetus with a heart defect.

The surge of interest in fetal cardiology has come at a time when major advances in diagnostic modalities, neonatal cardiac surgery, critical care, medical therapy, and interventional cardiology have also occurred. The major technologic improvement in ultrasonography has allowed for enhanced imaging of the fetal heart. New generation two-dimensional and Doppler ultrasound equipment provides superior resolution and excellent color and spectral Doppler display for accurate diagnosis. In a tiny fetus, it is possible to identify most cardiac and contiguous vessel anatomy.

FACTORS AFFECTING FETAL CARDIAC IMAGING

The ability to accurately diagnose a fetal cardiac anomaly depends on several factors (Table 60-1).

Diagnostic images can usually be sufficiently obtained starting at 16–18 weeks gestational age. If necessary, transvaginal ultrasonography can be performed between 12 and 16 weeks. The amniotic fluid facilitates effective transmission of ultrasound, thus resulting in optimal images. An adequate amount of amniotic fluid relative to fetal mass begins at 16–18 weeks gestational age until

**FACTORS THAT AFFECT THE QUALITY
OF IMAGING THE FETAL HEART**

1. Imaging equipment
2. Gestational age
3. Maternal obesity and abdominal scarring
4. Oligohydramnios or polyhydramnios
5. Uterine anomalies
6. Number of fetuses
7. Fetal position
8. Fetal extracardiac anomalies

approximately 24 weeks. In later gestational age (i.e., third trimester) echocardiographic images may be affected by the increased fetal mass, relative decrease in amniotic fluid, and the thicker fetal skeleton and soft tissues which the ultrasound beam has to penetrate. Obesity or abdominal scars (i.e., from prior Caesarian section) can create difficulty in imaging because of the thicker abdominal wall and the increased distance of the fetus from the ultrasound source. Excessive amount of amniotic fluid as seen in polyhydramnios may also result in suboptimal images because of the distance of the fetus from the ultrasound source. Fetuses with oligohydramnios have minimal or no amniotic fluid required for adequate ultrasound transmission. Uterine anomalies, as seen in bicornuate uterus or a large fibroid, may result in poor imaging because of the thickened and irregular uterine mass and a fetus that may be placed in an unusual presentation. The presence of more than one fetus in the uterine cavity may result in the fetus being interrogated to be smaller or in a fetus being in an unusual position and location. The ideal position for fetal imaging is with the anterior fetal thorax in closest proximity to the ultrasound probe. Any other fetal position can create imaging difficulty because of the fetal spine and ribs that the ultrasound has to penetrate. Unfortunately, a fetus in the mid-second to early third trimester can change position easily and frequently, increasing the difficulty of the test. As the gestation reaches term, the fetus in a cephalic presentation may move into the

pelvic cavity, further increasing the distance of the heart from the transducer. Several noncardiac fetal anomalies can affect fetal cardiac imaging, including diaphragmatic hernia and large masses, by virtue of distortion of cardiac position.

EXAMINATION TECHNIQUE

There are certain aspects in cardiac imaging that are unique to the fetus. The heart is most easily imaged at 18–24 weeks age of gestational principally because of an optimal amniotic fluid volume/solid fetal mass ratio and a fetal skeleton that is not heavily calcified. The lungs are fluid filled, thus allowing for echocardiographic views that are different from postnatal examination. The fetal heart lies more horizontally in the thorax. The pulmonary arterial branches are small because of the small amount of pulmonary blood flow. The stomach is fluid-filled. In imaging the heart, the most crucial and very first step is determining the right-left orientation of the heart and the stomach. Two-dimensional echocardiographic imaging sweeps are then performed followed by color and spectral Doppler for flow assessment. Various transducer sweeps are applied to identify cardiac and vessels structures, including the venae cavae, pulmonary veins, atria, foramen ovale, atrioventricular valves, ventricles, outflow tracts, the great arteries with their valves and branches, ductus arteriosus, ductus venosus and the umbilical vessels (Figures 60-1 and 60-2).

Cardiac dimensions vary with gestational age. The right and left ventricular dimensions increase linearly with increasing gestation and with the fetal head's biparietal diameter. The right ventricle is slightly larger than the left ventricle (average ratio approximately 1.16:1). The right atrium is slightly larger than the left atrium (average ratio approximately 1.12:1). The aortic and pulmonary arterial sizes increase linearly with gestation and with the fetal head's biparietal diameter (average pulmonary artery/aortic ratio approximately 1.2:1). There is progressive tapering of the transverse aortic arch, with the smallest diameter being in the isthmus (that part of the aorta between the left subclavian artery and the ductus arteriosus). The right ventricular and

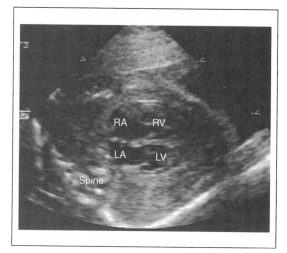

FIGURE 60-1

4 chamber view of the fetal heart (RA = right atrium, RV = right ventricle, LA = left atrium, LV = left ventricle).

left ventricular stroke volume and cardiac output increase exponentially with gestational age. The stroke volume of the right ventricle is larger than the left ventricle by about 28%. The physiologic increases in heart rate result in a decrease in ventricular size and stroke volume, with no change in ventricular output and shortening. Normal fetal

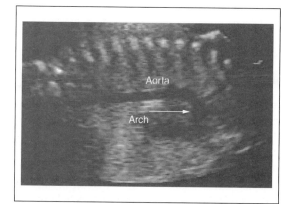

FIGURE 60-2

Fetal echocardiogram demonstrating the aorta and the aortic arch.

shortening fraction is 32–36%. The fetal ventricle is less compliant than the neonatal ventricle, probably because of decreased contractile elements in the fetal myocardium. This is evidenced by decreased passive Doppler filling velocities and higher filling velocities contributed by atrial contraction. In the neonate, child and adult, the passive Doppler filling velocities are much higher than the filling velocities contributed by atrial systole.

INDICATIONS FOR FETAL ECHOCARDIOGRAPHY

Fetal echocardiography is indicated when fetal, maternal, or familial factors are present that could result in higher risk for occurrence of fetal heart disease.

Table 60-2 lists the various fetal factors associated with an increased risk of detecting fetal heart disease.

Detection, accurate diagnosis, and management of fetal arrhythmia are important because of the association with higher perinatal and neonatal mortality, higher incidence of congenital heart disease and higher incidence of fetal distress. The fetal heart rate is faster than that of infants and children, averaging 130–140 beats per minute, falling to 125–130 beats per minute towards term. Fetal bradycardia is a heart rate less than 100 beats per minute. Fetal tachycardia is heart rate greater than 180 beats per minute. It is also the duration of abnormal heart rate that determines the presence of

TABLE 60-2

FETAL FACTORS ASSOCIATED WITH AN INCREASED RISK OF HEART DISEASE

1. Cardiac arrhythmia
2. Intrauterine growth retardation
3. Abnormal karyotype
4. Cardiac structural anomaly suspected during an obstetric screening ultrasonography
5. Noncardiovascular structural anomalies
6. Fetal distress, heart failure or hydrops

symptoms, with sustained rates ≤60 beats per minute or ≥220 beats generally not tolerated.

Nonimmune hydrops fetalis is now more common than immune hydrops fetalis, and fetal arrhythmia has become the most common cause of nonimmune hydrops fetalis. A fetal electrocardiogram through the maternal abdomen is difficult to acquire because of the stronger voltages detected from the maternal heart. The pattern of Doppler spectral velocity waveforms and M-mode echocardiography are used to indirectly provide the electrophysiologic diagnosis of fetal rhythm disorders. Cardiac rhythm diagnosis from echocardiography is based on the mechanical performance of the atria and the ventricles and not on actual electrophysiologic phenomena. A new method that is not yet generally available is a fetal magnetocardiogram, a recording of the magnetic field generated by the electrical activity of the fetal heart. This recording actually has the same waveforms found in the electrocardiogram—P waves, QRS complexes, T waves and measurable intervals. Fetal magnetocardiography may allow the accurate electrophysiologic diagnosis of arrhythmias.

Structural heart disease occurs in 6–15% of fetuses with arrhythmia. Slow fetal heart rates are caused by sinus bradycardia, blocked premature atrial contractions, second-degree atrioventricular block, or complete (third-degree) atrioventricular block. An irregular fetal heart rhythm may be from premature atrial or premature ventricular contractions. Fast fetal heart rates are caused by sinus tachycardia, supraventricular tachycardia, atrial flutter, chaotic atrial tachycardia or ventricular tachycardia.

Sinus bradycardia is usually a transient phenomenon observed during an ultrasound procedure owing to pressure on the uterus by the ultrasound probe. Premature atrial contraction is the most frequent type of arrhythmia seen. Rarely, premature atrial contractions may be associated with supraventricular tachycardia, but, in general, premature atrial contractions are benign and do not require any treatment. Premature ventricular contractions in the fetus are rare. They have been associated with cardiomyopathy, cardiac tumors, complete heart block with very slow ventricular escape beats, long QT syndrome and structural cardiac anomalies.

Second-degree atrioventricular block is a rare diagnosis in utero. Cases have been reported of this rhythm disorder that evolved into complete atrioventricular block, usually in the presence of maternal lupus erythematosus. Complete atrioventricular block or third-degree atrioventricular block is one of the leading causes of nonimmune hydrops fetalis. A poor prognosis is observed if the heart rate is ≤55 beats per minute. Structural heart disease is seen in about 40%, the most common of which are corrected transposition of great arteries and common atrioventricular canal defect. Common atrioventricular canal associated with complete heart block has a 96% mortality rate; however, there is an 83% survival for complete heart block if the heart is structurally normal. Asymptomatic mothers of fetuses with isolated complete heart block should be evaluated for collagen vascular disease because of the high association with the presence of anti-Ro (SS-A) and anti-La (SS-B) antibodies. These mothers may be at risk for the occurrence of frank symptoms of collagen vascular disease later.

An abnormally fast heart rate may be from sinus tachycardia, atrioventricular reentry tachycardia, atrial flutter/fibrillation or ventricular tachycardia. Sinus tachycardia in the fetus (usually between 180 and 200 beats per minute) is usually a result of an underlying abnormality such as hypoxia, acidosis, infection, distress, myocarditis, or maternal drug ingestion. Sinus tachycardia does not usually result in hydrops and is managed by treating the underlying cause. The other forms of tachycardia may result in various degrees of fetal hydrops including pericardial or pleural effusion, ascites, or generalized edema. Reentry types of supraventricular tachycardia commonly present with a fast heart rate (220–300 beats per minute) with little variability, abrupt onset and cessation, and a one to one atrioventricular conduction which may be sustained or nonsustained. Occasionally, Wolf-Parkinson-White syndrome may be documented in a fetal magnetocardiogram. Fetal atrioventricular reentry tachycardia usually occurs in an otherwise structurally normal heart, but has been associated with Ebstein anomaly, corrected transposition of great arteries, and cardiac tumors crossing the atrioventricular groove. Atrial flutter is characterized by a faster rate (400–500 beats per minute) and variable atrioventricular block (atrial rate faster than the ventricular rate). Ventricular tachycardia is relatively rare and has been seen in myocarditis, cardiac tumors, and in association with complete atrioventricular block.

Pharmacologic agents to treat fetal tachycardia can be delivered transplacentally (orally or intravenously through the mother) or by direct fetal administration. Medications that have been used include: digoxin, flecainide, verapamil, procainamide, quinidine, amiodarone, propranolol, and sotalol. Delivery and postnatal therapy is the treatment of choice for term babies or for near-term fetuses with documented fetal lung maturity. Prematurity in the presence of hydrops contributes to the morbidity and mortality. Delivery before 35 weeks age of gestation is indicated if there is progressive heart failure and inability to convert the tachycardia in spite of aggressive therapy, or if there are signs of fetal distress.

The presence of intrauterine growth retardation (Table 60-3) is an indication for fetal cardiac evaluation. Intrauterine growth retardation may be the result of the interplay of maternal, fetal, or environmental conditions associated with a higher risk for occurrence of structural or functional fetal cardiac disorders. Growth retardation may be a reflection of the competency of the fetoplacental unit. Chronic uterine insufficiency has been shown to present with certain echocardiographic parameters. Decreased or absent diastolic flow velocity in the aorta and umbilical artery indicates increased placental vascular resistance. Reversed flow signals in the inferior vena cava may be seen, compared with the near-continuous flow velocity seen normally. If these Doppler profiles are observed, early delivery may be indicated.

Another fetal risk factor for cardiac defects is documentation of an abnormal fetal karyotype. A fetal karyotype is determined from cell samples taken from the amniotic fluid or from the chorionic villus. Amniocentesis and karyotyping are advised in the presence of advanced maternal age (≥35 years of age), abnormal maternal serum markers, a history of previous chromosomal abnormalities, a family history of cardiac abnormalities, other fetal ultrasound abnormalities, and recurring spontaneous abortions. Advanced maternal age is the most common indication for prenatal cytogenetic diagnosis. Although chromosomal abnormalities occur in offspring of mothers of all ages, the frequency of trisomic offspring increases with age, rising exponentially after age 35. The cause is unknown. Prenatal diagnosis should be offered to all women who will be ≥35 year at delivery. Abnormal maternal serum markers (alpha-fetoprotein, human chorionic gonadotropin, and unconjugated estriol) indicate an increased risk of carrying a fetus with Down syndrome (low alpha-fetoprotein, low estriol, and high chorionic gonadotropin) or trisomy 18 (low alpha-fetoprotein, low estriol, and low human chorionic gonadotropin). There is an increased risk of chromosomal abnormalities, that may be associated with the occurrence of a fetal heart defect, when chromosomal abnormalities are seen in a previous child or a parent or when a couple has had a child with physical anomalies and unknown chromosomal status; thus, prenatal karyotype analysis is advised. Parental chromosomal abnormalities are most often diagnosed during evaluation for recurrent spontaneous abortions (habitual abortions), children with malformations, or a history of infertility.

TABLE 60-3

CAUSES OF INTRAUTERINE GROWTH RETARDATION ASSOCIATED WITH AN INCREASED RISK OF FETAL CARDIAC DISEASE

1. Maternal causes
   a. Multiple fetuses in same pregnancy
   b. Abnormalities of placental blood supply
   c. Maternal cardiovascular disease (hypertension, toxemia, diabetes)
   d. Maternal infection (rubella)
2. Fetal causes
   a. Chromosomal/genetic abnormalities (Turner, Down, and so forth)
   b. Twin-twin transfusion/TRAP (twin reversed arterial perfusion)
   c. Cardiac defects
3. Environmental
   a. Alcohol
   b. Cocaine
   c. Warfarin
   d. Phenytoin

There is a high association between congenital heart disease and an abnormal karyotype (Chapter 11). Likewise certain genetic syndromes are associated with congenital abnormalities.

Fetal echocardiography is also advised in the presence of a noncardiovascular structural anomaly in the fetus. Fetal extracardiac abnormalities have a 25–45% chance of having an associated structural cardiac anomaly. Anomalies of the renal system have a 50% risk, while central nervous system anomalies have only a 2–5% risk for heart defects. Certain specific extracardiac anomalies may be associated with heart defects such as left-sided diaphragmatic hernia with hypoplastic left heart syndrome, and duodenal atresia with an endocardial cushion defect. Likewise, specific cardiac lesions can be associated with extracardiac malformations: atrial septal defect (51–74%), atrioventricular canal (36–43%), ventricular septal defect (29–43%), tetralogy of Fallot (28–31%), coarctation of aorta (19–26%), truncus arteriosus (14–48%) and hypoplastic left heart syndrome (12–14%).

Fetal echocardiography is the tool used to document the presence of fetal heart failure. A normal fetal heart circumference is approximately half the circumference of the thorax. Cardiac size is the best predictor of outcome in fetal heart failure, with zero survival when the chamber size is above the 95th percentile. Prolonged cardiomegaly can lead to fetal lung compression and pulmonary hypoplasia. A depressed ventricular function may also be seen. When hydrops fetalis does occur, there may be subcutaneous edema (skin thickness ≥5 mm), pleural or pericardial effusion, ascites, polyhydramnios and placental thickening.

The finding of signs of fetal hydrops necessitates a careful and comprehensive search for its etiology. One important cause is exposure to indomethacin. Indomethacin is occasionally used as a tocolytic agent in patients with premature labor and to decrease amniotic fluid volume in polyhydramnios; however, because the ductus arteriosus can be responsive to this prostaglandin synthetase inhibitor, fetal ductal constriction or even closure could occur. This may result in acute right ventricular failure and even hydrops fetalis. Fortunately,

the effect is often reversible, and echocardiography can be used to monitor therapy.

Echocardiography is indicated in certain maternal and familial conditions (Table 60-4). While the risk of having a heart defect is 8 in 1000 live births, the risk of occurrence of fetal heart defect for subsequent pregnancy increases to 1.5–3% depending on the anomaly involved (Chapter 11).

The recurrence risk of heart defect is increased if either the mother or father is affected (Table 60-5). There is a higher risk if the mother is affected, suggesting the influence of mitochondrial or ribosomal DNA that have a maternal source.

The presence of acquired maternal cardiovascular heart diseases such as rheumatic heart disease,

---

TABLE 60-4

MATERNAL AND FAMILIAL FACTORS ASSOCIATED WITH AN INCREASE OF HEART DISEASE

1. History of congenital heart disease
2. Genetic syndromes
3. Maternal diabetes
4. Exposure to known cardiac teratogens
5. Collagen vascular disease
6. Certain maternal infections

TABLE 60-5

RECURRENCE RISK FOR CONGENITAL HEART DEFECT GIVEN ONE AFFECTED PARENT

	Percent Risk	
	Mother Affected	Father Affected
Aortic stenosis	13–15	3
Atrial septal defect	4–4.5	1.5
Atrioventricular canal	14	1
Coarctation of aorta	4	2
Patent ductus arteriosus	3.5–4	2.5
Pulmonary stenosis	4–5.5	2
Tetralogy of Fallot	2.5	1.5
Ventricular septal defect	6–10	2

TABLE 60-6

POTENTIAL CARDIAC TERATOGENS

Drugs	Frequency of Cardiac Malformation (%)	Type of Cardiac Malformation
Alcohol	25–30	VSD, PDA, ASD
Amphetamines	5–10	VSD, PDA, ASD, TGA
Phenytoin	2–5	PS, VSD, AS, ASD
Trimethadione	15–30	TGA, TOF, HLHS
Lithium	10	Ebstein
Retinoic acid	10	VSD
Thalidomide	5–10	TOF, VSD, ASD, Truncus arteriosus

hypertension, or cardiomyopathy should be considered for fetal cardiac evaluation because of the effect of these diseases on the fetoplacental well-being and the possibility of fetal effect by the maternal medications.

Maternal diabetes mellitus is a common reason for referral for fetal cardiac evaluation. Congenital cardiac malformation may be seen in about 5% of infants of diabetic mothers but echocardiographic evidence of hypertrophic cardiomyopathy may be observed in as many as 30% of fetuses. Structural malformations are more frequently seen in those with preexisting diabetes mellitus than in true gestational diabetes. Congenital malformation rates are not increased among offspring of women with true gestational diabetes in whom metabolic disturbances are not present during organogenesis. The most frequent cardiac anomalies include ventricular septal defect and transposition of great arteries. Other defects involving the great arteries, including truncus arteriosus and double outlet right ventricle, are also prevalent. The relative risk for hypertrophic cardiomyopathy increases if the mother has gestational diabetes and develops poor control or insulin resistance in the third trimester. Fetal hypertrophic cardiomyopathy, frequently manifesting as a disproportionately hypertrophied ventricular septum, is an anabolic result of fetal hyperinsulinemia triggered by maternal hyperglycemia during the third trimester. Cardiac septal

hypertrophy correlates with maternal glycosylated haemoglobin levels. Neonatal hypertrophic cardiomyopathy usually resolves within six months.

As has been discussed, maternal collagen vascular disease may result in fetal complete heart block. Fetal cardiomyopathy with fetal hydrops could also occur. Maternal phenylketonuria is associated with a five-fold increase in incidence of tetralogy of Fallot. Certain maternal infections may affect the fetal heart. Rubella infection is known to cause peripheral pulmonary arterial stenosis and postnatal persistence of the ductus arteriosus. Coxsackie virus infection may result in fetal myocarditis. Human parvovirus infection (Fifth disease) may result in myocarditis, pericardial effusion, gross hydrops fetalis, and even still-birth.

Certain drugs taken during pregnancy increase the chance of congenital heart disease (Table 60-6).

ACCURACY OF DIAGNOSIS

As imaging technology became more refined with the advent of high frequency transducers, the ability to zoom on distant structures without losing resolution, and the availability of color, pulsed and continuous-wave Doppler, the diagnosis of fetal heart abnormalities has become consistently accurate. There are very few false positive diagnoses of congenital heart disease. False negative findings may be seen in total anomalous pulmonary venous connection (because of close proximity of the common pulmonary venous chamber to left atrium), coarctation of aorta, and certain lesions that are difficult to distinguish from normal such as a patent foramen ovale, atrial septal defect, postnatal patent ductus arteriosus, tiny ventricular septal defect, minor valvar anomalies, and peripheral pulmonary stenosis. There are also lesions that can progress beyond the time of ultrasonographic examination. These include valvar anomalies (aortic and pulmonary stenosis), coarctation of aorta, cardiac tumor, ventricular hypoplasia, hypertrophic cardiomyopathy, and dilated cardiomyopathy.

ADVANTAGES OF DETECTION

Accurate antenatal diagnosis of the heart can now be provided. Fetal cardiology has allowed for a far greater understanding of the intrauterine spectrum of the natural course of heart defect. It is now known that those fetuses diagnosed to have cardiac defects have a higher incidence of spontaneous intrauterine death and a higher risk for chromosomal or genetic abnormality. Knowledge of preexisting cardiac disease permits optimum chance of infant survival. Options for in utero or immediate postnatal therapy or intervention can be implemented. Expectant delivery and possible resuscitation can be planned with delivery in institutions with the appropriate personnel available. Knowledge of carrying a child with heart disease gives parents the option of terminating the pregnancy in the presence of severe heart disease. Mothers prepared for the birth of a child with a heart defect appear emotionally better able to deal with the situation. Parents of fetuses in whom a heart defect is ruled out feel great relief. Finally, parental advice and counseling regarding future pregnancies can be properly undertaken during the fetal evaluation.

Because of advances in the field of fetal cardiac imaging and obstetric and cardiologic therapy and intervention, a fetus suspected to have a cardiac disease should be referred to an expert in fetal cardiology for proper advice, workup and treatment.

Suggested Readings

Allan L, Hornberger LK, Sharland G (eds): *Textbook of Fetal Cardiology*. London, UK, Greenwich Medical Media, 2000.

Allen HD, Gutgesell HP, Clark EB, Driscoll DJ (eds): *Moss and Adams' Heart Disease, in Infants, Children and Adolescents*. Baltimore, MD, Lippincott Williams & Wilkins, 2001, Chap. 24 (Maternal diseases and therapies affecting the fetal cardiovascular system by Rosemary E. Reiss, pp. 551–568) and Chap. 25 (Congenital heart disease and arrhythmias in the fetus by Daniel G. Rowland and John J. Wheller, pp. 569–581).

APPENDIX: PHARMACOLOGY IN PEDIATRIC CARDIOLOGY

INOTROPIC AND VASOPRESSOR AGENTS

Amrinone

INOCOR

Onset: 2–5 min

Mode of action: Myocardial cAMP phosphodiesterase inhibitor, increase intracellular cAMP resulting in better myocardial function, pulmonary and systemic vasodilation

Route	Dose	Frequency
Infusion	Load: 0.5 mg/kg may be repeated q20 min Maintenance: 5–20 μg/kg/min	

Side effects: Arrhythmia, thrombocytopenia
Caution: Bleeding disorder, hypertrophic cardiomyopathy, hypotension

Calcium Chloride

Onset: Rapid

Mode of action: Enhances contractility through regulation of action potential

Route	Dose	Frequency
IV	Hypocalcemia: 10–20 mg/kg	q10 min

Side effects: Bradycardia, hypotension, peripheral vasodilation, hypercalcemia, hypermagnesemia, hyperchloremic acidosis
Caution: Central venous line administration ONLY. Maximum concentration is 20 mg/mL infusion. May precipitate arrhythmia in digitalized patient. Extravasation may lead to tissue necrosis (use local hyaluronidase if this occurs).
Contraindication: Hypercalcemia, ventricular fibrillation

Adapted from: The Pediatric Cardiology Pharmacopeia By: Ra'id Abdulla, Sharon Young and Steve Barnes Published in *Pediatric Cardiology*, vol. 18, no. 3, 1997.

Calcium Gluconate

Onset: Rapid

Mode of action: Enhances contractility through regulation of action potential

Route	Dose	Frequency
PO, IV	Hypocalcemia: 50–125 mg/kg, max = 4 g	qid

Side effects: Bradycardia, hypotension, peripheral vasodilation, hypercalcemia, hypermagnesemia
Caution: Central venous line administration ONLY. Maximum concentration is 20 mg/mL infusion. May precipitate arrhythmia in digitalized patient. Extravasation may lead to tissue necrosis (use local hyaluronidase if this occurs).
Contraindication: Hypercalcemia, ventricular fibrillation

Digoxin

LANOXIN, LANOXICAPS

Onset: PO: 1–2 h, IV: 5–30 min

Mode of action: Inhibition of Na^+-K^+ pump resulting in increase Ca^{2+} intracellular influx

Route	Dose	Frequency
PO	Loading: 10 μg/kg max = 375 μg Maintenance: 5 μg/kg, max = 125 μg Premature infants should receive 1/2 loading and maintenance doses	q6 h × 4
IV	75% of PO doses	bid

Side effects: Sinus bradycardia, AV block, fatigue, headache, nausea, anorexia, neuralgias, blurred vision, photophobia
Caution: Renal failure. Cardioversion or calcium infusion may cause VF in patients receiving digoxin (pretreatment with Lidocaine may be helpful)
Therapeutic level: 0.8–2 ng/mL, not reliable in neonates, since they may have falsely elevated levels (because of maternal digoxin like substances in serum)
Contraindication: Ventricular arrhythmia, AV block, IHSS, constrictive pericarditis

Dobutamine

DOBUTREX

Onset: Rapid

Mode of action: Stimulates beta-adrenergic receptors, resulting in increase myocardial contractility and heart rate

Route	Dose	Frequency
Infusion	2–20 μg/kg/min max = 40 μg/kg/min	

Side effects: Ventricular arrhythmias, hypertrophic cardiomyopathy, tachycardia, hypertension, angina, palpitation, headache
Caution: Patient should be euvolemic
Contraindication: IHSS, tachycardia, arrhythmias, hypertension

Dopamine

INTROPIN

Onset: Rapid

Mode of action: Through norepinephrine by stimulating adrenergic and dopaminergic receptors, selective renal vasodilation

Route	Dose	Frequency
Infusion	Renal dose: 2–5 μg/kg/min Inotropic dose: 5–15 μg/kg/min	

Side effects: Tachyarrhythmias, premature beats, hypertension, headache, nausea
Caution: Correct hypovolemia. Extravasation will cause tissue necrosis, phentolamine should be infiltrated around the extravasation to minimize necrosis. Do *not* use discolored solution, high doses (>15 μg/kg/min causes decrease renal perfusion)
Contraindication: Infusion through UAC, pheochromocytoma, ventricular fibrillation

Epinephrine HCl

ADRENALINE

Onset: 1–5 min

Mode of action:

Inotropy: Beta-adrenergic receptor stimulation

Vasoconstriction: Alpha-adrenergic receptor stimulation

Route	Dose	Frequency
IV, ETT	Bradycardia/hypotension: 1:10,000 0.1 mL/kg	q3–5 min
Infusion	1–10 μg/kg/min	q3–5 min

Side effects: Tachyarrhythmias, hypertension, headache, nervousness, nausea, vomiting, decrease renal flow
Caution: Hyperthyroidisim, hypertension, arrhythmias. Do *not* use discolored solution. Extravasation will cause tissue necrosis, phentolamine should be infiltrated around the extravasation to minimize necrosis
Contraindication: Acute coronary artery disease, angle closure glaucoma

Milrinone

PRIMACOR

Onset: Rapid

Mode of action: Myocardial cAMP phosphodiesterase inhibitor, increase intracellular cAMP resulting in better myocardial function, pulmonary and systemic vasodilation

Route	Dose	Frequency
Infusion	Load: 50 μg/kg, over 10–15 min Maintenance: 0.1–1 μg/kg/min	

Side effects: Arrhythmia, headache, hypotension, thrombocytopenia rarely reported
Caution: Renal dysfunction
Contraindication: Severe pulmonary or aortic obstructive disease

Phenylephrine HCl

NEO-SYNEPHRINE

Onset: Rapid

Mode of action: Alpha-adrenergic receptors stimulant

Route	Dose	Frequency
IV	5–20 μg/kg, max = 0.5 mg	q10–15 min
Infusion	0.1–0.5 μg/kg/min, max = 4 μg/kg/min	

Side effects: Tremor, insomnia, palpitation, hypertension, angina, excitability, headache, tremors, bradycardia
Caution: Hypertension, hyperthyroidism, arrhythmia, hyperglycemia. Extravasation will cause tissue necrosis, phentolamine should be infiltrated around the extravasation to minimize necrosis
Contraindication: Pheochromocytoma, severe hypertension, ventricular tachyarrhythmias, severe coronary artery disease

Norepinephrine

LEVOPHED

Onset: Rapid

Mode of action: Stimulates alpha- and beta-adrenergic receptors (predominantly alpha effect)

Route	Dose	Frequency
Infusion	0.05–0.1 μg/kg/min, max = 2 μg/kg/min	

Side effects: Arrhythmias, palpitation, hypertension, angina, headache, anxiety, vomiting, uterine contractions, respiratory distress, diaphoresis
Caution: Hypertension, arrhythmia, occlusive vascular disease. Extravasation will cause tissue necrosis, phentolamine should be infiltrated around the extravasation to minimize necrosis
Contraindication: Pheochromocytoma, severe hypertension, ventricular tachyarrhythmias, severe coronary artery disease

ANTIARRHYTHMIC AGENTS

Adenosine

ADENOCARD

Onset: Very rapid

Mode of action: Slows AV node conduction

Route	Dose	Frequency
IV, rapid push	0.1 mg/kg Increase by 0.05 mg increments every 2 min to a max of 0.25 mg/kg, max = 12 mg/dose	Rapid IV push q2 min prn

Side effects: Palpitations, flushing, headache, dyspnea, nausea, chest pain, lightheadedness, bradycardia
Caution: Bronchospasm in asthmatics
Contraindication: AV block or sick sinus syndrome, unless pacemaker placed
Drug interactions: Potentiates effects of dipyridamole. Carbamazepine may increase heart block. Theophylline antagonizes effect of adenosine

Amiodarone

CORDARONE

Onset: 3 days–3 weeks

Mode of action: Class III, inhibits alpha- and beta-adrenergic receptors, prolongs action potential and refractoriness

Route	Dose	Frequency
PO	Loading: 10–15 mg/kg max = 1600 mg Maintenance: 2.5–5 mg/kg, max = 800 mg	qd × 7–14 days
Infusion	Load: 5–7 mg/kg over 20–30 min Maintenance: 10–20 mg/kg/day	qd

Side effects: Long half life. Pulmonary fibrosis, alters thyroid (hypothyroidism) and liver dysfunction. Worsening AV block and bradycardias. Anorexia, nausea, vomiting, dizziness, paresthesia, ataxia and tremor, corneal deposits, blue discoloration of skin, photosensitivity
Caution: Increases digoxin (reduce dose by 1/2), warfarin, flecainide, procainamide, quinidine and phenytoin serum levels, thyroid disease
Therapeutic level: 0.5–2.5 mg/L
Contraindications: AV block, sinus node dysfunction, sinus bradycardia

Atenolol

TENORMIN

Onset: 60–120 min

Mode of action: Class II antiarrhythmic agent, long acting selective β_1 blocker

Route	Dose	Frequency
PO	0.8–2 mg/kg	qd

Side effects: Hypoglycemia, hypotension, nausea, vomiting, depression, weakness, less bronchospam than propranolol, heart block, bradycardia, negative inotropic effect
Caution: Congestive heart failure (CHF), adjust dose in renal failure
Contraindication: Cardiogenic shock, pulmonary edema

Bretylium Tosylate

BRETYLOL

Onset: IV: 6–20 min, IM: <2 h

Mode of action: Class III antiarrhythmic agent, sodium channel blocker, inhibits norepinephrine release

Route	Dose	Frequency
IV, IM	5–10 mg/kg	qid

Side effects: Hypertension followed by hypotension, PVC, arrhythmias, increased sensitivity to digitalis and catecholamines, nausea, vomiting, vertigo, confusion, lethargy
Caution: Pulmonary hypertension, aortic stenosis, renal dysfunction
Contraindication: Digitalis induced arrhythmias

Disopyramide

NORPACE

Onset: Minutes

Mode of action: Class Ia antiarrhythmic agent, sodium channel blockers depresses myocardial excitability

Route	Dose	Frequency
PO	2.5–5 mg/kg	qid

Side effects: Negative inotropic effect, prolong QRS and QT durations, ventricular arrhythmias, anticholinergic effect (dry mouth, urinary retention, constipation), nausea, vomiting, hypoglycemia, cholestasis, syncope
Caution: Already prolonged QRS or QT durations, CHF, renal dysfunction
Contraindication: Already reduced myocardial contractility, AV block
Drug interactions: Increase disopyramide effect: erythromycin because of decrease in metabolism. Decrease disoparymide effect: Hepatic inducing agents, phenobarbital, phenytoin, rifampin

Esmolol

BREVIBLOC

Onset: Rapid

Mode of action: Class II. Selective β_1 blocker

Route	Dose	Frequency
Infusion	Loading: 0.5 mg/kg Maintenance: 50 μg/kg/min, increase by 50 μg/kg increments to a maximum of 300 μg/kg/min. Reload with each increase. Titrate to effect	Over 1 min

Side effects: Hypoglycemia, hypotension, nausea, vomiting, depression, phlebitis, bronchospam at higher doses, heart block, bradycardia, negative inotropic effect
Caution: Skin necrosis may occur with extravasation, maximum concentration: 10 mg/mL because of hyperosmolarity. May increase digoxin or theophylline serum levels
Contraindication: Cardiogenic shock, heart block, severe asthma

Flecainide

TAMBOCOR

Onset: Rapid

Mode of action: Class Ic antiarrhythmic agent, sodium channel blocker, cell membrane depression

Route	Dose	Frequency
PO	1–2 mg/kg max = 100 mg	tid

Side effects: Negative inotropic effect, arrhythmias, rash
Caution: Heart failure, heart block, hepatic impairment, reduce dose by 25–50% in renal failure
Contraindication: 2nd or 3rd degree AV block
Therapeutic level: 0.2–1 μg/mL

Lidocaine

XYLOCAINE

Onset: Rapid

Mode of action: Class Ib antiarrhythmic agent, sodium channel blocker, local anesthetic depressing myocardial irritability

Route	Dose	Frequency
IV	0.5–1.0 mg/kg	Repeat after 5 min, prn
Infusion	20–50 μg/kg/min	

Side effects: Hypotension, shock, nausea, seizures, respiratory depression, anxiety, euphoria, drowsiness, agitation
Caution: Hepatic disease, heart failure
Contraindication: AV block
Therapeutic level: 2–5 μg/mL

Phenytoin

DILANTIN

Onset: Minutes

Mode of action: Not well defined

Route	Dose	Frequency
PO	2.5–5 mg/kg	bid
IV	Load: 1.25 mg/kg	
(Arrhythmia dose)	Maintenance: 2.5–5 mg/kg, max = 250 mg	bid

Side effects: Gingival hyperplasia, hirsutisim, exfoliative dermatitis, osteomalacia, ataxia, drowsiness, blood dyscrasias, systemic lupus erythmatosus (SLE) like syndrome, Stevens-Johnson syndrome, peripheral neuropathy, lymphadenopathy, hepatitis, nystagmus, hypotension, bradycardia, folic acid deficiency
Caution: Oral absorption reduced in neonates, serum levels are increased by cimetidine, chloramphenicol, INH, sulfonamide, trimethoprim. Rapid injection may cause hypotension and bradycardia
Contraindication: Heart block or sinus bradycardia

Procainamide

PRONESTYL, PROCAN SR

Onset: IV: Rapid PO: 2–4 h, IM: 10–30 min

Mode of action: Class Ia antiarrhythmic agent, sodium channel blocker depressing myocardial excitability and conduction

Route	Dose	Frequency
PO	4–12 mg/kg max = 1g	q3–6 h
IV	Load: 5–15 mg/kg max = 100 mg	over 30 min
Infusion	Maintenance: 20–80 μg/kg/min, max = 6 mg/min	

Side effects: Hypotension, prolongs QRS and QT durations, SLE like symptoms, fever, positive coomb's test, thrombocytopenia, rash, myalgia, arrhythmias, GI symptoms, confusion
Caution: Toxicity when QRS >0.2 s
Therapeutic level: 4–10 mg/L of procainamide, or 10–30 mg/L of procainamide and NAPA levels combined
Drug interactions: PA and NAPA levels are increased with: cimetidine, ranitidine, amiodarone, beta-blockers, trimethoprin. Anticholinergic agents enhance effect
Contraindication: Myasthenia gravis, complete heart block

Propafenone

RHYTHMOL

Onset: Rapid

Mode of action: Class Ic antiarrhythmic agent, also blocks sodium channels and beta blocker effect

Route	Dose	Frequency
PO	2–3 mg/kg	tid
IV	1–2 mg/kg	
Infusion	4–8 μg/kg/min	

Side effects: AV block, palpitations, bradycardia, CHF, conduction disturbances, dizziness, drowsiness, dry mouth, altered taste, dyspnea, flatulence, blurred vision, dyspepsia
Caution: Recent MI, CHF, hepatic or renal dysfunction
Contraindication: Cardiogenic shock, bronchospastic disorder, conduction disorder

Propranolol

INDERAL

Onset: PO: 40–120 min, IV: Rapid

Mode of action: β blocker, class II antidysrhythmic agent

Route	Dose	Frequency
PO	0.5–1 mg/kg	qid
IV	0.01–0.15 mg/kg,	qid, prn
(over 10 min)	max = 1 mg/dose	

Side effects: Hypo or hyperglycemia, hypotension, nausea, vomiting, depression, weakness, bronchospasm, heart block, bradycardia, negative inotropic effect

Caution: In lung disease, heart, hepatic or renal failure. Barbiturates, rifampin or indomethacin will increase clearance, cimetidine, hydralazine, chlorpromazine, or verapamil cause decrease in clearance and enhanced effect

Contraindication: Asthma. Cardiogenic shock and heart block

Quinidine

Onset: Gluconate: IV 30–60 min, PO 4–8 h, Sulfate: 1 h

Mode of action: Class Ia antidysrhythmic agent, sodium channel blocker, depressing atrial and ventricular excitability. Vagolytic

Route	Dose	Frequency
PO	Gluconate: 4–10 mg/kg, max = 600 mg	tid
	Sulfate: 6 mg/kg	qid
	max = 600 mg	
IV, IM	Gluconate: 2–10 mg/kg	q3–6 h, prn
	max = 400 mg	

Side effects: GI symptoms, hypotension, tinnitus, thrombotic thrombocytpenic purpura, rash, heart block, blood changes, widen QRS complex, prolongs QT, ventricular arrhythmia, thrombocytopenia, anemia

Caution: Toxicity is indicated by QRS interval >0.02 s. Causes increase of digoxin serum level (reduce digoxin by 1/2). Quinidine's effect is enhanced by amiodarone or cimetidine. Quinidine's effect is reduced by rifampin, phenytoin or barbiturates. Atrial flutter may conduct 1:1 when quinidine is used alone, owing to enhancement of AV conduction

Therapeutic level: 2–7 mg/L

Contraindication: AV block

Tocainide

TONOCARD

Onset: 10–20 min

Mode of action: Sodium channel blocker, local anesthetic depressing myocardial irritability

Route	Dose	Frequency
PO	9–13 mg/kg max = 700 mg	tid

Side effects: Rash, nausea, arrhythmias, dizziness, vertigo, blood changes
Therapeutic level: 4–10 μg/mL

Verapamil

ISOPTIN, CALAN, VERELAN

Onset: PO: 60–120 min, IV: Rapid

Mode of action: Class IV calcium channel blocker

Route	Dose	Frequency
PO	1.5–3.5 mg/kg max = 160 mg	tid
IV over 2–3 min	<1 year: 0.1–0.2 mg/kg, >1 year: 0.1–0.3 mg/kg max = 5 mg/dose	q30 min prn If stable: tid, bid

Side effects: Negative inotropic effect, constipation, hypotension, dizziness, fatigue
Caution: Extreme caution in infants and in WPW, may cause apnea, bradycardia, or hypotension. Do not use with other negative inotropes (e.g., beta-blockers). To reverse hypotension use calcium, isopreternol, and IV volume. Reduce digoxin by 1/3 to 1/2
Contraindication: CHF, hypotension, shock, AV block, right-to-left shunt lesions, atrial fibrillation, sinus bradycardia
Drug interactions: May increase serum level of digoxin, quinidine, carbamazepine, cyclosporin. Phenobarbital and rifampin may increase metabolism of verapamil

VASODILATORS

Captopril

CAPOTEN

Onset: 15–30 min

Mode of action: Angiotensin converting enzyme inhibitor

Route	Dose	Frequency
PO	Neonates:	tid
	0.05–0.1 mg/kg	
	Infants and children:	tid
	Initially: 0.15–0.3 mg/kg, then titrate to a max	
	of 2 mg/kg	
	Adolescents and adults:	tid
	12.5–25 mg, increase weekly by 25 mg/dose	
	max = 150 mg/dose	

Side effects: Hypotension, rash, proteinurea, neutropenia, tachycardia, cough, diminution of taste, reduce aldosterone production causing increase potassium renal absorption causing hyperkalemia
Caution: Adjust with renal dysfunction, administer 1 h prior to meals
Drug interactions: NSAIDs, e.g., indomethacin, may decrease the antihypertensive effect of captopril. Potassium sparing agents will potentiate hyperkalemic effect

Diazoxide

HYPERSTAT

Onset: Rapid

Mode of action: Vasodilator

Route	Dose	Frequency
IV, rapid	1–3 mg/kg	q5–15 min prn,
injection over 30 s	max = 150 mg	then q4–24 h

Side effects: Hyponatremia, salt and water retention, arrhythmia, hypotension, GI disturbances, ketoacidosis, rash, hyperuricemia, hyperglycemia, flushing, tachycardia, dizziness, phlebitis
Caution: Diabetes mellitus, renal or hepatic disease
Contraindication: Coarctation of the aorta, AV shunts, dissecting aortic aneurysm

Enalapril

VASOTEC

Onset: PO: 30–60 min, IV: 10–15 min

Mode of action: Angiotensin converting enzyme inhibitor

Route	Dose	Frequency
PO	0.1 mg/kg max = 40 mg/day	qd, bid
IV, slow over 5 min	5–10 μg/kg max = 1.25 mg	qid

Side effects: Nausea, diarrhea, headache, dizziness, hypotension rash, diminishing of taste, neutropenia, hyperkalemia, hypoglycemia, chronic cough
Caution: Reduce dose in renal failure
Drug interactions: NSAIDs, e.g., indomethacin, may decrease the antihypertensive effect. Potassium sparing agents will potentiate hyperkalemic effect

Hydralazine

APRESOLINE

Onset: PO: 10–30 min, IV: 5–20 min

Mode of action: Peripheral vasodilator

Route	Dose	Frequency
PO	0.3–1.5 mg/kg max = 25 mg	bid, qid
IV, IM	0.1–0.2 mg/kg max = 20 mg	q4–q6 h

Side effects: SLE like syndrome (reversible), palpitation, flushing, rash hematologic changes. Hypotension, tachycardia, headache, anorexia, nausea
Caution: Severe renal failure and cardiac disease, CVA
Contraindication: Coronary artery disease, dissecting aortic aneurysm, mitral valve rheumatic heart disease

Metoprolol

LOPRESSOR

Onset: 15–30 min

Mode of action: selective β_1 blocker

Route	Dose	Frequency
PO	0.5–2.5 mg/kg, max = 225 mg	bid
IV	0.1–0.3 mg/kg, over 1 h	

Side effects: Hypoglycemia, hypotension, nausea, vomiting, abdominal pain, CNS symptoms (depression, weakness, dizziness) bronchospasm, heart block, bradycardia, negative inotropic effect
Caution: In lung disease, heart, hepatic or renal failure
Drug interactions: Barbiturates, rifampin will increase clearance of metoprolol. Metoprolol metabolism decreases with cimetidine, amiodarone, diltiazem, propafenone, quinidine, hydralazine, chlorpromazine, or verapamil
Contraindication: Asthma, heart block with concurrent use of verapamil

Nifedipine

ADALAT, PROCARDIA

Onset: PO 20–30 min, sublingual 1–5 min

Mode of action: Calcium channel blocker

Route	Dose	Frequency
PO, sublingual	0.25–0.5 mg/kg max = 10 mg	tid, qid

Side effects: Hypotension, flushing, tachycardia, headaches, dizziness, nausea, palpitation, bone marrow suppression, arthralgia, shortness of breath
Caution: Heart failure, aortic stenosis
For sublingual administration: Puncture capsule and express fluid sublingually
(conc. = 10 mg/0.34 mL)

Nitroglycerine

TRIDIL, NITRO-BID

Onset: Rapid

Mode of action: Vasodilation, venous more than arterial

Route	Dose	Frequency
Infusion	Initial: 0.25–0.5 μg/kg/min Then: 0.5–10 μg/kg/min, usual dose 1–3 μg/kg/min	
Ointment	1–2 cm	q2–4 h

Side effects: Flushing, headache, hypotension, tachycardia, nausea, perspiration, tolerance
Caution: Increase ICP, hypovolemia
Contraindication: Glaucoma, severe anemia

Nitroprusside

NIPRID, NITROPRESS

Onset: Rapid

Mode of action: Peripheral vasodilator

Route	Dose	Frequency
Infusion	0.5–10 μg/kg/min, usual dose is 3 μg/kg/min neonates max = 6 μg/kg/min	

Side effects: Profound hypotension, metabolic acidosis, weakness, psychosis, headache, increased ICP, thyroid suppression, nausea, sweating, cyanide and thiocyanate toxicity
Caution: Monitor thiocyanate level, if used >48 h. Keep level <35 mg/L
Contraindication: Reduced cerebral perfusion, coarctation of the aorta, AV shunts

Prazosin HCl

MINIPRESS

Onset: 1–3 h

Mode of action: Vasodilator, α_1 adrenergic receptor blocker

Route	Dose	Frequency
PO	Initially: 5 μg/kg as test dose, then titrate to 25 μg/kg max = 4 mg/dose	qid

Side effects: Orthostatic hypotension, syncope, tachycardia, dizziness, headache, fluid retention, nausea, dry mouth, nasal congestion, urinary frequency

Caution: "First dose phenomenon": orthostasis, syncope, usually within 90 min of first dose

DIURETIC AGENTS

Bumetanide

BUMEX

Onset: PO: 30–60 min, IV: 5–10 min

Mode of action: Loop diuretic, prevent reabsorption of chloride at ascending loop of Henle

Route	Dose	Frequency
IV, IM, PO	0.015–0.1 mg/kg, max = 2 mg	qd
Infusion	0.01–0.025 mg/kg/h	

Side effects: Hypotension, dizziness, weakness, vertigo, nausea, muscle cramps, hypoglycemia, increase serum creatinine, hyperurecemia, hypokalemia, hypocalcemia, hyponatremia, hypochloremia, hypercalciurea. Metabolic alkalosis

Caution: Sulfonamide hypersensitivity owing to cross-reaction

Chlorothiazide

DIURIL

Onset: 1–2 h

Mode of action: Inhibits renal tubular reabsorption

Route	Dose	Frequency
PO	10–20 mg/kg	bid
IV	1–4 mg/kg	bid

Side effects: Hypokalemia, hypochloremia, alkalosis, hypotension, dizziness, vertigo, hyperlipidemia, cholestasis, muscle weakness, parasthesia, prerenal azotemia, hyperurecemia, hyperglycemia, blood dyscrasias, allergic reaction
Caution: Sulfonamide hypersensitivity

Ethacrynic Acid

EDECRIN

Onset: PO: 10–30 min, IV: rapid

Mode of action: Potent loop diuretic, prevent reabsorption of chloride at ascending loop of Henle

Route	Dose	Frequency
PO	1–3 mg/kg, max = 25 mg	bid
IV	1 mg/kg	bid, tid

Side effects: Hypovolemia, hypokalemia, hypochloremic alkalosis, pre-renal azotemia, hyperurecemia, 8th cranial nerve damage (deafness), abnormal LFTs, agranulocytosis or thrombocytopenia, anorexia, dysphagia, GI bleeding, GI irritation, rash, hypotension, vertigo, hyponatremia, hyperglycemia, hepatotoxicity, ototoxic, tinnitus, hematuria, hypomagnesemia
Drug interactions: Potentiate potassium wasting with other loop diuretics. Increase risk for ototoxicity when used with aminoglycosides. Increase effect of Warfarin because it displaces warfarin from protein binding
Caution: Renal dysfunction

DRUGS USED IN CARDIAC EMERGENCIES

Atropine

Onset: Rapid

Mode of action: Blocks acetylcholine activity

Route	Dose	Frequency
IV, ET	0.01–0.02 mg/kg, min = 0.1 mg max = 1 mg	prn

Side effects: Dry mouth, blurred vision, tachycardia, dry hot skin, restlessness, fatigue, difficult micturition, impaired GI motility, CNS symptoms, hyperthermia, palpitation, delirium, headache, tremor
Contraindication: Glaucoma, tachycardia, thyrotoxicosis, GI obstruction, uropathy

Diphenhydramine

BENADRYL

Onset: PO: 20–40 min, IV: 10–20 min

Mode of action: Histamine 1 receptor antagonist

Route	Dose	Frequency
PO, IV, IM	1–2 mg/kg max = 50 mg	qid

Side effects: Sedation, drowsiness, insomnia, vomiting, anorexia, constipation, diarrhea, anticholinergic effect, hypotension, palpitation, tachycardia, paradoxic excitement, fatigue, photosensitivity, rash, dry mouth, urinary retention, blurred vision, thickened bronchial secretions
Caution: Peptic ulcers, hyperthyroidism
Contraindication: Angle closure glaucoma, GI or urinary tract obstruction

Bretylium Tosylate

BRETYLOL

Onset: Rapid

Mode of action: Sodium channel blocker, inhibits postganglionic norepinephrine release

Route	Dose	Frequency
IV	1st dose: 5 mg/kg Repeat doses: 10 mg/kg Total dose = 30 mg	q10–20 min

Side effects: Hypertension followed by hypotension, PVC, arrhythmias, increased sensitivity to digitalis and catecholamines, nausea, vomiting, hyperthermia, nasal congestion, conjunctivitis, diaphoresis
Caution: Renal dysfunction, severe hypotension
Contraindication: Digitalis induced arrhythmias

Calcium Chloride

Onset: Rapid

Mode of action: Enhances contractility through regulation of action potential

Route	Dose	Frequency
IV	Cardiac arrest: 20 mg max = 500 mg (5 mL)	q10 min prn

Side effects: Bradycardia, hypotension, peripheral vasodilation, hypercalcemia, hypomagnesemia, hyperchloremic acidosis, hypercalcemia
Caution: Central venous line recommended. Maximum concentration is 20 mg/mL infusion. May precipitate arrhythmia in digitalized patient. Extravasation may lead to tissue necrosis (use local hyaluronidase if this occurs).
Contraindication: Hypercalcemia, ventricular fibrillation

Epinephrine Hydrochloride

1:10,000

ADRENALINE

Onset: Rapid

Mode of action: Stimulates alpha, beta 1 and 2 adrenergic receptors

Route	Dose	Frequency
IV, ET	0.01 mg/kg max = 1 mg	prn

Side effects: Anxiety, tremor, headache, tachycardia, hypertension, arrhythmias

Lidocaine

XYLOCAINE

Onset: Rapid

Mode of action: Class Ib antiarrhythmic agent, sodium channel blocker, local anesthetic depressing myocardial irritability

Route	Dose	Frequency
IV, ET	0.5–1.0 mg/kg	q5 min, prn
Infusion	20–50 μg/kg/min	

Side effects: Hypotension, shock, nausea, seizures, respiratory depression, anxiety, euphoria, drowsiness, agitation
Caution: Hepatic disease, heart failure
Contraindication: AV block
Therapeutic level: 2–5 μg/mL

Sodium Bicarbonate

Onset: IV rapid

Mode of action: Alkalization

Route	Dose	Frequency
IV, ET	Cardiac arrest: 0.5–1 meq/kg	

Side effects: Increased oxygen affinity to Hgb, alkalosis, edema, hyperosmolality, hypernatremia cerebral hemorrhage, hypokalemia, hypocalcemia
Caution: In infants under 3 months, use concentration of 0.5 meq/mL. Do not mix with calcium salts or catecholamines. Extravasation may cause tissue necrosis, infiltrate with hyalurunidase to minimize tissue necrosis
Contraindication: Inadequate alveolar ventilation

Pancuronium

PAVULON

Onset: Rapid

Mode of action: Postsynaptic acetylcholine receptor blocker

Route	Dose	Frequency
IV	0.1 mg/kg	prn

Side effects: Tachycardia
Caution: Secure airway prior to administration. Effect increased by hypothermia, acidosis, decreased renal function, volatile anesthetics, succinycholine, hypokalemia, and aminoglycoside

Vecuronium Bromide

NORCURON

Onset: Rapid

Mode of action: Postsynaptic acetylcholine receptor blocker

Route	Dose	Frequency
IV	0.1 mg/kg	prn

Caution: Hepatic impairment, neuromuscular disease. Longer recovery period in infant less than 1 year. Potency and duration of effect may be prolonged by volatile anesthetics, aminoglycoside, metronidazole, tetracycline, bacitracin, and clindamycin
Antidotes: Neostigmine, pyridostigmine, or edrophonium

SEDATIVES

Chloral Hydrate

NOCTEC

Onset: 10–20 min

Mode of action: CNS depressant

Route	Dose	Frequency
PO, PR	20–100 mg/kg max = 2000 mg	q6–8 h prn

Side effects: Irritates mucosa causing upset GI, laryngospasm if aspirated. Myocardial and respiratory depressant. CNS depression
Contraindications: Hepatic or renal impairment
Caution: Heart disease

Chlorpromazine

THORAZINE

Onset: Rapid

Mode of action: Tranquilization, central dopaminergic antagonist, and post-synaptic adrenergic blocker

Route	Dose	Frequency
IM, IV, PO	0.5–2 mg/kg max = 50 mg	q4–6 h prn

Side effects: Alpha blocking, hypotension, jaundice, lower seizure threshold, extrapyramidal symptoms, agranulocytosis, leukopenia, hepatotoxicity
Contraindications: Narrow angle glaucoma, severe liver and cardiac disease
Caution: Patients with cardiac disease, seizure disorder
ECG changes: Prolonged PR, flattened T, ST depression

Diazepam

VALIUM

Onset: Rapid

Mode of action: CNS depression through enhanced GABA at the limbic system

Route	Dose	Frequency
IM, IV	0.04–0.25 mg/kg	prn
PO	0.04–0.25 mg/kg Q8	q8 h, prn

Side effects: Hypotension, CNS and respiratory depression, physical dependence
Contraindications: Narrow angle glaucoma
Caution: Glaucoma, shock, depression, hypoalbuminemia, hepatic dysfunction. No faster than 1–2 mg/min (IV)

Fentanyl

SUBLIMAZE

Onset: Rapid

Mode of action: Semisynthetic opiate analgesic

Route	Dose	Frequency
IV, IM	1–3 μg/kg	q2 h, prn
Infusion	1–5 μg/kg/h	

Side effects: Respiratory depression (beyond period of analgesia). Chest wall rigidity with large bolus doses. Bradycardia, functional ileus., physical dependence
Contraindications: Increase ICP and IOP
Caution: IV dose over 3–5 min, hepatic and renal insufficiency, respiratory disease

Ketamine

KETALAR

Onset: Rapid

Mode of action: Dissociative anesthesia by direct action on the cortex and limbic system

Route	Dose	Frequency
IV	0.5–2 mg/kg	q2 h prn
PO	6–10 mg/kg	q2 h prn
IM	3–7 mg/kg	q2 h prn
Infusion	0.5–2 mg/kg/h	q2 h prn

Side effects: Hypertension, tachycardia, respiratory depression, laryngospasm, hypersalivation, delirium. CNS symptoms (dream-like state, confusion, agitation)
Contraindications: Elevated ICP, thyrotoxicosis, CHF, angina, and psychosis disorder
Caution: Must be used in conjunction with antisialagouge because of increased secretions

Meperidine

DEMEROL

Onset: Rapid

Mode of action: Semisynthetic opiate analgesic

Route	Dose	Frequency
IM, IV, SC, PO	1–2 mg/kg max = 100 mg	q3–4 h prn

Side effects: Nausea, vomiting, respiratory depression, smooth muscle spasm, physical dependence, seizures, constipation and lethargy, tachycardia
Contraindications: Cardiac arrhythmia, asthma, increased ICP, renal failure
Caution: Potentiated by MAO inhibitors, phenothiazines and other CNS depressants, biliary colic

Midazolam

VERSED

Onset: IV: Rapid, IM: 5–15 min, PO/PR: 15–30 min

Mode of action: CNS depression by inducing GABA at limbic system

Route	Dose	Frequency
IV	0.05–0.1 mg/kg	prn
	max = 2.5 mg	
IN	0.2 mg/kg	prn
PO	0.3–0.75 mg/kg	prn
IM	0.1–0.2 mg/kg	prn
PR	0.5–1.0 mg/kg	prn
Infusion	0.05–0.5 mg/kg/h	

Side effects: Respiratory depression, hypotension, bradycardia, myclonic jerking in neonates
Contraindications: Narrow angle glaucoma, shock, physical dependence
Caution: Lower dose by 25% when used with narcotics, cimetidine or anesthetic agents. Care should be observed in the postoperative open-heart patient, and with hemodynamic instability

Morphine Sulfate

DURAMORPH, CENTIN, ASTRAMORPH

Onset: IV: Rapid, PO: 15–30 min

Mode of action: Strongest narcotic analgesic. Unspecified aid with CHF, pulmonary edema, and anoxic spells

Route	Dose	Frequency
IV, IM, SC	0.05–0.2 mg/kg	q2–4 h, prn
	max = 10 mg/dose	
Infusion	0.01–0.1 mg/kg/h	

Side effects: Physical dependence, CNS and respiratory depression, bronchospam, nausea, vomiting, constipation, hypotension, bradycardia, increases ICP, meiosis, biliary or urinary spasm
Contraindications: Increase ICP and IOP (unless ventilated), shock
Caution: Hepatic failure, renal failure

Naloxone

NARCAN

SEDATIVE REVERSAL AGENT

Onset: Rapid

Mode of action: Opioid antagonist

Route	Dose	Frequency
IV, IM, SC, ET Infusion	0.01–0.1 mg/kg, max = 2 mg Last effective dose over 1 h, then decrease by 50% every hour for 6–12 h	q3 min prn

Side effects: Narcotic withdrawal symptoms in opioid dependence, with abrupt reversal of narcotic may cause nausea, vomiting, diaphoresis, tachycardia, hypertension, and tremulousness
Caution: Chronic cardiac disease

Promethazine

PHENERGAN

Onset: Rapid

Mode of action: Antihistaminic, antiemetic, phenothiazine

Route	Dose	Frequency
IV, IM, PR	0.5–1.0 mg/kg max = 50 mg	q4–6 h prn

Side effects: CNS depression, anticholinergic effect, antihistaminic effect, photosensitivity, extrapyramidal reaction
Contraindications: Increase IOP
Caution: Seizure, liver disease, CV disease

MISCELLANEOUS

Acetylsalicylic Acid

ASPIRIN

Mode of action: Inhibits prostaglandin synthesis which prevents thromboxane A_2 formation, leading to decrease platelet aggregation

Route	Dose	Frequency
PO	Antiplatelet: 3–10 mg/kg	qd
	Anti-inflammatory: 15–25 mg/kg	qd

Side effects: Rash, nausea, hepatotoxicity, GI bleeding, bronchospasm, GI distress, tinnitus
Caution: Renal dysfunction, erosive gastritis, peptic ulcer or gout
Contraindication: Hepatic failure, bleeding disorder, hypersensitivity to other NSAID, children <16 year with chicken pox or flu symptoms, because of the association with Reye's syndrome

Ammonium Chloride

Mode of action: Chloride supplementation in severe hypochloremic metabolic alkalosis, as seen with loop diuretics

Route	Dose	Frequency
PO, IV	12.5–25 mg/kg Or (0.2)(wt. in kg)(103-Cl level)(0.5) = meq needed	q6–8 h prn

Side effects: Bradycardia, phlebitis and necrosis with infiltration, headache, hyperammonemia, GI irritation, hyperventilation
Caution: Maximum concentration for infusion: 0.2 meq/kg/h peripheral and 0.4 meq/mL central; maximum rate of infusion 1 meq/kg/h (53 mg of NH_4Cl = 1 meq of Cl)
Contraindication: Severe hepatic or renal dysfunction

Argeninine HCl (10%)

R-GENE

Mode of action: Chloride supplementation in severe hypochloremic metabolic alkalosis, as seen with loop diuretics

Route	Dose	Frequency
PO, IV	(0.4)(wt. in kg)(103-Cl level)(0.5) = mL needed	q6 h prn

Side effects: Flushing and headache with rapid infusion, hyperglycemia, hyperkalemia, GI upset, phlebitis, necrosis with infiltration
Caution: Maximum rate of infusion 1 gm/kg/h
Contraindication: Renal or hepatic failure

Dexamethasone

DECADRON

Mode of action: Anti-inflammatory effect by suppression of migration of polymorphonuclear leukocytes and reversal of increased capillary permeability

Route	Dose	Frequency
PO, IV	Airway edema: 0.1–0.5 mg/kg Anti-inflammatory: 0.02–0.07 mg/kg	qid × 4 before extubation qid

Side effects: Hypertension, headache, vertigo, psychosis, heart failure, adrenal suppression, hyperglycemia, hypokalemia, Cushing's syndrome, gastric ulceration, muscle weakness, osteoporosis, fractures, cataract, glaucoma
Caution: Active infections, hypertension, CHF, liver failure, hypothyroidism, thromboembolic disease

Heparin

Onset: IV rapid

Mode of action: Potentiates antithrombin III which inactivates thrombin and prevents the conversion of fibrinogen to fibrin

Route	Dose	Frequency
IV Infusion	50–100 U/kg, max = 5,000–10,000 U Maintenance: 10–25 U/kg/h, adjust according to PTT max = 800–1600 U/h	q4 h

Side effects: Bleeding, allergy, alopecia, thrombocytopenia, fever, headache, chills, urticaria, increased LFTs
Caution: Adjust dose to desired clotting time. Use preservative free heparin in neonates
Antidote: Protamine sulfate
Contraindication: Severe thrombocytopenia, suspected intracranial hemorrhage
Drug interactions: Increase susceptibility to bleeding with other anticoagulants

Ibuprofen

ADVIL, MOTRIN

Mode of action: Nonsteroidal anti-inflammatory agent (inhibits PG synthesis)

Route	Dose	Frequency
PO	Analgesic and antipyretic: 4–10 mg/kg	q6–8 h
	Anti-inflammatory: 10–15 mg/kg	q6–8 h

Side effects: Drowsiness, fatigue, headache, GI irritation, inhibition of platelet aggregation, hepatitis, acute renal dysfunction, blood dyscrasias
Caution: CHF, renal disease, hepatic disease
Drug interaction: May increase digoxin, methotrexate lithium serum levels. May decrease effect of furosemide and bumetanide
Contraindication: Active GI bleeding, GI ulcers, platelet dysfunction

Indomethacin

INDOCIN

Onset:

Mode of action: Prostaglandin synthesis inhibitor

Route	Dose	Frequency
IV	Closure of ductus arteriosus: 0.1–0.25 mg/kg	q12–24 h For PDA closure: 3 dose course may be used

Side effects: Decrease platelet aggregation, GI disease: ulcers, diarrhea, blood dyscrasias, GI bleeding, hypertension, oligurea, renal failure, somnolence, hyperkalemia, hypoglycemia, hepatitis, tinnitus
Caution: Monitor renal and hepatic function. Keep urine output >0.6 mL/kg/h
Contraindication: Neonates with blood urea nitrogen (BUN) >30 mg/dL, Cr >1.8 mg/dL, thrombocytopenia, recent IVH, NEC, or active bleeding

Isoproterenol

ISUPREL

Onset: 30–60 s

Mode of action:

Chronotropy: Beta-adrenergic receptor stimulation

Route	Dose	Frequency
IV infusion	0.025–2 μg/kg/min	

Side effects: Tachyarrhythmias, hypertension, myocardial ischemia, hypotension, dizziness, headache, vertigo, nausea, tremor, sweating
Caution: Do not use discolored solution
Contraindication: Angina, ventricular arrhythmia, narrow-angle glaucoma, digitalis intoxication, IHSS

Prostaglandin E$_1$

PROSTIN

Onset: 1.5–3 h

Mode of action: Direct effect on vascular smooth muscles causing pulmonary, systemic and ductus arteriosus vasodilation

Route	Dose	Frequency
Infusion	Initial: 0.05–0.1 μg/kg/min Maintenance: 0.01–0.04 μg/kg/min	

Side effects: Hypotension, flushing, tachycardia, fever, seizure like activity, apnea, hypocalcemia, diarrhea, hypoglycemia, inhibition of platelet aggregation, cortical hyperostosis (chronic therapy)
Caution: Apnea occur in 10–12% of neonates, usually appear in first hour of therapy

Protamine Sulfate

Onset: 5 min

Mode of action: Forms a stable salt with Heparin, thus neutralizing its effect

Route	Dose	Frequency
IV	1 mg for each 90–100 units heparin max dose = 50 mg	prn

Side effects: Hypotension, bradycardia, flushing, pulmonary hypertension, nausea, dyspnea
Caution: Known allergic reaction to fish or previous exposure to protamine
Max infusion rate: 5 mg/min

Streptokinase

STREPTASE, KABIKINASE

Onset: Rapid

Mode of action: Converts plasminogen to plasmin, thus promoting thrombolysis

Route	Dose	Frequency
IV	Initial: 3500–4000 units/kg over 30 min Maintenance: 1000–1500 units/kg/h	

Side effects: Hypotension, arrhythmia, flushing, fever, urticaria, bleeding, bronchospasm
Caution: Avoid IM injection
Contraindication: Major surgery within 10 days, GI bleeding, recent trauma, severe hypertension, internal bleeding, CVA (within 2 months), intracranial or intraspinal surgery, brain carcinoma

Tolazoline HCl

PRISCOLINE

Onset: Minutes, peak effect 30 min

Mode of action: Alpha adrenergic receptor antagonist, peripheral vasodilation is mediated by histamine-like action

Route	Dose	Frequency
IV	Test dose: 1–2 mg/kg	Over 10 min
Infusion	Neonates: 0.5–1 mg/kg/h Children: 1–2 mg/kg/h	

Side effects: Hypotension, flushing, tachycardia, hypochloremic metabolic alkalosis, increased secretions, nausea, diarrhea, gastric bleeding, thrombocytopenia, agranulocytosis, mydriasis, oligurea, pulmonary hemorrhage

Urokinase

ABBOKINASE

Onset: Rapid

Mode of action: Direct activation of plasminogen to plasmin, thus causing thrombolysis

Route	Dose	Frequency
IV	Occluded IV catheter: 5000 U/mL conc. Instill a volume equal to that of the catheter in each lumen and leave for 1–4 h, then aspirate catheter, *do not* flush	prn
Infusion	DVT, pulmonary emboli: 4400 U/kg over 10 min, then 4400 U/kg/h for 12–72 h	

Side effects: Allergic reaction, fever, rash, bronchospasm, bleeding
Caution: Avoid IM injection
Contraindication: Bleeding, AV malformation, history of CVA or recent trauma, brain carcinoma, intracranial or intraspinal surgery

Vitamin K (phytonadione)

AQUA MEPHYTON, MEPHYTON

Onset: PO 6–12 h, IV 1–2 h

Mode of action: Cofactor in the synthesis of the clotting factors II, VII, IX, and X

Route	Dose	Frequency
PO	2.5–5 mg/day	qd
IV, IM	1–2 mg/dose	

Side effects: Flushing, hypotension, dizziness, GI upset, changes in taste, sweating, anaphylactoid-like reaction with IV administration
Caution: IV administration should be restricted for emergencies only, since risk of severe adverse reaction could occur. Do not use in patients with prosthetic valves

Warfarin

COUMADIN, SOFARIN

Onset: 36–72 h

Mode of action: Inhibits hepatic synthesis of vitamin K-dependent factors (I, VII, IX, X)

Rute	Dose	Frequency
PO	Loading: 0.2 mg/kg, max = 15 mg	qd
	Maintenance: 0.05–0.35 mg/kg, max = 10 mg	qd

Side effects: Fever, skin lesions, anorexia, hemorrhage, hemoptysis

Caution: Adjust to desired PT, INR, fever, skin lesions with necrosis, anorexia, hemorrhage, hemoptysis. Give 0.1 mg/kg loading dose with impaired liver function

Drug interactions: Warfarin effect increases with ethacrynic acid, indomethacin, mefenamic acid, phenylbutazone, aspirin,

Antidote: Vitamin K

Contraindication: Bleeding, liver or renal failure, malignant hypertension

INDEX

Page numbers followed by italic *f* or *t* denote figures or tables, respectively.